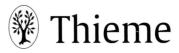

Endoscopic Ultrasound

An Introductory Manual and Atlas

Christoph F. Dietrich, MD
Professor
Department of Internal Medicine 2
Caritas Hospital
Bad Mergentheim, Germany

With contributions by
Hubert Allgayer, Paolo G. Arcidiacono, Thomas Beyer,
Barbara Braden, Eike Burmester, Silvia Carrara, Christoph F. Dietrich,
Ralf Eberhardt, Siegbert Faiss, Wolfgang Fischbach, Holger Frey,
Marc Giovannini, Christian Greis, Felix J.F. Herth, Michael Hocke,
Stephan Hollerbach, Jan Janssen, Christian Jenssen, Nicolas Kahn,
Peter H. Kann, Mark Krasnik, Thomas Leineweber, Michael Mayr,
Joachim C. Mertens, Frank Meyer, Kathleen Moeller, Jens Niehaus,
Dieter Nuernberg, Carlos Ortiz-Moyano, Anand V. Sahai, Marco Sailer,
Mario Sarbia, Hans Seifert, Hans-Werner Sudholt, Theodoros Topalidis,
Peter Vilmann, Stephan Wagner, Uwe Will, Jonathan M. Wyse

2nd edition

1280 illustrations

Thieme
Stuttgart · New York

Library of Congress Cataloging-in-Publication Data

Dietrich, Christoph Frank.
Endoscopic ultrasound : an introductory manual and atlas /
[edited by] Christoph Frank Dietrich ; with contributions by
Hubert Allgayer ... [et al].
    p. ; cm.
  Includes bibliographical references and index.
  ISBN 978-3-13-143152-3 (alk. paper)
    1. Endoscopic surgery. 2. Endoscopic ultrasonography. 3. Operative
ultrasonography. I. Dietrich, Christoph Frank. II. Allgayer, H. (Hubert)
    [DNLM: 1. Endosonography. WN 208]
  RD33.53.E637 2011
  616.07'543-dc22

                                                     2011006489

Translator (DVD): Gertrud Champe, Surry, Maine, USA

© 2011 Georg Thieme Verlag,
Rüdigerstrasse 14, 70469 Stuttgart, Germany
http://www.thieme.de
Thieme New York, 333 Seventh Avenue,
New York, NY 10001, USA
http://www.thieme.com

Cover design: Thieme Publishing Group
Typesetting by primustype Hurler, Notzingen, Germany
Printed in Italy by L.E.G.O. S.p.A., Vicenza

ISBN 978-3-13-143152-3   1 2 3 4 5 6

Foreword

Ultrasound has gained diagnostic and therapeutic acceptance throughout the world. In most countries in continental Europe, ultrasound is practiced by clinicians—in contrast to the UK and the USA. The diagnostic accuracy of conventional abdominal ultrasound has markedly improved with the use of color and contrast enhancement. Endoscopic ultrasound (EUS) has become extremely important for detecting lesions in various organs and for cancer staging. Miniprobes, now available in many endoscopy units, make it possible to assess extremely small lesions in the vicinity of the endoscope.

Christoph F. Dietrich is the author and editor of several books published in German on ultrasound, including EUS, that have met with an enthusiastic response among German gastroenterologists and endoscopists. He has now collaborated with a group of international gastroenterologists and endoscopists in preparing the present volume in English, covering the specific field of EUS. I feel sure the book will be as successful internationally as his best-selling books on conventional and contrast ultrasound have been in German-speaking countries.

The book is well-structured, taking a practical clinical approach and providing tips and tricks and a large number of excellent illustrations. It covers many specialized aspects of EUS, such as three-dimensional linear EUS, sonoelastography, EUS-guided biopsy, miniprobes, EUS-guided neurolysis of the celiac plexus, laparoscopic ultrasound scanning, and EUS-guided endosurgery.

The successful first edition has now led to a markedly improved second international edition, containing a learning DVD with didactically excellent video sequences and video examples. This book is, to my knowledge, the only EUS-teaching book presenting the new techniques of real-time elastography and contrast-enhanced low mechanical index endoscopic ultrasound (CELMI-EUS) for the clinical routine.

The illustrations are of excellent quality. The new edition also covers the new therapeutic EUS-techniques including EUS-cholangiodrainage and others, as well as possible complications, taking into consideration a thorough analysis of the literature.

The authors are experts in EUS from all over Europe and Canada. I have already learned a great deal from the book for my own everyday work and will use it in teaching fellows and residents.

I am convinced that readers will be able to improve their knowledge and skills in EUS with this excellent new edition.

Professor Wolfgang F. Caspary, MD
Department of Medicine I, Frankfurt University Hospital, Frankfurt am Main, Germany

Preface to the Second Edition

Endoscopic ultrasound (EUS) has developed in recent years to become not only an impressive diagnostic tool, but even more importantly a challenging therapeutic method. EUS has now been incorporated into the major international guidelines. With the growing preference for low-risk interventions, a shift has been taking place toward minimally invasive procedures, as a consequence of which surgical interventions are increasingly being carried out only when percutaneous and EUS-guided maneuvers are not indicated or have been unsuccessful.

Endosonography is making a substantial contribution to interdisciplinary planning and treatment not only in patients with pancreatic pseudocysts, abscesses, and necroses, but also in those with pancreatic duct obstruction (using EUS-guided pancreatic duct drainage, which can be carried out with a rendezvous maneuver) due to strictures caused by pancreatic stones, for example, and in patients with papillary conditions in which retrograde insertion into the papilla is not possible with conventional endoscopic retrograde cholangiopancreatography. Other fascinating recent developments in endoscopic ultrasound have included EUS-guided cholangiodrainage in patients with common bile duct stenosis and previously unsuccessful endoscopic retrograde cholangiography, rendezvous procedures, and minimally invasive indications. The new therapeutic techniques can only be carried out by examiners who have a high level of training and anatomic expertise, and the present volume is designed to provide instruction in the abilities and skills required. The original main diagnostic indications—for examining the walls of the upper and lower gastrointestinal tract and the hepatobiliary and pancreatic system—have been updated in this second edition.

Curved linear-array instruments using Doppler techniques, elastography, and new contrast-enhanced ultra-sound applications have improved over the years and are now being used for diagnostic and therapeutic purposes. Radial instruments are still often used in everyday routine work, but they do not provide any treatment options.

However, a bewildering variety of materials, including biopsy needles and drainage systems, are currently available to the clinician. This book also presents an overview of the devices and materials currently available, to allow the most reliable results to be achieved with the lowest level of complications. Although the book presents the findings of published studies, it is also important to take the interventionist's personal experience into account, as this can also influence the choice of device.

This practically oriented textbook and atlas has been updated by an international group of gastroenterologists and surgeons to provide instruction in the basics of the method. It also includes tips and tricks for educational purposes in the form of teaching videos. An additional aim in the book has been to incorporate information about EUS into general clinical algorithms in a comprehensive way. The second edition is therefore not only intended as a specialist text for endoscopists and ultrasonographers, but is also designed to provide information for the medical profession in general.

I would like once again to cordially thank all those who have contributed to the book, including those who are not directly mentioned in the text—especially the team at Thieme Medical Publishers, including Annie Hollins, Elisabeth Kurz, and Angelika Findgott—for their invaluable support of the project.

Christoph F. Dietrich

Contributors

Hubert Allgayer, MD
Professor
Department of Oncology
Rehabilitation Clinic Ob der Tauber
Bad Mergentheim
Germany

Paolo G. Arcidiacono, MD
Gastroenterology and
Gastrointestinal Endoscopy Unit
IRCCS San Raffaele Hospital
Vita Salute San Raffaele University
Milan
Italy

Thomas Beyer, MD
Clinic for Lung Diseases Ballenstedt/Harz gGmbH
Ballenstedt
Germany

Barbara Braden, MD
Professor
Consultant Gastroenterologist
John Radcliffe Hospital
Oxford
UK

Eike Burmester, MD
Department of Gastroenterology and Hepatology
SANA Clinics Lübeck AG
Lübeck
Germany

Silvia Carrara, MD
Gastroenterology and Gastrointestinal Endoscopy Unit
IRCCS San Raffaele Hospital
Vita Salute San Raffaele University
Milan
Italy

Christoph F. Dietrich, MD
Professor
Department of Internal Medicine 2
Caritas Hospital
Bad Mergentheim
Germany

Ralf Eberhardt, MD
Department of Pneumology and Internal Medicine
Thorax Clinic at the University of Heidelberg
Heidelberg
Germany

Siegbert Faiss, MD
Department of Medicine 3
(Gastroenterology/Hepatology)
Barmbek General Hospital
Hamburg
Germany

Wolfgang Fischbach, MD
Professor
Department of Medicine II
Clinic Aschaffenburg
Aschaffenburg
Germany

Holger Frey
Böhmenkirch
Germany

Marc Giovannini, MD
Endoscopic Unit
Paoli-Calmettes Institute
Marseilles
France

Christian Greis, PhD
Bracco Imaging Deutschland GmbH
Constance
Germany

Felix J.F. Herth, MD
Professor
Department of Pneumology and Internal Medicine
Thorax Clinic at the University of Heidelberg
Heidelberg
Germany

Michael Hocke, MD
Department of Internal Medicine II
Clinic Meiningen GmbH
Meiningen
Germany

Stephan Hollerbach, MD
Professor
Department of Gastroenterology and Hemato-oncology
Allgemeines Krankenhaus Celle
Celle
Germany

Jan Janssen, MD
Professor
Helios Klinikum Wuppertal
Wuppertal
Germany

Christian Jenssen, MD
Department of Internal Medicine and Gastroenterology
Märkisch Oderland Hospital GmbH
Strausberg, Wriezen
Germany

Nicolas Kahn
Department of Pneumology and Internal Medicine
Thorax Clinic at the University of Heidelberg
Heidelberg
Germany

Peter H. Kann MD
Professor
Division of Endocrinology and Diabetology
Philipps University
Marburg
Germany

Mark Krasnik, MD
Department of Cardiothoracic Surgery
Gentofte Hospital
Hellerup
Denmark

Thomas Leineweber, MD, MBA
Department of Gastroenterology
Asklepios Clinic North – Heidberg
Hamburg
Germany

Michael Mayr, MD
Department of Internal Medicine and Gastroenterology
Gastroenterological Practice
Berlin
Germany

Joachim C. Mertens, MD
Research Fellow
Gastroenterology Basic Research Center
Mayo Clinic
Rochester, MN
USA

Frank Meyer, MD
Department of Surgery
University Hospital
Magdeburg
Germany

Kathleen Moeller, MD
Department of Internal Medicine and Gastroenterology
SANA Clinics AG
Berlin
Germany

Jens Niehaus, MD
Department of Gastroenterology and Hepatology
SANA Clinics AG
Lübeck
Germany

Dieter Nuernberg, MD
Professor
Ruppin Clinics GmbH
Department of Medicine B
Neuruppin
Germany

Carlos Ortiz-Moyano, MD, PhD
Division of Medical Gastroenterology
Hospital Universitario Virgen Macarena
Seville
Spain

Anand V. Sahai, MD
Professor
Department of Gastroenterology
Centre Hospitalier de l'Universite de Montreal
Montreal
Canada

Marco Sailer, MD
Professor
Department of Surgery
Bethesda – Allgemeines Krankenhaus GmbH
Bergedorf, Hamburg
Germany

Mario Sarbia, MD
Professor
Practice for Pathology
Munich
Germany

Hans Seifert, MD
Professor
Department of Gastroenterology
Municipal Hospitals
Oldenburg
Germany

Hans-Werner Sudholt, MD
Department of Internal Medicine
Municipal Hospital Wertheim/Main
Wertheim
Germany

Theodoros Topalidis, MD
Cytology Laboratory
Hannover
Germany

Peter Vilmann, MD, DSc, HC
Department of Surgical Gastroenterology
Copenhagen University Hospital Herlev
Endoscopic Unit at Gentofte Hospital
Hellerup
Denmark

Stephan Wagner, MD
Institute for Pathology
Königs Wusterhausen
Germany

Uwe Will, MD (Dr. med. habil.)
Professor
SRH Wald-Klinikum Gera gGmbH
Medical Clinic 3
Gera
Germany

Jonathan M. Wyse, MD
Assistant Professor of Medicine
Division of Gastroenterology
Jewish General Hospital
Montreal
Canada

Contents

I Techniques

8   Sonoelastography: a New Ultrasound Modality for Assessing Tissue Elasticity
C.F. Dietrich, H. Frey

II   Diagnostic Imaging and Interventions

9   EUS-Guided Biopsy: Equipment and Technique
H.W. Sudholt, P. Vilmann

10   EUS-Guided Biopsy—Indications, Problems, Pitfalls, Troubleshooting, and Clinical Impact
C. Jenssen, K. Moeller, M. Sarbia, S. Wagner

11   Tips and Tricks for Fine-Needle Puncture
T. Beyer, T. Topalidis

12   Complications of Endoscopic Ultrasound: Risk Assessment and Prevention

C. Jenssen, M. Mayr, D. Nuernberg, S. Faiss

III Gastrointestinal Tract

13   Esophagus, Stomach, Duodenum

C.F. Dietrich, S. Faiss

14   Endoscopic Ultrasound in Subepithelial Tumors of the Gastrointestinal Tract

C. Jenssen, C.F. Dietrich

15   Endosonographic Diagnosis and Treatment Planning in Gastrointestinal Lymphoma

W. Fischbach, C.F. Dietrich

16   Endoscopic Ultrasound in Chronic Pancreatitis

C. Jenssen, C.F. Dietrich

17   Pancreatic Adenocarcinoma: the Role of Endoscopic Ultrasonography

P.G. Arcidiacono, S. Carrara

18   Benign and Malignant (Cystic) Tumors of the Pancreas

C.F. Dietrich, C. Jenssen

19   Pancreatic Interventions
H. Seifert, C.F. Dietrich

20   Endosonography of the Hepatobiliary System
C.F. Dietrich, M. Hocke, H. Seifert

21   Endoscopic Ultrasound Imaging of the Adrenals
C.F. Dietrich, P.H. Kann

22   Contrast-Enhanced EUS
M. Hocke, C.F. Dietrich

23   Incidental Findings in the Surrounding Organs (Miscellaneous)
C.F. Dietrich

24   Endoanal and Endorectal Sonography

M. Sailer, H. Allgayer, C.F. Dietrich

25   Three-Dimensional Endorectal Ultrasound and Rectal Cancer

M. Giovannini

26   Endoscopic Ultrasound of the Colon

C.F. Dietrich, J.C. Mertens

IV   Lung and Mediastinum

27   Mediastinum from the Esophagus

C.F. Dietrich, M. Hocke, F.J.F. Herth

28   Endobronchial Ultrasound with Miniprobe Radial Scanning
F.J.F. Herth, N. Kahn, R. Eberhardt

29   Endobronchial Ultrasound
F.J.F. Herth, R. Eberhardt

V   Additional Applications

30   EUS-Guided Neurolysis of the Celiac Plexus
S. Hollerbach

31   EUS-Guided Biliary Drainage
E. Burmester, J. Niehaus

I Techniques

I Techniques

1 Basics of Radial Endoscopic Ultrasound

M. Hocke, C.F. Dietrich

Endoscopic ultrasound today demands the highest level of expertise from physicians working in endoscopy. The method requires a combination of familiarity with endoscopic techniques and experience in ultrasound. When it is properly performed and critically assessed, it makes extensive diagnostic and therapeutic applications possible.

However, newcomers to the field often find themselves facing a multitude of problems, even when they have sufficient knowledge of endoscopy and sonography. The consequent frustration can result in this valuable method being abandoned. This chapter therefore aims to simplify the examination technique so that it can be carried out successfully after a little practice.

Firstly, we can introduce the "ten golden rules of endoscopic ultrasound," established by the endoscopic ultrasound specialist Dr. Uwe Will and confirmed in practice by other experienced endosonographers. These rules should be remembered when difficulties arise during an examination (in both radial and longitudinal ultrasound), and they make it possible to regain orientation:

1. If you can't see anything, withdraw.
2. Always turn the instrument clockwise.
3. No air, always use suction.
4. Use your knowledge of anatomy for orientation.
5. Stay at the back of the stomach.
6. Only make small movements.
7. Do nothing.
8. Use water.
9. Is there any other method that would be better than endoscopic ultrasound?
10. When in doubt, trust those with more experience.

■ Notes

1. During an endoscopic ultrasound examination, you will often find yourself with an image in which no anatomical structures are recognizable. In this situation, you should gradually pull the scope back until a recognizable marker appears. From this position, you will be able to continue with the examination.
2. To keep the papilla of Vater in the same position, especially when examining the descending duodenum, it may be necessary to make a slight clockwise turn with the scope. This can also help avoid slippage of the scope from the duodenum into the stomach (this technique is also used in endoscopic retrograde cholangiopancreatography).
3. Air is the enemy of the endoscopic ultrasound; suction should be applied continually throughout the examination.
4. Problems can occur when you first orient yourself visually using specific structures and then start trying to construct an ultrasound image. The air needed for good visibility will prevent the ultrasound from working and there will be a large discrepancy between the visual appearance of the structure and the ultrasound image. It is always preferable to locate a structure on a purely endoscopic ultrasound image, using anatomical markers for orientation.
5. Positioning the instrument at the back wall of the stomach can often help when orientation has been lost, as the best-known markers (the retroperitoneal and mesenteric vessels) are easy to recognize from this location.
6. The biggest mistake made by beginners is to move the scope too far in one go. Large movements lead to some anatomic markers being missed and therefore to a loss of orientation during the examination.
7. Not moving the instrument does not mean keeping it in one place. The peristaltic movements alone result in a gradual change of view through the different levels, without any action on the part of the operator. This provides time for the markers to be noted as they become visible.
8. In hollow, air-filled organs, such as the gastric body and fundus regions, filling with water can produce unexpectedly effective images. However, a few practitioners do not believe this is necessary.
9. When endoscopic ultrasound is carried out correctly, the practitioner will quickly begin to grasp how wide its range of possible applications is.
10. Experience colors vision; two examiners looking at the same image may interpret what they see very differently.

Patient Preparation

The patient should be made aware of the risks and effectiveness of the procedure beforehand. Endoscopic ultrasound is not suitable as a screening method and should only be used to answer specific questions.

Light sedation (with midazolam or propofol) is recommended for the examination, which should be performed with the patient lying on the left side.

Examination Procedures

In principle, the procedure used in the examination depends on the question being posed. For the newcomer, the easiest phenomena to examine and diagnose are protuberances in the digestive tract and surface tumors. The instrument is positioned directly in front of the relevant area, and the examination takes place under continuous suction. However, although this process is easy to carry out in the duodenum, antrum, and esophagus, the presence of air and the many folds in the gastric body and fundus regions make it more difficult there. The most difficult areas to examine are the angular notch and the fundus region.

Small protuberances in the gastrointestinal tract are often difficult to image with the balloon method alone. The examiner should be aware that mucosal masses may be "flattened out" with the balloon and therefore remain hidden. These should preferably be examined using the miniprobe method, which makes it possible to locate lesions more precisely.

The most difficult endoscopic ultrasound procedure is examining extraintestinal organs and structures. Success here depends on excellent knowledge of ultrasound anatomy, so that pathological structures can be detected by recognizing markers.

As a rule, the operator should make sure that the radial endoscopic ultrasound instruments are standardized for the "CT view"—i.e., viewing the patient from underneath. This can best be seen in the mediastinum. It is essential to remember that when the descending aorta and the spine are at the bottom edge of the picture, the image will appear mirrored: the right main bronchus appears on the left side of the image, the left main bronchus on the right.

To maintain orientation during the imaging process, it is necessary to identify a series of standard ultrasound cross-sections in the gastrointestinal tract. This should be performed during every examination. Each cross-section and the best technique for locating it are described below.

◼ Cross-Section of the Descending Duodenum

To produce images of extraintestinal structures, one should start by positioning the scope in the descending duodenum by sight in the same way as in endoscopic retrograde cholangiopancreatography (ERCP), and then straighten it slowly. Using the water-filled balloon is recommended in order to improve the contact (preferred by

one of the present authors, M.H.), but as mentioned before, some practitioners do not consider this necessary (preferred by C.F.D.). The left hand is used to maintain continuous suction and also to angle the tip of the scope to optimize contact with the intestinal wall. Sideways movements are made by turning the instrument with the right hand, or by turning the whole instrument at the shaft. The small wheel is not usually used for positioning.

As the scope is pulled back slowly from this relatively blind position, two anatomic markers become visible: the inferior vena cava and aorta on the left side of the screen and the superior mesenteric vein on the right side. These two markers form a "V" shape, which surrounds parts of the pancreas. This is the first recognizable image to appear while the scope is being withdrawn from the descending duodenum; the view of the pancreas opens up—the "golden V"—when this position has been reached (**Fig. 1.1**).

◼ Cross-Section of the Papilla of Vater

From this section in the descending duodenum, the instrument should be pulled back while the shaft is turned slightly to the right. The markers are the common bile duct (close to the scope) and the pancreatic duct, which lead to the papilla of Vater (**Fig. 1.2**). When these two markers have been correctly identified, imaging and examination of the papilla of Vater can be carried out, using slow forward and backward movements.

◼ Cross-Section of the Duodenal Bulb, including the Porta Hepatis and Gallbladder

After examining the papilla of Vater, one should stop turning the instrument to the right, hold the common bile duct in the center of the image, and then turn the instrument at the shaft slightly to the left. This movement allows the tip of the scope slowly to relocate itself into the duodenal bulb (as in ERCP). The instrument repositions itself in such a way that the common bile duct lets itself be untwisted lengthways, and eventually an image is produced that should be recognizable from percutaneous ultrasound. In this position, the common bile duct courses away from the hepatic duct bifurcation near the ultrasound transducer and is accompanied by the portal vein in the distant part of the image. The extrahepatic bile ducts can be examined optimally from this position. A small forward movement with the scope will provide a new image of the papilla region, perpendicular to the previous view. Near the middle of the common bile duct, the bifurcation of the cystic duct can be seen. This leads to the gallbladder. The gallbladder can be examined from the duodenal bulb or from the distal stomach (**Fig. 1.3**).

I Techniques

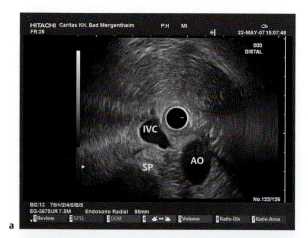

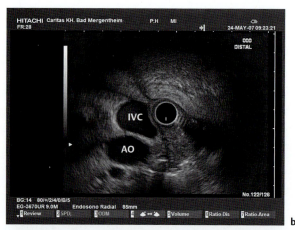

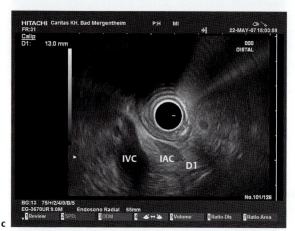

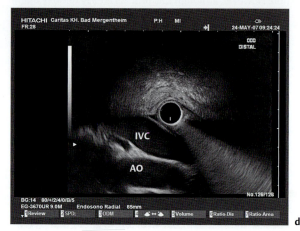

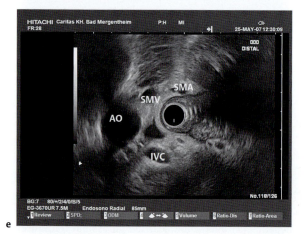

Fig. 1.1a–e The aorta (AO) and inferior vena cava (IVC) can be seen from the lower duodenum as parallel structures coursing in front of the spine, either horizontally (**a, b**) or vertically (**c, d**). (▶ Videos 1.1a–c; in Video 1.1c, the interaortocaval lymph node [IAC] is visible between the two markers. The uncinate process of the pancreas can be seen on the right.) The distance to which the scope needs to be inserted in order to reach this cross-section depends on whether the patient is lying on the left side or on the stomach, the angle of the scope tip, and other factors. Interaortocaval lymph nodes between the two major vessel structures can be imaged to a size of 17 mm (**c**). *Note:* The scope makes an arc around the inferior vena cava through the series of images (**a–d**). In (**e**) (and ▶ Video 1.1 d), the aorta and inferior vena cava appear on one side of the image (the transducer is producing an almost horizontal cross-section) and the superior mesenteric artery appears on the other. When the tip of the scope is angled upward and the scope is pulled back, the uncinate process of the pancreas can be identified (▶ Video 1.1e). SMA, superior mesenteric artery; AO, aorta; IAC, interaortocaval lymph node; IVC, inferior vena cava; SMV, superior mesenteric vein, SP, spine.

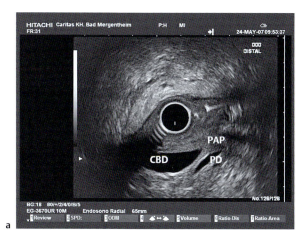

a

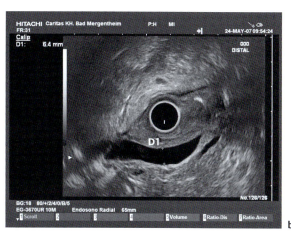

b

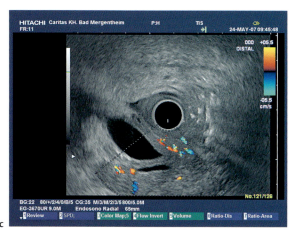

c

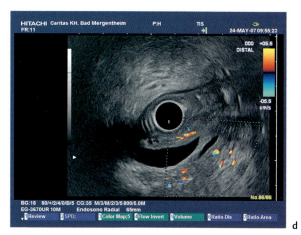

d

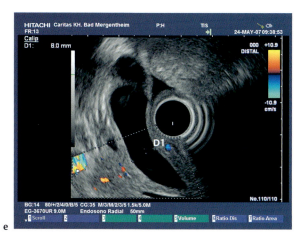

e

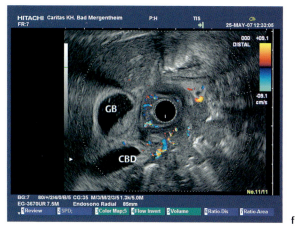

f

Fig. 1.2a–f Papilla of Vater, standard cross-section. The common bile duct (CBD) and pancreatic duct (PD, Wirsung duct) are seen close to the papilla (PAP) and in relation to the duodenum using B-mode ultrasound (**a, b**) and color Doppler (**c–e**). Pulling the scope back into the duodenal bulb makes it possible to follow the common bile duct to the porta hepatis and to examine the gallbladder (GB, **f**) (▶ Videos 1.2 f, g). The videos correspond to the still images and demonstrate the image adjustment process (▶ Videos 1.2a–g).

I Techniques

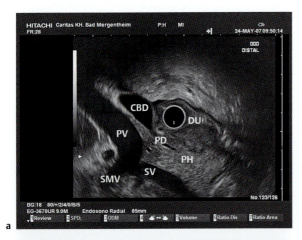

a

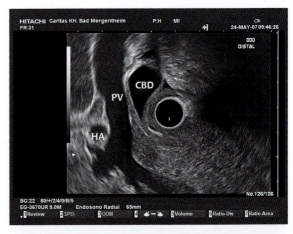

b

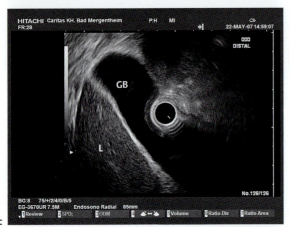

c

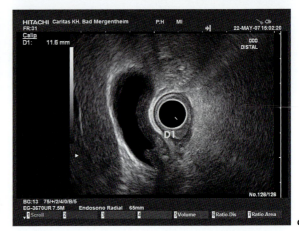

d

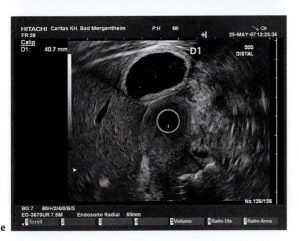

e

Fig. 1.3a–e Imaging of the bile duct and portal vein from the papilla to the hilum (**a, b**). Further withdrawal produces an image of the gallbladder (**c–e**). Sludge can be distinguished from gallstones (**d, e**). HA, hepatic artery proper; DU, duodenum; CBD, common bile duct; PD, pancreatic duct; GB, gallbladder; L, liver; PH, head of the pancreas; PV, portal vein; SV, splenic vein; SMV, superior mesenteric vein. The videos demonstrate the examination procedure (▶ Videos 1.3a–d).

Cross-Section of the Stomach, Including the Body of the Pancreas

When the scope is pulled gently back, the body of the pancreas should become visible at the bottom of the image (on the left), easily recognized by the dorsally positioned splenic vein. This section is easy to interpret, as it is similar to percutaneous ultrasound diagnosis. The left liver lobe, which appears at the top of the image, is an important aid to orientation. Loosening the large wheel and straightening the tip of the scope by twisting clockwise and anticlockwise at the shaft make it possible to see the entire body and tail end of the pancreas, as well as a large part of the pancreatic head. The spleen rounds off the image on the right side (**Fig. 1.4**).

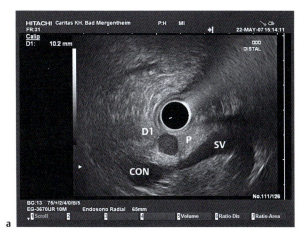

a

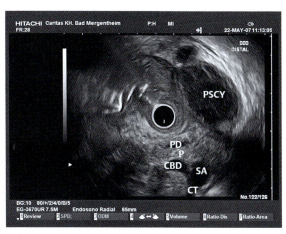

b

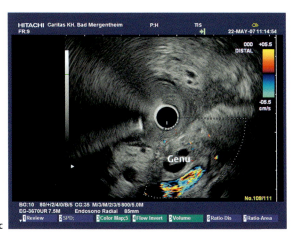

c

Fig. 1.4a–c Stomach, view of the body of the pancreas (P). The body of the pancreas is bordered by the splenic vein (SV) from its confluence (CON) to the pancreatic tail, shown here in a patient with a pancreatic tumor (12 mm) (**a**). Another anatomic marker is the celiac trunk, shown here in a patient with chronic pancreatitis and development of a pseudocyst (**b**). The point at which the body of the pancreas meets the pancreatic head has to be located carefully, with the ultrasound head in continuous contact; the pancreatic duct is often difficult to follow in the region of the uncinate process and can only be distinguished from the blood vessels by using color Doppler ultrasound (**c**). SA, splenic artery; CBD, common bile duct; PD, pancreatic duct; CON, confluence; P, pancreas; PSCY, pseudocyst; CT, celiac trunk; SV, splenic vein. The corresponding videos show the topography (▶ Video 1.4a–c).

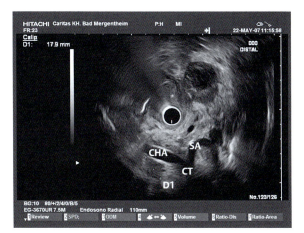

Fig. 1.5 View of the mesenteric vessel branches from the stomach. A normal lymph node is shown between the markers in the ventral hepatoduodenal ligament next to the hepatic artery. CHA, common hepatic artery; SA, splenic artery; CT, celiac trunk. ▶ Video 1.5a shows the corresponding topography. ▶ Video 1.5b shows the celiac artery and its branches from the duodenum directly next to the portal vein and the common bile duct.

■ Cross-Section of the Para-Aortic Region

Withdrawing further leaves the upper pancreas behind, and the abdominal aorta is relatively easily found as a marker at the bottom of the image. The angle of view makes the junctions of the large abdominal vessels difficult to recognize; in good conditions, however, the confluence of the celiac artery with the splenic artery and hepatic artery can be seen (**Fig. 1.5**).

■ Cross-Section of the Adrenal Glands

From this position at the confluence of the large abdominal vessels, the scope should be pushed back in, while twisting slightly clockwise at the shaft. This movement makes it possible to return via the fundus region to the tail of the pancreas. First the spleen can be seen on the right, and then, as the scope is pulled back to a distance of approximately 45 cm from the incisors, the kidney can be found, also on the right side of the image. The left adrenal gland can be found above the kidney, framed by the splenic

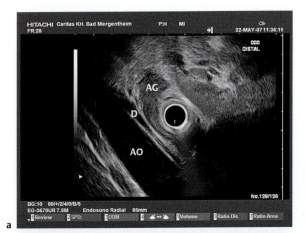

a

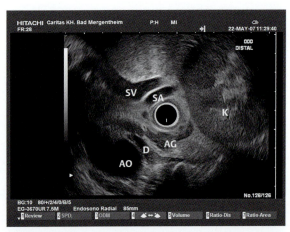

b

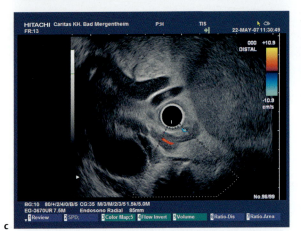

c

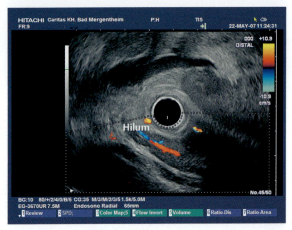

d

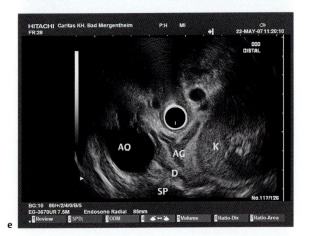

e

Fig. 1.6a–e Adrenal gland (AG) on the left. The anatomic markers for locating the left adrenal gland are the kidney (K), spleen and splenic vessels (SA, SV: splenic artery, splenic vein), as well as the aorta (AO), the diaphragm (D), and the spine (SP). It is sometimes possible to see the pancreatic tail as well. The angle of the cross-section depends on the position of the scope in the stomach and may be more sagittal (**a**) or more transverse (**b–e**). The vessels of the adrenal glands can be seen using color Doppler ultrasound (**c, d**).
▶ Videos 1.6a–f correspond to the figures and show the topography in real time. ▶ Video loop 1.6 g additionally shows the relative location of the spleen.

artery and splenic vein. The position of the scope may vary widely here, and the adrenal glands can have very different appearances depending on the angle from which they are seen, as illustrated in the following still images and ▶ video sequences (**Fig. 1.6**). The adrenal gland vessels can be visualized using color Doppler ultrasound.

■ Cross-Section of the Lower Mediastinum

All of the structures surrounding the upper gastrointestinal tract have now been examined. An examination of the mediastinum should now form the conclusion to the procedure. Thanks to the anatomic markers, this is one of the easiest tasks, along with the examination of changes on

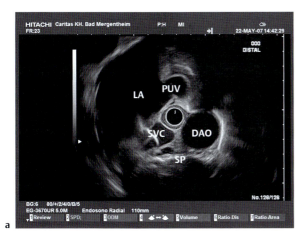
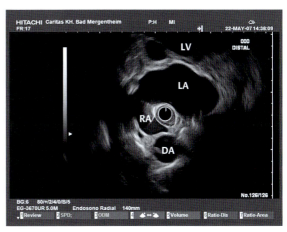

a / b

Fig. 1.7a, b The lower mediastinum, at the atrium level (**a, b**). The image shows the left atrium (LA) with the inflow of the pulmonary vessels (PUV), the descending aorta (DAO), the superior vena cava (SVC) with a central venal catheter producing a bright echo pattern, the inflow of the superior vena cava into the right atrium (RA), as well as the mitral valve, left ventricle (LV), and spine (SP). The corresponding video loops show the topography. In the videos (▶ Video 1.7), the brachiocephalic vein in front of the spine and the mitral valve (MV) are also marked.

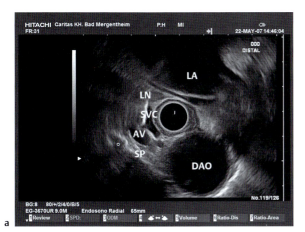
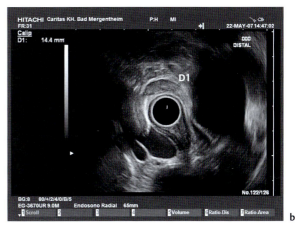

a / b

Fig. 1.8a, b Central mediastinum. The anatomic markers are the descending aorta (DAO), running in front of the spine (SP), the azygos vein (AV), and the superior vena cava (SVC), shown here with a central venous catheter. The subcarinal region lies ventrally, with the corresponding group of lymph nodes (LN) adjacent to the left atrium (LA) (**a**). A subcarinal lymph node is visible between the markers (**b**). ▶ Video loop 1.8 shows the topography.

the surface of the gastrointestinal tract (**Fig. 1.7**). It is advisable to carry out the examination with the spine and descending aorta at the lower edge of the image as standard, so that mediastinal organs can always be located in the same positions. After the scope has been pulled back, the left atrium should be visible as a marker at the top edge of the image.

■ Cross-Section of the Central Mediastinum

Another tubular structure, the azygos vein, is visible on the left of the image, next to the spine (**Fig. 1.8**).

■ Cross-Section of the Upper Mediastinum

As the scope is withdrawn further, the confluence of the ascending aorta and descending aorta in the aortic arch can be seen, with the cervical and brachial vessels leading off it (**Fig. 1.9**).

These cross-sections are designed to help the examiner maintain orientation in the difficult radial anatomy of the upper gastrointestinal tract and to help him or her return to a recognizable structure when orientation is occasionally lost.

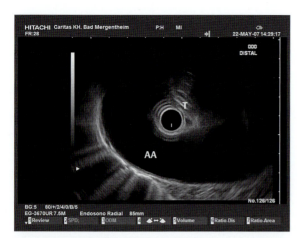

Fig. 1.9 Upper mediastinum, showing the aortic arch (AA). The trachea (T) can be recognized opposite the aortic arch by the reverberating echoes (▶ Video 1.9).

Rating Levels of Skill in the Endoscopic Ultrasound Method

It is extremely important to be able to judge one's own ability in endoscopic ultrasound critically, in order to recognize opportunities for diagnostic improvement using this powerful method. Practitioners can match their own achievements against the learning stages involved and assess their results accordingly. Four stages of learning are generally recognized.

1. Justified lack of confidence. This can be recognized by complete reliance on the instructor. Independent diagnosis at this stage is almost impossible. Problems often occur even when bringing the instrument into the descending duodenum. Finding the papilla section marker is unsuccessful 75% of the time. In comparison with percutaneous ultrasound, the results of endoscopic ultrasound are often poorer. These problems are common when fewer than 50 examinations have been carried out.

2. Unjustified confidence. After a few successes, practitioners tend to overrate their own ability. It is in the interests of the method and of patients to recognize this phase quickly and to keep it as short as possible. Clear signs of this stage are attempts to diagnose the malignancy of masses that are beyond the range of this image-based method. Other signs are, for example, not recognizing cholangiolithiasis, which is then diagnosed with ERCP, or failing to notice surface lesions 5–10 mm in size in the gastrointestinal tract. A lack of perspective is common in this phase; practitioners focus exclusively on structures that they recognize and have no overview of the surroundings. This stage is often found in those who have performed up to 100 independent examinations.

3. Unjustified lack of confidence. Several misdiagnoses can cause practitioners to lose faith in both themselves and the method. Many give up on the method at this point, although their own experience is much more advanced than they realize. This phase can be recognized by a tendency only to describe what is being seen and to avoid making a working or hypothetical diagnosis. Practitioners are heavily reliant on other image-based diagnostic methods (such as computed tomography and percutaneous ultrasound) and base their results on these, even when they do not quite match the impression provided by endoscopic ultrasound. This stage is usually found in those who have carried out around 150 independent examinations.

4. Justified confidence. After these first stages have been passed, the enormous potential of the method starts to become apparent. The practitioner is able to make confident diagnoses and, when necessary, to prescribe interventional therapy (e.g., correct diagnosis of an infected pancreatic pseudocyst followed by endoscopic ultrasound cyst drainage). Practitioners who regularly check their results and assess them critically will find that the potential of this method is almost unlimited.

2 Longitudinal EUS Anatomy

J. Janssen

Introduction

Endoscopic ultrasonography (EUS) started in the 1980s with mechanical radial scanners, which provide a circumferential overview of the gastrointestinal wall and surrounding structures. This specific imaging method was quickly accepted, and reports about difficult anatomic orientation were rare—probably due to the resemblance of the images to those provided by computed tomography (CT). Some 10 years later, longitudinal electronic scanners were developed, allowing biopsies to be taken and EUS interventions to be performed with real-time guidance. Despite the high resolution and good image quality provided, these systems had, and are still having, difficulty in becoming accepted as routine diagnostic instruments as well. The main obstacle is the impression that anatomic orientation is more difficult, resulting in a longer learning curve.

The image produced with linear EUS is similar to that in conventional ultrasound images. To make it easier to recognize images familiar from abdominal ultrasound, the image orientation on the monitor should be analogous: oral (= cranial) on the left side of the screen and anal (= caudal) on the right side.

The lack of a circumferential view has to be compensated by 360° rotation with the echoendoscope. Skilled ultrasonographers and endoscopists, including those with experience in endoscopic retrograde cholangiopancreatography (ERCP), are therefore likely to succeed more easily with linear EUS.

Since the very beginnings of longitudinal EUS, several groups have been concerned with the issues involved in education and training in EUS.[1-4] Workshops and meetings provide an opportunity to learn the examination technique, as well as useful tricks, from experts. However, hands-on training requires a familiar setting and cannot be offered in workshops.

When various EUS centers are compared, it is surprising to see how many different approaches to linear EUS there are, each represented by successful experts. The technique presented in this chapter thus describes only one of several ways of performing linear EUS.

The Philosophy of the Examination

The underlying idea is to develop EUS anatomy along landmarks and guiding structures. The need for endoscopic control is negligible; the exact position of the tip of the echoendoscope is of no interest.

Introduction of the Echoendoscope

As the tip of a longitudinal echoendoscope is stiff and relatively long, it might be difficult to insert the scope smoothly into the esophagus. In particular, the insertion of thicker therapeutic instruments might be challenging. After testing different approaches, the following EUS-guided procedure has proven to be most successful in our institution:Outside the patient, the tip of the scope is rectangularly deflected and inserted around the root of the tongue into the hypopharynx. From this moment, the wall of the hypopharynx can be visualized endosonographically. Often the wall is folded and the tip of the scope could violate or even penetrate the wall when being pushed forward (**Fig. 2.1a**). By slight rotation of the probe, the dorsal wall can be coupled on parallel with the scanner and is displayed horizontally (**Fig. 2.1b**). The scope can now easily be moved forward into the esophagus. Any force must be avoided to prevent perforation.

EUS Landmarks

The *long axis* in the chest and abdomen is represented by the *thoracic and abdominal aorta,* which can be imaged from the esophagus and stomach. The *pancreas* is the *transverse axis* in the abdomen. The third guiding structure (which is of lesser importance) is the *inferior vena cava* (IVC), which can be imaged from the descending part of the duodenum.

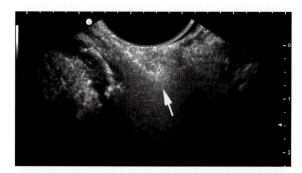 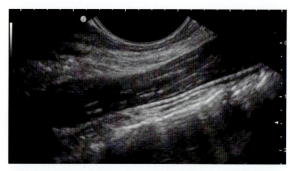

Fig. 2.1a, b The deflected tip of the echoendoscope is introduced into the hypopharynx, but the wall layers cannot be identified due to folds and interposed gas (arrow) (**a**). After slight rotation of the tip toward the dorsal wall and partial reversion of the deflection, the wall layers can be displayed horizontally (**b**). The probe can now easily be moved into the esophagus.

The Examination Sequence

As the aorta is used as the main longitudinal anatomic axis, it seems reasonable to pick up this structure as early as possible while introducing the scope. As the aorta is followed, further anatomic structures become visible, as described in detail later. Thus, the examination starts orally and subsequently extends to the aboral areas. Usually, the region of interest is imaged repeatedly, with the instrument being moved forward and backward while the scope is rotated, as appropriate. Until the pylorus has to be passed, there is normally no need for endoscopic guidance, except to examine small mural lesions. Air insufflation is therefore not necessary, and close contact between the probe and the gastrointestinal wall is established more easily.

 Whenever the echoendoscope cannot be moved easily, endoscopic guidance is mandatory to avoid injuring or even perforating the gastrointestinal wall.

Deep introduction of the echoendoscope into the duodenum is not required for several EUS indications, such as the staging of esophageal cancer. Intubation of the duodenum is necessary to visualize the anatomic area around the pancreatic head or common bile duct, or both.

Special Linear EUS Anatomy

■ EUS Anatomy Displayed from the Esophagus

After the echoendoscope has been introduced, the first anatomic structure seen is the aortic arch, at ≈ 22 cm from the incisors. The branching of the left subclavian artery can be detected immediately, or after turning the scope slightly to the left (**Fig. 2.2a**). Continuing the rotation in a counterclockwise direction along the aortic arch leads to the descending thoracic aorta (**Fig. 2.2b**), which can easily be followed caudally by pushing the scope and adjusting the wheels to adapt the probe to the longitudinal axis of the aorta (▶ Video 2.1a).

The aortopulmonary window, covering level 4 L lymph nodes according to the American Thoracic Society (ATS) map, can also be depicted starting at the aortic arch, with the instrument now being rotated clockwise and moved slightly forward (**Fig. 2.2c**, ▶Video 2.1c). **Figure 2.2 d** is a diagram illustrating the aortopulmonary window.

The trachea is found ≈ 18–25 cm from the incisors by rotating the probe to the front (≈ 180° when starting from the descending aorta). It is sonographically characterized by a bright line with dorsal reverberating artifacts, which are caused by the intratracheal air (**Fig. 2.3a**, ▶ Video 2.2). As the scope is moved forward, the line will end at the carina of the trachea (▶ Video 2.2). The infracarinal area is the region of the posterior level 7 lymph nodes according to the ATS map, which is easily accessible for EUS-guided puncture. For visualization of the right main bronchus, the instrument has to be rotated clockwise (**Fig. 2.3b**). For the left main bronchus, the imaging procedure is reversed. **Figure 2.3c** is a diagram illustrating the trachea and infracarinal lymph node stations.

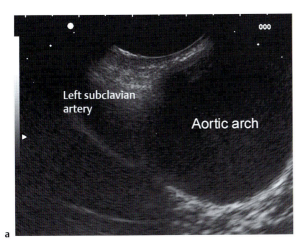

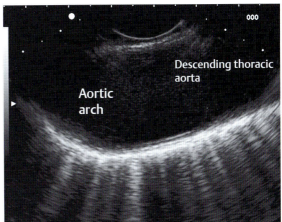

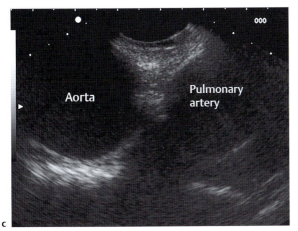

Fig. 2.2a–d **a** The aortic arch and left subclavian artery are seen at 22 cm from the incisors.
b When the scope is turned counterclockwise, the arch can be followed into the descending thoracic aorta.

c When the instrument is rotated clockwise and pushed slightly, the aortopulmonary window becomes visible.
d The anatomic outline of the aortopulmonary window. LN: level 4L lymph node (American Thoracic Society map).

> **!** If one scans *to the front* (e.g., trachea/bronchi), the scope has to be rotated *equivocally* (e.g., to the right) to display a structure lateral to the starting point (e.g., on the right side). If the probe is directed *dorsally*—e.g., toward the aorta—the instrument has to be rotated *unequivocally* to visualize structures on one or the other side of the aorta.

The azygos vein is located at the right side of the aorta and ventral to the thoracic spine. Starting from the aorta, it can be visualized by counterclockwise rotation of the scope (**Fig. 2.4a,b**, ▶ Video 2.3). The vein can be followed close to the oral opening into the superior caval vein by retracting the probe along the azygos vein (▶ Video 2.3).

As the instrument is pushed forward, the left atrium of the heart is seen as a dominant cardiac structure close to the esophagus (**Fig. 2.5a**, ▶ Video 2.4a). Modifying the direction of the scanner in accordance with the individual situation is helpful for inspecting more distant parts of the heart (aortic and mitral valve, left ventricle) and the associated large vessels (ascending thoracic aorta, pulmonary trunk, pulmonary veins) (**Fig. 2.5a–c**, ▶ Video 2.4b).

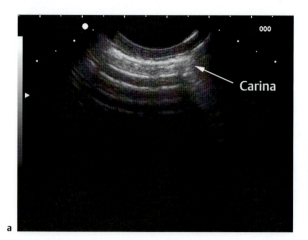

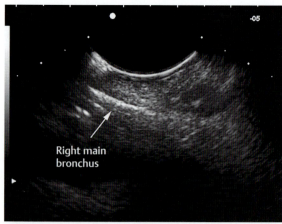

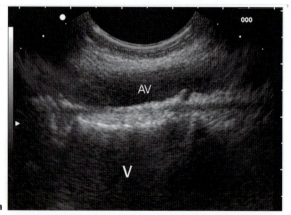

Fig. 2.3a–c a Gas filling in the trachea produces a bright line with dorsal reverberation artifacts.
b Clockwise rotation and some angulation of the probe are necessary for visualization of the right main bronchus.
c Diagram of the trachea and infracarinal lymph-node area.
LN: posterior level 7 lymph node (American Thoracic Society map).

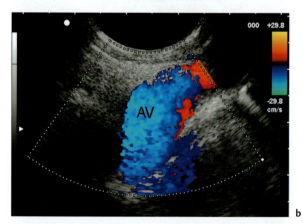

Fig. 2.4a, b The azygos vein (AV) is imaged by counterclockwise rotation of the probe when starting from the upper descending thoracic aorta (**a**). V: vertebra. The vessel can be followed by retract-ing the probe up to the region close to the opening into the superior vena cava (**b**).

■ EUS Anatomy Imaged from the Stomach

As the descending thoracic aorta is followed (**Fig. 2.6a**, ▶ Video 2.1a), the left crus of the diaphragm is seen as a hypoechoic structure ventral to the aorta (**Fig. 2.6b**, ▶ Video 2.5a). This marks the transition into the abdomen. As the stomach is entered, it is important to deflect the probe to maintain close contact with the dorsal gastric wall. In this way, the descending aorta can be followed continuously from the thorax into the abdomen. Intra-abdominally, the cranial abdominal aortic branches, celiac trunk, and superior mesenteric artery (SMA) can usually be seen (**Fig. 2.6c, d**, ▶ Video 2.5a).

The SMA is the decisive landmark for finding the pancreatic body, which is always located ventral to the SMA (**Fig. 2.6 d**, ▶ Video 2.5b).

The pancreas is scanned longitudinally in a craniocaudal direction. With clockwise rotation and slight retraction of the scope toward the spleen, the pancreatic body and the

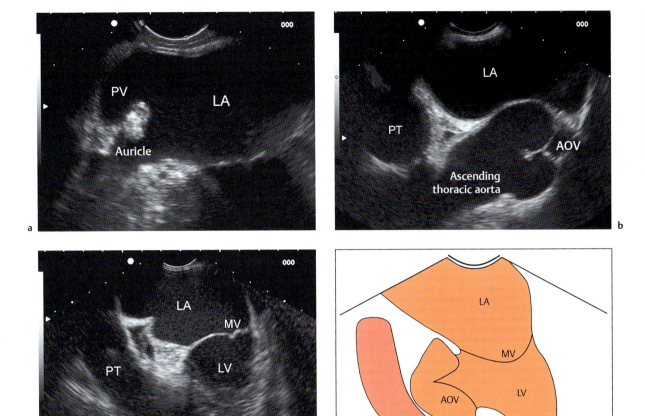

Fig. 2.5a–d EUS anatomy of the heart. The left atrium (LA) is the dominant structure close to the esophagus. Small movements of the probe make it possible to visualize the mitral valve (MV), left ven- tricle (LV), aortic valve (AOV), ascending thoracic aorta, and pulmo- nary trunk (PT). d Diagram showing the most prominent cardiac structures. PV: pulmonary vein.

tail are imaged. In most cases, the left adrenal gland is simultaneously visualized at the left side of the aorta (Figs. 2.6e and 2.7a, ▶ Video 2.6). The adrenal crura can be elaborated by slight movements of the scope tip (Fig. 2.7b, ▶ Video 2.6). Advancing the probe caudally will reveal the left kidney (Fig. 2.6e).

After one has returned to the SMA and continued the counterclockwise rotation, the right part of the pancreatic body and the cranial parts of the pancreatic head, includ- ing the portal venous confluence and the common bile duct outside the pancreas, are examined (Fig. 2.8, ▶ Video 2.7).

This procedure ensures a fast and complete examination of the pancreas, except for the caudal parts of the pancre-

atic head. It is important to carry out the rotations slowly and to ensure that the complete craniocaudal extent of the organ is imaged. There is no need to produce the classic cross-sectional images of the pancreas familiar from trans- cutaneous ultrasonography and radial EUS.

It is always possible to scan through the left liver lobe from the oral lesser curvature of the stomach (Fig. 2.9). When the probe is rotated and angulated as appropriate, the left hepatic vein running into the IVC (Fig. 2.9a, ▶ Video 2.8), the left hepatic duct (Fig. 2.9b), and the left branch of the portal vein including the hepatoumbilical ligament (Fig. 2.9c) can be visualized.

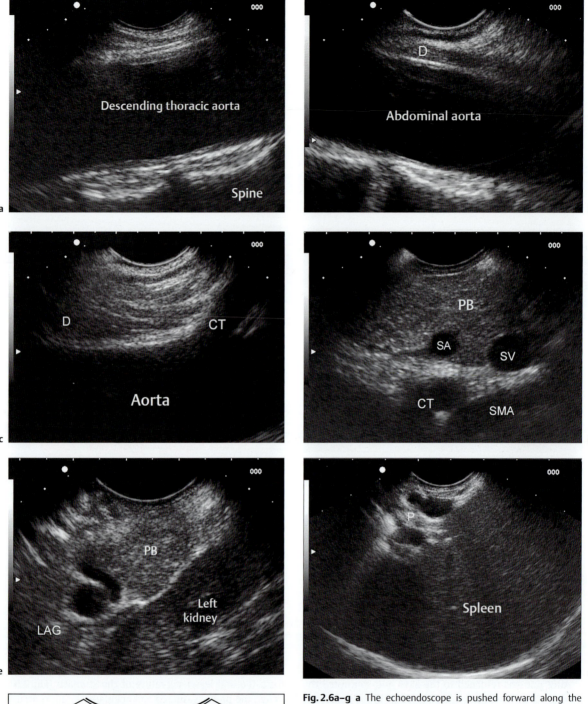

Fig. 2.6a–g a The echoendoscope is pushed forward along the descending thoracic aorta into the abdomen.

b The entrance is marked by the hypoechoic left crus of the diaphragm (D).

c, d This is followed by the cranial aortic branches, the celiac trunk (CT), and the superior mesenteric artery (SMA in **d**). PB, pancreatic body; SA, splenic artery, SV, splenic vein.

e Clockwise rotation and slight retraction of the probe allow visualization of the pancreatic body (PB), left adrenal gland (LAG) and left kidney, and finally the splenic hilum (**f**).

g Diagram of the anatomic structures that can usually be located from the abdominal aorta. SA, splenic artery; SV, splenic vein; SMA, superior mesenteric artery.

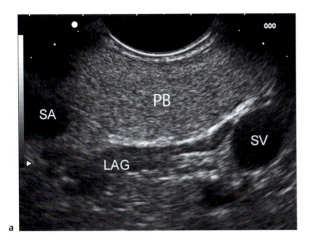

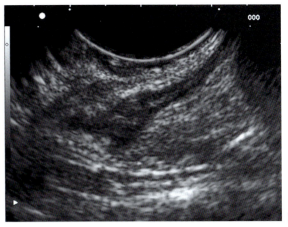

a
b

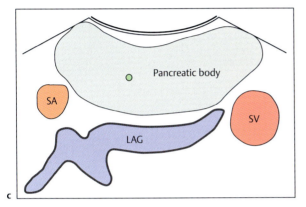

c

Fig. 2.7a–c a The left adrenal gland (LAG) is located at the left side of the aorta and is imaged by slight clockwise rotation of the instrument, starting at the aorta along the pancreatic body (PB). SA, splenic artery; SV, splenic vein.
b The substructure of the adrenal gland—i.e., the hypoechoic cortex and the hyperechoic medulla—is easily differentiated.
c Outline of the anatomic relationship between the pancreatic body and the left adrenal gland. LAG, left adrenal gland; SA, splenic artery; SV, splenic vein.

◼ EUS Anatomy Imaged from the Duodenum

For exploration of the entire pancreatic head, the papilla of Vater, and the distal common bile duct, it is necessary for the scope to pass into the descending duodenum under endoscopic guidance. The instrument is straightened in the same way as in ERCP. We prefer to place the patient in the prone position if the focus of the examination is on the periampullary region or the distal common bile duct. The probe is adherent to the duodenal wall at the minor side. If the insertion depth of the instrument is correct, the caudal pancreatic head and the uncinate process can be seen (**Fig. 2.10**, ▶ Video 2.9). The scope is slowly retracted step by step. At each step, rotation of the instrument is necessary to scan through the entire pancreatic head, thus compensating for the absence of a radial view with the linear probe. The superior mesenteric vessels can be imaged behind the pancreatic head in a precise horizontal section. The vein is seen closer to the probe, while the artery is more distant (**Fig. 2.10b**, ▶ Video 2.9a).

The papilla of Vater is identified as a small hypoechoic structure (**Fig. 2.10c**, ▶ Video 2.9b), which can often be differentiated from pancreatic tissue during the procedure described above, except in very hypoechoic (young) organs. If it is difficult to find the papilla, it is advisable to couple to it under endoscopic guidance.

The common bile duct and the pancreatic duct each run into the papilla of Vater. The two ducts can be followed by thorough retraction of the scope, with the wheels being adjusted and the instrument rotated under guidance from the ultrasound image (**Fig. 2.11**, ▶ Video 2.10). It may be difficult to detect small ducts within a hypoechoic pancreas. EUS imaging conditions improve whenever the ducts are dilated.

The IVC is found by turning the echoendoscope dorsally. The cranial pole of the right kidney is often seen in this position as well. The right adrenal gland is located behind the IVC and can be imaged by pulling the scope back and following the IVC cranially toward the superior duodenal flexure (**Fig. 2.12**).

As one moves back into the duodenal bulb, the probe can be directed cranially to allow inspection of the structures of the liver hilum. Color Doppler imaging facilitates correct identification of the vessels (**Fig. 2.13a**, ▶ Video 2.11). Further retraction of the instrument is needed to visualize the gallbladder (**Fig. 2.13b**).

I Techniques

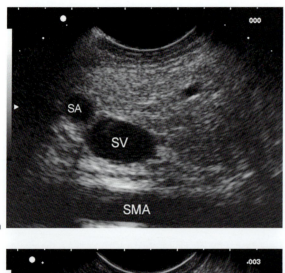

a

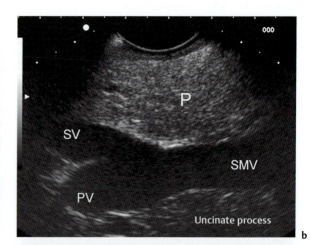

b

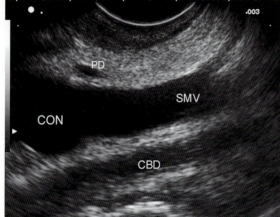

c

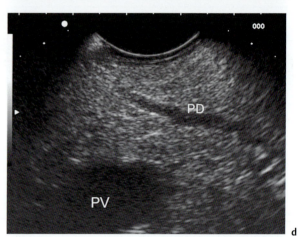

d

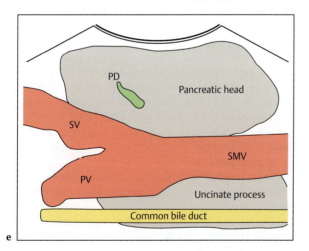

e

Fig. 2.8a–e Starting at the longitudinal image of the superior mesenteric artery (SMA in **a**), counterclockwise rotation of the probe results in imaging of the portal venous confluence (CON in **c**) and the cranial pancreatic head (P in **b**). Dorsally, the common bile duct (CBD) is seen. PD, pancreatic duct; PV, portal vein; SA, splenic artery; SMV, superior mesenteric vein; SV, splenic vein. **d** Angulation of the probe allows visualization of the pancreatic duct (PD), which crosses the confluence ventrally. PV, portal vein. **e** The diagram summarizes the details within and around the pancreatic head, displayed from the stomach. PD, pancreatic duct; PV, portal vein; SV, splenic vein; SMV, superior mesenteric vein.

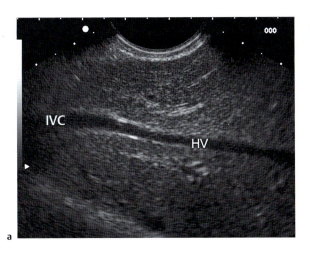

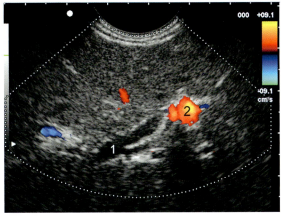

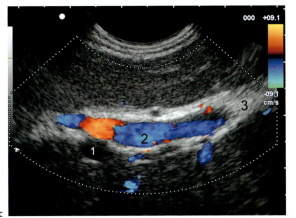

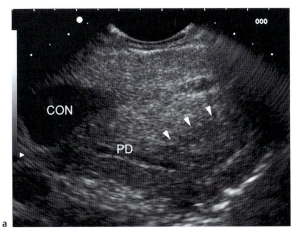

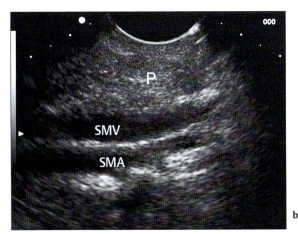

Fig. 2.9a–d Imaging of the left liver lobe from the lesser gastric curvature.
a The left hepatic vein (HV) and the inferior vena cava (IVC).

b, c The left hepatic duct (1), the left branch of the portal vein (2), and the hepatoumbilical ligament (3) can be inspected.
d Diagram.

Fig. 2.10a–d The pancreatic head imaged in the endoscopic retrograde cholangiopancreatography (ERCP) position after straightening of the instrument.
a The ventral pancreas (arrowheads) is hypoechoic, contrasting with the more hyperechoic dorsal pancreas. CON, portal venous confluence; PD, pancreatic duct.

b With precise horizontal scanning, the superior mesenteric vessels are visualized behind the pancreatic head. SMA, superior mesenteric artery: P, pancreatic head; SMV, superior mesenteric vein.

Fig. 2.10c, d ▷

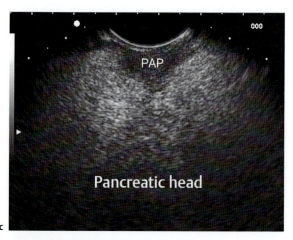

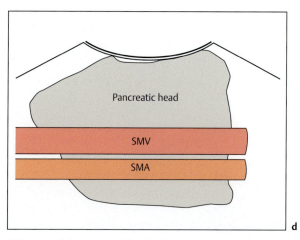

Fig. 2.10c, d (continued)
c The papilla of Vater (PAP) is a small hypoechoic structure that can usually be differentiated from the pancreatic tissue.

d Diagram of the pancreatic head and superior mesenteric vessels, imaged from the descending duodenum. SMV, superior mesenteric vein; SMA, superior mesenteric artery.

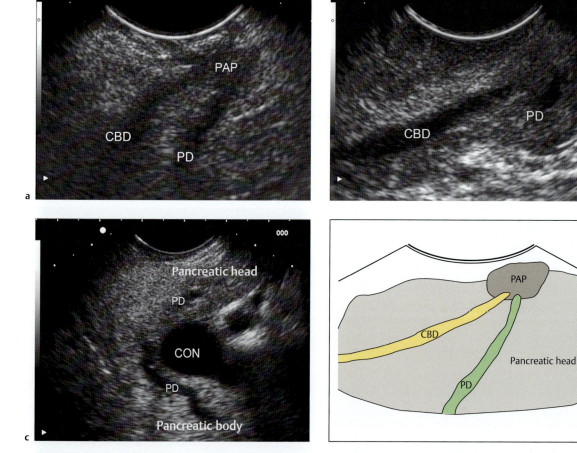

Fig. 2.11a–d a The common bile duct (CBD) and pancreatic duct (PD) are imaged by small movements after visualization of the papilla of Vater (PAP).
b The two ducts can be followed separately by retracting the echoendoscope and adjusting the orientation of the tip. CBD, common bile duct; PD, pancreatic duct.

c The image of the pancreatic duct here is complementary to the image from the stomach shown in **Fig. 2.8 d**. CON, confluence; PD, pancreatic duct.
d The typical periampullary anatomy. CBD, common bile duct; PAP, papilla of Vater; PD, pancreatic duct.

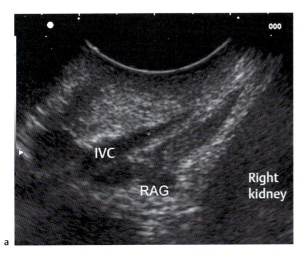

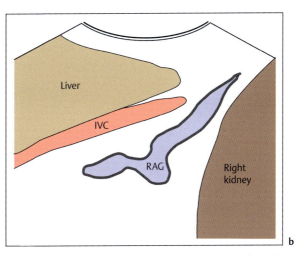

Fig. 2.12a, b a The right adrenal gland (RAG) is best found by retracting the probe along the inferior vena cava (IVC).

b The position of the right adrenal gland at the top of the right kidney and behind the inferior caval vein. IVC, inferior vena cava; RAG, right adrenal gland.

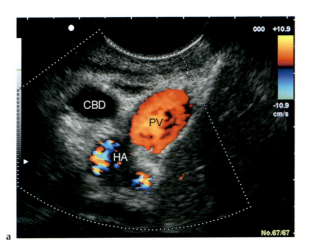

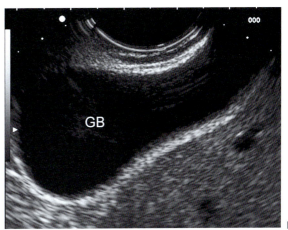

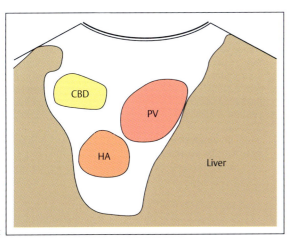

Fig. 2.13a–c a Turning the probe cranially allows inspection of the vessels of the liver hilum. Color Doppler helps identify the vessels. CBD, common bile duct; HA, hepatic artery; PV, portal vein.
b After retraction, the gallbladder (GB) is seen.
c Diagram illustrating the anatomy of the liver hilum. CBD, common bile duct; HA, hepatic artery; PV, portal vein.

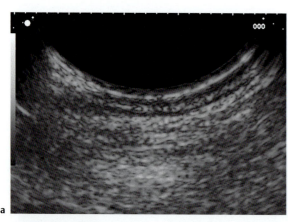

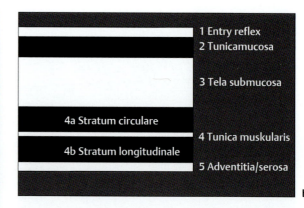

1 Entry reflex
2 Tunicamucosa

3 Tela submucosa

4a Stratum circulare

4 Tunica muskularis

4b Stratum longitudinale

5 Adventitia/serosa

Fig. 2.14a, b a Imaging of the gastric wall layers with conventional linear EUS (10 MHz) without water filling or a balloon. **b** The endosonographic wall layers correlate with the histological ones.

Examination of the Gastrointestinal Wall

Lesions in the gastrointestinal wall are examined endo-sonographically as a specially targeted issue after endoscopy. It is therefore hardly ever necessary to scan the complete wall of the upper gastrointestinal tract in a screening fashion.

Large lesions are found with EUS alone, whereas small ones can be identified under endoscopic guidance more quickly. To investigate the mural layers without compression, it is advisable to fill the lumen with water. Nevertheless, an experienced endosonographer is able to adapt the linear probe to the wall with as little pressure as necessary, thus imaging five or even seven layers of the normal or infiltrated gastrointestinal wall (**Fig. 2.14a,b**, ▶ Video 2.12). As the near scanning field has improved significantly in modern probes, water filling of a mounted balloon is not necessary.

It is important to scan the gastrointestinal wall vertically to image the true thickness of the wall. Oblique scanning leads to overestimation of the thickness and may suggest an infiltrating process.

Conclusion

In our experience, the approach to linear EUS anatomy described here helps beginners find their way through the anatomic forest of EUS. Concentrating on the ultrasound image instead of the endoscopic image makes it easier to adapt the course of the examination to the individual anatomy and pathological findings. Sooner or later, each examiner is able to find his or her own way of performing EUS, modifying and unifying the examination strategies suggested by different experts.

References

1. Janssen J, Greiner L. Examination technique and general principles. In: Rösch T, Will U, Chang KJ, eds. Longitudinal endosonography: atlas and manual for use in the upper gastrointestinal tract. Berlin: Springer; 2001:11–19.
2. Burmester E, Leineweber T, Hacker S, Tiede U, Hütteroth TH, Höhne KH. EUS meets Voxel-Man: three-dimensional anatomic animation of linear-array endoscopic ultrasound images. Endoscopy 2004;36(8):726–730.
3. Bhutani MS, Hoffman BJ, Hawes RH. A swine model for teaching endoscopic ultrasound (EUS) imaging and intervention under EUS guidance. Endoscopy 1998;30(7):605–609.
4. Sorbi D, Vazquez-Sequeiros E, Wiersema MJ. A simple phantom for learning EUS-guided FNA. Gastrointest Endosc 2003;57(4):580–583.

I Techniques

3 EUS meets VOXEL-MAN: a Software-Based Training System for Longitudinal EUS

T. Leineweber, E. Burmester

The indications for endoscopic ultrasound (EUS) have changed fundamentally in recent years. Starting with the interpretation of B-mode images, the range of indications has expanded to include more invasive diagnostic and therapeutic techniques. It was always possible to obtain convincing B-mode images with radial scanners, but the advent of invasive techniques required longitudinal echoendoscopes allowing optimal monitoring of the instruments inserted through the working channel into the ultrasound scanning area.

There are two different techniques in EUS imaging (**Fig. 3.1**):

- *Radial scanning* (radial EUS). The radial instrument produces a 360° image with a 90° angle to the axis of the endoscope (**Fig. 3.1**, right side). This results in a cross-sectional imaging modality when the instrument is adapted to the sagittal axis of the human body—e.g., in the esophagus. Anatomic orientation is easier with a radial instrument, as the images match the viewing patterns of other cross-sectional modalities such as computed tomography (**Fig. 3.2**).
- *Longitudinal scanning* (longitudinal EUS). This instrument produces a longitudinal sagittal sector image parallel to the axis of the endoscope (**Fig. 3.1**). It is challenging to understand these anatomical sections, as they are not comparable to the usual scans produced in computed tomography (CT) or magnetic resonance imaging (MRI). The examiner therefore needs to have excellent skills to achieve the correct orientation. Because of the

flexible tip of the endoscope, multiple sections are available, which cannot be found in an anatomical atlas. For these reasons, longitudinal EUS is more difficult to learn than radial EUS (**Fig. 3.3**).

For a considerable period, the main indication for endoscopic ultrasound was imaging of the wall of the gastrointestinal tract. High-frequency scanners allowed high-resolution imaging of the wall layers, with improved staging of tumors in the wall. Longitudinal echoendoscopes provide a new range of invasive diagnostic indications,

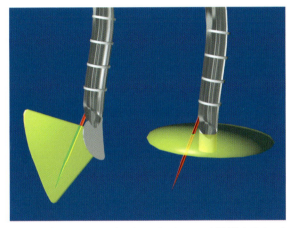

Fig. 3.1 The two types of endoscopic ultrasound (EUS). *Left:* longitudinal EUS; *right:* radial EUS.

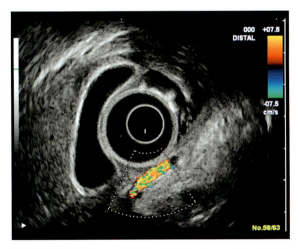

Fig. 3.2 Radial EUS image of the body of the liver and the gallbladder.

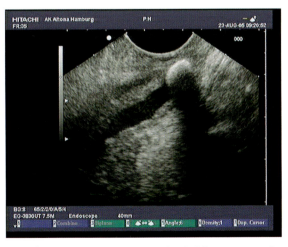

Fig. 3.3 Longitudinal EUS image of the head of the pancreas, with a migrated gallstone in the dilated pancreatic duct.

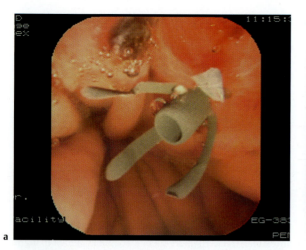
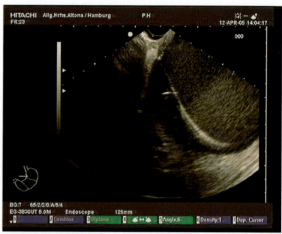

Fig. 3.4a, b Optical (**a**) and longitudinal (**b**) EUS images of pancreatic pseudocyst drainage.

such as EUS-guided fine-needle aspiration (EUS-FNA), and invasive therapeutic indications, such as EUS-guided drainage of pancreatic pseudocysts (**Fig. 3.4**).

The crucial aspect in invasive procedures is to control each step with endoscopic ultrasound. Only longitudinal echoendoscopes offer needle control, as the transducer has the same orientation as the axis of the endoscope, so that the needle moves within the ultrasound field (**Fig. 3.1**).

Outstanding familiarity with the anatomy is important for recognizing the relationship between vessels and organs and minimizing the risk of injuring sensitive structures during invasive procedures.

EUS meets VOXEL-MAN simulates the movements of a longitudinal endosonographic transducer in the human body on a Windows-based operating system. It is a learning tool for the complex anatomical relationships encountered in longitudinal EUS. The software program makes an important contribution to minimizing the risk for patients.

EUS meets VOXEL-MAN

EUS meets VOXEL-MAN consists of three main parts[1–6]:
- An anatomic simulation of longitudinal EUS—the VOXEL-MAN module
- A comparative atlas of longitudinal VOXEL-MAN anatomy and ultrasound anatomy
- Video sequences of real-time examinations, with integrated VOXEL-MAN simulation

The anatomic simulation shows the cross-sectional anatomy using the VOXEL-MAN model.[1,2] This three-dimensional anatomic model is based on the U.S. National Library of Medicine's Visual Human Project data. All parts of *EUS meets VOXEL-MAN* are now available in both image orientations—cranial left and cranial right.

VOXEL-MAN module. The anatomical scenes were calculated for six reference positions in the esophagus, stomach, and duodenum using a QuickTime video format. Users can simulate two basic movements of the endoscope—rotation and angulation using the PC's mouse within the scenes. The transducer can be rotated over 360° and angulated over 20° on the longitudinal axis. Within the six reference positions, all of the crucial anatomical landmarks in longitudinal endoscopic ultrasound can be depicted. Most of the landmarks are vessels, which have to be identified precisely. The integrated knowledge base lists all of the anatomic structures in the model and allows the user to look for these structures and annotate them in three languages (German, English, and Latin).

Atlas. Each anatomical image (**Fig. 3.5**) shows:
- A three-dimensional overview, with the position of the scanner head in the human body and its relationship to the most important anatomical landmarks (left side).
- The corresponding anatomical section, with a mask overlay depicting only the representation of real endoscopic ultrasound (right side).

The atlas shows striking parallelism between the VOXEL-MAN anatomy and real endoscopic ultrasound images (**Fig. 3.6**).

Video sequences. The videos demonstrate real-time longitudinal anatomy and the steps of an examination in order to "translate" the VOXEL-MAN anatomy into the real-time examination.

EUS meets VOXEL-MAN thus provides an interactive simulation of longitudinal endoscopic ultrasound using a detailed computer-based three-dimensional anatomic model.[3–6]

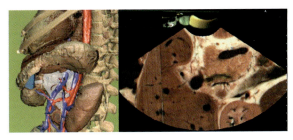

Fig. 3.5 VOXEL-MAN anatomy

▇ Systematic Approach to an EUS Examination

Familiarity with the reference positions and their corresponding anatomical landmarks is crucial for every EUS examination. It is not necessary to adhere closely to the reference positions in their numbered order during the examination (from cranial to caudal or caudal to cranial), as each examination may have its own different emphasis.

These are the reference positions and their corresponding anatomic landmarks:

- Reference position 1: upper esophagus, descending aorta (**Fig. 3.7**), aortic arch, azygos vein
- Reference position 2: middle esophagus, heart (**Fig. 3.8**), right pulmonary artery, trachea (**Fig. 3.9**), bronchus, and aortopulmonary window
- Reference position 3: gastric fundus, abdominal aorta (part IV) with exiting celiac trunk (**Fig. 3.10**), splenic artery and splenic vein with pancreatic body and tail (**Fig. 3.11**), splenoportal confluence (**Fig. 3.12**), left lobe of the liver
- Reference position 4: duodenal bulb, portal hilum (**Fig. 3.13**), gallbladder (**Fig. 3.14**), common bile duct
- Reference position 5: papilla region, mesenteric vessels, head of the pancreas with pancreatic duct (**Fig. 3.15**), common bile duct, cystic duct
- Reference position 6: deep parts of the duodenum, abdominal aorta (part V), and inferior vena cava (**Fig. 3.16**)

For more information, see http://www.eus-meets-voxel-man.de.

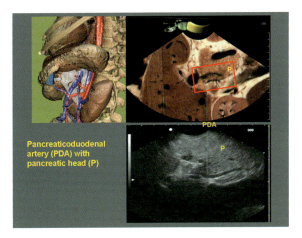

Pancreaticoduodenal artery (PDA) with pancreatic head (P)

Fig. 3.6 Parallelism between VOXEL-MAN and ultrasound anatomy: the pancreaticoduodenal artery (PDA) and pancreatic head (P).

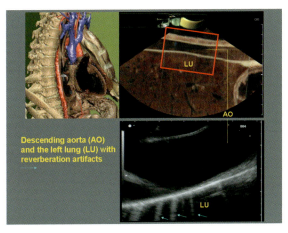

Descending aorta (AO) and the left lung (LU) with reverberation artifacts

Fig. 3.7 Atlas image of the descending aorta (AO) and left lung (LU), with reverberation artifacts (arrows).

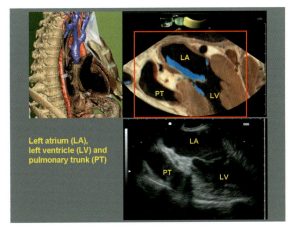

Left atrium (LA), left ventricle (LV) and pulmonary trunk (PT)

Fig. 3.8 Atlas image of the left atrium (LA) of the heart, left ventricle (LV), and pulmonary trunk (PT).

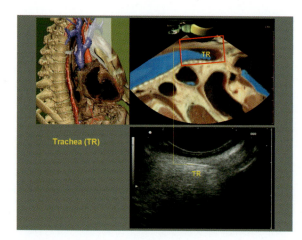

Fig. 3.9 Atlas image of the trachea (TR).

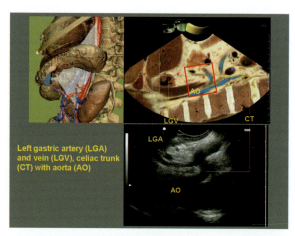

Fig. 3.10 Atlas image of the left gastric artery (LGA) and vein (LGV), with the celiac trunk (CT) and aorta (AO).

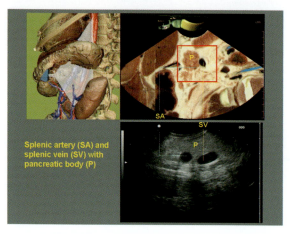

Fig. 3.11 Atlas image of the splenic artery (SA) and vein (SV), with the pancreatic body (P).

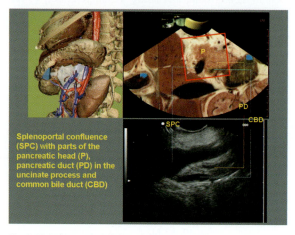

Fig. 3.12 Atlas image of the splenoportal confluence (SPC), with parts of the pancreatic head (P), the pancreatic duct (PD) in the uncinate process, and common bile duct (CBD).

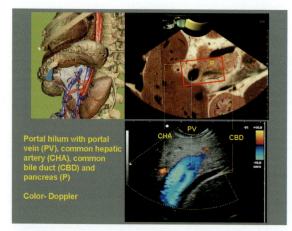

Fig. 3.13 Atlas image of the portal hilum with the portal vein (PV), common hepatic artery (CHA), common bile duct (CBD), and pancreas (P). The vessels are shown with color Doppler imaging.

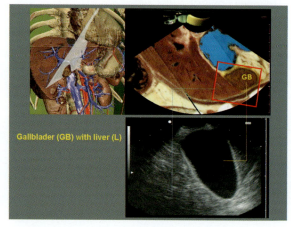

Fig. 3.14 Atlas image of the gallbladder (GB) with the liver.

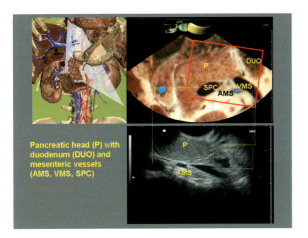

Fig. 3.15 Atlas image of the pancreatic head (P) with the duodenum (DUO) and mesenteric vessels. AMS, superior mesenteric artery; VMS, superior mesenteric vein; SPC, splenoportal confluence.

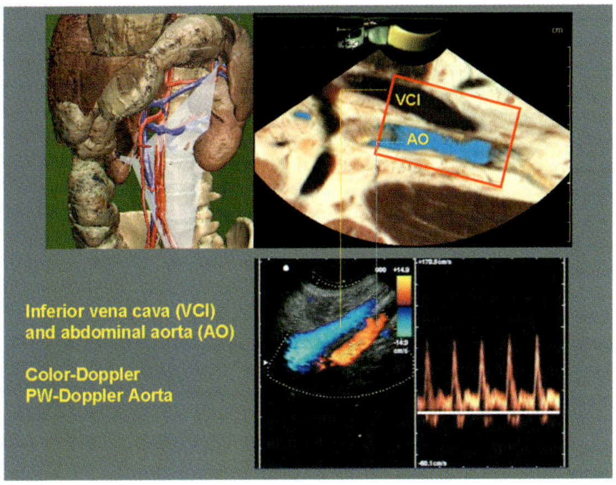

Fig. 3.16 Atlas image of the inferior vena cava (VCI) and abdominal aorta (AO), with color Doppler and pulsed-wave Doppler imaging of the aorta.

References

1. Höhne KH, Pflesser B, Pommert A, et al. VOXEL-MAN 3 D navigator: inner organs. Regional, systemic and radiological anatomy. Heidelberg: Springer; 2000 (3 CD-ROMs, ISBN 3–540–14759–4).
2. Pommert A, Höhne KH, Pflesser B, et al. Creating a high-resolution spatial/symbolic model of the inner organs based on the Visible Human. Med Image Anal 2001;5(3):221–228.
3. Hacker S, Tiede U, Burmester E, Leineweber T, Höhne KH. Ein virtuelles Trainingssystem für endoskopische Longitudinal-Ultraschalluntersuchungen. In: Meiler M, Saupe D, Kruggel F, eds. Bildverarbeitung für die Medizin 2002. Algorithmen—Systeme—Anwendungen. Proceedings des Workshop vom 10.–12. März 2002 in Leipzig. Informatik Aktuell. Berlin: Springer; 2002:149–152.
4. Hacker S, Tiede U, Burmester E, Leineweber T, Höhne KH. A virtual training system for linear-type endoscopic ultrasonography. In: Lemke HU, Vannier MW, Inamura K, Farman AG, Doi K, Reiber JHC, eds. CARS 2002: computer-assisted radiology and surgery. Proceedings of the 16th International Congress and Exhibition, Paris, June 26–29, 2002. Heidelberg: Springer; 2002:1–5.
5. Burmester E, Hollerbach S. Report on the working session "Endoscopic Ultrasound" of the German Society for Digestive and Metabolic Diseases in Bonn, 11. 9. 2002. [Article in German] Z Gastroenterol 2003;41(4):362–367.
6. Burmester E, Leineweber T, Hacker S, Tiede U, Hütteroth TH, Höhne KH. EUS Meets Voxel-Man: three-dimensional anatomic animation of linear-array endoscopic ultrasound images. Endoscopy 2004;36(8):726–730.

4 Miniprobes

H. Seifert, C.F. Dietrich

During the last 15 years, endoscopic ultrasound (EUS) has gained wide acceptance as the method of choice for the local staging of gastrointestinal tumors. It allows visualization of the intestinal wall and of surrounding structures with a resolution unequaled by other imaging modalities. However, EUS continued for a long time to be a specialty requiring expensive equipment, echoendoscopes dedicated to the technique, and special training of examiners. With the advent of flexible high-frequency miniprobes that can be introduced through the working channel of any endoscope, EUS became available as an additional and very powerful diagnostic tool during routine endoscopic procedures. While conventional transabdominal ultrasonography (TUS) using the most sophisticated techniques provides excellent images of almost every anatomical region in the abdomen, miniprobes can be directed to very small structures of interest that can only be targeted under direct endoscopic guidance. It is thought that structures missed on TUS can be identified with miniprobes and vice versa, making the two methods ideal and complementary partners in modern gastrointestinal imaging.

After a discussion of a few technical considerations and practical remarks, useful applications of EUS miniprobes (see **Table 4.1**) and future perspectives for the technique are discussed below, on the basis of the available published evidence and the authors' experience. Examples are given in various other chapters.

Technical Considerations and Practical Remarks

Miniprobes for routine diagnostic use are usually high-frequency mechanical scanners with a diameter of 1.7–3.4 mm that can be introduced through the working channel of any flexible endoscope. Frequently asked questions regarding the clinical application of miniprobes include the following.

Which frequency should be used? The available miniprobes cover a frequency range of 12–30 MHz, with higher frequencies corresponding to lesser penetration depth. There have been no systematic studies comparing miniprobes of different frequencies for a single application. In the authors' experience, 20-MHz probes are most useful for all applications. With lower frequencies, visualization of the extramural anatomy and staging of advanced tumors may be easier. However, for the extramural anatomy, conventional EUS with radial or longitudinal scanners provides similar frequencies (7.5–12 MHz) and superior image quality, and for advanced tumors, EUS local staging seems of limited relevance. With higher frequencies (30 MHz), fine resolution of the intestinal wall would be excellent, but with the drawback of losing sight of almost any external structure. As long as there is at best very limited evidence correlating ultrasound morphology with histology, 20 MHz appears to provide the ideal compromise between excellent local resolution and visualization of the relevant surrounding anatomy. At this frequency, with a penetration depth of ≈ 2 cm, a considerable

Table 4.1 Applications of miniprobes in the gastrointestinal tract

Application	Targets	Examples
Examination of structures within or adjacent to the intestinal wall	• Mucosal neoplasias • Submucosal tumors • Myogenic tumors, GIST • Paraesophageal or paragastric lymph nodes • Vascular formations (varices) • All organs within 2 cm of the intestine	• Cancer staging (EEC, EGC, endoscopic mucosal resection) • Differentiation of unknown structures (e.g., cystic vs. solid) • Focal pancreatic lesions
IDUS	Bile duct and pancreatic duct with surrounding tissue	Small pancreatic and biliary tumors, stones, staging of CCC
EDUS	Distal bile duct and pancreatic duct	Small CBD stones Small periampullary tumors

CBD, common bile duct; CCC, cholangiocarcinoma; EDUS, extraductal ultrasound; EEC, early esophageal cancer; EGC, early gastric cancer; IDUS, intraductal ultrasound; GIST, gastrointestinal stromal tumor.

part of the abdominal anatomy can be seen. This perigastric and periduodenal (and sometimes also pericolonic) volume of 2 cm comprises the periesophageal area and part of the mediastinal lymph nodes, the aorta, pericardial and pleural fluid, infradiaphragmatic and perigastric lymph nodes, the splenic hilum, celiac trunk, splenic artery and vein, part of the pancreas and pancreatic duct, the left adrenal gland, the distal common bile duct (CBD), and sometimes liver hilum, part of the gallbladder, and free abdominal fluid. In addition, the intestinal wall with adherent lesions is seen with superior resolution. This is true of both intraluminal and intraductal applications; for lesions in the pancreatic or the bile duct, a periductal cylinder of 1–2 cm correctly represents the region of interest.

Diameter, rigidity and shape: are they important? Theoretically, a minimal diameter would be most desirable. It would allow easy introduction even through narrow working channels and atraumatic cannulation of the papilla of Vater for pancreatic or biliary intraductal ultrasonography (IDUS). Rigidity of the tip should be minimal to allow steering with the Albarrán lever without breaking the transducer. The tip should be rounded and smooth, as otherwise it could be trapped by mucosal folds, leading to injury to the mucosa and damage to the probe. Alternatively, probes with a guide wire port at their tip are very useful for wire-guided IDUS, but are also restricted to this technique. In the authors' experience, very slim probes (<2 mm) are easy to handle, but at the cost of inferior image quality. For most universal use, a 2.5-mm probe with a flexible, blunted tip appears at present to be the best compromise.

How is sonographic coupling to the wall accomplished? Is a balloon required? Although balloons are available, sonographic coupling to the intestinal wall is better obtained by direct contact between the probe and the mucosal surface or, for small superficial lesions, by injecting some saline or tap water. The use of large-channel endoscopes that allow instillation as well as aspiration of water while the miniprobe is inserted can therefore be recommended. Using a balloon sheath increases the diameter of the probe from 2.5 or 2.0 mm to 3.6 mm, thereby preventing effective suction even with a large-channel endoscope (3.7 mm). For endobronchial ultrasonography (EBUS), balloons are necessary to obtain adequate coupling.[1,2]

What about durability and price? The durability of different miniprobes has improved considerably in recent years. However, they can still easily be damaged by one mistake—trapping them with the duodenoscope's elevator. Most often, they lose functionality due to small breaks in the plastic sheath close to the tip, leading to air bubbles disturbing the image. In some miniprobes, the plastic sheath can be exchanged—a very cost-effective repair. We believe that miniprobes should be available at a reasonable price, as part of the advanced endoscopic arma-

mentarium. If they were capable of replacing conventional EUS for many of its applications, then even now they would represent a cost-effective alternative. The lack of adequately defined reimbursement for EUS in some countries should not lead to the disappearance of a powerful diagnostic tool such as this.

Before physicians embark on miniprobe EUS, it is recommended that they compare the latest developments from different companies with regard to image quality, possible applications, and price. If handled properly, a miniprobe should last for at least 80–100 applications (including IDUS) (**Table 4.1**).

Miniprobe Applications in the Gastrointestinal Tract

■ Examination of Structures within and Adjacent to the Intestinal Wall

Miniprobe EUS has been reported to be valuable for the staging of colorectal neoplasms (T staging accuracy 90%), cholangiocellular carcinoma (T staging accuracy 89%, N staging 60%), lymphoma, and esophageal and pancreatic tumors.[3–9] The literature is summarized in **Table 4.2**.[4,7,9–15]

In stenosing esophageal tumors, EUS staging with miniprobes appears to be recommendable, as passage is always possible without prior bougienage or balloon dilation of the stenosis. As long as any form of therapy other than endoscopic palliation is intended, this type of traumatic approach to a tumor contradicts the principles of oncology. In addition, in advanced esophageal tumors, the value of EUS staging appears to be questionable. Most stenosing tumors of the esophagus can be expected to be T3 N1[16]—all the more so when the tumor boundaries are beyond the reach of the miniprobe (i.e., 20 mm).

In "submucosal" tumors, myogenic lesions are easily differentiated from submucosal or intramucosal ones. Vascular lesions such as gastric angiodysplasia or eroded vessels after ulcer bleeding are clearly visualized, and there may be substantial therapeutic implications.

In comparison with conventional endosonography using 7.5-MHz large-diameter instruments, miniprobe ultrasonography allows safe passage through high-grade malignant esophageal strictures; higher accuracy rates for T staging; and similar rates for N staging.[7]

After endoscopic mucosal resection (EMR) became an important therapeutic option for early esophageal and gastric cancer, miniprobe EUS staging was found to be the most valuable method of preinterventional local staging.[11] In 46 patients with gastric cancers, the miniprobe EUS findings were compared with histopathological findings after treatment. The total accuracy of miniprobe EUS relative to the depth of tumor invasion was 71.7% (33 of 46

Table 4.2 Miniprobe ultrasound in the evaluation of various diseases

Method	Disease	Accuracy (%)	Sensitivity (%)	Specificity (%)	PPV	NPV	Reference
IDUS	Biliary obstruction	89.1	91.1	80	n.a.	n.a.	[4]
EUS	Biliary obstruction	75.6	75.7	75	n.a.	n.a.	[4]
UMP	Gastric cancer	71.7	n.a.	n.a.	n.a.	n.a.	[4]
EUS	Esophageal carcinoma	62	n.a.	n.a.	n.a.	n.a.	[7]
MPS	Esophageal carcinoma	86.8	n.a.	n.a.	n.a.	n.a.	[7]
MPS	Gastric cancer with lymph-node involvement	80	73	89	n.a.	n.a.	[10]
MPS	Esophageal cancer	90	n.a.	n.a.	n.a.	n.a.	[10]
MPS	Esophageal cancer with lymph-node involvement	78	75	80	n.a.	n.a.	[10]
MPS	Gastric cancer	82	n.a.	n.a.	n.a.	n.a.	[10]
MPS	Gastric cancer all tumors	61	n.a.	n.a.	n.a.	n.a.	[11]
MPS	Gastric cancer T1	72	n.a.	n.a.	n.a.	n.a.	[11]
MPS	Gastric cancer T2–4	40	n.a.	n.a.	n.a.	n.a.	[11]
MPS	Gastric cancer nodal staging, overall	69	n.a.	n.a.	n.a.	n.a.	[11]
MPS	Gastric cancer N0	86	n.a.	n.a.	n.a.	n.a.	[11]
MPS	Gastric cancer N1	25	n.a.	n.a.	n.a.	n.a.	[11]
MPS	Gastric cancer N2	14	n.a.	n.a.	n.a.	n.a.	[11]
IDUS	Papillary adenocarcinoma	90	89	90	n.a.	n.a.	[12]
IDUS	Bile duct cancer	76	89	50	n.a.	n.a.	[13]
IDUS	Pancreatic carcinoma	n.a.	75	67	n.a.	n.a.	[14]
ERCP	Pancreatic carcinoma	n.a.	37	67	n.a.	n.a.	[14]
CT	Pancreatic carcinoma	n.a.	37	33	n.a.	n.a.	[14]
EUS	Pancreatic carcinoma	n.a.	50	67	n.a.	n.a.	[14]
IDUS	Biliary tract tumor	n.a.	89	89	n.a.	n.a.	[14]
ERCP	Biliary tract tumor	n.a.	78	88	n.a.	n.a.	[14]
CT	Biliary tract tumor	n.a.	33	60	n.a.	n.a.	[14]
EUS	Biliary tract tumor	n.a.	33	75	n.a.	n.a.	[14]
EUS	Pancreatic cancer	n.a.	92.9	58.3	n.a.	n.a.	[15]
CT	Pancreatic cancer	n.a.	64.3	66.7	n.a.	n.a.	[15]
ERP	Pancreatic cancer	n.a.	85.7	66.7	n.a.	n.a.	[15]
IDUS	Pancreatic cancer	n.a.	100	91.7	n.a.	n.a.	[15]

CT, computed tomography; ERCP, endoscopic retrograde cholangiopancreatography; ERP, endoscopic retrograde pancreatography; EUS, endoscopic ultrasonography; IDUS, intraductal ultrasonography; MPS, miniprobe sonography; n.a., data not available; NPV, negative predictive value; PPV, positive predictive value; UMP, ultrasound miniprobe.

patients). The accuracy for T1m tumor diagnosis was 75.7% (22 of 29 patients). For T1sm lesions, it was 76.9% (10 of 13 patients), but the accuracy for T2 tumor diagnosis was low due to ultrasound attenuation. When the analysis was performed on the basis of the size of tumor, the accuracy was 50.0% (nine of 18 patients) for all tumors larger than 20 mm in diameter and 85.7% (24 of 28 patients) for all tumors smaller than 20 mm.[17]

Gastric mucosa-associated lymphoid tissue (MALT) lesions have been accurately visualized with miniprobe EUS.[6] During the follow-up period after therapy, in patients with normal miniprobe ultrasonography findings (n = 15), the histological examination confirmed complete remission in all patients. Hypoechoic thickening of the mucosa or submucosa, or both, was seen in nine patients. Endoscopic biopsies in four of these nine patients revealed recurrent lymphoma.[6]

In 63 patients with tumors of the colon or rectum, miniprobe ultrasonography revealed carcinoma in five of 30 broad-based polyps, although adenomas were diagnosed on endoscopy. Correct assessment of lymph-node involvement was obtained in 47 of 55 patients. On the basis of the miniprobe ultrasonography findings, management was modified in seven of the 63 patients.[3]

Despite the excellent resolution of small anatomical structures provided, miniprobe EUS is not a substitute for histological analysis. In ulcerated or polypoid lesions, malignancy must be confirmed or excluded by biopsy; this applies in particular to the follow-up situation after radiotherapy or chemotherapy.

Extraductal Ultrasonography

Extraductal ultrasound (EDUS), as opposed to intraductal ultrasound (IDUS; see Chapter 5) is defined as endoscopic ultrasound with miniprobes visualizing the distal CBD from the duodenal, extraductal position. EDUS is a non-invasive application of miniprobes, without the need to cannulate the ostium and without altering the organ of interest. The distal CBD and in many instances also the distal pancreatic duct can be visualized in an unaltered state. EDUS allows excellent visualization of the distal common bile duct and detects small stones with a sensitivity of 94% and a specificity of 99%.[9]

Future Developments

Linear miniprobes with electronic scanners (no mechanical parts). Three-dimensional display and the ability to review endoluminal ultrasound data interactively may improve the staging of gastrointestinal tumors.[18] In a small series of patients with cholangiocellular carcinoma, three-dimensional intraductal ultrasonography allowed accurate assessment of tumor invasion of the right hepatic artery in 88% of cases, the portal vein in 100%, and pancreatic parenchyma in 100%.[12] These preliminary data are encouraging for further evaluation of this technique. Spatial three-dimensional reconstructions of high-resolution IDUS images combined with cholangioscopic images and histopathology or cytopathology findings obtained via percutaneous transhepatic access may become a powerful diagnostic technique for planning differential therapy of cholangiocarcinoma.

Conclusions

The preliminary results show that miniprobe ultrasonography can in many cases enhance the examination of structures within and adjacent to the intestinal wall. This technique is easily performed during routine endoscopy, and is therefore helpful in everyday routine conditions due to the view beyond the gastrointestinal wall that it provides.

References

1. Hürter T, Hanrath P. Endobronchial sonography: feasibility and preliminary results. Thorax 1992;47(7):565–567.
2. Herth F, Becker HD, Manegold C, Drings P. Endobronchial ultrasound (EBUS)—assessment of a new diagnostic tool in bronchoscopy for staging of lung cancer. Onkologie 2001; 24(2):151–154.
3. Hünerbein M, Totkas S, Ghadimi BM, Schlag PM. Preoperative evaluation of colorectal neoplasms by colonoscopic miniprobe ultrasonography. Ann Surg 2000;232(1):46–50.
4. Menzel J, Poremba C, Dietl KH, Domschke W. Preoperative diagnosis of bile duct strictures—comparison of intraductal ultrasonography with conventional endosonography. Scand J Gastroenterol 2000;35(1):77–82.
5. Tamada K, Nagai H, Yasuda Y, et al. Transpapillary intraductal US prior to biliary drainage in the assessment of longitudinal spread of extrahepatic bile duct carcinoma. Gastrointest Endosc 2001;53(3):300–307.
6. Lügering N, Menzel J, Kucharzik T, et al. Impact of miniprobes compared to conventional endosonography in the staging of low-grade gastric malt lymphoma. Endoscopy 2001; 33(10):832–837.
7. Menzel J, Hoepffner N, Nottberg H, Schulz C, Senninger N, Domschke W. Preoperative staging of esophageal carcinoma: miniprobe sonography versus conventional endoscopic ultrasound in a prospective histopathologically verified study. Endoscopy 1999;31(4):291–297.
8. Ariyama J, Suyama M, Satoh K, Wakabayashi K. Endoscopic ultrasound and intraductal ultrasound in the diagnosis of small pancreatic tumors. Abdom Imaging 1998; 23(4):380–386.
9. Seifert H, Wehrmann T, Hilgers R, Gouder S, Braden B, Dietrich CF. Catheter probe extraductal EUS reliably detects distal common bile duct abnormalities. Gastrointest Endosc 2004;60(1):61–67.
10. Hünerbein M, Ghadimi BM, Haensch W, Schlag PM. Transendoscopic ultrasound of esophageal and gastric cancer using miniaturized ultrasound catheter probes. Gastrointest Endosc 1998;48(4):371–375.
11. Akahoshi K, Chijiiwa Y, Sasaki I, et al. Pre-operative TN staging of gastric cancer using a 15 MHz ultrasound miniprobe. Br J Radiol 1997;70(835):703–707.
12. Tamada K, Kanai N, Tomiyama T, et al. Prediction of the histologic type of bile duct cancer by using intraductal ultrasonography. Abdom Imaging 1999;24(5):484–490.
13. Tamada K, Kanai N, Ueno N, et al. Limitations of intraductal ultrasonography in differentiating between bile duct cancer in stage T1 and stage T2: in-vitro and in-vivo studies. Endoscopy 1997;29(8):721–725.
14. Menzel J, Domschke W, Konturek JW, Gillessen A, Foerster E. Intraductal ultrasound in the pancreaticobiliary duct system. [Article in German] Dtsch Med Wochenschr 1997; 122(3):41–49, discussion 50.
15. Furukawa T, Tsukamoto Y, Naitoh Y, Hirooka Y, Hayakawa T. Differential diagnosis between benign and malignant localized stenosis of the main pancreatic duct by intraductal ultrasound of the pancreas. Am J Gastroenterol 1994; 89(11):2038–2041.
16. Vickers J, Alderson D. Influence of luminal obstruction on oesophageal cancer staging using endoscopic ultrasonography. Br J Surg 1998;85(7):999–1001.

17. Okamura S, Tsutsui A, Muguruma N, et al. The utility and limitations of an ultrasonic miniprobe in the staging of gastric cancer. J Med Invest 1999;46(1-2):49–53.

18. Hünerbein M, Ghadimi BM, Gretschel S, Schlag PM. Three-dimensional endoluminal ultrasound: a new method for the evaluation of gastrointestinal tumors. Abdom Imaging 1999;24(5):445–448.

5 Intraductal Ultrasound

B. Braden, H. Seifert, C.F. Dietrich

Following initial reports on the intravascular use of high-frequency filiform miniprobes, biliary and pancreatic intraductal ultrasonography (IDUS) led to impressive imaging of these ducts and to valuable diagnostic information complementary to endoscopic retrograde cholangiopancreatography (ERCP), especially in patients with intraductal papillary tumors—further enhancing the potential of endoscopic ultrasonography.[1-3] Although there are some features that are typical of malignant lesions, there are no criteria sufficiently reliable to allow differentiation between benign and malignant biliary or pancreatic lesions.

Miniprobes with outer diameters of only 2–3 mm can be inserted through the instrument channel of standard endoscopes and provide high-frequency ultrasound images. The flexibility and small diameter of miniprobes allow intraductal ultrasonography (IDUS) in the biliary tract and pancreatic duct, as well as in the endobronchial system.

High-frequency endoscopic ultrasound (EUS) probes are not well suited for screening examinations. The high resolution of miniprobes is useful for further differentiation and characterization of pathological structures that have been identified with other imaging methods (e.g., endoscopy or transabdominal ultrasound) or to answer specific clinical questions (e.g., suspected choledocholithiasis).

Due to wear on the instruments, miniprobes have a short lifespan when used intraductally, and this is still a drawback with this endosonographic technique. No cost–benefit analyses have so far been published.

Technical Developments

In comparison with conventional endosonography, miniprobes work at substantially higher frequencies (12–30 MHz). This results in a high resolution (0.07–0.18 mm) that allows precise differentiation of the discrete wall layers in the esophagus, stomach, and bowel. Electronic miniprobes have a ring at the top that incorporates 64 transducer elements, which produce a 360° image. Electronic miniprobes are highly flexible, but have the disadvantage of restricted lateral resolution. In contrast, mechanical systems produce a 360° image with significantly better resolution, with a rotating transducer at the top of the probe.

New miniprobe developments, with controlled automated retraction over a defined distance, allow three-dimensional reconstruction after complex image processing.

Continuing research on probe design, which may improve the durability of the instruments and extend the depth of penetration, may encourage more widespread use of this novel technology.

Intraductal Ultrasound of the Hepatobiliary System

Small-caliber miniprobes can be inserted into the bile duct during ERCP. Prior papillotomy makes insertion easier, but may not be essential. Wire-guided miniprobes allow cannulation of the bile duct in nearly 100% of cases without previous sphincterotomy.[4] Miniprobes can also be placed in specific intrahepatic bile ducts over a selectively placed guide wire. The position of the probe can be controlled radiographically during endoscopic retrograde cholangiography (ERC).

IDUS prolongs the examination time only marginally (≈5–10 minutes). It has been reported that it does not increase the complication rate with ERCP (one case of mild pancreatitis in 400 patients).[5]

Biliary IDUS provides a high-resolution display of structures in the hepatoduodenal ligament (portal vein, hepatic artery, and lymph nodes) (**Fig. 5.1**).[6] Close to the papilla of Vater, IDUS depicts the surrounding pancreatic parenchyma with a penetration depth of 2 cm. In the intrahepatic position, the miniprobe shows parallel branches of the portal vein and the surrounding liver parenchyma.

IDUS distinguishes three layers of the normal wall of the bile duct. The fine inner and more echogenic layer corresponds to the transition echo. The next layer, less echogenic, matches the mucosa and muscularis propria (fibromuscular layer). The outer more echogenic layer corresponds to the fatty tissue of the subserosa, the serosa, and the transition echo to neighboring organs.[7]

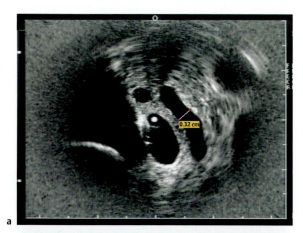

a

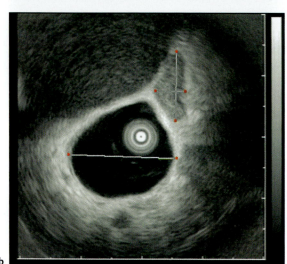

b

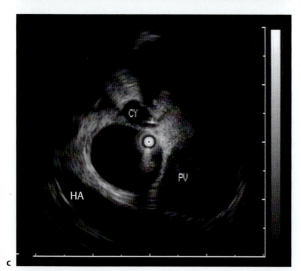

c

Fig. 5.1a–c Anatomy of the bile duct.
a Intraductal (common bile duct) imaging of the pancreatic duct close to the papilla.
b A lymph node in the hepatoduodenal ligament close to the cystic duct.[6]
c The origin of the cystic duct. PV, portal vein; HA, hepatic artery; CY, cystic duct.

Choledocholithiasis

With both transabdominal ultrasonography and computed tomography, it can sometimes be difficult to detect gallstones in the bile duct. Interpreting magnetic resonance imaging (MRI) of the bile duct is still a sophisticated exercise. ERCP is therefore still the gold standard in the diagnosis and treatment of choledocholithiasis. However, even on ERCP, small stones may be overlooked, and it is difficult to distinguish between aerobilia and small stones. Conventional endosonography from a duodenal position has a high sensitivity of 95% for detecting choledocholithiasis, similar to that of ERCP.[8]

The best results reported for detecting choledocholithiasis were obtained with IDUS of the bile duct.[9,10] In a prospective study by Palazzo, 97% of bile duct stones were detected with the miniprobe, 81% during ERCP, 61% with intravenous cholangiography, and 45% by transabdominal ultrasonography.[11] Particular advantages of IDUS are that it makes it easier to distinguish between air, sludge, and stones and that it provides high resolution even of small stones (<5 mm in diameter). IDUS of the bile duct can therefore be a valuable tool for diagnosing choledocholithiasis. If (wire-guided) IDUS of the bile duct is negative, sphincterotomy can be avoided. In contrast to invasive IDUS, we prefer extraductal ultrasound (EDUS; see also Chapter 20 on EUS of the hepatobiliary system) in most cases[12] (see below).

Review of the Literature

IDUS is useful for detecting small residual bile duct stones during endoscopic balloon sphincteroplasty when stones are fragmented by mechanical lithotripsy, or when there is evidence of a dilated bile duct (>10 mm).[13] In 62 patients with suspected bile duct stones, the accuracy of ERC combined with IDUS for diagnosing bile duct stone and/or sludge was higher than that of ERC alone (97% versus 87%; $P<0.05$). With dilated bile ducts, the diagnostic accuracy of ERC combined with IDUS was also higher than that of ERC alone (95.5% versus 72.7%; $P<0.05$). Additional diagnostic information provided by IDUS included identification of cystic duct stones in five patients, characterization of bile duct strictures in two patients, and choledochal varices in one patient.[14] In 65 patients in whom there was a strong suspicion of choledocholithiasis, the IDUS probe was inserted by means of the duodenoscope into the bile duct without a sphincterotomy. All stones identified by IDUS or retrograde cholangiography were removed after endoscopic sphincterotomy. The final diagnosis was choledocholithiasis in 59 patients. The bile duct diameter ranged from 0.6 to 2.3 cm, and the stone size from 2 mm to 2 cm. IDUS successfully identified all stones in these patients.[15]

IDUS is also helpful for confirming complete stone clearance after endoscopic stone removal, thereby decreasing the rate of early recurrence of common bile duct stones.[16,17] Examples are shown in **Figs. 5.2** and **5.3**; by contrast, adenoma of the papilla with intraductal growth is illustrated in **Fig. 5.4**.

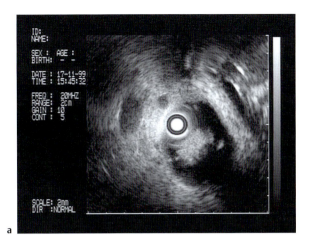

Fig. 5.2a–c Choledocholithiasis.
a Intraductal ultrasonography, showing choledocholithiasis and the accompanying acoustic shadow.
b The corresponding endoscopic retrograde cholangiogram.
c The corresponding endoscopic image.

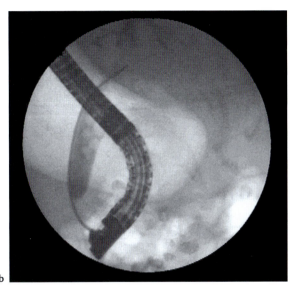

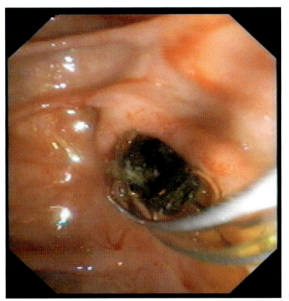

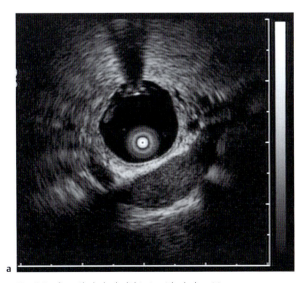

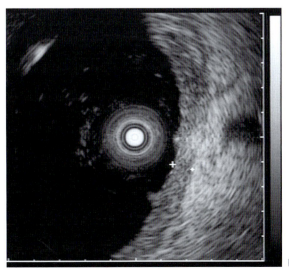

Fig. 5.3a, b a Choledocholithiasis with cholangitis.

b Wall thickening is seen between the markers (scale: 2 mm).

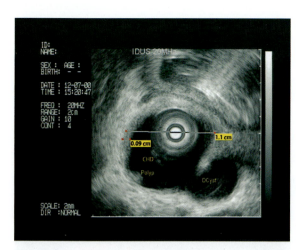

Fig. 5.4 Adenoma of the papilla with intraductal growth. Intraductal ultrasound is particularly helpful for detecting intraductal growth (polyps) and therefore indicates when surgery is required. CHD, common hepatic duct; DCyst, ductal cyst.

■ Bile Duct Strictures

IDUS can help to distinguish between benign and malignant bile strictures. The criteria for malignancy are fewer echogenic lesions extending beyond the borders of the organ, irregular ductal surfaces, interruption of the typical ultrasound wall layering, and a heterogeneous echo pattern.

High-grade stenoses may require dilation of the bile duct using balloon catheters before the miniprobe can pass.

In comparison with conventional endoscopic ultrasound, IDUS has proved to be superior for predicting the benign or malignant status of biliary structures and the resectability of biliary tumors.[18] When ERCP was supplemented with IDUS, the accuracy of correct differentiation between malignant and benign strictures increased significantly to 88% and was superior to that of magnetic resonance cholangiopancreatography (MRCP).[19]

It may be possible to distinguish scarred strictures after cholecystectomy and in patients with Mirizzi syndrome from tumor stenosis of invasive cancers (although this is a controversial issue).

If polypoid structures are detected adhering to the biliary wall, a histological examination should be performed. The likelihood of malignancy increases with the size of the polypoid lesion (> 8 mm).

Primary sclerosing cholangitis is characterized by multifocal concentric strictures. In 40 patients with primary sclerosing cholangitis and a dominant bile duct stricture, IDUS identified cholangiocarcinoma with 87% sensitivity and 91% specificity[20] and was superior to ERCP alone. However, the diagnostic dilemma in ultrasonography is that it is difficult to distinguish between inflammatory conditions and tumor infiltration[21] (**Fig. 5.5**).

■ Cholangiocellular Carcinoma

Cholangiocellular carcinoma expands along the ductal structures. IDUS is able to determine the longitudinal extension of bile duct tumors, which is crucial for predicting resectability. Tumor invasion of the surrounding organs and blood vessels can be detected with IDUS, as well as infiltration of the pancreatic parenchyma, the portal vein, or the hepatic artery.

The limited depth of penetration restricts the diagnostic power of IDUS in determining the expansion of the tumor and the infiltration of lymph nodes beyond the hepatoduodenal ligament. IDUS is not capable of assessing the M and N stages. A thickening of the biliary wall can be caused by inflammation or tumor infiltration. Endosonography cannot provide any certainty in differentiating between inflammation and neoplastic infiltration, and is therefore inaccurate for predicting the T stage. Normally, inflammation causes symmetric wall thickening, while neoplastic wall alterations have an asymmetrical appearance (**Fig. 5.6**). Papillary adenomatosis is regarded as benign in most cases, but malignant transformation is possible (**Fig. 5.7**).

Review of the Literature

It is not possible to distinguish between strictures or inflammatory or neoplastic lesions.[22] IDUS cannot reliably distinguish between bile duct cancer in stage T1 and that in stage T2.[23] EUS is useful in assessing portal vein invasion by cholangiocarcinomas at the middle and distal common bile duct (with an accuracy of 91%), but is less accurate (57%) in assessing invasion at the proximal bile duct.[24–26] While IDUS proved useful for assessing the extent of bile duct cancer invasion into the right hepatic artery, it did not demonstrate the hepatic artery proper or the left hepatic artery sufficiently for diagnosing vascular involvement.[24–26]

In 18 patients with extrahepatic bile duct cancer, the accuracy of IDUS, EUS, and angiography in assessing pancreatic parenchymal invasion was 100%, 78%, and 61%, respectively. However, IDUS was not capable of assessing pancreatic capsular invasion.[27]

In 62 patients with presumed malignant strictures of the bile duct, IDUS was performed using an ultrasonic probe (diameter 2.0 mm, frequency 20 MHz). Following IDUS, a bile duct biopsy was performed. The IDUS images of the tumor were classified as polypoid lesions, localized wall thickening, intraductal sessile tumors, sessile tumor outside of the bile duct, or absence of apparent lesions. The IDUS findings were compared with the histological findings and clinical course. Multiple regression analysis showed that the presence of a sessile tumor (intraductal or outside of the bile duct; $P < 0.05$), tumor size greater than 10 mm ($P < 0.001$), and an interrupted wall structure ($P < 0.05$) were independent variables predictive of malignancy. It was concluded that IDUS criteria can predict malignancy when biopsy fails.[28] Probably, with the techniques currently available, optimal planning of hepatobiliary surgery for cholangiocellular carcinoma requires a combination of ERC or percutaneous cholangiography and cholangioscopy, IDUS, transabdominal ultrasonography (TUS), and possibly MRCP and angiography. Assessment of the surgical margins with IDUS alone was found to be inaccurate in some cases.[29]

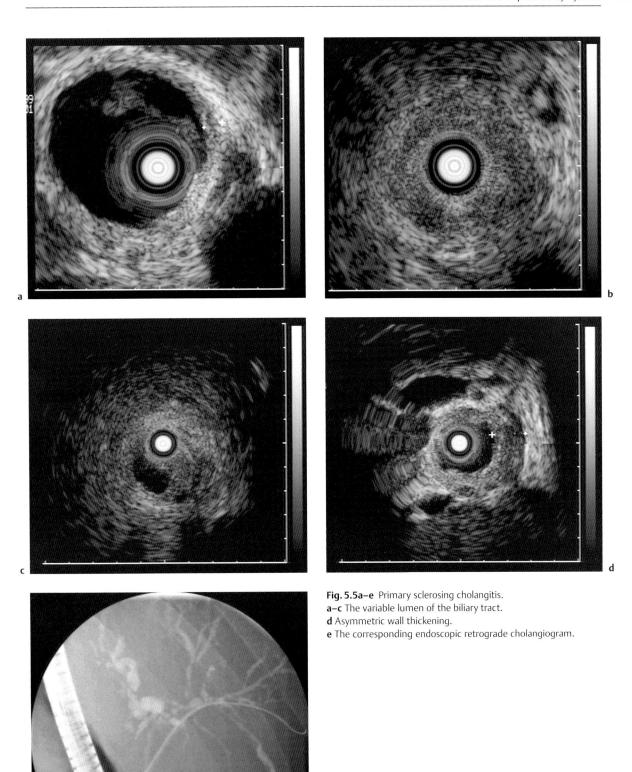

Fig. 5.5a–e Primary sclerosing cholangitis.
a–c The variable lumen of the biliary tract.
d Asymmetric wall thickening.
e The corresponding endoscopic retrograde cholangiogram.

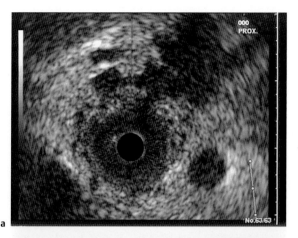

a

Fig. 5.6a–c a Cholangiocellular carcinoma. The lesion is characterized by destructive growth and invasion, but neoplastic changes are difficult to distinguish from inflammatory reactions.
b The position of the miniprobe in the corresponding endoscopic retrograde cholangiogram.
c ERCP.

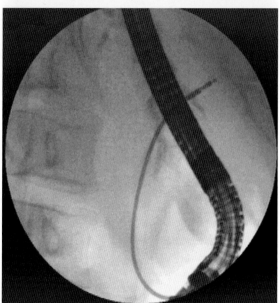

b

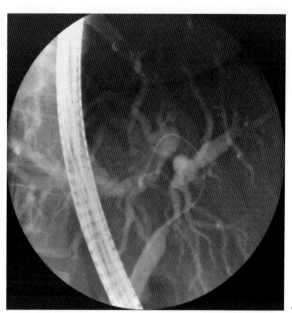

c

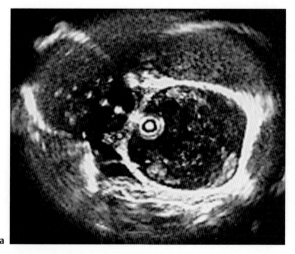

a

Fig. 5.7a, b Biliary tract papillomatosis. This is a benign and rare condition.
a Intraductal ultrasonography.
b Endoscopic retrograde cholangiography.

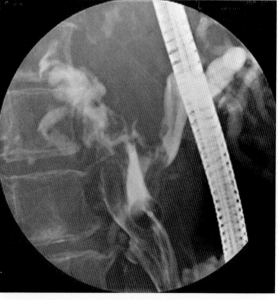

b

IDUS of the Pancreatic Ducts

Conducting IDUS of the pancreatic duct involves a risk of inducing acute pancreatitis. Although the risk is considered to be fairly low (< 1%),[30,31] it may depend on the examiner's level of experience as well as on patient selection.

Although miniprobes can often be inserted into the pancreatic duct without prior sphincterotomy, the contorted course of the duct may make further intubation difficult. The investigation often has to be stopped at the genu.

Using a 20-MHz miniprobe, the boundary of the pancreatic duct appears as a hyperechoic layer. Higher-frequency miniprobes (30 MHz) depict three layers—two hyperechoic layers and an intermediate hypoechoic layer.

IDUS can be helpful for differentiating between benign and malignant strictures of the pancreatic duct. IDUS can depict the signs of chronic pancreatitis (calcifications, fibrosis, pancreatic lithiasis, small cysts). According to studies by Furukawa et al.,[31] IDUS can distinguish between strictures of the pancreatic duct caused by focal pancreatitis and tumor stenosis with an accuracy of 90%. In addition, IDUS can assess tumor infiltration into the splenic, mesenteric, and portal veins.

IDUS may also be useful in the differential diagnosis of cystic pancreatic tumors (serous cystadenoma, mucinous cystadenoma, mucinous cystadenocarcinoma, intraductal papillary mucinous cystic tumor). Early identification of these lesions is important, as the management and outcome differ from those for ductal pancreatic adenocarcinoma.

Neuroendocrine tumors of the pancreas (gastrinoma, insulinoma, glucagonoma, VIPoma, somatostatinoma) are rare neoplasms that may arise sporadically or in association with a hereditary endocrine neoplasia syndrome. They require precise imaging and localization for the planning of resection.

Even intraoperatively, up to 20% of insulinomas and up to 50% of gastrinomas are difficult to find. Results of initial studies indicate that IDUS may be able to improve the localization of neuroendocrine tumors in the pancreas in comparison with conventional methods (such as EUS and octreotide receptor scintigraphy).[32] Even tiny lesions can be detected using the high resolution provided by miniprobes.[33] In a few cases, the additional information provided by the IDUS results may allow organ-preserving enucleation instead of pancreatic resection.

Table 5.1 Indications for intraductal ultrasonography (IDUS)

Biliary tract
Suspected choledocholithiasis (?)
Differentiating between benign and malignant biliary strictures (?)
Local tumor staging (?)
Pancreas
Differentiating between benign and malignant pancreatic strictures (?)
Local tumor staging (?)
Characterization of cystic tumors (?)
Localization of neuroendocrine tumors not detectable on EUS (?)

Review of the Literature

In the diagnosis of 239 patients with pancreatic disease (including 48 cancers, 90 mucin-producing tumors, seven islet cell tumors, two metastatic pancreatic tumors, seven serous cystadenomas, one pancreatic teratoma, three solid cystic tumors, 49 cases of chronic pancreatitis, 25 cases of focal pancreatitis, and seven cases of pancreatolithiasis), IDUS was able to image the entire cross-section of the portal vein and other large veins. IDUS was useful in detecting carcinoma in situ and small tumors, in assessing the intraductal spread of the tumor and its pancreatic parenchymal invasion in mucin-producing tumors of the main duct, and in assessing the indications for surgery by revealing mural nodules in mucin-producing tumors of the ductal branches. IDUS was also useful in evaluating the feasibility of partial resection of the tumor in mucin-producing tumors of the ductal branches and pancreatic islet cell tumors, in accurately locating multiple lesions in pancreatic islet cell cancer, and in differentiating between benign and malignant cases of localized stenosis of the main pancreatic duct related to pancreatic stenting. With IDUS, it was possible to identify the site of pancreatic stones to assess the need for endoscopic treatment. Acute pancreatitis as a complication occurred in one of the 239 patients who underwent IDUS (0.4%).[31] Very small neuroendocrine pancreatic tumors were diagnosed by pancreatic IDUS[32] (**Table 5.1**).

IDUS in Patients with Tumors of the Papilla and with Sphincter of Oddi Dysfunction

In contrast to pancreatic carcinoma, tumors of the papilla of Vater can usually be resected and therefore have a better prognosis. Adenomas in the papilla of Vater are premalignant conditions. The choice of the resection method depends on the presence of intraductal growth. Intraductal extension of the tumor requires pylorus-preserving pancreatoduodenectomy (the Whipple operation), while extraductal adenoma can be resected endoscopically. IDUS allows visualization of the papilla of Vater, including the sphincter of Oddi. IDUS depicts papillary tumors and detects neoplastic intraductal growth or infiltration of the surrounding structures. In contrast to other imaging methods such as computed tomography (CT) and EUS, IDUS has a high level of sensitivity. However, IDUS may overlook lymph-node infiltration by papillary carcinoma, due to its limited depth of penetration.

In 21 patients with suspected biliary sphincter of Oddi dysfunction, IDUS of the papilla was technically feasible and safe, but could not be used as a substitute for sphincter of Oddi manometry.[34]

Conclusion

Intraductal endosonography is particularly valuable for diagnosing stenoses of unknown origin in the common bile duct. It must be borne in mind that IDUS (like other ultrasound methods, as well as CT and MRI) is not able to differentiate reliably between benign and malignant lesions. In most cases, extraductal EUS techniques are sufficient.

References

1. Furukawa T, Naitoh Y, Tsukamoto Y, et al. New technique using intraductal ultrasonography for the diagnosis of diseases of the pancreatobiliary system. J Ultrasound Med 1992; 11(11):607–612.
2. Furukawa T, Tsukamoto Y, Naitoh Y, Hirooka Y, Katoh T. Evaluation of intraductal ultrasonography in the diagnosis of pancreatic cancer. Endoscopy 1993;25(9):577–581.
3. Furukawa T, Tsukamoto Y, Naitoh Y, Mitake M, Hirooka Y, Hayakawa T. Differential diagnosis of pancreatic diseases with an intraductal ultrasound system. Gastrointest Endosc 1994;40(2 Pt 1):213–219.
4. Tamada K, Nagai H, Yasuda Y, et al. Transpapillary intraductal US prior to biliary drainage in the assessment of longitudinal spread of extrahepatic bile duct carcinoma. Gastrointest Endosc 2001;53(3):300–307.
5. Levy MJ, Vazquez-Sequeiros E, Wiersema MJ. Evaluation of the pancreaticobiliary ductal systems by intraductal US. Gastrointest Endosc 2002;55(3):397–408.
6. Dietrich CF, Lee JH, Herrmann G, et al. Enlargement of perihepatic lymph nodes in relation to liver histology and viremia in patients with chronic hepatitis C. Hepatology 1997;26(2):467–472.
7. Noda Y, Fujita N, Kobayashi G, et al. Comparison of echograms by a microscanner and histological findings of the common bile duct, in vitro study. [Article in German] Nippon Shokakibyo Gakkai Zasshi 1997;94(3):172–179.
8. Palazzo L, Girollet PP, Salmeron M, et al. Value of endoscopic ultrasonography in the diagnosis of common bile duct stones: comparison with surgical exploration and ERCP. Gastrointest Endosc 1995;42(3):225–231.
9. Linghu EQ, Cheng LF, Wang XD, et al. Intraductal ultrasonography and endoscopic retrograde cholangiography in diagnosis of extrahepatic bile duct stones: a comparative study. Hepatobiliary Pancreat Dis Int 2004;3(1):129–132.
10. Moon JH, Cho YD, Cha SW, et al. The detection of bile duct stones in suspected biliary pancreatitis: comparison of MRCP, ERCP, and intraductal US. Am J Gastroenterol 2005;100(5):1051–1057.
11. Palazzo L. Which test for common bile duct stones? Endoscopic and intraductal ultrasonography. Endoscopy 1997;29(7):655–665.
12. Seifert H, Wehrmann T, Hilgers R, Gouder S, Braden B, Dietrich CF. Catheter probe extraductal EUS reliably detects distal common bile duct abnormalities. Gastrointest Endosc 2004;60(1):61–67.
13. Ohashi A, Ueno N, Tamada K, et al. Assessment of residual bile duct stones with use of intraductal US during endoscopic balloon sphincteroplasty: comparison with balloon cholangiography. Gastrointest Endosc 1999;49(3 Pt 1):328–333.
14. Das A, Isenberg G, Wong RC, Sivak MV Jr, Chak A. Wire-guided intraductal US: an adjunct to ERCP in the management of bile duct stones. Gastrointest Endosc 2001;54(1):31–36.
15. Tseng LJ, Jao YT, Mo LR, Lin RC. Over-the-wire US catheter probe as an adjunct to ERCP in the detection of choledocholithiasis. Gastrointest Endosc 2001;54(6):720–723.
16. Tsuchiya S, Tsuyuguchi T, Sakai Y, et al. Clinical utility of intraductal US to decrease early recurrence rate of common bile duct stones after endoscopic papillotomy. J Gastroenterol Hepatol 2008;23(10):1590–1595.
17. Ang TL, Teo EK, Fock KM, Lyn Tan JY. Are there roles for intraductal US and saline solution irrigation in ensuring complete clearance of common bile duct stones? Gastrointest Endosc 2009;69(7):1276–1281.
18. Menzel J, Poremba C, Dietl KH, Domschke W. Preoperative diagnosis of bile duct strictures—comparison of intraductal ultrasonography with conventional endosonography. Scand J Gastroenterol 2000;35(1):77–82.
19. Domagk D, Wessling J, Reimer P, et al. Endoscopic retrograde cholangiopancreatography, intraductal ultrasonography, and magnetic resonance cholangiopancreatography in bile duct strictures: a prospective comparison of imaging diagnostics with histopathological correlation. Am J Gastroenterol 2004;99(9):1684–1689.
20. Tischendorf JJ, Meier PN, Schneider A, Manns MP, Krüger M. Transpapillary intraductal ultrasound in the evaluation of dominant bile duct stenoses in patients with primary sclerosing cholangitis. Scand J Gastroenterol 2007;42(8):1011–1017.
21. Hirche TO, Russler J, Braden B, et al. Sonographic detection of perihepatic lymphadenopathy is an indicator for primary sclerosing cholangitis in patients with inflammatory bowel disease. Int J Colorectal Dis 2004;19(6):586–594.
22. Tamada K, Kanai N, Tomiyama T, et al. Prediction of the histologic type of bile duct cancer by using intraductal ultrasonography. Abdom Imaging 1999;24(5):484–490.
23. Ueno N, Nishizono T, Tamada K, et al. Diagnosing extrahepatic bile duct stones using intraductal ultrasonography: a case series. Endoscopy 1997;29(5):356–360.
24. Tamada K, Ido K, Ueno N, et al. Assessment of hepatic artery invasion by bile duct cancer using intraductal ultrasonography. Endoscopy 1995;27(8):579–583.
25. Tamada K, Ido K, Ueno N, et al. Assessment of portal vein invasion by bile duct cancer using intraductal ultrasonography. Endoscopy 1995;27(8):573–578.
26. Tamada K, Ido K, Ueno N, Kimura K, Ichiyama M, Tomiyama T. Preoperative staging of extrahepatic bile duct cancer

with intraductal ultrasonography. Am J Gastroenterol 1995;90(2):239–246.

27. Tamada K, Ueno N, Ichiyama M, et al. Assessment of pancreatic parenchymal invasion by bile duct cancer using intraductal ultrasonography. Endoscopy 1996;28(6):492–496.

28. Tamada K, Tomiyama T, Wada S, et al. Endoscopic transpapillary bile duct biopsy with the combination of intraductal ultrasonography in the diagnosis of biliary strictures. Gut 2002;50(3):326–331.

29. Dietrich CF, Seifert H, Schreiber-Dietrich D, Caspary WF, Wehrmann T. Benigne Papillomatose der Gallenwege: Eine sonographische Blickdiagnose? [abstract] [Article in German] Ultraschall Med 1998;19:88.

30. Menzel J, Domschke W. Intraductal ultrasonography (IDUS) of the pancreato-biliary duct system. Personal experience and review of literature. Eur J Ultrasound 1999;10 (2-3):105–115.

31. Furukawa T, Oohashi K, Yamao K, et al. Intraductal ultrasonography of the pancreas: development and clinical potential. Endoscopy 1997;29(6):561–569.

32. Menzel J, Domschke W. Intraductal ultrasonography may localize islet cell tumours negative on endoscopic ultrasound. Scand J Gastroenterol 1998;33(1):109–112.

33. Yamao K, Okubo K, Sawaka A, et al. Endoluminal ultrasonography in the diagnosis of pancreatic diseases. Abdom Imaging 2003;28(4):545–555.

34. Wehrmann T, Stergiou N, Riphaus A, Lembcke B. Correlation between sphincter of Oddi manometry and intraductal ultrasound morphology in patients with suspected sphincter of Oddi dysfunction. Endoscopy 2001;33(9):773–777.

6 Radial EUS, Linear EUS, or Ultrasound Miniprobe: Which Is the Most Suitable Device in Gastrointestinal EUS?

J. Janssen, C.F. Dietrich

The Development of EUS: a Short Historical Survey

Shortly after ultrasound first became available as a diagnostic imaging method in medicine,[1] its use was expanded by Wild et al., who presented an intracavitary rectal application in 1957.[2] The principle of using a blind, rigid probe has been maintained and further improved for vaginal and rectal ultrasonography (**Fig. 6.1a**).

Endoscopic ultrasonography (EUS) with flexible instruments has developed quickly since the early 1980s[3] and is now accepted as an indispensable tool in gastroenterology and associated fields. Apart from other indications, EUS is essential for the pretherapeutic local staging of gastrointestinal tumors. It is the method of choice for determining the origin and type of submucosal lesions. The use of longitudinal systems makes it possible to carry out fine-needle biopsy of lesions close to the gastrointestinal tract and local interventions guided by real-time EUS.

The development of flexible echoendoscopes started with mechanical radial scanners (5 MHz, 360°), which were mounted on top of a conventional endoscope.[3] Soon after this, prototype echoendoscopes based on the radial mechanical technique were manufactured by the Olympus Corporation.[4] Subsequent models worked with a frequency range of 5–12 MHz and dominated clinical applications for some 10 years. Most of the relevant studies on diagnostic EUS were conducted using this type of instrument.

At the beginning of the 1990s, a novel longitudinally scanning echoendoscope was presented and produced in series (Hitachi/Pentax FG-32UA).[5] This instrument had an electronic scanner at frequencies of 5–10 MHz and allowed vessels to be examined using pulsed Doppler and color Doppler (**Fig. 6.1b**). In comparison with the mechanical devices, electronic scanners provided significantly better spatial resolution and higher imaging quality, especially in the near field. The fundamental advantage of the linear scanner is that it allows real-time controlled EUS-guided biopsy and interventions. Needles can be introduced through a working channel, and their tip is moved forward into the tissue within the scanning plane.[6] The combination of these interventional instruments with color flow Doppler imaging reduces the risk of bleeding during puncture and transmural insertion of drains. Nowadays, modern radial scanners also work electronically, incorporating Doppler facilities and providing better spatial resolution.

The ultrasound miniprobe was also developed at the same time as longitudinal scanners. The miniprobe is characterized by its small caliber and high ultrasound frequency (7.5–30 MHz), which provides high resolution, but at the expense of penetration depth. These probes were initially used in intracoronary ultrasonography,[7–9] and the applications were later extended to the gastrointestinal field.[10] The miniprobe is inserted into the working channel of a standard endoscope; endoscopy and EUS can thus be combined in a single examination. The small caliber of the instrument makes it possible to explore narrow tumor stenoses and allows intraductal biliary or pancreatic ultrasonography. Miniprobes usually work mechanically and produce a radial 360° image. The main

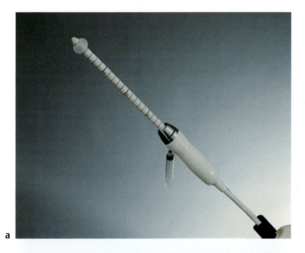

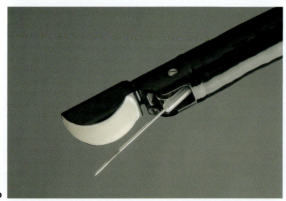

Fig. 6.1a, b The modern rigid rectal probe (**a**) and flexible longitudinal echoendoscope (**b**) for diagnostic and interventional endoscopic ultrasonography.

disadvantage of these devices is their small penetration depth (2–3 cm) at frequencies of 20–30 MHz. Their use is therefore limited when the focus of the examination is on the surroundings of the gastrointestinal wall—e.g., for exploring lymph nodes and the pancreas (reviewed in[11]).

The main obstacles to the widespread use of EUS are its limited (although still expanding) range of indications and the high initial costs and operating costs. It depends on the structure of local departments whether the purchase of one or more types of EUS instrument is economically justifiable. If only one system is to be bought, the choice of the correct type of EUS unit is also an issue.

In centers with low annual numbers of examinations, it is economically mandatory for the basic ultrasound unit to be usable for transabdominal, vascular, and cardiac ultrasonography as well. All EUS equipment manufacturers now offer variable-use systems. The initial costs for a standard echoendoscope are about $ 60 000–90 000. Experience shows that the lifetime of an instrument used at a frequency of 500 examinations per year is ≈ 3 years. Purchasing a second echoendoscope is profitable above a frequency of three or four examinations per day. The lifetime of a miniprobe is highly dependent on the examiner's level of experience and the care taken with the instrument, and on the uses to which it is put (e.g., esophageal applications versus intraductal ultrasonography). Reports on the average number of examinations conducted with one probe vary from 10 to 90. The price of a miniprobe is about $ 2000–4000.

During the last 10 years, the quality of all of the EUS systems available on the market has significantly improved. However, there are specific differences between the systems. The following sections provide general comparisons between linear and radial standard EUS systems and ultrasound miniprobes, without concentrating on specific instruments that are currently available.

Miniprobe Versus Conventional EUS

The indisputable advantage of miniprobe ultrasonography is that it makes it possible to carry out endoscopy and EUS during a single session. An ideal indication for this method is the evaluation of submucosal tumors or unclear external impressions.[11] The only precondition for this is that the basic ultrasound unit should be immediately available, rather than being used for routine examinations by another physician in a different room.

High-frequency miniprobe ultrasonography is limited by its low penetration depth. Systematic exploration of the pancreas and lymph-node areas or other structures more distant from the gastrointestinal wall is therefore not generally possible, although it has been done successfully in several cases. The second disadvantage is that it is not possible to carry out real-time controlled fine-needle aspiration biopsy (FNAB) with the miniprobe.

The outer diameter of standard echoendoscopes is ≈ 12.5–14.5 mm. In contrast to the miniprobe, these instruments are not able to pass high-grade tumor stenoses and do not allow intraductal ultrasound (IDUS) examinations. However, the unresectability of a stenosing esophageal cancer can often be confirmed with conventional EUS just by scanning the oral end of the tumor; bougienage is therefore not necessary in these cases. If passage is mandatory to determine the exact stage of the tumor, bougienage can precede EUS. The perforation risk is low with this procedure.[12,13]

Miniprobes are often preferred in the staging of early gastrointestinal cancer before endoscopic treatment. Studies have reported good results with high-frequency miniprobes in this setting (see Chapter 4), but there have as yet been no studies prospectively comparing the miniprobe with modern electronic conventional EUS systems. These new-generation instruments, working at 10–12 MHz, provide excellent spatial resolution including the near field, which in our opinion is comparable with the quality of miniprobe imaging (**Fig. 6.2**). Irrespective of the EUS system used, problems resulting from concomitant inflammation, causing overstaging, or due to the location of the tumor (e.g., in the cardia) have not been solved. It therefore seems unnecessary to debate whether one system or another is preferable, since the ultimate assessment of the tumor stage, and of whether oncological surgery is needed due to deep submucosal infiltration, is made by the pathologist after endoscopic resection.

In conclusion, the only *specific* indications that cannot be investigated with conventional EUS in comparison with miniprobe ultrasonography are those involving IDUS. Nevertheless, advocates of the miniprobe appreciate the high resolution it provides and its rapid availability in connection with endoscopy.

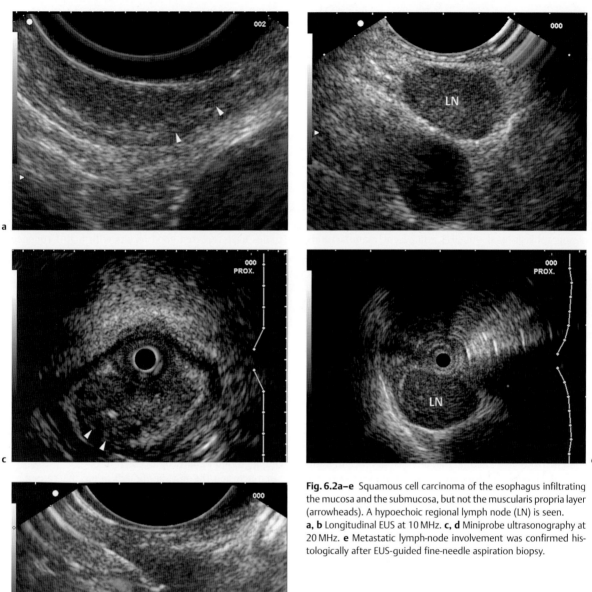

Fig. 6.2a–e Squamous cell carcinoma of the esophagus infiltrating the mucosa and the submucosa, but not the muscularis propria layer (arrowheads). A hypoechoic regional lymph node (LN) is seen. **a, b** Longitudinal EUS at 10 MHz. **c, d** Miniprobe ultrasonography at 20 MHz. **e** Metastatic lymph-node involvement was confirmed histologically after EUS-guided fine-needle aspiration biopsy.

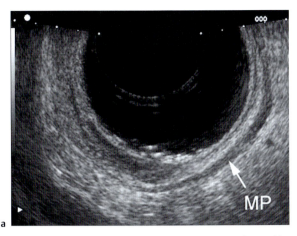
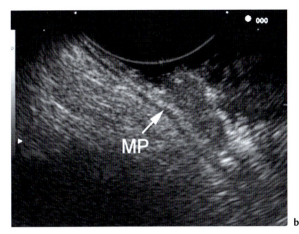

Fig. 6.3a, b A malignant rectal polyp in the mucosa, with no infiltration into the submucosa. The same result is convincingly demonstrated with both rigid radial EUS (**a**) and flexible longitudinal EUS (**b**). MP, muscularis propria.

Conventional Radial EUS Versus Conventional Longitudinal EUS

Most data on the accuracy of EUS in the staging of gastrointestinal tumors are derived from studies conducted with radial scanners in the 1980s. The number of studies dealing with the diagnostic capabilities of linear EUS is still small. The quality of radial and linear EUS is probably comparable in the staging of pancreatic cancer,[14] the evaluation of suspected pancreatic disease,[15] and the detection of bile duct stones.[16,17] Although longitudinal EUS is widely used for the staging of gastrointestinal wall tumors, there has only been one prospective study demonstrating that linear and radial EUS are equivalent in the staging of esophageal cancer.[18] In contrast to the 1980s, only early-stage esophageal and rectal carcinomas are primarily operated on nowadays. If EUS reveals a locally advanced tumor stage, patients primarily undergo neoadjuvant therapy. The conditions for conducting studies comparing EUS results and the pathological tumor stage have therefore significantly changed. Nevertheless, the few data currently available suggest that linear EUS is not poorer than radial EUS in the assessment of gastrointestinal wall tumors.

The decisive difference between radial and longitudinal EUS is that the linear technique allows biopsies to be taken and interventions to be carried out with real-time EUS guidance. Many studies have shown that EUS-guided FNAB of lymph nodes, pancreatic lesions, the left adrenal gland, and other structures close to the gastrointestinal tract is safe and highly accurate.[19–21] The frequency of punctures is ≈ 20–30% of all EUS examinations in centers offering this method. The complication risk is low. The short distances between the tip of the instrument and the targeted lesion minimize the risk of tract metastases. Lymph nodes as small as 3–5 mm can be reliably punctured, and the question of whether there is metastatic nodal disease in pancreatic carcinoma can be explored before surgery. Lymph nodes and tumors in the dorsal mediastinum can be evaluated histologically. As the more invasive method, mediastinoscopy can be replaced in a significant proportion of patients.

EUS was initially performed in large university medical centers, from which initial experience was reported and the development of the radial EUS examination technique was promoted and spread. Examiners who have learnt EUS in these centers and left to work in peripheral hospitals are most familiar with the radial technique. Consequently, longitudinal scanners are still not used for diagnostic EUS in many centers, mainly because of the different orientation and examination technique, which is thought to be more difficult. Longitudinal EUS is often carried out for biopsy in addition to previous diagnostic radial EUS.

Our experience shows that the learning curve for linear EUS can be shortened through structured training and by taking a systematic approach toward EUS anatomy.[22] We therefore believe that the conventional linear probe is an all-round instrument that has no significant disadvantages in comparison with the radial system (**Fig. 6.3**).

Figures 6.4, 6.5, 6.6, 6.7, 6.8 present comparisons of EUS systems in different organ systems. In all of the patients, longitudinal and radial scanning were of similar value, whereas the miniprobe was advantageous in the gastrointestinal wall.

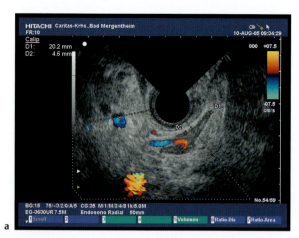
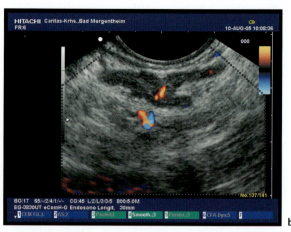

Fig. 6.4a, b A normal adrenal gland (between the markers), displayed with radial scanning (**a**) and longitudinal scanning (**b**). The adrenal hilum and adrenal vessels are delineated with both methods.

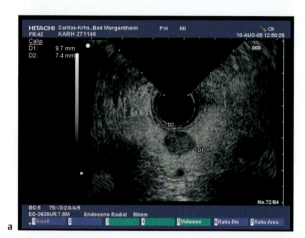
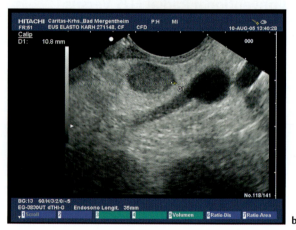

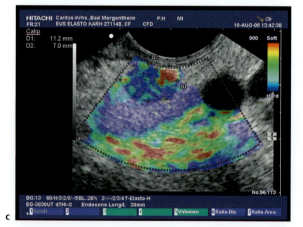

Fig. 6.5a–c A pancreatic metastasis in a patient with adrenal gland carcinoma, displayed with the radial (**a**) and longitudinal (**b**) techniques. **c** Elastography is also possible with both techniques; the longitudinal technique is illustrated here, indicating inhomogeneous elasticity.

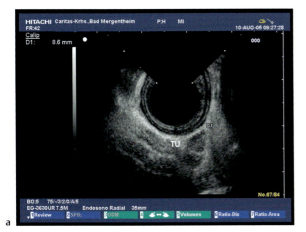

a

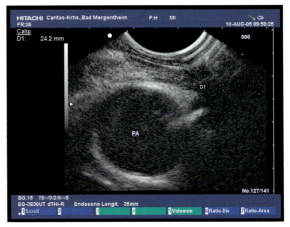

b

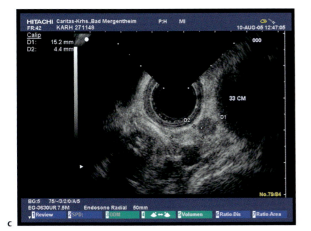

c

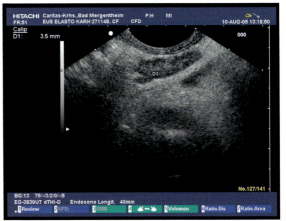

d

Fig. 6.6a–d Subcarinal lymph nodes. Normal subcarinal lymph nodes can be displayed with the radial (**a**) and longitudinal (**b**) techniques. Pathological lymph-node infiltration (about 4 mm) can also be displayed with both methods (**c**, **d**), whereas tumor puncture is only possible with the longitudinal scanner. PA, pulmonary artery; TU, tumor.

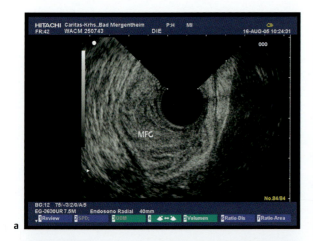

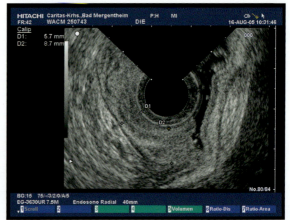

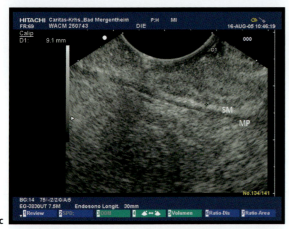

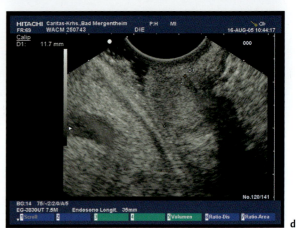

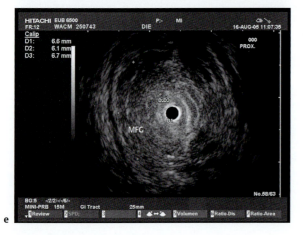

Fig. 6.7a–e Large fold gastritis associated with *Helicobacter pylori* infection, displayed using radial scanning (**a, b**) longitudinal scanning (**c, d**), radial techniques (**b**), and miniprobe technology via the longitudinal echoendoscope (**e**). MFG, large mucosal fold gastritis. MP, muscularis propria; SM, submucosa.

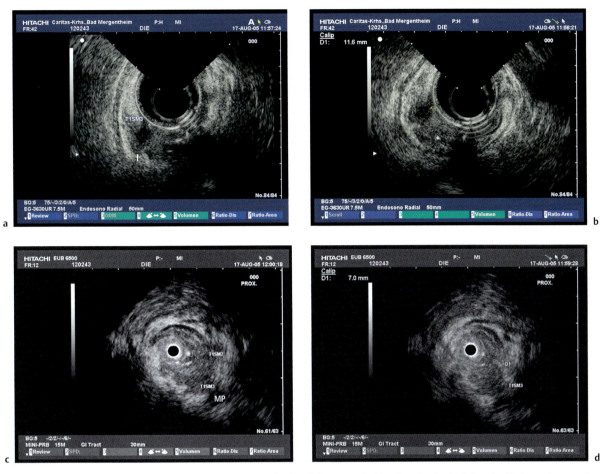

Fig. 6.8a–d Rectal carcinoma with T1sm3 infiltration, displayed with radial scanning (**a**, **b**) and miniprobe (**c**, **d**). Longitudinal scanning was of less value. MP, muscularis propria.

Which Is the EUS Technique of the Future?

As EUS-guided FNAB is indispensable for all EUS examiners, one can conclusively recommend linear probes as all-round instruments for users who only want to purchase a single system. This is particularly so since longitudinal EUS is equivalent to, or even better than, radial EUS for plain diagnostic imaging. Special indications that require miniprobes (e.g., stenoses, IDUS) are relatively rare and can be dealt with after bougienage or with extraductal ultrasonography using the standard linear probe. However, miniprobes are a useful addition to the EUS equipment if affordable and if the specific indications are encountered in the department. Only large EUS centers will be able to justify the purchase of all three of the EUS systems described.

References

1. Howry DH, Bliss WR. Ultrasonic visualization of soft tissue structures of the body. J Lab Clin Med 1952;40(4):579–592.
2. Wild JJ, Reid JM. Progress in techniques of soft tissue examination by 15 MC pulsed ultrasound. In: Kelly-Fry E, ed. Ultrasound in biology and medicine: a symposium sponsored by the Bioacoustics Laboratory of the University of Illinois and the Physiology Branch of the Office of Naval Research, held at Robert Allerton Park, Monticello, Illinois, June 20–22, 1955. Washington, DC: American Institute of Biological Sciences, 1957:30–45.
3. Strohm WD, Phillip J, Hagenmüller F, Classen M. Ultrasonic tomography by means of an ultrasonic fiberendoscope. Endoscopy 1980;12(5):241–244.
4. Lux G, Heyder N, Lutz H, Demling L. Endoscopic ultrasonography—technique, orientation and diagnostic possibilities. Endoscopy 1982;14(6):220–225.
5. Vilmann P, Khattar S, Hancke S. Endoscopic ultrasound examination of the upper gastrointestinal tract using a curved-array transducer. A preliminary report. Surg Endosc 1991;5(2):79–82.
6. Vilmann P, Hancke S, Henriksen FW, Jacobsen GK. Endosonographically-guided fine needle aspiration biopsy of malignant lesions in the upper gastrointestinal tract. Endoscopy 1993;25(8):523–527.
7. Meyer CR, Chiang EH, Fechner KP, Fitting DW, Williams DM, Buda AJ. Feasibility of high-resolution, intravascular ultrasonic imaging catheters. Radiology 1988;168(1): 113–116.
8. Gussenhoven WJ, Essed CE, Frietman P, et al. Intravascular echographic assessment of vessel wall characteristics: a correlation with histology. Int J Card Imaging 1989;4 (2-4):105–116.
9. Yock PG, Linker DT, Angelsen BA. Two-dimensional intravascular ultrasound: technical development and initial clinical experience. J Am Soc Echocardiogr 1989;2(4): 296–304.
10. Engström CF, Wiechel KL. Endoluminal ultrasound of the bile ducts. Surg Endosc 1990;4(4):187–190.
11. Menzel J, Domschke W, Brambs HJ, et al. [Mini-probe ultrasound of the upper gastrointestinal tract—1995 state of the art and perspectives. Workshop on Mini-Probe Ultrasound in Gastroenterology, Münster, 28 October 1995]. Ultraschall Med 1996;17(3):143–148.
12. Pfau PR, Ginsberg GG, Lew RJ, Faigel DO, Smith DB, Kochman ML. Esophageal dilation for endosonographic evaluation of malignant esophageal strictures is safe and effective. Am J Gastroenterol 2000;95(10):2813–2815.
13. Wallace MB, Hawes RH, Sahai AV, Van Velse A, Hoffman BJ. Dilation of malignant esophageal stenosis to allow EUS guided fine-needle aspiration: safety and effect on patient management. Gastrointest Endosc 2000;51(3):309–313.
14. Gress F, Savides T, Cummings O, et al. Radial scanning and linear array endosonography for staging pancreatic cancer: a prospective randomized comparison. Gastrointest Endosc 1997;45(2):138–142.
15. Kochman ML, Elta GH, Bude R, Nostrant TT, Scheiman JM. Utility of a linear array ultrasound endoscope in the evaluation of suspected pancreatic disease. J Gastrointest Surg 1998;2(3):217–222.
16. Kohut M, Nowakowska-Duława E, Marek T, Kaczor R, Nowak A. Accuracy of linear endoscopic ultrasonography in the evaluation of patients with suspected common bile duct stones. Endoscopy 2002;34(4):299–303.
17. Lachter J, Rubin A, Shiller M, et al. Linear EUS for bile duct stones. Gastrointest Endosc 2000;51(1):51–54.
18. Siemsen M, Svendsen LB, Knigge U, et al. A prospective randomized comparison of curved array and radial echoendoscopy in patients with esophageal cancer. Gastrointest Endosc 2003;58(5):671–676.
19. Janssen J, Johanns W, Luis W, Greiner L. [Clinical value of endoscopic ultrasound-guided transesophageal fine needle puncture of mediastinal lesions]. Dtsch Med Wochenschr 1998;123(47):1402–1409.
20. Dietrich CF, Wehrmann T, Hoffmann C, Herrmann G, Caspary WF, Seifert H. Detection of the adrenal glands by endoscopic or transabdominal ultrasound. Endoscopy 1997; 29(9):859–864.
21. Fritscher-Ravens A, Sriram PV, Bobrowski C, et al. Mediastinal lymphadenopathy in patients with or without previous malignancy: EUS-FNA-based differential cytodiagnosis in 153 patients. Am J Gastroenterol 2000;95(9): 2278–2284.
22. Janssen J, Greiner L. Examination technique and general principles. In: Rösch T, Will U, Chang KJ, eds. Longitudinal endosonography: atlas and manual for use in the upper gastrointestinal tract. Berlin: Springer; 2001:11–19.

7 Ultrasound Contrast Agents and Contrast-Enhanced Ultrasonography

C. Greis, C.F. Dietrich

Imaging the internal organs is crucially important for identifying diseases and for treatment and follow-up. Diagnostic imaging has made tremendous technological progress in recent years, making possible ever more advanced and more detailed examinations of anatomy and physiology. In addition to techniques such as multislice computed tomography (CT), whole-body magnetic resonance imaging (MRI), and positron-emission tomography (PET), which require large and expensive machines, there is still a substantial need for easily available, patient-friendly, and inexpensive methods such as ultrasonography. However, the technique needs to fully meet the standards of modern diagnostic imaging in all respects.

These requirements have become substantially more demanding over the years. Following the introduction of contrast agents, the original simple imaging of anatomical structures was extended to imaging of the blood supply (vessels and perfusion) and, most recently, the imaging of molecular structures (molecular imaging) with the aid of tissue-specific contrast agents. All such investigations can in principle be performed with sonography as well. This chapter provides an overview of the contrast agents currently available, with their most important properties, and of contrast-specific sonographic techniques that allow selective imaging of contrast agent signals.

The basis of all sonographic examinations is B-mode sonography, which uses differences in echogenicity in tissue to produce detailed high-resolution images of anatomic structures. In addition, Doppler sonography allows imaging of the blood flow in vessels and the derivation of spectra for the quantitative determination of blood flow over time. However, Doppler sonography has serious limitations: it only functions at fairly high flow rates (greater than the wall motion), for flow in a defined direction toward or away from the transducer, and for adequate flow volumes. Imaging of capillary flow (small volumes, very slow speeds), particularly in tumors with complex vascular architecture, is not possible using this technique. For this purpose, contrast agents that allow the imaging of blood on the basis of specific parts of the contrast signal are required.

Ultrasound contrast agents were originally developed to improve the contrast of weak (noisy) echo signals, but a combination with contrast-specific scanner techniques made a completely new application available: B-mode imaging of very small quantities of contrast agent (equivalent to blood volumes) in tissue (parenchyma). This requires sensitive detection (right down to the individual microbubbles) and selective detection (to distinguish between tissue signals and noise) of the contrast agent, making it possible to image the blood supply in tissue.

This type of contrast-specific sonography firstly allows the imaging of vascularity and vessel geometry in organs (capillary volume); and secondly, can image and quantify the passage of a contrast agent bolus through the vascular system in real time (capillary flow). Capillary volume and capillary flow are the determinants of parenchymal perfusion.

Historical Background

The principle of ultrasound contrast agents has been known for more than 30 years, since Gramiak and Shah observed strong ultrasound echo signals in blood following the injection of indocyanine green.[1] The signals were formed as a result of air bubbles that were co-administered during the rapid bolus injection. Since that time, the intentional creation of air or gas bubbles of this type has been used to produce echogenic solutions that make the hypoechoic blood visible using ultrasound.

Home-made ultrasound contrast agents of this type were prepared, for example, through vigorous shaking of physiological saline or viscous infusion solutions, or by sonicating radiographic contrast agents. As their lack of stability inhibited pulmonary passage, they were mainly used for shunt diagnosis[2,3] or to image myocardial perfusion after intracoronary administration.[4,5]

Since 1991, standardized ultrasound contrast agents have been available for right-heart diagnosis (Echovist) and, since 1995, ultrasound contrast agents that are stable on passage through the lungs (Levovist) have been commercially available. Since 2001, second-generation contrast agents containing gases with low solubility in water have been on the market (SonoVue) and have substantially increased the stability and duration of the contrast.

Classification of Ultrasound Contrast Agents

■ Blood-Pool Contrast Agents

The original objective in developing standardized ultrasound contrast agents was to obtain products that pass through the lungs, making contrast imaging of the entire vascular system possible after intravenous injection (blood-pool agents). Most products available or in development today fall into this category. Ideally, blood-pool contrast agents should be transported freely in the bloodstream without leaving the vascular bed or accumulating in specific tissues (**Table 7.1**).

Some of these contrast agents do not move perfectly freely with the bloodstream, but have some tissue-specific affinity. This means that they accumulate in specific tissues—e.g., the reticuloendothelial cells in the liver and spleen—at the end of the vascular phase. This effect has been described for Levovist[6,7] and Sonazoid[8,9] and can be used diagnostically to identify functional liver tissue in the late, liver-specific, phase (i.e., after the end of the vascular phase). Care needs to be taken to ensure that the late-phase examination is not recorded too soon, to avoid overlap with the portal venous phase.

■ Tissue-Specific Contrast Agents

These are contrast agents that have a high affinity to specific tissues or molecular structures and which therefore accumulate specifically in these tissues. In principle, this includes the above blood-pool contrast agents with liver-specific late phases. In the narrower sense, however, it is taken to mean contrast agents with a shell containing structures with high molecular affinities (e.g., antibody fragments).

Currently, no tissue-specific contrast agents are available for use in humans, but several substances are in preclinical development.[10–14] Contrast agents of this type make it possible to detect neoangiogenesis, intravascular thrombi, plaques, or inflammation, for example.

■ Drug-Delivery Systems

The shells of ultrasound contrast agents can be used not only for the transport of gases or air, but can also transport drugs in the body. The release of these drugs then takes place locally, either through nonspecific rupture of the shell after specific binding to the target tissue (target-specific microbubbles) or by selective local rupture of the freely circulating microbubbles in the target area (e.g., by exposure to ultrasound). Systems of this type can be used for the transport of conventional drugs or even of DNA or RNA fragments (e.g., antisense molecules).[15,16] After initial in vitro and in vivo experiments with stains and marker DNA, studies are now underway with functional DNA and have already resulted in measurable clinical effects in animal studies. It is helpful that ultrasound can be used not just to release the active substance, but also allows penetration into the tissue (sonoporation). Products of this type are already in preclinical testing.

■ Intracavitary Contrast Agents

These were generally developed as blood-pool contrast agents; however, the administration route is not intravenous, but rather by catheter or needle into a body cavity. Established indications are contrast hysterosalpingosonography to assess the patency of the tubes when investigating fertility,[17] and voiding urosonography to investigate vesicoureterorenal reflux, particularly in children.[18]

Table 7.1 Ultrasound contrast agents: overview of products

Name	Manufacturer	Shell	Gas	Approved
Echovist[a]	Bayer Schering Pharma	Galactose	Air	1991
Albunex[b]	Molecular Biosystems	Albumin	Air	1993
Levovist	Bayer Schering Pharma	Galactose	Air	1995
Optison	GE Healthcare	Albumin	Perfluoropropane	1998
SonoVue	Bracco	Phospholipids	Sulfur hexafluoride	2001
Luminity[c]	Lantheus Medical Imaging	Phospholipids	Perfluoropropane	2001
Sonazoid[d]	Daiichi Sankyo	Phosphatidylserine	Perfluorobutane	2006

[a] Does not pass pulmonary circulation.
[b] No longer marketed.
[c] Marketed in U.S. as Definity.
[d] Marketed only in Japan.

◼ Oral Contrast Agents

These are actually negative contrast agents, as they do not produce echogenicity, but eliminate the interfering echogenicity in the gastrointestinal tract caused by the presence of air. At present, the sole product approved for this purpose is only available in the United States (SonoRx). The drinkable liquid contains cellulose fibers that adsorb the air that causes interference, thus allowing overlap-free examination of organs behind the gastrointestinal tract.[19]

Mode of Action of Ultrasound Contrast Agents

◼ Structure

The basic principle of ultrasound contrast agents is the creation of many small interfaces with high echogenicity. This is ideally achieved using gaseous microbubbles. To increase the stability of microbubbles in the blood and achieve a standardized size, the bubbles are surrounded by a shell. There are products with hard shells (e.g., galactose microparticles, denatured albumin) and products with flexible shell membranes (e.g., phospholipid shells). In terms of the gas, a distinction is made between products containing air (first-generation products) and those with low-solubility gases (second-generation products) (**Fig. 7.1**). The latter produce longer-lasting contrast, as the gas they contain only dissolves slowly in the surrounding blood.

   The microbubbles usually have a diameter of 2–10 µm, which is about the size of the red blood cells. Unlike common CT and MRI contrast agents, therefore, they do not pass into the interstitial fluid, but remain confined to the vascular system (blood-pool contrast agents). This substantially simplifies the assessment of tissue perfusion, as the contrast agent distribution can be considered equivalent to the distribution of the blood. Luckily, the resonance frequency of microbubbles of this size is in the region of the sound frequencies used for diagnostic imaging, which makes it possible to generate a harmonic response.

◼ Echogenic Properties

When sound waves strike the microbubbles, they are reflected from the surface. More precisely, the process is known as backscattering. The backscattered sound waves have the same wavelength as the emitted sound waves. This backscattering behavior is referred to as the linear

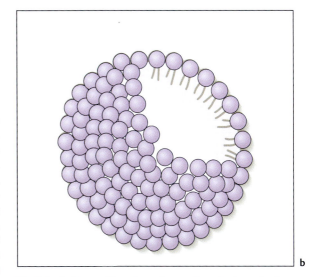

Fig. 7.1a, b Composition of an ultrasound contrast agent microbubble. Microscopic image (**a**) and schematic configuration (**b**) of SonoVue microbubbles. A flexible outer shell of phospholipids surrounds the enclosed SF_6 gas. The phospholipids form a monolayer, with the lipid side facing inward (toward the gas) and the hydrophilic side pointing outward (toward the blood).

behavior of the microbubbles. The microbubbles in ultrasound contrast agents are very effective backscatterers. They increase the signal intensity by more than 30 dB,[20] which corresponds to a factor of 1000 in the received sound intensity.

   However, as the sound pressure increases, nonlinear behavior of the microbubbles becomes increasingly prominent. The bubbles first start to oscillate, sending out harmonic oscillations,[21,22] and then, as the sound pressure increases further, the microbubbles become unstable, start to split up, and finally break down. In the process, they send out a brief high-energy signal (stimulated acoustic emission, SAE)[23,24] (**Fig. 7.2**).

   In principle, all ultrasound contrast agents show this behavior, but the absolute level of sound energy at which the harmonic response and the rupture of the microbubbles sets in varies from one contrast agent to another.

I Techniques

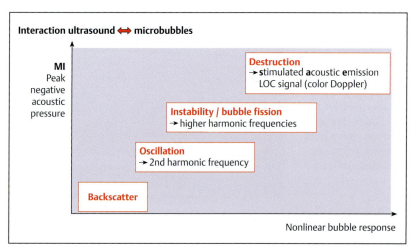

Interaction ultrasound ⬌ microbubbles

MI
Peak negative acoustic pressure

Destruction
→ **s**timulated **a**coustic **e**mission
LOC signal (color Doppler)

Instability / bubble fission
→ higher harmonic frequencies

Oscillation
→ 2nd harmonic frequency

Backscatter

Nonlinear bubble response

Fig. 7.2 Behavior of microbubbles as a function of insonation pressure. The behavior of microbubbles in the acoustic field depends primarily on the insonation pressure. If the acoustic pressure is very low, passive backscattering of the input signal occurs. At somewhat higher acoustic pressures, the microbubbles start to oscillate at their resonance frequency. If the acoustic pressure is too high, the microbubbles break down. LOC, loss of correlation; MI, mechanical index.

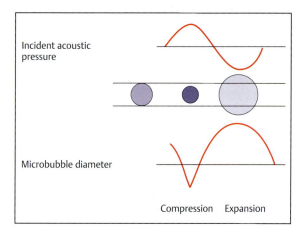

Incident acoustic pressure

Microbubble diameter

Compression   Expansion

Fig. 7.3 Oscillation of microbubbles in a sound field. Compression of the microbubbles during the high-pressure phase (against the internal gas pressure) is less than expansion in the low-pressure phase. The fluctuation in the diameter of the microbubbles is therefore asymmetrical and is not a linear function of pressure fluctuation—a nonlinear response.

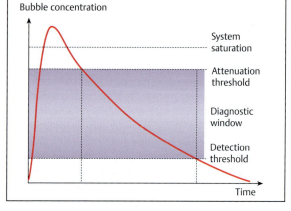

Bubble concentration

System saturation

Attenuation threshold

Diagnostic window

Detection threshold

Time

Fig. 7.4 Course of the microbubble concentration in blood after bolus administration. After bolus injection, there is a rapid increase in the contrast-agent concentration up to a maximum (peak intensity), followed by a somewhat slower wash-out phase. If the attenuation threshold or even system saturation is reached at the maximum, artifacts such as shadowing or blooming can occur.

Microbubbles with flexible shells start to oscillate at low sound energies and show pronounced harmonic behavior. Hard-shelled contrast agents, on the other hand, give a very good SAE signal on rupture.

During oscillation, the microbubbles produce a nonlinear echo signal.[25] This is because the compression of the microbubbles against the pressure of the inner gas content is less than the expansion. This leads to asymmetrical fluctuation of the bubble diameter, which is no longer linearly dependent on the sound pressure (**Fig. 7.3**).

◼ Dosage and Administration

Ultrasound contrast agents are usually administered by intravenous bolus injection. To achieve the fastest and most complete possible wash-in of the contrast agent

bolus, flushing with 5–10 mL of physiological saline is recommended.[26] The injection should ideally be given in a large-volume arm vein, with the syringe connected to the indwelling cannula directly or via the straight part of a T connector. If there are compelling reasons for interposing an infusion tube, it must be as short as possible and the inner lumen should not be too tight. Particularly for measuring perfusion profiles (e.g., to characterize lesions), the injection has to be given rapidly to obtain sharp temporal separation.

After the bolus injection, there is a rapid increase in the microbubble concentration, followed by a slow wash-out over several minutes. Attention has to be given to three threshold values (**Fig. 7.4**):

- *System saturation.* This threshold is frequently reached right at the start of contrast wash-in and gives rise to saturation artifacts and (in color Doppler) blooming effects.

Table 7.2 Recommended doses of different ultrasound contrast agents

Product	Concentration	Dose
Levovist	200 mg/mL	10–16 mL
	300 mg/mL	5–10 mL
	400 mg/mL	5–8 mL
Optison		0.5–3.0 mL
SonoVue		(0.6–)1.2–2.4 mL

- *Attenuation threshold.* Above this threshold, there is a strong echo signal close to the transducer because of the high microbubble concentration; distal to this there is shadowing, like that seen behind hyperechoic tissue structures.
- *Detection threshold.* Below this threshold, the microbubble concentration is too low and the microbubbles can no longer be detected.

The diagnostic window within which the bubble concentration is optimal for imaging is located between the detection threshold and the attenuation threshold. The absolute level of these thresholds depends on the machine used, the contrast software installed, and the machine settings. Most machines now have presets suitable for contrast agents, allowing rapid selection of the most important parameters for optimal contrast imaging.

The signal strength (gray value or power Doppler intensity) is an approximately linear function of the bubble concentration, allowing quantitative assessment of the perfusion. However, this only applies at contrast agent concentrations that are not too high (below the attenuation threshold).

The optimal dose of contrast agent depends, among other things, on the technique used (B-mode, Doppler, harmonic mode, etc.), the settings and sensitivity of the ultrasound machine, the target organ, and the contrast enhancement required. With the newer second-generation contrast agents, doses of 1–5 mL are usually adequate. The quantity of gas they contain is very low (e.g., only 8 μL/mL in the case of SonoVue), which illustrates the high sensitivity of contrast agent imaging. The dosages shown **Table 7.2** are recommended as standard values. With the most recent scanner technology, even smaller doses down to less than 1 mL per injection are possible.

If longer contrast times with uniform contrast enhancement are required, a continuous infusion of microbubbles can be given.[26,27] The infusion rate has to be adjusted so as to provide uniform contrast without saturation artifacts. For longer infusion times, it should be noted that the microbubbles float toward the top of the carrier liquid over time and become concentrated on the surface of the liquid in the syringe. Regular, or preferably continuous, mixing of the solution is recommended (e.g., with special infusion pumps).

Artifacts Caused by Contrast Agents

■ Saturation Artifacts

The high amplitude of the backscattered signal can lead to saturation of the receiver electronics at high microbubble concentrations. In color Doppler, this takes the form of smearing of the color signal (color blooming), which also occurs at high color amplification or transmitter power.[28] This effect often occurs shortly after wash-in of the contrast agent and disappears as the microbubble concentration declines again.

■ Destruction Artifacts

At very high sound pressures, large quantities of microbubbles become unstable and finally break down. This gives rise to high energy signals (stimulated acoustic emission). If these signals mix with normal backscattered signals, they lead to an artificial echo image (bubble noise).[28] However, when such signals are generated deliberately, they can be used for imaging.

The destruction of microbubbles in regions of high sound pressure (e.g., close to the transducer in the focal plane) can also lead to attenuation phenomena that simulate lack of contrast enhancement. This can be avoided by reducing the sound energy and/or lowering the focal plane.

During sonography of regions with low blood-flow velocities (capillary beds), the section of the image affected only fills up again very slowly after destruction of the microbubbles. This can lead to bleaching of the contrast effect in tissue, which might be misinterpreted as an absence of contrast agent. In such cases, the perfusion can still be imaged by sonography at a reduced imaging rate (intermittent imaging).[29,30] Individual images (frames) are recorded and displayed as still images until the next frame is captured. The length of the delay is normally 1–10 seconds (i.e., one frame is recorded every 1–10 seconds), depending on the strength of the blood flow. Recording of the frames can also be synchronized with the cardiac pulse (triggered imaging). However, in more recent procedures, bubble rupture is usually avoided by reducing the transmission power (i.e., using a low mechanical index procedure).

■ Shadow Artifacts

If the microbubble concentration is too high, very strong echo signals are produced close to the transducer, leading to shadowing or attenuation of deeper-lying structures.[31] The effect corresponds to the attenuation phenomenon behind very echogenic structures. Increasing the signal intensity by administering higher doses of contrast agent is therefore only possible to a limited extent, so that it is better to use more sensitive, contrast-specific techniques.

■ Overestimated Flow Rates in Spectral Doppler

If the machine parameters are set correctly (i.e., amplification, wall filter, etc.), correct flow rates can also be measured with contrast-enhanced ultrasonography. If the signal is too strong, the Doppler gain may have to be reduced. There may be differences in the measured values in comparison with ultrasonography without contrast enhancement, if the maximum flow rate (i.e., the upper limit of the Doppler spectral curve) is not detected because the signal strength is too low.[28,32] This is often the case for pathological flow in small volumes (e.g., flow in a stenosis, reflux jet, or shunt flow). In this situation, contrast enhancement contributes to more reliable measurement.

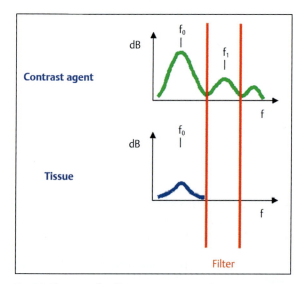

Fig. 7.5 The principle of harmonic imaging. In harmonic imaging, contrast-specific parts of the signal are separated from tissue signals using a frequency filter. However, this also suppresses nonlinear signals in the range of the fundamental frequency.

Contrast-Specific Imaging Procedures

Contrast-specific imaging procedures make use of the nonlinear behavior of the contrast-agent microbubbles for selective imaging of the ultrasound contrast agent, and thus of the blood volume.

There are numerous technical approaches to separating the (nonlinear) contrast-agent echo from the (linear) tissue echo and the artifact echoes (noise, speckle, clutter, motion artifacts in Doppler, etc.). The objective of each of these procedures is to optimize the contrast–tissue ratio and the contrast–noise ratio.

The proper separation of contrast-agent signals from background signals is a quality parameter for the contrast-specific imaging modality of the ultrasound scanner. Ideally, the contrast-specific image should be completely black before arrival of the contrast agent. Any background signals (e.g., from tissue) visible at baseline due to insufficient signal separation may be misinterpreted as perfusion.

■ Frequency Filter Procedures

In frequency filter procedures (harmonic imaging), the nonlinear signals in the region of the second harmonic frequency (i.e., twice the transmitted frequency) are separated out by means of a filter. Thus, only a part of the frequency spectrum that consists exclusively of nonlinear signals is used for imaging. The filter removes those parts of the signal at the fundamental frequency f_0, and only those signals in the region of the second harmonic frequency are used for imaging (**Fig. 7.5**).

The advantage of this procedure is that it reduces the tissue signal (although, because of the formation of harmonics during the propagation of the sound wave, the echoes are not completely suppressed) and provides a clear reduction in noise artifacts (e.g., clutter). The contrast signal is thus more intense in comparison with the tissue (signal–tissue ratio) and noise (signal–clutter ratio), but not completely selective. The disadvantage of harmonic imaging is the need to use narrow-band transducers with lower resolution (to avoid overlapping of the two frequency bands) and the high sound energy required (as the most intense part of the backscattered signal is not used for imaging). Harmonic imaging thus generally ruptures a relatively large proportion of the microbubbles.

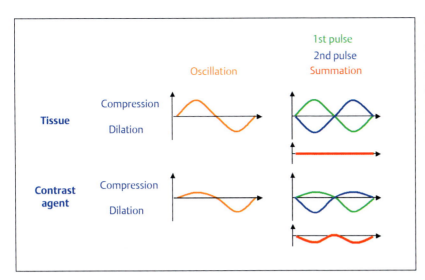

Fig. 7.6 The principle of the pulse summation procedure (pulse/phase inversion). In the pulse summation procedure, the contrast-specific parts of the signal are separated from the tissue signal by co-evaluation of several successive pulse sequences. This produces very good suppression of the tissue signal and high sensitivity for contrast-agent signals.

Harmonic Power Doppler

Color Doppler uses an autocorrelation procedure to calculate the Doppler signal—i.e., it compares two echoes recorded a short time apart and interprets changes as movement. As mentioned above, harmonic imaging uses high sound energies, rupturing a relatively large number of microbubbles. Color Doppler interprets the disappearance of the microbubbles (erroneously) as very rapid movement and displays the corresponding color-coded signal on the monitor. It thus gives rise to a microbubble-dependent "Doppler" signal of high intensity (and random direction). In regions of very low blood flow (such as capillary regions)—i.e., where there is no velocity-based Doppler signal—harmonic power Doppler can be used to image the distribution of microbubbles (perfusion imaging). In this case, high intensity (bright signal) means a large number of microbubbles and thus a high blood volume.

The advantage of this procedure is real-time subtraction of the background signal (tissue) and a color-coded image corresponding to the microbubble concentration (if the machine settings are correct). The disadvantage is high sensitivity to motion artifacts.

Pulse Summation Procedures

Pulse summation procedures (pulse/phase inversion, power modulation, or a combination of the two) use a completely different technique to separate nonlinear and linear signals (**Fig. 7.6**). Several consecutive sound waves from a single scan line are evaluated together. In the simplest case, a positive wave and a negative wave (with inverted phase) are subtracted from one another, resulting in cancellation of the signal. Linear signals are thus not displayed. On the other hand, nonlinear signals (formed

due to the different reactions of microbubbles to positive and negative waves) do not cancel out during this calculation and are displayed.[33,34]

Instead of simple pulse inversion, other mathematical techniques (e.g., doubling and subsequent halving of the amplitude, digital coding, etc.) can be used.

All of the main equipment manufacturers now offer one or more contrast-specific imaging procedures. However, all of the procedures are based on one of the two principles, or a combination of the two. A sequential summation image is sometimes also used, collecting signals from multiple subsequent frames and thus allowing reconstruction of the course of the microvessels from the paths of the microbubbles passing through. The manufacturers are constantly improving and further developing the techniques.

In general, all of the procedures either use high sound energy (high mechanical index procedures), with destruction of the microbubbles forming the basis of the signal specific to the contrast agent, or very low sound energy (low mechanical index procedures), in which the persistent oscillation of the microbubbles forms the basis of the contrast-specific signal. The choice of the optimal procedure depends on contrast agent used. Microbubbles with thick, rigid shells are more suitable for high mechanical index (MI) procedures, while those with thin, flexible shells are better for low-MI procedures. **Table 7.3** provides an overview of the contrast-specific procedures currently available.

The significant advantage of pulse summation procedures is that (in contrast to harmonic imaging) wideband transducers with better spatial resolution can again be used (**Fig. 7.7**). However, because several (short) pulses have to be transmitted per scan line, the frame rate is lower than for normal B-mode images.

As a result of the use of the entire frequency spectrum, the signal strength as a whole is higher than in classical harmonic imaging. In addition to the better spatial

Table 7.3 Contrast-specific imaging modalities (abdominal sonography)

Manufacturer	Machine platform	Name of the procedure*
Aloka	SSD Alpha 10	Extended pure harmonic detection (E-PHD)
	SSD Alpha 5	Extended pure harmonic detection (E-PHD)
	SSD-5500	Extended pure harmonic detection (E-PHD)
	ProSound Alpha 7	Extended pure harmonic detection (E-PHD)
B-K	Pro Focus	Power modulation
Esaote	MyLab 25	Contrast-tuned imaging (CnTI)
	MyLab 30	Contrast-tuned imaging (CnTI)
	MyLab 40	Contrast-tuned imaging (CnTI)
	MyLab 50	Contrast-tuned imaging (CnTI)
	MyLab 70	Contrast-tuned imaging (CnTI)
GE	Logiq E9	Amplitude modulation
	Logiq 9	Coded phase inversion (CPI)
	Logiq 7	Coded phase inversion (CPI)
	Logiq S6	Coded phase inversion (CPI)
Hitachi	EUB 8500	Dynamic contrast harmonic imaging (dCHI-W)
	EUB 6500	Dynamic contrast harmonic imaging (dCHI-W)
	HV 900	Dynamic contrast harmonic imaging (dCHI-W)
Philips	iU22	Power modulation/pulse inversion (PM/PI)
	HD 11	Pulse inversion (PI)
Siemens	S 2000	Cadence contrast pulse-sequencing (CPS)
	Acuson Sequoia	Cadence contrast pulse-sequencing (CPS) Cadence coherent contrast imaging (CCI)
	Antares	Cadence contrast pulse sequencing (CPS)
Toshiba	Aplio XG	Contrast harmonic imaging (CHI)
	Xario XG	Contrast harmonic imaging (CHI)

* Manufacturer's trade name

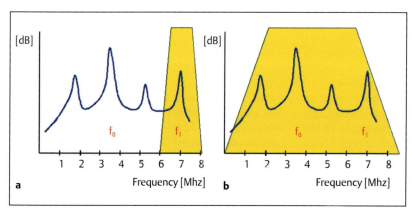

a   b

Fig. 7.7a, b Use of the full bandwidth in the pulse summation procedure (wide-band harmonic imaging). **a** Harmonic imaging (narrow-band). **b** Wide-band harmonic imaging. Because the pulse summation procedure does not use a frequency filter to separate contrast-agent signals from tissue signals, it is possible to use wide-band transducers with better spatial resolution, as in normal B-mode sonography. This is the origin of the term "wide-band harmonic imaging" (**b**), which is sometimes used in contrast to normal harmonic imaging with narrow-band transducers (**a**).

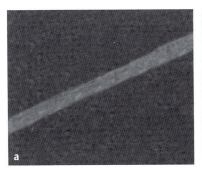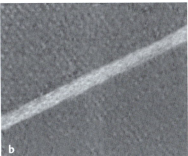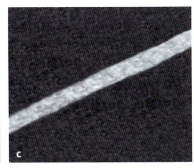

Fig. 7.8a–c The contrast–tissue ratio.
a In normal B-mode, the contrast signal from the blood is considerably enhanced, approximately to the level of the tissue signal. However, this sometimes gives rise to an anti-contrast effect—i.e., the blood and tissue signals reach a similar gray value that can no longer be differentiated. Advantages of B-mode: high spatial resolution and high frame rate; disadvantages: relatively weak contrast signal and no separation from the tissue signal.
b Harmonic imaging makes the contrast-agent signals relatively stronger and substantially suppresses the tissue signals. However,

nonlinear signals from the tissue created by propagation effects (known as tissue harmonics) appear in the image. Advantages of harmonic imaging (the frequency filter mode): strong contrast signal and high frame rate; disadvantages: reduced spatial resolution and only partial separation from the tissue signal.
c Pulse summation procedures provide optimal imaging of the contrast-agent signal, with almost complete suppression of tissue signals. Advantages of the pulse summation mode: strong contrast signal, full spatial resolution, and complete separation from the tissue signals; disadvantage: slightly reduced frame rate.

resolution, wide-band harmonic imaging produces a further improved contrast–tissue ratio (with virtually complete suppression of the tissue signal)[34] (**Fig. 7.8**).

■ Investigations at Very Low Insonation Power (Low-MI Imaging)

Because pulse summation procedures use the entire frequency spectrum for imaging, the energy backscattered from the microbubbles can be used substantially more effectively. It is therefore possible to use significantly lower transmitter powers than for harmonic imaging, which results in less destruction of the microbubbles. Particularly with newer products with flexible shells (e.g., SonoVue, Definity), it is possible to use minimal sound pressure (mechanical index < 0.1), at which microbubbles oscillate for a long time, emitting strong harmonic signals, without being destroyed. This makes it possible to image parenchymal blood flow with continuous transmission (real-time perfusion imaging).[35]

The transmitter power is nowadays normally shown on the machine monitor as the mechanical index (MI). The MI is calculated from the maximum negative sound pressure divided by the square root of the sound frequency. It should be noted that the actual local sound pressure in the sound field varies greatly because of the beam geometry and the increasing attenuation in deeper layers. In addition, the methods of calculation used by different machine manufacturers are not the same. The absolute MI values can therefore only be taken as indicative, and are not directly comparable from machine to machine.

As a general rule, the harmonic response of the microbubbles does increase with an increasing mechanical index (creating a more intense contrast signal), but (to an even greater extent) so do the harmonic components from the tissue (caused by propagation effects), so that the overall contrast–tissue ratio deteriorates. In addition, destruction of the microbubbles increases. Appropriate adjustment of the insonation power (MI) is therefore essential for good contrast imaging.

■ Flash Echo Imaging

In general, the objective of this contrast-specific imaging procedure is continuous imaging of the blood supply in tissue, as far as possible without destroying microbubbles. Despite this, in certain situations it may be desirable to briefly destroy all microbubbles in the insonation field during continuous imaging, using a pulse of high sound energy (a flash or burst).[36]

The brief destruction of the microbubbles during a continuous examination in low-MI mode allows imaging of the refilling of the capillary bed (replenishment) and thus the assessment of the dynamics of perfusion.[37] The blood flow in capillaries is so slow that replenishment with new microbubbles takes several seconds. The time until full contrast intensity is reached again (the slope of the replenishment curve) is a measure of the blood flow, whereas the intensity is a measure of the blood volume. Multiplying the two values together provides a parameter for assessing parenchymal perfusion (see the section on quantitative evaluation below).

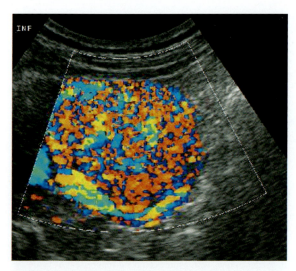

Fig. 7.9 Stimulated acoustic emission (SAE) imaging. In SAE, virtually all of the microbubbles are destroyed at the same time. This produces a very intense wide-band signal, which can be used as a brief flash for virtually all procedures. In color Doppler, the disappearance of the microbubbles is misinterpreted as rapid movement and therefore displayed as a (chaotic) velocity signal. However, longer-term imaging of the kinetics of the contrast agent is not possible with this method.

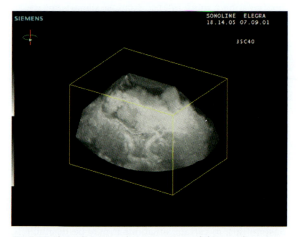

Fig. 7.10 Three-dimensional representation of the vascular geometry of a lesion. The vascular geometry of the afferent and efferent vessels and of the capillary network of a lesion in the spleen, infiltrated (mainly in the peripheral regions) by a T cell lymphoma.

■ SAE Imaging

This technique actually dates from the early days of perfusion imaging, when interference-free continuous examination with low sound energy was not possible. In SAE imaging, a rapid sweep of the tissue is performed with high sound energy (high MI) in color Doppler mode and stored in the digital image memory. In the process, virtually all microbubbles are ruptured simultaneously, pro-

ducing a very strong Doppler signal. Subsequent examination of the individual frames from the image memory reveals the original distribution of the microbubbles.[6,7] It should be noted that the SAE effect only occurs in areas of sufficiently high sound energy (in the near field); in deeper regions, the sound pressure may be too low to break the microbubbles. Although this is the most sensitive procedure for detecting microbubbles, it has largely lost its importance because of the technical advantages of real-time imaging (**Fig. 7.9**).

SAE imaging can be performed with any normal color Doppler machine and is technically very simple, as standardized machine settings can be used and image acquisition only has to be performed once, a few minutes after injection of the contrast agent. This means that the contrast agent can be administered in daylight, before the ultrasound examination is started. However, it is only ever possible to record an instantaneous image, and ultrasound loses its real-time character.

Qualitative Evaluation

■ Vascular Geometry

Contrast-enhanced B-mode sonography can image veins and arteries at a high spatial resolution without blooming and independent of direction. Panorama sweeps and three-dimensional reconstructions are possible[38] (**Fig. 7.10**). The imaging of afferent and efferent vessels and the capillary circulation makes it possible to image vascular abnormalities. Vascular geometry can make an important contribution to the characterization of focal lesions.

The possibility of destruction of microbubbles must be borne in mind when examining blood vessels with contrast-enhanced ultrasonography. In large-volume vessels or vessels with high flow rates, bubbles destroyed in the image plane are rapidly replenished, so that real-time imaging can be performed with relatively high sound energy. However, in small vessels with low flow rates (e.g., capillary beds), replenishment with fresh contrast agent is very slow, so either a reduced image rate (intermittent imaging) or very low sound energy (low-MI imaging) have to be used for examinations. These effects can be used to produce images with different weighting. Depending on the issue being investigated, it is possible to image just the afferent vessels with high flow rates (flow-based imaging) or the entire vasculature including capillaries (volume-based imaging).

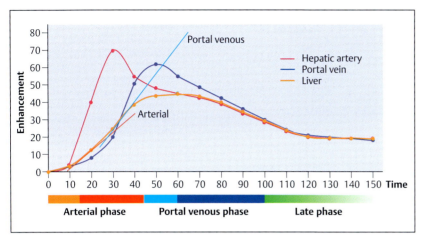

Fig. 7.11 Contrast phases in the liver. Because of the dual blood supply to the liver through the hepatic artery and portal vein, two separate sets of wash-in kinetics can be observed at different times. Initially, there is contrast enhancement due to wash-in from the hepatic artery (the arterial phase) and then, approximately 30–40 seconds later, contrast enhancement due to wash-in from the portal vein is seen. Because the normal liver parenchyma is mainly supplied by the portal vein, the contrast enhancement in liver tissue is substantially stronger in the portal venous phase.

Perfusion Abnormalities (Hyperperfusion/Hypoperfusion)

The optimal approach for examining parenchymal perfusion is real-time imaging, using low sound energy (low-MI imaging). Intermittent imaging should only be used when a suitable low-MI technique is not available or when extremely high sensitivity is required to detect the tiniest perfusion signals (e.g., to image perfusion in hypovascular metastases). This has to be borne in mind, of course, when interpreting the results, and the description of the vascularity must always be performed in comparison with the surrounding normal tissue. A more sensitive technique would never change a hypovascular lesion into a hypervascular lesion, even if it did reveal the presence of contrast agent.

Using low sound energy (low-MI imaging), continuous examination of a region is possible, allowing the assessment of a certain region at different time points. This allows unlimited examination of the organ (e.g., the liver) throughout the period of contrast enhancement, making it possible to detect and simultaneously characterize lesions, and greatly simplifying the course of the examination (**Fig. 7.11**).

The continuous examination allows easy assessment of contrast-agent dynamics in tissue. Contrast ultrasonography has the advantage that the examination can be performed continuously from the start of the injection, so that all phases of perfusion can be observed (even the very early, rapid processes). This should always be used. In very slow, late processes (e.g., in hemangiomas), the examination should be interrupted after ≈ 1 minute for periods of ≈ 30–60 seconds to avoid significant microbubble destruction and to give both the patient and the examiner a rest. When the various flow phases are being examined in liver tissue, it is easy to recognize abnormal uptake of contrast agent in focal lesions and use it diagnostically. The results are comparable with phase images in computed tomography, although with a much clearer depiction of vascular structures due to the absence of extravasation of ultrasound contrast microbubbles.

Quantitative Evaluation

Bolus Kinetics

The wash-in and wash-out kinetics of the contrast agent after a bolus injection can also be measured quantitatively. To do this, a region of interest (ROI) is generally specified, and the total pixel intensity in that region is recorded as a function of time. The measurement can be carried out off-line from the video signal, or preferably from the digital dataset in memory. Care must be taken to ensure that no distortion of the measured values occurs during postprocessing in the ultrasound equipment (particularly when using the video signal).

The recording of bolus kinetics follows the principle of indicator dilution theory. For a homogeneous distribution of microbubbles in blood, the height of the wash-out curve is a measure of the blood volume and the wash-out time is a measure of the blood flow. However, exact application of this principle requires an exact bolus time point, which is not strictly obtained following an intravenous injection. However, the small injection volume with modern contrast agents is an advantage here.

The major advantage of ultrasound contrast agents and their microbubbles is that they represent a genuine intravascular marker which, unlike other contrast agents (e.g., in CT, MRI, or with nuclear tracers), do not pass into the interstitial space or the intracellular fluid. The contrast distribution and wash-in/wash-out kinetics thus exactly reflect the behavior of the blood.

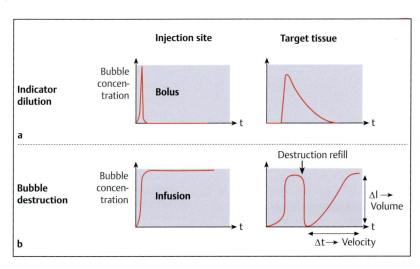

Fig. 7.12 a, b Bolus and replenishment kinetics.
a In classical bolus kinetics, the change in contrast in the target tissue is recorded after a fast bolus injection. However, cardiopulmonary passage after an intravenous injection always results in the bolus diffusing apart and being diluted, which adversely affects the temporal resolution.
b In replenishment kinetics, the increase in the signal occurs as a result of replenishment directly from the afferent vessels after local destruction of the microbubbles in the sound field directly, so that a very high level of temporal resolution is achieved.

Transit Time Analysis

In transit time analysis, a simultaneous continuous measurement is performed in the afferent and efferent vessels of an organ. The exact time of onset of contrast wash-in is recorded. The transit time—i.e., the time required for blood to flow through an organ—can be determined from the time difference between inflow and outflow. The transit time can be regarded as a measure of the general perfusion of an organ. It is increased in generalized hypoperfusion and shortened in the presence of arteriovenous shunts. Transit time analysis can therefore be used to look for occult hepatic lesions (with arteriovenous shunts).

Replenishment Kinetics

A fundamental problem with using bolus kinetics is the prolonged wash-in time following intravenous injection, which is due to venous pooling and to the bolus drifting apart during passage through the heart and lungs. This limits the diagnostic value of the method for rapid wash-in profiles, despite the intravascular character of the microbubbles. The ability to use a single flash to rupture virtually all microbubbles in a capillary bed within fractions of a second opens up fresh scope for this principle.

Instead of wash-in and wash-out of a bolus injection, replenishment after rupture of the microbubbles can be investigated starting from a constant contrast level. This technique is also known as the negative bolus technique. The initial level of contrast agent can be kept constant—for example, through continuous infusion.

In replenishment kinetics, the intensity is a measure of the blood volume in tissue, and the time taken to return to the previous intensity (or the slope of the refill curve) is a measure of the flow rate. Multiplication of these two parameters provides a measure of perfusion in the tissue. To determine the absolute perfusion (mL/min/g), this value would have to be standardized by weighting it for the tissue in the measured area (**Fig. 7.12**).

Depletion Kinetics

If the destruction of the microbubbles is arranged so that only some of the bubbles in the sound field are destroyed during the recording of one image frame (by adjusting the insonation energy and image rate), fractional signal breakdown is achieved over several frames. The number of frames required until all the microbubbles are destroyed (i.e., until the signal is completely quenched) depends on the amount of contrast agent present (i.e., the blood volume) and the amount of replenishment between two frames (i.e., the blood flow). The quenching time thus reflects the local perfusion and can be used to investigate relative differences in perfusion. The advantage of this method is the short measurement time (only ≈ 1 second) for the complete kinetics. It is thus possible to measure several sets of kinetics (e.g., in several focal planes) after a simple bolus injection (at the inflow maximum).

Parametric Imaging

Parametric imaging is based on the measurement of wash-in or replenishment curves of this type and the calculation of characteristic, curve-specific parameters (e.g., time to peak, slope of the peak, half-life, area under the curve, etc.). However, the calculation is not performed for a large region of interest, but separately for each individual pixel. The corresponding curve parameters can be color-coded for each pixel. Thus, for example, flow rate images or volume images can show regions of high flow or volume in brighter colors. Parametric images of this type make it possible to document the complete contrast-agent dynamics on a single image.[39]

Clinical Indications for Contrast-Enhanced Ultrasonography

■ Doppler Signal Enhancement (Vascular Flow)

Originally, ultrasound contrast agents were developed both to image body cavities to improve the delineation of contours (e.g., identification of the endocardium in echocardiography) and especially to enhance the Doppler signal—so they are still often known as signal enhancers, even though their uses now extend far beyond that. Enhancement of the Doppler signal is always necessary if the signal without contrast agent is too weak, or rather if the signal–noise ratio is too poor (otherwise it would be simpler to increase the amplifier setting on the machine). The crucial point is that the contrast agent (the signal enhancer) selectively enhances the useful signal, but not the noise. However, the better the ultrasound machine used, the less need there is for this type of Doppler signal enhancement. Modern high-end color Doppler machines can usually provide an adequate Doppler signal without contrast enhancement.

However, when the signal–noise ratio is inadequate for an unambiguous diagnosis in individual cases, injection of a signal enhancer is the method of choice. This may occur in regions with very low flow volumes (e.g., residual volume in a severe stenosis) or very slow flow (e.g., aneurysms). When there is vascular occlusion, the signal enhancer increases the diagnostic accuracy, because the absence of a flow signal could also be caused by too low a signal strength (below the noise filter) or an unfavorable vessel angle (e.g., in a bend in the vessel).

Signal enhancers are very important in organs that are difficult to examine with ultrasonography, such as the brain. Cerebral ultrasonography is only possible through an acoustic window in the skull (transcranial ultrasound), and the sound cone is substantially attenuated. In this case, signal enhancers usually allow examinations with a high diagnostic value.

■ Diagnosis of Ischemia

In contrast to the large vessels, both the signal strength and the flow rate of blood in the capillary beds are too low to produce a detectable Doppler signal. In this case, an ultrasound contrast agent is necessary to allow any imaging of the blood volume at all. The contrast agent does not just function as an image enhancer, but also as a marker, the passage of which through the organ can be observed as a function of time. This allows dynamic assessment of the blood supply (perfusion).

With the aid of additional quantitative techniques, as described above, it is possible to identify and assess regional or global hypoperfusion. For example, it is possible to detect stenosis in the afferent artery as relative ischemia in the upstream parenchyma. This allows hemodynamic quantification of stenoses (e.g., in the renal artery, coronary arteries, etc.). If necessary, functional examinations can be performed as well—e.g., after administration of a vasoactive substance.

■ Diagnosis of Traumatic Lesions

Blunt traumatic injuries can lead to structural defects in organs that are difficult or impossible to detect with noncontrast ultrasonography, particularly if the capsule is still intact and there is little or no free fluid. After administration of the contrast agent, it is generally possible to recognize all disturbances of the microvascular system clearly. Tissue ruptures appear as a black line in contrasted parenchyma and hematomas as extensive unperfused areas.

■ Detection of Focal Lesions

Focal lesions are detected either by identifying hyperperfusion or hypoperfusion in comparison with the surrounding tissue, or through changes in the wash-in kinetics of the contrast agent. The classification as hyperperfused or hypoperfused is thus made in comparison with the surrounding normal tissue and is always related to a particular time point. An early arterial hyperperfused lesion may appear hypoperfused during the portal venous phase.

Hyperperfused lesions can generally be seen during the arterial phase as regions of high contrast enhancement (white spots). On high-intensity sonography (bubble destruction), the high flow rates mean that they show intense contrast at short delay times. On the other hand, hypoperfused lesions can be detected in the portal venous phase as black spots against the clearly contrasted normal liver tissue.

Focal lesions of nonhepatic tissue (e.g., metastases from extrahepatic tumors) can be detected by the absence of accumulation of liver-specific contrast agents (e.g., Levovist). Lesions of this type appear as accumulation defects in the late-phase images. Usually, there is a coincidence between absence of accumulating reticuloendothelial cells and absence of portal-venous vessels, so that imaging of contrast agent accumulation as well as imaging of portal-

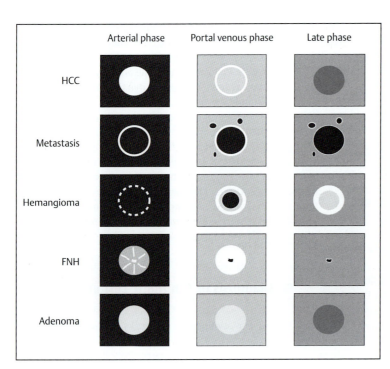

	Arterial phase	Portal venous phase	Late phase
HCC			
Metastasis			
Hemangioma			
FNH			
Adenoma			

Fig. 7.13 Characteristic contrast patterns in hepatic lesions. Focal hepatic lesions show characteristic remodeling of the vascular supply, which may include arterialization. The increased arterial supply is usually followed by a reduction in the portal venous supply. This results in temporal and geometric changes in the wash-in profile of the lesion, which can be used for characterization. FNH, focal nodular hyperplasia; HCC, hepatocellular carcinoma.

venous contrast agent distribution both result in the same appearance of liver metastases as black spots in late phase.

Characterization of Focal Lesions

In the first place, contrast-enhanced ultrasonography can be used to assess whether a lesion is strongly perfused or not. Modern ultrasound equipment has excellent contrast resolution and can identify even slightly altered regions of the liver (e.g., regional fatty changes) as suspect regions. Such findings are often obtained incidentally in routine examinations and show no symptoms. If no increased arterial perfusion can be seen in such regions, a benign process can usually be assumed.

Because of the double blood supply via the portal vein and the hepatic artery, focal lesions in the liver often do not display general hyperperfusion or hypoperfusion, but a complex temporal and spatial pattern of hyperenhancement and hypoenhancement, depending on the phase of flow. Some lesions have a characteristic vascular pattern (e.g., wheel spokes) or perfusion pattern (e.g., halo contrast, iris diaphragm phenomenon), which makes it possible to characterize the lesion.[40] However, not all lesions show the typical aspects of the particular lesion type, due to hemorrhagic or deteriorating changes. Nevertheless, if a characteristic perfusion pattern is observed and if it corresponds to the patient's clinical picture, a definitive diagnosis can usually be made (**Fig. 7.13**).[41–45]

Monitoring of Interventions and Treatment Follow-Up

Contrast-enhanced ultrasonography is an excellent method for monitoring and follow-up of percutaneous ablation therapy (alcohol injection, radiofrequency therapy, laser ablation, etc.). Vital and nonvital tissue are very easy to distinguish on the basis of the vascularization. Because monitoring can be performed during the intervention itself, any necessary further treatment can be initiated immediately, in the same session. Because of the gas artifacts formed during thermoablation, a pause is required between the end of treatment and checking the results. In general, however, an initial assessment of the position and size of the necrotic area is possible 5–10 minutes after the end of treatment.

With hyperperfused lesions (e.g., hepatocellular carcinomas), care has to be taken to ensure complete ablation of the hyperperfused tissue. However, hyperemic regions around the ablated area as a result of the treatment must not be misinterpreted as hyperperfused tissue. With hypoperfused lesions (e.g., metastases) only indirect assessment of the necrotic area is possible. The contrast defect in the portal venous phase must be larger than the original lesion (≈ 0.5–1.0 cm as a safety distance).

It is also possible to monitor the outcome of radiotherapy or chemotherapy. Regression of the vascularization allows earlier assessment of the onset of treatment success than is possible simply by assessing the reduction in size. Particularly with selective antitumor therapies (e.g., antiangiogenic treatment), the vascular response can be monitored with a high degree of accuracy and early assessment of the individual patient's response to therapy is possible.[46] Initial clinical studies showed that the early vascular response measured 2 weeks after the start of therapy is even able to predict survival in the following years.[47]

Safety Aspects

There are four major risks associated with ultrasound contrast agents: the toxicological risk, the embolic risk, the anaphylactic risk, and the generation of biological effects due to ultrasound-induced cavitation.

Ultrasound contrast agents are made up of air or an inert gas and a shell of nontoxic material. They do not contain any components with toxic potential, and are only administered in very small quantities. No toxic effects are known, nor has clinical use revealed any toxic side effects of clinical significance. In most cases, the injection is tolerated extremely well.

The embolic risk is also negligible, as commercial ultrasound contrast agents consist of microbubbles with a standardized size distribution and pass freely through the capillaries. No signs of induced ischemia have been observed in functional clinical studies of the heart and brain. Even highly sensitive electroencephalography was only found to show mild alerting reactions (caused by the audible pulse sounds of the transducer) with contrast agents and ultrasonography, and no pathological signs.[48,49] An assessment by the European Committee for Medical Ultrasound Safety (ECMUS) concluded that the toxic and embolic potential of ultrasound contrast agents is of no clinical significance.[50]

In general, the injection of macromolecular substances and colloidal/particulate solutions involves a certain risk of anaphylactic reactions (triggered by corresponding antibodies) or anaphylactoid reactions (triggered by interaction with mediators, such as histamine).[51] Macromolecular substances are contained in ultrasound contrast agents as components of the shell (e.g., albumin) and/or as excipients to adjust the osmotic value (e.g., macrogol). In isolated cases, pseudoallergic reactions have been observed after administration of an ultrasound contrast agent. Such pseudoallergic reactions may be comparatively harmless (sensation of warmth, flushing) or even very dramatic (dyspnea, bradycardia, hypotension, anxiety). In such cases, the patient must be treated symptomatically[52,53] (e.g., with H_1/H_2-blockers, glucocorticosteroids, epinephrine if necessary). In patients with severely impaired cardiac function (e.g., coronary heart disease, acute or chronic heart failure) the fall in blood pressure as a result of pseudoallergic reactions can lead to complications, with transient myocardial ischemia. Although pseudoallergic reactions of this type are very rare, the examiner should be prepared for them and appropriate emergency equipment should be available.

One potential risk of ultrasound contrast agents is ultrasound-induced cavitation.[54] In the low-pressure phase of the sound wave, the fluid in the blood can be pulled away from the microbubbles, so that a free gas bubble is formed. In the subsequent high-pressure phase, this gas bubble collapses, releasing a large amount of energy in a small area, which leads to a large rise in temperature. This can lead to the formation of free radicals, electromagnetic radiation (sonoluminescence), and lysis of neighboring cells.[50]

The induction of biological effects of this type has been demonstrated many times in vitro,[55–61] but in conditions that do not correspond to the situation in vivo—using very high contrast agent concentrations (> 0.2%), very long transmitter pulse times (> 2 µs), very high sound energies (MI > 1.9), and/or nonphysiological hematocrit values. No significant biological effects have yet been observed with clinically relevant values for these parameters.[60,62]

Numerous experiments have been conducted to detect such biological effects in vivo as well. In most cases, no cavitation was observed, even after the injection of saline containing air bubbles. No endothelial damage was observed.[50] However, transient pores in the endothelium, which close again after a short time (< 1 second), may form. During this time, substances and/or blood components can pass into the tissue. In unfavorable conditions, this could lead to petechial hemorrhage. The extent of this endothelial perforation is directly proportionate to the microbubble concentration (i.e., the contrast-agent dose) and the insonation energy used. The use of low doses of contrast (with a gas volume of only a few microliters) and low sound energies (low-MI imaging) substantially reduces this risk. Therapeutically, this effect—known as sonoporation—can be used for targeted drug delivery. The optimal insonation energies, frequencies, pulse sequences, and microbubble concentrations for this are currently being investigated in several preclinical studies.

Free radicals are only formed in the blood, and not (as in radiography) in tissue. In the blood, they only survive for a few milliseconds and are captured by blood components. In one experiment in mice, low-grade hemolysis was observed, but it was only < 4% and had virtually no clinical significance.[63]

At clinically relevant sound pressures (0.6–1.6 MPa), microbubbles are ruptured relatively slowly (in the order of 1 millisecond), and cavitation effects only occur after multiple pulses of high intensity.[64] There is a clear sound-energy threshold for the occurrence of such biological effects. This has led to the introduction of parameters and upper limits for the energy emitted by ultrasound equipment. The best known is the mechanical index (MI),[65] which is shown on the monitor of most machines.

The safety of contrast-enhanced ultrasonography was demonstrated in numerous clinical studies during approval procedures for the contrast agents. No significant changes in the blood or laboratory values have been found after contrast-enhanced examinations. A critical evaluation of the available results by the European Committee for Medical Ultrasound Safety (ECMUS) showed that, although it appears possible for microbubbles or non-degassed saline to increase the probability of ultrasound-induced cavitation, the clinical significance of this effect is small.[50] It was, however, recommended that treatment with high-energy therapeutic ultrasound or lithotripsy should not be performed within 1 day of the administration of an ultrasound contrast agent.

References

1. Gramiak R, Shah PM. Echocardiography of the aortic root. Invest Radiol 1968;3(5):356–366.
2. Nemec JJ, Marwick TH, Lorig RJ, et al. Comparison of transcranial Doppler ultrasound and transesophageal contrast echocardiography in the detection of interatrial right-to-left shunts. Am J Cardiol 1991;68(15):1498–1502.
3. Kasper W, Geibel A, Tiede N, Just H. Patent foramen ovale in patients with haemodynamically significant pulmonary embolism. Lancet 1992;340(8819):561–564.
4. Feinstein SB, Lang RM, Dick C, et al. Contrast echocardiography during coronary arteriography in humans: perfusion and anatomic studies. J Am Coll Cardiol 1988;11(1):59–65.
5. Sabia PJ, Powers ER, Jayaweera AR, Ragosta M, Kaul S. Functional significance of collateral blood flow in patients with recent acute myocardial infarction. A study using myocardial contrast echocardiography. Circulation 1992;85(6):2080–2089.
6. Blomley MJ, Albrecht T, Cosgrove DO, et al. Improved imaging of liver metastases with stimulated acoustic emission in the late phase of enhancement with the US contrast agent SH U 508A: early experience. Radiology 1999;210(2):409–416.
7. Albrecht T, Blomley MJ, Heckemann RA, et al. [Stimulated acoustic emissions with the ultrasound contrast medium levovist: a clinically useful contrast effect with liver-specific properties]. Rofo 2000;172(1):61–67.
8. Needlemann L, Blomley M, Albrecht T, Hoffmann CW, Olstad MA, Leen EL. Liver parenchyma contrast-enhanced ultrasound: preliminary results of a multi-center study for liver lesion detection. [abstract] Radiology 2000;217(Suppl):305.
9. Leen EL, Albrecht T, Harvey CJ, Goldberg BB, Olstad MA, Cosgrove DO. Multicenter study of Sonazoid-enhanced pulse inversion harmonic imaging in the characterisation of focal hepatic lesions: preliminary results. [abstract] Radiology 2000;217(Suppl):458.
10. Lanza GM, Wallace KD, Scott MJ, et al. A novel site-targeted ultrasonic contrast agent with broad biomedical application. Circulation 1996;94(12):3334–3340 [published erratum in Circulation 1997;95:2458].
11. Klibanov AL, Hughes MS, Marsh JN, et al. Targeting of ultrasound contrast material. An in vitro feasibility study. Acta Radiol Suppl 1997;412:113–120.
12. Lanza GM, Wallace KD, Fischer SE, et al. High-frequency ultrasonic detection of thrombi with a targeted contrast system. Ultrasound Med Biol 1997;23(6):863–870.
13. Lanza GM, Trousil RL, Wallace KD, et al. In vitro characterization of a novel, tissue-targeted ultrasonic contrast system with acoustic microscopy. J Acoust Soc Am 1998;104(6):3665–3672.
14. Unger EC, McCreery TP, Sweitzer RH, Shen D, Wu G. In vitro studies of a new thrombus-specific ultrasound contrast agent. Am J Cardiol 1998;81(12A):58G–61G.
15. Price RJ, Skyba DM, Kaul S, Skalak TC. Delivery of colloidal particles and red blood cells to tissue through microvessel ruptures created by targeted microbubble destruction with ultrasound. Circulation 1998;98(13):1264–1267.
16. Shohet RV, Chen S, Zhou YT, et al. Echocardiographic destruction of albumin microbubbles directs gene delivery to the myocardium. Circulation 2000;101(22):2554–2556.
17. Hamilton JA, Larson AJ, Lower AM, Hasnain S, Grudzinskas JG. Routine use of saline hysterosonography in 500 consecutive, unselected, infertile women. Hum Reprod 1998;13(9):2463–2473.
18. Darge K, Troeger J, Duetting T, et al. Reflux in young patients: comparison of voiding US of the bladder and retrovesical space with echo enhancement versus voiding cystourethrography for diagnosis. Radiology 1999;210(1):201–207.
19. Lev-Toaff AS, Langer JE, Rubin DL, et al. Safety and efficacy of a new oral contrast agent for sonography: a phase II trial. AJR Am J Roentgenol 1999;173(2):431–436.
20. Kaps M, Schaffer P, Beller KD, Seidel G, Bliesath H, Wurst W. Phase I: transcranial echo contrast studies in healthy volunteers. Stroke 1995;26(11):2048–2052.
21. Schrope BA, Newhouse VL. Second harmonic ultrasonic blood perfusion measurement. Ultrasound Med Biol 1993;19(7):567–579.
22. Burns PN. Harmonic imaging with ultrasound contrast agents. Clin Radiol 1996;51(Suppl 1):50–55.
23. Burns PN, Fritzsch T, Weitschies W, Uhlendorf V, Hope-Simson D, Powers JE. Pseudo-Doppler shifts from stationary tissue due to stimulated emission of ultrasound from a new microsphere contrast agent. [abstract] Radiology 1995;197:402.
24. Blomley MJ, Albrecht T, Cosgrove D, et al. Stimulated acoustic emission imaging ("sono-scintigraphy") with the ultrasound contrast agent Levovist: a reproducible Doppler ultrasound effect with potential clinical utility. Acad Radiol 1998;5(Suppl 1):S236–S239, discussion S252–S253.
25. de Jong N, Frinking PJ, Bouakaz A, et al. Optical imaging of contrast agent microbubbles in an ultrasound field with a 100-MHz camera. Ultrasound Med Biol 2000;26(3):487–492.
26. Becher H, Burns PN. Contrast agents for ultrasound. In: Becher H, Burns PN, eds. Handbook of contrast echocardiography. Berlin: Springer; 2000:5–16.
27. Correas JM, Burns PN, Lai X, Qi X. Infusion versus bolus of an ultrasound contrast agent: in vivo dose-response measurements of BR1. Invest Radiol 2000;35(1):72–79.
28. Forsberg F, Liu JB, Burns PN, Merton DA, Goldberg BB. Artifacts in ultrasonic contrast agent studies. J Ultrasound Med 1994;13(5):357–365.
29. Porter TR, Xie F. Transient myocardial contrast after initial exposure to diagnostic ultrasound pressures with minute doses of intravenously injected microbubbles. Demonstration and potential mechanisms. Circulation 1995;92(9):2391–2395.
30. Wei K, Skyba DM, Firschke C, Jayaweera AR, Lindner JR, Kaul S. Interactions between microbubbles and ultrasound: in vitro and in vivo observations. J Am Coll Cardiol 1997;29(5):1081–1088.

31. Bos LJ, Piek JJ, Spaan JA. Effects of shadowing on the time-intensity curves in contrast echocardiography: a phantom study. Ultrasound Med Biol 1996;22(2):217–227.
32. Strauss AD, Beller KD. Arterial parameters under echo contrast enhancement. Eur J Ultrasound 1997;5:31–38.
33. Bauer A, Hauff P, Lazenby J, et al. Wideband harmonic imaging: a novel contrast ultrasound imaging technique. Eur Radiol 1999;9(Suppl 3):S364–S367.
34. Burns PN, Wilson SR, Simpson DH. Pulse inversion imaging of liver blood flow: improved method for characterizing focal masses with microbubble contrast. Invest Radiol 2000;35(1):58–71.
35. Wilson SR, Burns PN, Muradali D, Wilson JA, Lai X. Harmonic hepatic US with microbubble contrast agent: initial experience showing improved characterization of hemangioma, hepatocellular carcinoma, and metastasis. Radiology 2000;215(1):153–161.
36. Kamiyama N, Moriyasu F, Mine Y, Goto Y. Analysis of flash echo from contrast agent for designing optimal ultrasound diagnostic systems. Ultrasound Med Biol 1999;25(3):411–420.
37. Wei K, Jayaweera AR, Firoozan S, Linka A, Skyba DM, Kaul S. Quantification of myocardial blood flow with ultrasound-induced destruction of microbubbles administered as a constant venous infusion. Circulation 1998;97(5):473–483.
38. Dietrich CF. [3 D real time contrast enhanced ultrasonography, a new technique]. Rofo 2002;174(2):160–163.
39. Ignee A, Jedrejczyk M, Schuessler G, Jakubowski W, Dietrich CF. Quantitative contrast enhanced ultrasound of the liver for time intensity curves-Reliability and potential sources of errors. Eur J Radiol 2010;73(1):153–158.
40. Schuessler G, Ignee A, Hirche T, Dietrich CF. [Improved detection and characterisation of liver tumors with echo-enhanced ultrasound]. Z Gastroenterol 2003;41(12):1167–1176.
41. Claudon M, Cosgrove D, Albrecht T, et al. Guidelines and good clinical practice recommendations for contrast enhanced ultrasound (CEUS) - update 2008. Ultraschall Med 2008;29(1):28–44.
42. Dietrich CF. Comments and illustrations regarding the guidelines and good clinical practice recommendations for contrast-enhanced ultrasound (CEUS)–update 2008. Ultraschall Med 2008;29(Suppl 4):S188–S202.
43. Dietrich CF, Mertens JC, Braden B, Schuessler G, Ott M, Ignee A. Contrast-enhanced ultrasound of histologically proven liver hemangiomas. Hepatology 2007;45(5):1139–1145.
44. Dietrich CF, Schuessler G, Trojan J, Fellbaum C, Ignee A. Differentiation of focal nodular hyperplasia and hepatocellular adenoma by contrast-enhanced ultrasound. Br J Radiol 2005;78(932):704–707.
45. Dietrich CF, Ignee A, Trojan J, Fellbaum C, Schuessler G. Improved characterisation of histologically proven liver tumours by contrast enhanced ultrasonography during the portal venous and specific late phase of SHU 508A. Gut 2004;53(3):401–405.
46. Lassau N, Lamuraglia M, Chami L, et al. Gastrointestinal stromal tumors treated with imatinib: monitoring response with contrast-enhanced sonography. AJR Am J Roentgenol 2006;187(5):1267–1273.
47. Lamuraglia M, Escudier B, Chami L, et al. To predict progression-free survival and overall survival in metastatic renal cancer treated with sorafenib: pilot study using dynamic contrast-enhanced Doppler ultrasound. Eur J Cancer 2006;42(15):2472–2479.
48. Seidel G, Kaps M, Verleger R, Meyrer R, Greis C. Einfluss eines Spherosomenhaltigen Echokontrastmittels (BY963) auf die EEG-Aktivität während der transkraniellen Duplex-sonographie. [abstract] [Article in German] Akt Neurol 1996;23(Suppl):S49.
49. Seidel G, Kaps M, Verleger R, Greis C. Improvement of color-coded duplex sonography in patients with insufficient acoustic bone window using the new echo contrast agent BY963: a safety study. [abstract] Cerebrovasc Dis 1996;6(Suppl 3):37.
50. Rott HD; European Committee for Medical Ultrasound Safety. Safety of ultrasonic contrast agents. Eur J Ultrasound 1999;9(2):195–197.
51. Ring J, Brockow K, Behrendt H. History and classification of anaphylaxis. Novartis Found Symp 2004;257:6–16, discussion 16–24, 45–50, 276–285.
52. Walther A, Böttiger BW. [Out-of-Hospital treatment of anaphylactoid reactions]. Internist (Berl) 2004;45(3):296–304.
53. Thomsen HS, Morcos SK; Contrast Media Safety Committee of European Society of Urogenital Radiology. Management of acute adverse reactions to contrast media. Eur Radiol 2004;14(3):476–481.
54. Mornstein V. Cavitation-induced risks associated with contrast agents used in ultrasonography. Eur J Ultrasound 1997;5:101–111.
55. Miller DL, Thomas RM, Williams AR. Mechanisms for hemolysis by ultrasonic cavitation in the rotating exposure system. Ultrasound Med Biol 1991;17(2):171–178.
56. Williams AR, Kubowicz G, Cramer E, Schlief R. The effects of the microbubble suspension SH U 454 (Echovist) on ultrasound-induced cell lysis in a rotating tube exposure system. Echocardiography 1991;8(4):423–433.
57. Holland CK, Roy RA, Apfel RE, Crum LA. In vitro detection of cavitation induced by a diagnostic ultrasound system. IEEE Trans Ultrason Ferroelectr Freq Control 1992;39(1):95–101.
58. Miller DL, Thomas RM. Ultrasound contrast agents nucleate inertial cavitation in vitro. Ultrasound Med Biol 1995;21(8):1059–1065.
59. Miller DL, Thomas RM. Contrast-agent gas bodies enhance hemolysis induced by lithotripter shock waves and high-intensity focused ultrasound in whole blood. Ultrasound Med Biol 1996;22(8):1089–1095.
60. Miller DL, Gies RA, Chrisler WB. Ultrasonically induced hemolysis at high cell and gas body concentrations in a thin-disc exposure chamber. Ultrasound Med Biol 1997;23(4):625–633.
61. Everbach EC, Makin IR, Francis CW, Meltzer RS. Effect of acoustic cavitation on platelets in the presence of an echo-contrast agent. Ultrasound Med Biol 1998;24(1):129–136.
62. Uhlendorf V, Hoffmann C. Nonlinear acoustical response of coated microbubbles in diagnostic ultrasound. Proc IEEE Ultrasonics Symp 1994;3:1559–1562.
63. Dalecki D, Raeman CH, Child SZ, et al. Hemolysis in vivo from exposure to pulsed ultrasound. Ultrasound Med Biol 1997;23(2):307–313.
64. Shi WT, Forsberg F, Tornes A, Ostensen J, Goldberg BB. Destruction of contrast microbubbles and the association with inertial cavitation. Ultrasound Med Biol 2000;26(6):1009–1019.
65. Meltzer RS. Food and Drug Administration ultrasound device regulation: the output display standard, the "mechanical index," and ultrasound safety. [editorial] J Am Soc Echocardiogr 1996;9(2):216–220.

8 Sonoelastography: a New Ultrasound Modality for Assessing Tissue Elasticity

C.F. Dietrich, H. Frey

It is well known that inflammatory conditions and tumors lead to an alteration of the normal tissue structure, causing hardening of the tissue and a change in its elasticity. The elasticity modulus is a measure of the stress that is applied to tissue structures relative to the strain or deformation produced. **Figure 8.1** shows a graph of the elasticity coefficient for different breast tissues.[1]

Assessing and visualizing tissue elasticity provides the clinician with potentially important information that can be used in the diagnosis of tumors and inflammatory conditions. Various ultrasound techniques have been developed and experimentally evaluated in recent years for visualizing the elastic properties of tissue.

Figure 8.2 demonstrates the different effects of compression on hard and soft tissue. Soft tissues are compressed more than hard tissue structures under the same pressure. This deformation can be detected from the ultrasound data and can be displayed. The sonoelastography modality described here uses standard ultrasound probes, and there is no requirement for additional equipment such as pressure or vibration measurement systems. The procedure is similar to that in conventional color Doppler examination. Measurements of tissue elasticity are acquired in real time and presented as a color overlay on the conventional B-mode image.

Technical Characteristics

Conventional ultrasound images (B-mode images) are constructed from ultrasound signals that are reflected back from tissue boundaries within the body. The ultrasound signal is also attenuated by tissues to an extent that depends on the tissue density. The returning signals are reconstructed and displayed. Because tumors often have a similar echogenicity to that of the adjacent tissue, it can be very difficult or even impossible to delineate a tumor with conventional B-mode imaging. However, malignancies are often associated with a change in tissue hardness. Sonoelastography is an ultrasound technique that is capable of displaying tissue hardness to provide the clinician with important additional diagnostic information. The technique is especially useful in lesions that are not easily palpated—providing tissue differentiation by quantifying the tissue elasticity.

A technique known as the extended combined autocorrelation method provides the mathematical basis for the sonoelastography method described below. The returning radiofrequency echo patterns are compared over time. If the transducer has not moved during a given time and no pressure is applied to the scanned tissues, the received echo patterns will be the same, provided there is no respiratory or cardiac motion. If gentle pressure is applied to the tissues, the radiofrequency echo patterns will change. If the distance between two reflectors remains the same, it is a "harder" tissue area. If this distance decreases, then it

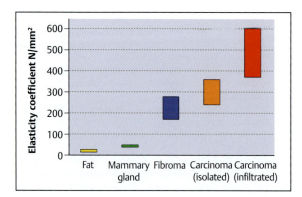

Fig. 8.1 Coefficients of elasticity in various tissues in the breast (adapted from[1]).

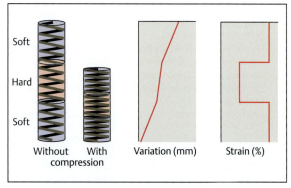

Fig. 8.2 The elasticity characteristics of various tissues under compression, based on a spring-coil model. When the same pressure is applied, a soft (more elastic) spring coil is compressed to a greater extent than a hard spring.

represents elastically deformable tissue (**Fig. 8.3**). The echo patterns in the adjacent tissue areas are also analyzed in order to detect possible lateral displacement of the compressed tissue area.

For example, a round echogenic tissue structure moves vertically under compression, and if it is a hard, nondeformable structure without lateral displacement, it remains as a circular image with the same diameter. However, if the same structure is displaced laterally with compression, it is detected as a circular structure but with a smaller diameter.

With the extended combined autocorrelation method, it is possible to acquire measurements in real time and display them simultaneously on various ultrasound systems from different manufacturers. Using this technology, large displacements can be analyzed very quickly and accurately in comparison with conventional autocorrelation methods. An accurate mathematical explanation of the sonoelastography mode based on the extended combined autocorrelation method is described by Yamakawa and Shiina.[2]

The strain field is calculated from the displacement, allowing conclusions to be drawn regarding the elasticity of the tissue area examined. Areas characterized as soft tissue appear as areas of high strain, whereas hard tissue structures appear as areas with lower elasticity.

As sonoelastography developed, it became apparent that the procedure had to be integrated into a routine examination procedure using standard linear or curved transducers, as well as specialist transducers for endovaginal, endorectal, laparoscopic, and endoscopic applications. The method was also developed without any need for additional equipment (for example, to induce pressure or vibration in the tissues), providing a user-friendly system for routine clinical use.

The tissue elasticity distribution is calculated using a three-dimensional tissue phantom together with a 3D finite element method (3D-FEM). The finite element method (FEM) is a type of mathematical analysis that is used in engineering science to develop complex statistical components for calculating stress deformation and also complex flow fields and flow processing. Using this technique, complex geometrical structures are divided into small components (finite elements). The deformation of a structure such as a cube is well known, and the power that is introduced at the edge of the cube can be calculated. The calculation can be done first for each cube and then for the structure as a whole.

In the sonoelastography mode described below, the finite element method is used inversely. The structure being examined is divided in up to 30 000 equal cubes. Before compression, it is assumed that the tissue elasticity (measured using the modulus of elasticity or Young's modulus, E) is constant throughout. After compression, the resulting displacement is measured for each finite element (cube), and the deformation of the edges of the cube can be calculated and the strain evaluated. The FEM confirms

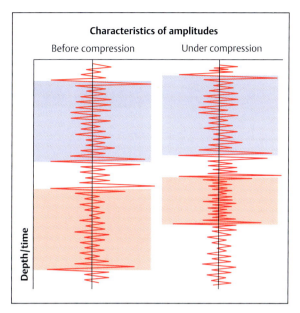

Fig. 8.3 Radiofrequency signals for an ultrasound vector before compression (left) and under compression (right). Compression in hard tissue areas is shown as blue and compression in soft tissue areas is red.

the tissue elasticity of each individual cube. The iterative process depends on different variables (e.g., the power, velocity, duration, and surface distribution of the induced compression). This iterative process is repeated until predefined thresholds are reached. The exact mathematical process involved in calculating tissue elasticity is described by Nitta et al.[3] and Yamakawa and Shiina.[4]

Research Results

The performance of real-time sonoelastography using the extended combined autocorrelation method and the 3D finite element method have been investigated using phantoms and in vivo experiments. **Figure 8.4a** shows a phantom containing a gelatin cube that has been used to mimic a tumor. The stellate tumor contains a concentration of 30% gelatin, while the surrounding tissue has a concentration of 10%. The materials are made of polyethylene dust. **Figure 8.4b** shows the phantom in B-mode imaging. It is not possible to visualize the simulated tumor clearly, as its echogenicity is similar to that of the surrounding gelatin. **Figures 8.4c** and **d** show the same structure in sonoelastography mode, with the stellate structure clearly visible in the deformation image and elasticity image.

To provide better visualization of tumors and to characterize them, the elastogram is displayed in color and provided as a transparent overlay on the conventional

I Techniques

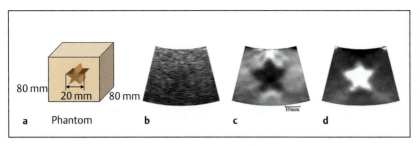

Fig. 8.4a–d a A tissue elasticity phantom, with an inclusion mimicking a star-shaped tumor.
b The B-mode image of the stellate inclusion. The structure is very difficult to visualize. By contrast, the stellate inclusion is easily seen in the deformation image (**c**) and elasticity image (**d**).

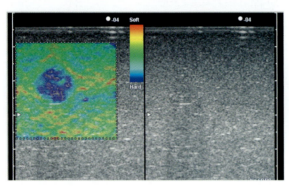

Fig. 8.5 A tissue elasticity image (left), with hard tissue areas shown in blue and soft tissue areas in red/green. The right side of the monitor image shows the corresponding B-mode display.

B-mode image. Hard tissue structures are displayed in blue, and soft structures are encoded in red (**Fig. 8.5**). Sonoelastography is a real-time method. E.g., using the Hitachi EUB-8500 system, the frame rate varies from 10 to 35 images per second, depending on the size of the area analyzed (the region of interest).

In addition, quantification of the color display can be provided using several algorithms. At present, this is still performed "offline," using digital video scans. Real-time quantification that accurately determines the elasticity values is currently being developed and will soon be incorporated into the system. Elastography is a widely discussed topic in the current literature.[5–18]

Sonoelastography in the Clinical Setting

Conventional ultrasound endoscopes are used for sonoelastography of the mediastinal and peri-intestinal lymph nodes, pancreas, and anorectum. Electronic longitudinal ultrasound endoscopes or fiberoptic or electronic radial endoscopes can all be used. The advantage of using endoscopic ultrasound with elastography is that aspiration can be carried out immediately in any suspicious area. The gentle curvature on the surface of the longitudinal endoscope is particularly well adapted for applying uniform pressure on tissues.

To perform sonoelastography, the ultrasound endoscope is positioned in the same way as for a conventional endosonography examination. The area to be evaluated is defined by a region of interest (ROI) in exactly the same way as in a color Doppler examination. For sonoelastography, little additional compression is required, as the pressure from the pulsation of the surrounding vessels is normally sufficient. A sensitive system setting is required. The ROI has to be sufficiently large, with the area of the lesion being no more than 50% of the size of the ROI, to allow the sonoelastography image to display the elasticity of the lesion relative to the surrounding tissues. Research aiming to allow accurate definition of elasticity is currently in progress. If the ROI is too small, the relative elasticity differences within the lesion are displayed and the hardness of the lesion relative to the normal surrounding tissue is not seen.

Clinical Applications

■ EUS Evaluation of Lymph Nodes

Review of the Literature

Endoscopic ultrasound (EUS) elastography was first described by Giovannini and co-workers in 2006, with very promising results for evaluating benign and malignant lymph nodes and pancreatic tumors.[19] It was hypothesized that the diffuse and focal organ changes caused by lymphadenopathy might have specific elastographic qualities that would make it possible to establish the correct diagnosis noninvasively, or at least allow the disease to be classified as benign or malignant. It should be borne in mind that malignant lymph node infiltration often starts in a microscopic and circumscribed form, independently of the size of the lymph node that has been infiltrated. Some 20–50% of malignant lymph node infiltration (depending on the part of the gastrointestinal tract examined) is therefore observed in lymph nodes <5 mm in size—which also means that it is difficult to detect the affected lymph nodes using EUS.[20]

The aim in a subsequent study was to test the feasibility of elastography-guided EUS of the mediastinum by comparing the elastographic patterns of lymph nodes with results from EUS-guided fine-needle aspiration biopsy (FNAB).[21] The accuracy of EUS-guided FNAB exceeds 90% for mediastinal masses (see Chapter 9). False-positive results are rarely reported, and the risk of false-negative findings related to malignant disease—i.e., the probability of missing a malignancy in lymph nodes found to be benign at the histologic examination—has been shown to be low.

Fifty consecutive patients undergoing EUS-guided FNAB of at least one mediastinal (paraesophageal) lymph node were included in the study. The indication for EUS-guided FNAB was based on computed-tomographic assessment of enlarged mediastinal lymph nodes. The lymph nodes were selected for FNA following the recognized B-mode criteria for malignancy (round, echo-poor, > 10 mm, sharp border), and each lymph node was recorded in the protocol. Each of the targeted lymph nodes was also examined elastographically.

The following classification of elastographic types was used: type 1, relatively homogeneous coloring; type 2, areas with two or three different colors; and type 3, honeycomb pattern. The elastographic colors were marked by letters: A, blue (hard tissue); B, green/yellow (intermediate); and C, red (soft). The letters were added to the type number in declining sequence of the proportion of color they represented within the region of interest. The elastographic types were later compared with the histology results from EUS-guided FNAB. Only lymph nodes with positive proof of lymphatic tissue or well-defined malignancy or benign disease were therefore accepted for data analysis. The elastographic classification was subsequently tested by two blinded reviewers. Sixty-six lymph nodes were explored; 37 lymph nodes were found to be benign and 29 were found to have malignant tissue at the histologic evaluation. Interobserver agreement was excellent ($\kappa = 0.84$). EUS elastography of mediastinal lymph nodes can be performed reliably. The results are good for a noninvasive technique, but they do not exceed the success rate of EUS-guided FNAB. The method might occasionally be useful for targeting the most suitable lymph nodes for FNAB.

Good elastographic records were obtained for all of the lymph nodes. Thirty-one of the 37 benign lymph nodes showed a homogeneous pattern of intermediate elasticity, while predominantly hard tissue with variable patterns was found in 23 of the 29 malignant lymph nodes.

Impulse Generation

In the mediastinum, "internal" compression by pulsatile excursions of the aorta and the heart induce sufficient changes to deform the paraesophageal lymph nodes, making it possible to calculate and differentiate their stiffness; a balloon technique is almost never needed.

Elastographic Patterns of Benign and Malignant Lymph Nodes

A homogeneous green pattern is almost characteristic for benign lymph nodes, and elastograms that are predominantly blue are indicators for malignancy, irrespective of the pattern type. Using the elastographic criteria described above, two blinded reviewers achieved an accuracy of 83.3% and 81.8%, respectively, for benign lymph nodes, and both had an 86.4% accuracy rate for malignant lymph nodes. The kappa coefficient of 0.84 indicates excellent interobserver agreement between the primary investigator and the two subsequent blinded reviewers, and the method is more accurate than using B-mode criteria for malignancy.

The detailed results show that 31 of the 37 benign lymph nodes (**Table 8.1**) were homogeneously colored green, indicating intermediate stiffness (type 1B). One lymph node in a patient who had undergone radiotherapy for a mediastinal lymphoma was homogeneously blue, i.e., hard (type 1A), whereas five lymph nodes showed areas with two or three different colors, representing areas of different elasticity (type 2A/B, n = 2; type 2B/A, n = 2; type 2A/B/C, n = 1). The honeycomb pattern (type 3) was not seen in benign lymph nodes. **Table 8.1** shows that the pattern distributions of type 1 versus type 2 elastograms were similar in benign lymph nodes up to 25 mm in size (n = 26) and benign lymph nodes larger than 25 mm (n = 11), and also in the nine lymph nodes affected by sarcoidosis compared with the other 28 benign lymph nodes.

The elastographic patterns in malignant lymph nodes were less uniform (**Table 8.2**): a homogeneous pattern was seen in 10 lymph nodes (type 1A, n = 8; type 1B, n = 2); a type 2 pattern with areas of different elasticity in 11 lymph nodes (type 2A/B, n = 8; type 2B/A, n = 2; type 2B/C, n = 1), and the honeycomb pattern in eight lymph nodes (type 3A/B, n = 7; type 3B/A, n = 1). In 23 of the 29 malignant lymph nodes, the elastographic image was predominantly

Table 8.1 Elastographic types of the 37 lymph nodes with benign histology after EUS-guided fine-needle aspiration biopsy. Differentiation of subgroups

Elastographic type	All benign lymph nodes	Size ≤ 25 mm	Size > 25 mm	Sarcoidosis
1A	1	1	0	0
1B	31	22	9	7
2A/B	2	1	1	1
2B/A	2	1	1	1
2A/B/C	1	1	0	0
3A/B	0	0	0	0
3B/A	0	0	0	0

Table 8.2 Elastographic types of the 29 lymph nodes with malignant histology after EUS-guided fine-needle aspiration biopsy. Differentiation of subgroups

Elastographic type	All malignant lymph nodes	Size ≤ 25 mm	Size > 25 mm
1A	8	8	0
1B	2	2	0
2A/B	8	4	4
2B/A	2	1	1
2B/C	1	1	0
3A/B	7	0	7
3B/A	1	0	1

a blue color, which represents relatively hard tissue (types 1A, 2A/B, 3A/B). Four of the six lymph nodes that were not predominantly blue were found to contain necrotic material at the histologic examination. None of the 13 malignant lymph nodes larger than 25 mm was assigned to elastographic type 1, consisting of homogeneous coloring; the honeycomb type 3 was only found in eight of these 13 large lymph nodes (62%).

The study thus showed that EUS elastography can help identify malignant lymph nodes that are suitable for effective FNA. The data are in accordance with those reported by Săftoiu et al.[22] and confirm that real-time EUS elastography can be applied with technical success to mediastinal lymph nodes and produces plausible results.

Săftoiu et al. examined lymph nodes in the entire upper gastrointestinal tract with EUS elastography. Using similar criteria to differentiate between benign and malignant lymph nodes, they reported an accuracy of 92.9% for an examiner using qualitative analysis and an accuracy of 95.2% using an "elasticity ratio" based on histogram analysis of the green and blue channels. Their results catch up with those of EUS-guided FNAB. The differences between the two studies may have been due to the different methods used for data analysis and/or differences in the composition of the patient groups.[22]

Chronic inflammation—caused by sarcoidosis or chemoradiotherapy, for example—induces fibrosis in benign and malignant lymph nodes, leading to a blue (hard) encoding at elastography. This phenomenon may make it impossible to use elastography to predict tumor disappearance following chemoradiotherapy for malignant lymph nodes. Tumor infiltration may be accompanied by a desmoplastic reaction, leading to the honeycomb pattern. Small malignant metastatic islands within the lymph nodes may not change either the B-mode appearance or the elastographic image in comparison with healthy lymph nodes and may also be missed during EUS-guided FNAB.

Elastography does not yet represent an adequate replacement for histologic examination or for FNAB. The method's limitations appear to be due to the overlapping of similar mechanical properties in normal tissue and in tissue affected by benign or malignant disease, rather than to technical shortcomings. Further research will be needed in order to assess whether computer-based analysis is superior to an examiner-based approach.

■ Pancreas

Review of the Literature

As mentioned above, EUS elastography was introduced by Giovannini and co-workers in the evaluation of 24 patients with pancreatic tumors.[19] The authors reported that all malignant lesions were correctly identified by EUS elastography (sensitivity 100%); however, the results were marred by a high rate of misclassified benign lesions (specificity 67%). Similar, although slightly less impressive, results in a subsequent European multicenter trial confirmed the findings.[23]

Janssen et al. investigated the feasibility of EUS elastography of the pancreas in a prospective single-center study and described elastographic patterns in the normal pancreas and in pancreata affected by inflammatory and focal disease in 73 patients—20 patients with a normal pancreas, 20 with chronic pancreatitis, and 33 with a focal pancreatic lesion (histologically confirmed in 32). Adequate elastographic recordings were obtained in all 73 patients. Patients with a hypoechoic or intermediately echogenic normal pancreas had a relatively homogeneous elastographic pattern. Thirty-one focal lesions including, 30 neoplasms and most of the chronically inflamed pancreata, had a honeycomb pattern dominated by hard strands. This pattern was analogous to the histologic structure of 10 resected tumors. Other patients with chronic pancreatitis and those with a hyperechoic healthy pancreas had miscellaneous elastographic appearances. It was concluded that EUS elastography of the pancreas is feasible and produces plausible results. The examination of homogeneous tissue was impaired by the relative scale used. It was not possible to distinguish between chronic pancreatitis and hard tumors using elastography, probably due to their similar fibrous structure.[21]

Another prospective study enrolled 70 patients with unclassified solid lesions of the pancreas and 10 control individuals with a healthy pancreas.[24] Elastography recordings were compared with cytological and histological findings as the gold standard in all of the patients. Adequate EUS elastography of the pancreas was performed in all of the healthy control individuals, but only in 56% of patients with solid pancreatic lesions. The main limitation of elastographic image acquisition was incomplete delineation of the border of lesions with a diameter of more than 35 mm (39%) or of lesions at some distance from the transducer (10%). The elastographic recordings were also hampered by the fact that the surrounding tissue, which is used as an internal reference standard for strain calculation, was insufficiently displayed in the case of larger lesions. The reduced ratio of target to surrounding tissue resulted in the formation of color artifacts and impaired reproducibility. By contrast, the majority of lesions smaller than 35 mm in diameter were adequately and reproducibly evaluated using EUS elastography (91%). The clinical value of the method for differential diagnosis, however, was limited, as strain images from all types of pancreatic mass were found to be harder than the surrounding tissues, irrespective of the underlying nature of the lesion (i.e., whether it was malignant or benign). EUS elastography predicted the nature of pancreatic lesions with poor diagnostic sensitivity (41%), specificity (53%), and accuracy (45%). In contrast to the initially disappointing data regarding the differential diagnosis of benign and malignant pancreatic disease, however, the results for detecting autoimmune pancreatitis (AIP) are much more promising (see below).[24,25]

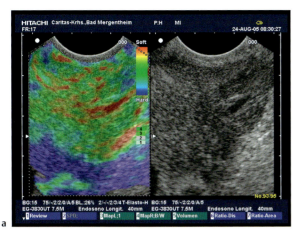

a

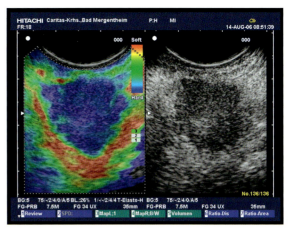

b

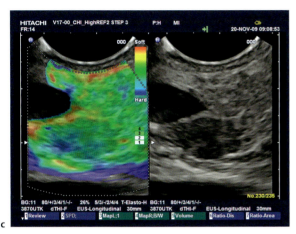

c

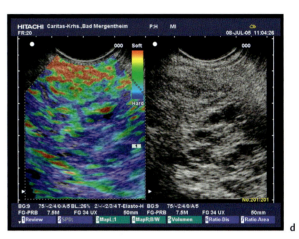

d

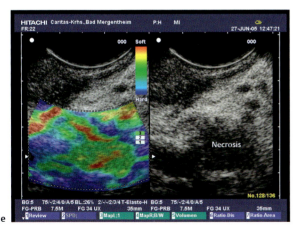

e

Fig. 8.6a–e a Normal intermediate (green) homogeneous pancreatic parenchyma in the dorsal and ventral anlage, excluding a tumor of the uncinate process.
b A hard (blue) T1 ductal adenocarcinoma of the pancreas.
c A benign intermediate (green) insulinoma (13 mm) of the pancreatic head, only detected by EUS.
d A large serous microcystic adenoma of the pancreas, with stiff (blue) septa.
e Soft (green, red) pancreatic necrosis.

Impulse Generation

Impulses mainly generated by the body itself—i.e., arterial pulsation and respiratory movements—are sufficient to deform the pancreas and thus allow strain calculations. External compression is not generally needed. We often use manipulation with the probe (although others do not).

Elastographic Pattern of the Pancreas

Normal Pancreas

Elastographic registration of the normal pancreas is characterized by a uniform, homogeneous green color distribution (representing intermediate stiffness) throughout the organ, and the reproducibility of the signal is comparatively good (**Fig. 8.6a–e**).

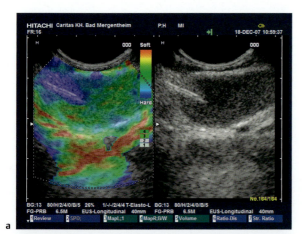

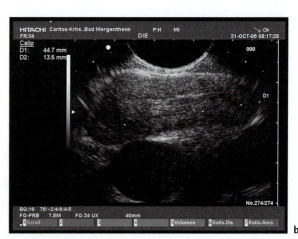

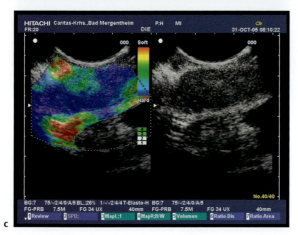

Fig. 8.7a–c Early malignant carcinoma infiltration is often circumscribed (**a**), whereas large lymph nodes in inflammatory lymphadenopathy do not show destruction of the lymph-node architecture, as seen in this patient with sarcoidosis and a soft (green) hilar region, only visible on elastography (**b, c**).

Pancreatic Tumors

Elastographic imaging of most pancreatic tumors is consistent and largely dominated by blue/green (stiff) planes or strands with only minor heterogeneity (honeycomb pattern), including softer tissue colors, but with a normal elastographic pattern in the remaining pancreatic parenchyma if no calcifications or duct enlargement are found as signs of chronic obstructive pancreatitis. The fibrous tissue characteristic of desmoplastic pancreatic carcinomas and microcystic adenomas causes stiffness of the tumor and probably produces the corresponding elastographic appearance. Tumors without sclerosis (insulinomas and lipomas) are coded homogeneously green, like normal pancreatic tissue (**Fig. 8.7a–c**).

Chronic Pancreatitis

Chronic pancreatitis is a sclerosing condition in which septa form a strong fibrous framework, often also with calcifications—which explains the similar elastographic pattern in patients with chronic pancreatitis and neoplasia. Janssen et al. recently investigated the clinical application of sonoelastography in patients with inflammatory

pancreatic disease and in patients presenting with and without pancreatic lesions. Consistent with our recently published findings, the elastographic patterns of chronic pancreatitis and most pancreatic tumors were described as being similar, with a blue/green honeycomb pattern.

In contrast to patients with autoimmune pancreatitis, it is important to note that patients who have the classic form of chronic obstructive calcified pancreatitis and mass lesions in the pancreatic head typically show duct enlargement or parenchymal calcification and fibrous strands—an appearance that is different from the echo-rich parenchyma in patients with AIP without duct enlargement.[26]

Autoimmune Pancreatitis

The differential diagnosis of focal pancreatic lesions is extensive and includes both benign and malignant etiologies. Confirming the diagnosis can be difficult and usually requires invasive procedures. Since patients with autoimmune pancreatitis (AIP) are not candidates for surgery, it is important to identify this entity using imaging methods and clinical data.[27]

The aim of a recently published prospective evaluation was to investigate the role of real-time EUS elastography in

Table 8.3 Characteristics of patients with autoimmune pancreatitis

Patient	Size (mm)[a]	PD (mm)	CBD (mm)	Age	Sex
1	30	1	10	55	Male
2	35	1	8	46	Male
3	32	Ndl	8	51	Male
4	22	Ndl	9	65	Male
5	31	Ndl	13	26	Male

[a] size of the mass lesion. The tumors were located in the pancreatic head in all patients. CBD, common bile duct; Ndl, not delineated; PD, pancreatic duct in the body of the pancreas, at the level of the superior mesenteric artery.

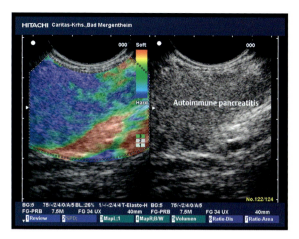

Fig. 8.8 Elastography in autoimmune pancreatitis. This example image shows a unique homogeneous hard (blue) elastographic pattern not only in the mass lesion, but also in the parenchyma located distal to the transducer and additionally throughout the entire organ, with normal B-mode echogenicity and no ductal enlargement.

the diagnosis of AIP. The pattern of elastographic images was compared with conventional EUS appearances and with histological findings obtained by transabdominal needle biopsy.[25] A recently published cohort of patients with ductal adenocarcinoma and healthy individuals served as controls.[24] The final diagnosis was achieved by histology using transabdominal (percutaneous) guided Tru-Cut puncture (18 G, 20 cm). A clinical follow-up period of at least 12 months was also mandatory.

All five patients with AIP (**Table 8.3**) presented with a mass lesion in the pancreatic head, dilation of the common hepatic bile duct, elevated enzymes indicating cholestasis, and—most importantly—a characteristic stiff elastographic pattern not only in the mass lesion but also in the complementary pancreatic tissue. This is unique and was not found in 17 patients with ductal adenocarcinoma or in 10 healthy individuals. It is of interest that the parenchyma of the distally located pancreatic tissue was homogenously echo-rich and that the pancreatic duct diameter was normal (<2 mm) in all of the patients. In 17 patients with ductal adenocarcinoma <30 mm and with no B-mode signs of chronic pancreatitis, the distally located parts of the pancreas showed a relatively homogeneous elastographic pattern, with a mainly green color distribution (representing intermediate stiffness).

EUS elastography of the pancreas shows a typical and unique finding, with homogeneous stiffness of the whole organ distinguishing AIP from the circumscribed mass lesions seen in ductal adenocarcinoma (**Fig. 8.8**). None of the five patients with mass lesions and AIP have undergone surgery—in contrast to recently published studies reporting that most patients with a final diagnosis of AIP received surgery.[25]

Kajiwara and co-workers reported on 160 patients with suspected pancreatic adenocarcinomas; 15 of the patients (9%) proved to have nonneoplastic pancreatic changes, while seven (4%) had AIP.[28] Other publications showed a 10% rate of benign lesions and a 3–5% rate of AIP among patients in a surgical population.[28–32]

In conclusion, EUS-guided real-time elastography of the pancreas has the potential to provide complementary information for improved tissue characterization that can

make it possible to avoid surgery, particularly when it is used to characterize AIP. The final diagnosis of AIP should be made using transcutaneous transabdominal biopsy, with the histological examination showing the typical signs of periductal inflammation and fibrosis, which cannot be demonstrated using fine-needle aspiration cytology. This approach needs to be confirmed by a prospective and controlled study.

Limitations

An assessment of the indications for and possible limitations of real-time tissue elastography using EUS in focal pancreatic disease[24] has shown that adequate and reproducible elastographic imaging of focal pancreatic disease is confined to lesions with a diameter of less than 30 mm. Elastographic delineation was incomplete in larger lesions. It is also important to note that adequate acquisition of elastographic images depends on examining the surrounding pancreatic parenchyma. For optimal elastographic image acquisition, the density of the region of interest needs to be compared with the surrounding tissue as a reference standard, with a ratio of displayed target tissue and surrounding parenchyma of approximately 1 : 1. If the region being analyzed only includes the target area, small variations in the hardness of the lesion itself will be emphasized, rather than its density in comparison with the normal surrounding parenchyma.

I Techniques

■ Anorectum

In a recently published study, real-time endosonographic elastography was performed in patients with fecal incontinence in order to further characterize the internal and external anal sphincters (IAS/EAS).[33] The second aim was to compare two quantification methods and correlate quantitatively obtained IAS/EAS elastographic color areas with clinical and functional parameters.[34] The main finding was that the IAS and EAS differed qualitatively and quantitatively with regard to their elastographic appearance, which is assumed to reflect underlying elastic and mechanical properties. The IAS contained more soft areas than the EAS, while conversely the EAS showed more hard areas than the IAS. The second finding was that the elastographic appearance of the IAS/EAS was independent of the underlying disease, as the major clinical characteristics and functional (manometric) parameters did not correlate significantly with the elastographic findings. There was also no correlation with gray-scale B-mode features. The last finding was that a visual assessment scale only showed moderate correlation with the computerized analysis for quantifying the elastic and mechanical properties of the anal sphincter. Although there was a general lack of correlation between the elastographic findings and clinical and functional parameters, there are still important questions relating to the underlying structural substrate for the elastographic differences between the IAS and EAS observed. Further problems include appropriate ways of quantifying elastographic information in terms of elastic and mechanical tissue properties, and the clinical relevance of elastography in patients with fecal incontinence in specific cases, such as following radiotherapy.[35] It has been shown in clinical and experimental trials that microcalcifications and fibrous tissue substantially contribute to the creation of hard signals, whereas vascular and parenchymal structures and edema may produce fairly soft signals; both of these features might help differentiate between benign and malignant tissue components. In skeletal muscles, additional factors such as muscular tension, isometric contraction, the condition of the extracellular matrix, shear stress, and strain distribution have also been shown to influence the sonographic and magnetic-resonance elastographic appearance. The general use of elastography[36] during diagnostic[37] and therapeutic[38] procedures has been rencently summarized.

■ DVD

Elastography videos are shown on the DVD as follows: Reproducibility of sonoelastography (▶ Video 8.1), tumor demarcation (gastrointestinal stromal tumor) (▶ Video 8.2), tumor demarcation (endorectal ultrasound, T2 tumor) (▶ Video 8.3), layer relationship (sphincter ani muscle) (▶ Video 8.4 and 8.5).

Summary

EUS elastography is a promising new imaging option, which—at least in our institution—appears to be capable of supplementing the information obtained with conventional ultrasound in almost all examinations. It may help distinguish between benign and malignant lesions, mainly in lymph nodes. The primary goal of elastography is not to replace tissue confirmation, but to potentially increase the yield of FNA and reduce the number of unnecessary biopsies. In addition, elastography may make it possible to identify autoimmune pancreatitis. Further studies with blinded examiners will be needed in order to determine the exact value of EUS elastography.

References

1. Krouskop TA, Wheeler TM, Kallel F, Garra BS, Hall T. Elastic moduli of breast and prostate tissues under compression. Ultrason Imaging 1998;20(4):260–274.
2. Yamakawa M, Shiina T. Strain estimation using the extended combined autocorrelation method. Jpn J Appl Phys 2001;40:3872–3876.
3. Nitta N, Yamakawa M, Shiina T, Ueno E, Doyley MM, Bamber JC. Tissue elasticity imaging based on combined autocorrelation method and 3-D tissue model. In: Schneider SC, Levy M, McAvoy BR, eds. Proceedings of the IEEE Ultrasonics Symposium 1998. Piscataway, NJ: Institute of Electrical and Electronics Engineers, 1998: 1447–1450.
4. Yamakawa M, Shiina T. Tissue elasticity reconstruction based on 3-dimensional finite-element model. Jpn J Appl Phys 1999;38:3393–3398.
5. Frey H. Realtime elastography. A new ultrasound procedure for the reconstruction of tissue elasticity. [Article in German] Radiologe 2003;43(10):850–855.
6. Ophir J, Céspedes I, Ponnekanti H, Yazdi Y, Li X. Elastography: a quantitative method for imaging the elasticity of biological tissues. Ultrason Imaging 1991;13(2):111–134.
7. Shiina T, Doyley MM, Bamber JC. Strain imaging using combined RF and envelope autocorrelation processing. In: Levy M, Schneider SC, McAvoy BR, eds. Proceedings of the IEEE Ultrasonics Symposium 1996. Piscataway, NJ: Institute of Electrical and Electronics Engineers, 1997: 1331–1336.
8. Lorenz A, Ermert H, Sommerfeld HJ, Garcia-Schürmann M, Senge T, Philippou S. Ultrasound elastography of the prostate. A new technique for tumor detection. [Article in German] Ultraschall Med 2000;21(1):8–15.

9. Céspedes I, Ophir J. Reduction of image noise in elastography. Ultrason Imaging 1993;15(2):89–102.

10. Bonnefous O, Pesqué P. Time domain formulation of pulse-Doppler ultrasound and blood velocity estimation by cross correlation. Ultrason Imaging 1986;8(2):73–85.

11. Konofagou E, Ophir J. A new elastographic method for estimation and imaging of lateral displacements, lateral strains, corrected axial strains and Poisson's ratios in tissues. Ultrasound Med Biol 1998;24(8):1183–1199.

12. Gao L, Parker KJ, Alam SK, Lernel RM. Sonoelasticity imaging: theory and experimental verification. J Acoust Soc Am 1995;97(6):3875–3886.

13. Srinivasan S, Kallel F, Ophir J. The effects of digitization on the elastographic signal-to-noise ratio. Ultrasound Med Biol 2002;28(11-12):1521–1534.

14. Srinivasan S, Kallel F, Souchon R, Ophir J. Analysis of an adaptive strain estimation technique in elastography. Ultrason Imaging 2002;24(2):109–118.

15. Maurice RL, Bertrand M. Speckle-motion artifact under tissue shearing. IEEE Trans Ultrason Ferroelectr Freq Control 1999;46(3):584–594.

16. Lubinski MA, Emelianov SY, O'Donnell M. Speckle tracking methods for ultrasonic elasticity imaging using short-time correlation. IEEE Trans Ultrason Ferroelectr Freq Control 1999;46(1):82–96.

17. Kallel F, Ophir J. A least-squares strain estimator for elastography. Ultrason Imaging 1997;19(3):195–208.

18. Ermert H, Lorenz A, Pesavento A. Elasticity imaging: new imaging modalities. Proceedings of the First European Medical and Biological Engineering Conference (EMBEC), Vienna, 4–7 November 1999. Med Biol Eng Comput 1999;37(Suppl 2 Pt II):954–955.

19. Giovannini M, Hookey LC, Bories E, Pesenti C, Monges G, Delpero JR. Endoscopic ultrasound elastography: the first step towards virtual biopsy? Preliminary results in 49 patients. Endoscopy 2006;38(4):344–348.

20. Jürgensen C, Dietrich CF. Role of endoscopic ultrasound (EUS) in the staging of rectal cancer. [Article in German] Z Gastroenterol 2008;46(6):580–589.

21. Janssen J, Dietrich CF, Will U, Greiner L. Endosonographic elastography in the diagnosis of mediastinal lymph nodes. Endoscopy 2007;39(11):952–957.

22. Săftoiu A, Vilmann P, Hassan H, Gorunescu F. Analysis of endoscopic ultrasound elastography used for characterisation and differentiation of benign and malignant lymph nodes. Ultraschall Med 2006;27(6):535–542.

23. Giovannini M, Thomas B, Erwan B, et al. Endoscopic ultrasound elastography for evaluation of lymph nodes and pancreatic masses: a multicenter study. World J Gastroenterol 2009;15(13):1587–1593.

24. Hirche TO, Ignee A, Barreiros AP, et al. Indications and limitations of endoscopic ultrasound elastography for evaluation of focal pancreatic lesions. Endoscopy 2008;40(11):910–917.

25. Dietrich CF, Hirche TO, Ott M, Ignee A. Real-time tissue elastography in the diagnosis of autoimmune pancreatitis. Endoscopy 2009;41(8):718–720.

26. Jenssen C, Dietrich CF. Endoscopic ultrasound in chronic pancreatitis. [Article in German] Z Gastroenterol 2005;43(8):737–749.

27. Dietrich CF, Jenssen C, Allescher HD, Hocke M, Barreiros AP, Ignee A. Differential diagnosis of pancreatic lesions using endoscopic ultrasound. [Article in German] Z Gastroenterol 2008;46(6):601–617.

28. Kajiwara M, Gotohda N, Konishi M, et al. Incidence of the focal type of autoimmune pancreatitis in chronic pancreatitis suspected to be pancreatic carcinoma: experience of a single tertiary cancer center. Scand J Gastroenterol 2008;43(1):110–116.

29. Hardacre JM, Iacobuzio-Donahue CA, Sohn TA, et al. Results of pancreaticoduodenectomy for lymphoplasmacytic sclerosing pancreatitis. Ann Surg 2003;237(6):853–858, discussion 858–859.

30. Abraham SC, Wilentz RE, Yeo CJ, et al. Pancreaticoduodenectomy (Whipple resections) in patients without malignancy: are they all 'chronic pancreatitis'? Am J Surg Pathol 2003;27(1):110–120.

31. Sasson AR, Gulizia JM, Galva A, Anderson J, Thompson J. Pancreaticoduodenectomy for suspected malignancy: have advancements in radiographic imaging improved results? Am J Surg 2006;192(6):888–893.

32. Kennedy T, Preczewski L, Stocker SJ, et al. Incidence of benign inflammatory disease in patients undergoing Whipple procedure for clinically suspected carcinoma: a single-institution experience. Am J Surg 2006;191(3):437–441.

33. Allgayer H, Ignee A, Dietrich CF. Endosonographic elastography of the anal sphincter in patients with fecal incontinence. Scand J Gastroenterol 2010;45(1):30–38.

34. Allgayer H, Dietrich CF, Rohde W, Koch GF, Tuschhoff T. Prospective comparison of short- and long-term effects of pelvic floor exercise/biofeedback training in patients with fecal incontinence after surgery plus irradiation versus surgery alone for colorectal cancer: clinical, functional and endoscopic/endosonographic findings. Scand J Gastroenterol 2005;40(10):1168–1175.

35. Dietrich CF. Anorectal sonoelastography. Tokyo: Medix; 2008:54–57.

36. Dietrich CF. Echtzeit-Gewebeelastographie. Anwendungsmöglichkeiten nicht nur im Gastrointestinaltrakt. Endoskopie Heute 2010;23:177–212.

37. Dietrich CF, Jenssen C. Evidenzbasierte Einsatzmöglichkeiten der Endosonografie. Z Gastroenterol 2011;49:1–23. In press.

38. Dietrich CF, Hocke M, Jenssen C. Interventional Endosonography. Ultraschall in Med 2011;32:8–25. In press.

II Diagnostic Imaging and Interventions

9 EUS-Guided Biopsy: Equipment and Technique

H.W. Sudholt, P. Vilmann

The development of endoscopic ultrasound scanning (EUS) began in the early 1980s with mechanical, radial-scanning transducers.[1-3] Despite excellent imaging resolution, the method did not gain widespread popularity until the development of EUS-guided fine-needle aspiration (EUS-FNA) biopsy.[4-8] For many years, efforts to characterize specific lesions and differentiate between them using EUS imaging alone postponed the necessary development of tissue sampling guided by endosonography. EUS-FNA is now performed routinely at many endoscopic centers, and the procedure is clearly having a major impact on the therapeutic management of patients by providing definitive tissue diagnosis of lesions outlined by endosonography. EUS-FNA is obviously by no means limited to the field of gastroenterology, since the gastrointestinal tract traverses through anatomical regions related to other medical specialties such as pulmonology, thoracic surgery, internal medicine, oncology, urology, gynecology, and endocrinology.[9-11] There is also considerable evidence that EUS-FNA in experienced hands can replace many other far more invasive and risky diagnostic procedures, such as mediastinoscopy, diagnostic laparoscopy, and even laparotomy or thoracotomy.[12-14]

One of the main strengths of EUS-FNA in comparison with radiographic imaging methods with percutaneous biopsy is the close proximity of the transducer to the regions of interest. This means that even minute lesions, down to a size of 5 mm, can be imaged and consequently biopsied. However, the technique is not easy to master, and considerable energy and effort need to be invested before an examiner's technique reaches an acceptable success rate comparable to that reported in the literature, at ≈90–95%, with an overall sensitivity and specificity of 90% and 100%, respectively. The aim of the present chapter is to describe the technique of EUS-guided biopsy in detail, based on a literature review and our extensive experience with this method.

Endoscopes

Table 9.1 and **Figs. 9.1, 9.2, 9.3, 9.4, 9.5** show the endoscopes that are currently commercially available for EUS-guided diagnostic fine-needle biopsy. Some of these devices have an Albarrán lever (elevator) to facilitate needle positioning. Several aspects need to be taken into consideration when one is choosing a biopsy instrument, including the Albarrán, the stiffness/flexibility and length of the distal part of the endoscope, the diameter of the distal end of the endoscope, the diameter of the working channel, and last but not least the quality of the ultrasound image. The final decision needs to be based on a compromise between these options.

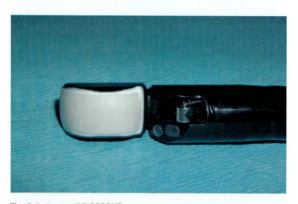

Fig. 9.1 Pentax EG-3830UT

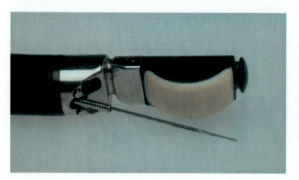

Fig. 9.2 Pentax FG-34UX

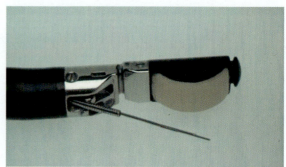

Fig. 9.3 Pentax FG-36UX

Table 9.1 Endoscopes currently commercially available for endoscopic ultrasound-guided diagnostic fine-needle aspiration biopsy

Pentax					
Fiberoptic ultrasound endoscopes					
Model	**Equipment diameter**	**Instrumentation channel (mm)**	**Working length (mm)**	**Angle (°)**	**Albarrán**
FG-34 UX	11.5	2.0	1250	105	No
FG-36UX	12.1	2.4	1250	105	Yes
FG-38UX	12.8	3.2 (therapy and biopsy)	1250	60	No
Video ultrasound endoscopes					
Model	**Equipment diameter**	**Instrumentation channel (mm)**	**Working length (mm)**	**Angle (°)**	**Albarrán**
EG-3630U	12.1	2.4	1250	130	Yes
EG-3830UT	12.8	3.8 (therapy and biopsy)	1250	120	Yes
Olympus					
Model	**Series**	**Short description**	**Albarrán**		
GF-UC160-OL5	EUS EXERA	Ultrasonic video gastroscope for FNA with 2.8-mm instrumentation channel	Yes		
GF-UCT160P-OL5	EUS EXERA	Ultrasonic video gastroscope for FNA and therapy with 3.7-mm instrumentation channel	Yes		
GF-UC140P-AL5	EUS	Ultrasonic video gastroscope for FNA with 2.8 mm instrumentation channel—compatible with Aloka systems	Yes		
GF-UCT140P-AL5	EUS	Ultrasonic video gastroscope for FNA and therapy with 3.7-mm instrumentation channel—compatible with Aloka systems	Yes		
Toshiba/Fujinon					
Model	**Series**	**Short description**	**Albarrán**		
EG 530 UT	EUS	Ultrasonic video gastroscope for FNA with 3.8-mm instrumentation channel	Yes		

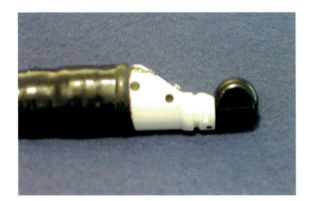

Fig. 9.4 Olympus GF-UC140P-AL5

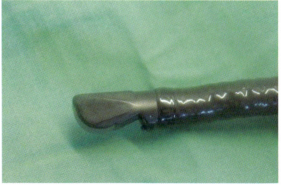

Fig. 9.5 Fujinon PEF-708FA

Biopsy Needles

In the early 1990s, special biopsy equipment was developed by one of the present authors (P.V.) and Søren Hancke in collaboration with the German accessory company GIP-Medizintechnik (now Medi-Globe), leading to the final breakthrough for the EUS-guided biopsy method.[15] A wide range of different needle systems is now available (**Table 9.2**). All of the other biopsy equipment for EUS-FNA that is currently available on the market is based on the same construction principles, so that the EUS-FNA procedure can be explained on the basis of the original design of the Hancke–Vilmann needle system.

The core of the biopsy instrument is a stiff steel needle 170 cm long. The needle is manipulated using a handle

Table 9.2 Biopsy needles

Manufacturer	Model	Needle	Special features	Adjustable length
Medi-Globe	Hancke–Vilmann	19–22 G	Reusable aluminum/steel instrument, disposable needle	No
Medi-Globe	SonoTip II	19–22 G	Disposable kit, metal spiral, Teflon-coated, round or filed stylet, laser structure	Yes
Olympus	EZ Shot 2 NA-220 H-8022	22 G	EUS-FNA-aspiration needle, disposable kit, with adjustable-length plastic tube	Yes
Olympus	EZ Shot 2 NA-220 H-8019	19 G	EUS-FNA aspiration needle, disposable kit, with adjustable-length plastic tube	Yes
Olympus	EZ Shot NA-200 H-8022	22 G	Disposable kit with plastic tube	Yes
Olympus	PowerShot NA-11 J-KB	22 G	EUS-FNA aspiration needle, disposable kit, with reusable metal tube, with power-shot function	Yes
Cook Endoscopy	EchoTip Ultra ECHO 1–22	22 G	Standard needle, disposable kit, with plastic tube	Yes
Cook Endoscopy	EchoTip Ultra ECHO-3–22	22 G	Same needle as above, but with Teflon-coated metal spiral	Yes
Cook Endoscopy	EchoTip Ultra ECHO-19	19 G	Disposable kit with plastic tube	Yes
Cook Endoscopy	EchoTip Ultra ECHO-25	25 G	Disposable kit, very thin and flexible	Yes
Cook Endoscopy	EUSN-19-QC Quick-Core	19 G	Tru-Cut histology needle with power-shot function	Limited

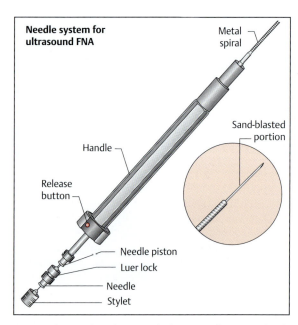

Fig. 9.6 The Hancke–Vilmann multiple-use needle system (Medi-Globe).

piston inside the biopsy handle (or outside it with the Olympus and Wilson-Cook systems) (**Fig. 9.6**). The handle piston with the needle transmits any movements made by the examiner directly to the needle tip without compressing the needle, so that it can even be used to penetrate hard tumors. The handle piston can be locked and un-

locked by means of a button (or screw) to avoid advancement of the needle during introduction and withdrawal of the biopsy assembly (**Fig. 9.7**).

The needle is supported by a stable metal spiral sheath, which is firmly connected to the aluminum handle. The handle can be firmly connected to the endoscope using a Luer lock. When the handle is screwed onto the endoscope's Luer connection, the metal spiral extends 4–5 mm out of the distal outlet of the working channel, so that the needle cannot damage the endoscope's instrument channel as it is being introduced.

Inside the needle, there is a stylet with the important feature (in the original version) of having a rounded tip, to avoid perforating the spiral and damaging the endoscope's working channel, requiring very expensive repairs. Nowadays the needle is also available with an optional beveled stylet (**Fig. 9.8**).

The instruments described above represent the conventional biopsy equipment developed by Vilmann and Hancke. In these instruments, the steel needle is disposable, while the other components can be reused several times. Due to the variety of customer requirements, Medi-Globe, Olympus, and Wilson-Cook have developed single-use plastic kits that can be disposed of completely (**Figs. 9.9, 9.10, 9.11, 9.12**). These innovations also make it possible to adjust the length of the needle sheaths to match the variable lengths of the endoscope working channels. However, many examiners still use the conventional biopsy equipment, which with its purely metal components provides a high degree of stability and guide precision, as

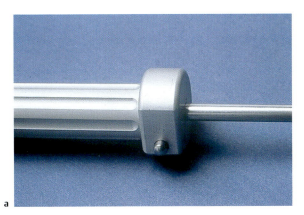

a

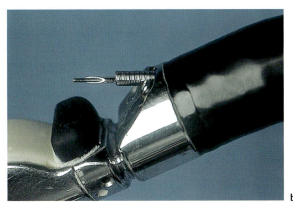

b

Fig. 9.7a, b a When the needle is completely retracted inside the sheath, the position can be fixed with a button to avoid accidental forward movement of the needle tip.

b The stylet is unprotected when the needle piston is unlocked. This may cause damage to the working channel during introduction of the needle assembly.

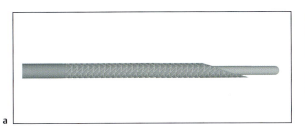

a

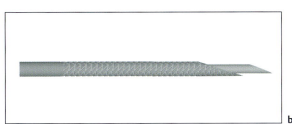

b

Fig. 9.8a, b Stylets can either be round (**a**) or beveled (**b**) at the distal end of the needle.

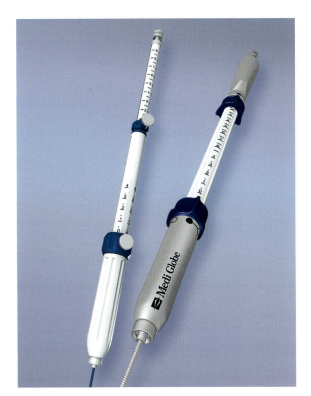

Fig. 9.9 The SonoTip II and SonoTip ProControl single-use system (by Medi-Globe).

this can be advantageous for biopsies of hard tumors. In addition to the aspiration needle equipment, the disposable kits also contain a syringe with a three-way stopcock that makes handling easier. An automatic spring-loaded biopsy system (Olympus PowerShot; **Fig. 9.13**) is also available; this has a metal spring that can forcefully shoot the needle out up to 3 cm (the depth is adjustable).

There is a wide range of different sheath designs, either consisting of metal rings with or without Teflon coating, or sheaths made entirely of Teflon or other plastic types (**Figs. 9.14** and **9.15**). Different sizes of sheath diameter are available; the larger sheath diameter sizes (Medi-Globe) are preferable for biopsies using large-channel endoscopes. The sheath diameters available from Medi-Globe are either 1.8 mm or 2.7 mm. To increase the visibility of the needle during EUS-FNA, the various manufacturers each have specific designs for the distal few centimeters of the needle tip, with different laser-produced marks in the metal (**Fig. 9.16**). In the authors' experience, there are no major differences between the various designs with regard to needle monitoring and visualization, but there are variations in the way they appear on the ultrasound image.

Only one histological Tru-Cut needle with a spring-loaded shot mechanism is currently available (the Quick-Core needle from Wilson-Cook) (**Fig. 9.17**).

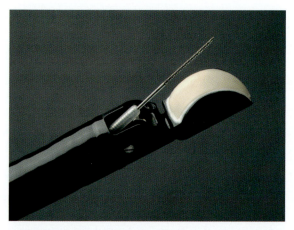

Fig. 9.10 Needle with reinforced metal sheath.

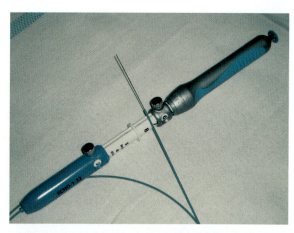

Fig. 9.11 Echo-Tip single-use system (Wilson-Cook).

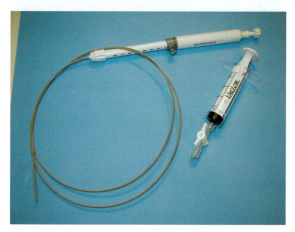

Fig. 9.12 EZ shot single-use system (Olympus).

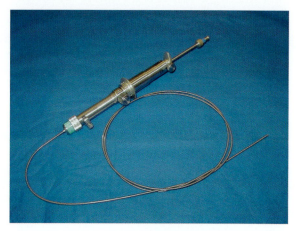

Fig. 9.13 Power Shot reusable spring-loaded needle system (Olympus).

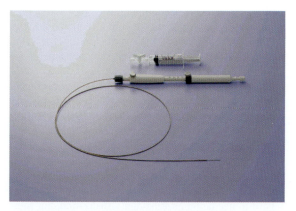

Fig. 9.14 Olympus EZshot2 (adjustable length).

	Sheath		Stylet	Needle
Order no.	French size	Design	Tip	Gauge
ECHO-1-22	5.2–4.5		Beveled	22
ECHO-3-22	5.2		2-mm ball tip	22
ECHO-19	5.2–4.0		2-mm ball tip	19
ECHO-25	5.2–4.5		2-mm ball tip	25
ECHO-20-CPN*	6.0		N/A	20

U.S. Patent Number: 5,081,997.

*Celiac plexus neurolysis
Cone-tip needle with side holes for injection of neurolysing agents.

Fig. 9.15 Different needle types and sheath designs (Wilson-Cook).

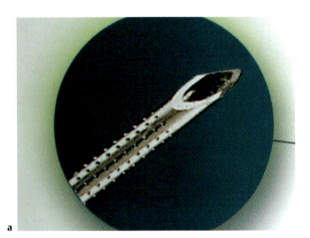
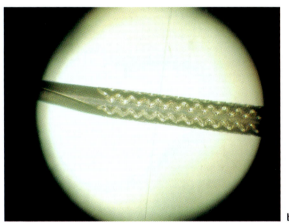

a   b

Fig. 9.16a, b Different laser-treated needle tips for enhanced ultrasonic needle visualization.

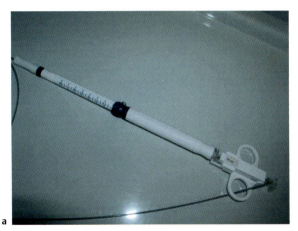
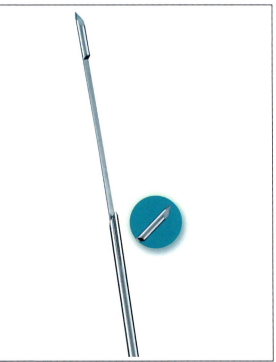

a

Fig. 9.17a, b The Quick-Core spring-loaded histological Tru-Cut needle (Wilson-Cook).

b

Examination Room

Due to the lengths of the instrument and other required equipment, the examination room should be sufficiently large. The stiff 170-cm needle has a high level of residual stress, so that carelessness in small rooms can result in injury to medical staff. Priority should be given to ensuring that there is sufficient space to place the endoscope, with a working surface nearby for the smear preparation.

The biopsy instrument should be used with sterile gloves as far as possible, to avoid iatrogenic infections with hospital germs.

Preparation of the Patient

EUS-FNA can be performed safely as an outpatient procedure in most cases. Laboratory tests are only necessary in selected patients—e.g., those receiving anticoagulation treatment or with known or potential bleeding disorders. As with all endoscopic procedures, the patient should fast for at least 2–4 hours. It is recommended that the examination should be conducted with the patient sedated as usual for endoscopy, with midazolam (3–6 mg) and fentanyl (50–100 µg). Low-dose midazolam (2–3 mg) in combination with low-dose propofol (30–50 mg) as required is used mainly in Germany. In most other European countries, only anesthesiologists are permitted to administer propofol.

Biopsy Procedure (Tables 9.3, 9.4, 9.5)

Before an EUS-guided biopsy procedure is started, several issues need to be taken into consideration. Firstly, the indication needs to be correct and patient safety should be considered. It is advisable for inexperienced examiners not to start with the most difficult types of biopsy. Contrary to what might be expected, the stomach wall is the most difficult area to biopsy, since the wall tends to move considerably along with the needle, and several of the indications in this location are submucosal tumors, which are difficult to diagnose with fine-needle aspiration (e.g., gastrointestinal stromal tumors and leiomyomas). **Table 9.3** lists the levels of difficulty of the various procedures in increasing order, based on our own experience. Our advice is that examiners should start with a biopsy of a large mediastinal tumor that is suspicious for lung cancer; in most cases, these lesions are very easy to target and the diagnosis is easy to obtain.

Cooperation by the patient is an important prerequisite for a complication-free biopsy procedure. Sudden movements have to be avoided to prevent injuries. Of course, the biopsy must not be performed when there is a vessel between the transducer and the tumor, or when the lesion cannot be properly positioned.

Firstly, the transducer has to be brought into a stable position in front of the lesion to be biopsied. As the prick angle is quite small, it is advantageous to position the lesion at the top margin of the image using the control device before introducing the needle (**Fig. 9.18**). The metal spiral (together with the retracted needle) is then introduced into the biopsy channel, and care must be taken to ensure that the needle piston is securely locked. Introducing the metal spiral with a needle that is sticking out by 1–2 mm at the distal end can severely damage the endoscope.

The spiral is fully inserted and the handle with the Luer lock is firmly screwed onto the biopsy channel (**Fig. 9.19**).

Two methods can be used to ensure that the sheath protects the entire length of the endoscope's working channel. Using the endoscope's lens, it can be observed that the sheath is extending from the distal end to a secure distance of 3–5 mm; alternatively, the position of the sheath can be checked by ultrasound. The latter technique is safe and advisable in experienced hands, but the first method should be used by those who are less experienced. However, ultrasound checking has the drawback that the transducer has to be lifted away from the mucosa and the ultrasound view of the lesion. A new firm contact then has to be made and the optimal transducer position has to be regained before the biopsy can be performed.

The needle should only be moved forward when the handle is firmly screwed onto the biopsy channel and

Table 9.3 Levels of difficulty of endoscopic ultrasound-guided fine-needle aspiration biopsy, in increasing order

1	Large mediastinal tumors
2	Mediastinal lymph nodes
3	Liver lesions
4	Adrenals
5	Perigastric lymph nodes
6	Pancreatic body and tail tumors
7	Peripancreatic lymph nodes
8	Pancreatic head tumors
9	Stomach wall (submucosal tumors)

Table 9.4 Biopsy recommendations

Establish firm transducer contact with the gastrointestinal wall
Straighten the endoscope
Use a four-hand procedure in difficult cases
Take multiple biopsies
Remove the stylet inside the lesion
Ensure full monitoring of the needle
Release the Albarrán when inside the lesion

Table 9.5 The biopsy procedure: tips and tricks

Preparation	
Before introducing the needle, check the biopsy equipment with this checklist	Make sure the needle and stylet are firmly screwed and connected
	Make sure the needle is not extending distally from the metal spiral
	Make sure the needle piston is locked firmly in the handle
After introducing the needle into the instrument channel	Is the handle firmly screwed and connected with the Luer lock on the endoscope's channel inlet? (Keep checking firm seating of this during the biopsy procedure)
Before advancing the needle	Is the metal spiral sheath visible in the endoscopic image?
Before the basic biopsy procedure	Check the precise positioning of the transducer in front of the biopsy target, which should be in the needle's potential pointing direction
	Exclude significant interposed vessels using color Doppler ultrasound or by assessing the tumor vascularization
Biopsy procedure	
	Advance the needle (after releasing the lock button) together with the stylet up to the inner surface of the gastrointestinal tract. The needle and insertion direction are now visible in the ultrasound image
	If using a round stylet, retract it ≈ 5 mm into the needle. A beveled stylet can be advanced together with the needle
	The needle is advanced into the lesion, with careful ultrasound monitoring; the stylet is reintroduced to exclude obstructing tissue plugs inside the needle tip and then completely removed and kept sterile
	Low pressure is created using a 10-mL syringe, and while the low pressure is maintained the needle is moved ≈ 5–10 times forward and back in the lesion
	The low pressure is slowly released while the needle is still inside the lesion
	If insufficient acoustic coupling is experienced in the duodenum initially during the biopsy procedure, fill the balloon shortly after needle contact with the duodenal wall
	If mounting of the biopsy instrument is difficult due to bending of the endoscope in the duodenum, withdraw the endoscope to the stomach and reenter after mounting the needle
	Release the elevator after EUS-guided tumor penetration, to reduce the resistance against the needle
	The entire needle assembly can only be removed from the endoscope after complete retraction of the needle into the sheath (note the lock position). If the needle is not retracted completely, it may damage the entire instrument channel
	The specimen is either expelled onto glass slides with air, using a syringe, or distributed evenly by reintroducing the stylet

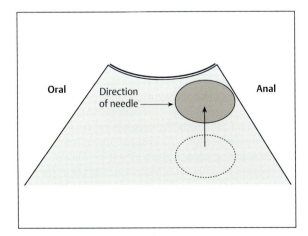

Fig. 9.18 Positioning the lesion at the top margin of the image.

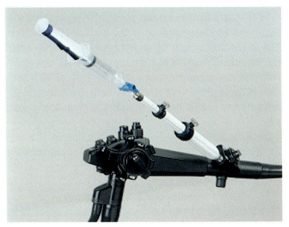

Fig. 9.19 A needle system firmly attached to the endoscope's biopsy inlet. A syringe with suction is mounted during the aspiration biopsy.

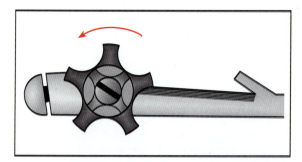

Fig. 9.20 Anticlockwise turning of the large control wheel, with deflection of the distal tip, lifts the lesion closer to the transducer.

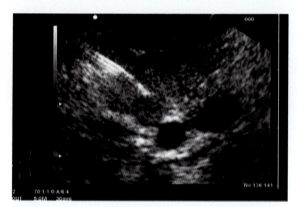

Fig. 9.21 Endoscopic ultrasound-guided biopsy of an insulinoma in the tail of the pancreas. The needle should be clearly visible during the entire biopsy procedure.

the sheath is visible at the distal end (**Figs. 9.7** and **9.19**). This is to avoid damage to the working channel due to unintended disconnection of the Luer lock connection during the biopsy.

Checking the ultrasound image, the examiner has to try to keep a very firm and stable contact between the transducer and the inner surface of the gastrointestinal tract. The endoscope should be straightened, especially when the pancreatic head is being punctured, as in the endoscopic retrograde cholangiopancreatography (ERCP) position, as these tumors are often very hard to biopsy and the resistance to needle movements should be as low as possible.

Once the position has been carefully adjusted, the needle with the attached stylet should be advanced until the biopsy direction can be estimated and the target of the biopsy can be reached easily.

An Albarrán is undoubtedly advantageous when very deep lesions have to be reached. However, it needs to be taken into account that the needle with the stylet is very stiff and that activating the Albarrán causes considerable strain on the sheath, biopsy needle, and stylet. Moreover, the flexion makes it more difficult to move the needle forward and backward during the biopsy procedure; when hard tumors are being penetrated, it even increases

the resistance, which is already quite high. In most cases, it is possible to adjust the direction of the biopsy needle insertion very precisely using the endoscope's conventional handle control buttons (**Fig. 9.20**).

The needle, still with the stylet, is then advanced up to the inner surface (mucosa) of the gastrointestinal tract. The next step depends on the type of stylet being used— either round or sharp (beveled). The round type leads to significantly less damage to the instrument channel and is preferable for those with less experience. When a biopsy is being performed with a beveled stylet, the needle can be advanced into a lesion immediately after it has been moved into position. If a round stylet is being used, it has to be retracted by a few millimeters (as it normally extends beyond the needle tip by 1–2 mm) before the actual penetration through the gut wall is performed. After the stylet has been retracted, the needle tip is exposed and can freely penetrate the tissue. Further retraction of the stylet should not be done, to avoid obstructive tissue plugs from superficial layers inside the biopsy needle. It is often unavoidable that a few cells from the gut wall (gastric mucosa, duodenal mucosa, esophageal mucosa) appear in the cytological material. Consequently, it is very important to provide the cytologist with precise information about the method and route of the biopsy.

With the stylet retracted but still inside the needle, the biopsy needle is now moved forward into the lesion under full ultrasound guidance (**Fig. 9.21**). It should be emphasized that complete monitoring of the needle tip is important whenever possible. There are a few cases in which a punch technique is the only way to penetrate a hard lesion. However, this technique should not be used as standard. After penetration into the middle of a lesion, the stylet is removed completely. One of the present authors (P.V.) always reintroduces the stylet into the needle before complete removal, to expel possible tissue plugs from superficial layers that are obstructing the needle lumen. This should of course only be done in cases in which there is no tumor interposed between the transducer and the target lesion, to avoid tumor seeding.

When hard tumors are being punctured, bending of the needle is sometimes observed; this may create problems with monitoring the needle tip and may potentially cause injury to the surrounding structures, particularly the vessels. If severe bending of the needle is experienced, a new needle should be chosen for a repeat biopsy. There is also a tendency during needle advancement for the transducer to be pushed away from the mucosa, so that the ultrasound image is lost. This occurs particularly during pancreatic biopsies. Loss of the ultrasound image and thus of ultrasound needle monitoring in these cases can be avoided to some extent by inflating the balloon immediately after initial mucosal contact with the needle.

When the optimal needle position is reached in the middle of the lesion, a 10-mL syringe with a locking device is firmly screwed onto the needle (the type of syringe usually used for Menghini biopsy has been found to be reliable for this). Pulling the syringe piston creates low pressure. The syringe piston is locked in this position for permanent suction. The needle is now moved to and fro 5–10 times inside the lesion with full ultrasound guidance. If considerable resistance is experienced when using the Albarrán during the biopsy, one should try to neutralize the Albarrán as soon as the needle tip is in the middle of the lesion. With the needle tip still in the lesion, suction is slowly released, and the needle is retracted (cautiously, as there is a danger of injury and contamination) inside the needle sheath and locked in a secure position. The complete needle assembly is now removed by disconnection from the inlet of the endoscope.

Consideration also needs to be given to the endoscope used when the type of needle is being selected. Biopsies can be safely taken with large-channel endoscopes. However, ultrasound control of the needle during biopsy is more difficult with standard needle systems, as there is a size difference between the needle sheath and the working channel. There is a tendency to lose sight of the needle on the ultrasound image when the needle sheath is floppy and unsupported by the endoscope working channel. This can be reduced using the Albarrán, which holds the sheath in a firm position. However, needles with an extended sheath size that fits the endoscope's working channel better are preferable.

If several lesions are present during an EUS examination, it has to be decided how many of the lesions, which lesions, and in which order they should be biopsied. Careful consideration is mandatory here, taking the TNM staging of each disease into account. It is obvious that a lesion that is suspected to be a distant metastasis should be biopsied before the local lymph nodes, with the primary lesion following last, in successive order, if the same needle is to be used. If this is not done, it is possible for false-positive up-staging of the disease to occur. If a new, more distant lesion is detected after an initial biopsy, a completely new needle should be chosen.

Preparing the Smear

In normal conditions after fine-needle aspiration biopsy, it is recommended that the biopsy material should immediately be expelled with air from the syringe onto the prepared specimen slides. Another method that can be recommended in EUS-FNA is to reintroduce the stylet into the needle and move it slowly forward. This creates high pressure in the needle, and the material can be expelled carefully and in a controlled way droplet by droplet onto the specimen slides. The decisive advantage of this method is that numerous specimens of the same quality can be prepared, whereas with the air expulsion method there is a risk of the material being expelled in an uncontrolled way. Stylet expulsion is particularly advantageous, as im-

munohistochemical stains are often necessary and are becoming more and more important. With this method, it is easy to identify cylinders that can be processed during histological analysis. However, the diagnostic benefit of histological specimens should not be overrated, as cytology also allows excellent immunohistochemical examination.

The smearing technique should be discussed with the cytopathologist. Personally, we smear the material with a second specimen slide that is placed smoothly on top of the first one and retracted, with a second specimen being obtained. Others recommend that, in addition to smearing of the material, a microhistological cylinder should be prepared, fixed with formalin, and processed into a cell block for histological evaluation.

The subsequent procedure, particularly fixation, should also be discussed with the cytologist. No general advice can be given here; basically, the specimen can be air-dried and fixed later, but some cytopathologists recommend immediate fixing and coloring of the smear. There is some evidence in the literature that it is preferable to have an attending cytopathologist in the examination room for immediate evaluation of the specimen. When a ready-to-use staining liquid is applied, it is possible to assess and evaluate the adequacy of the specimen even after only a few minutes. However, in the authors' experience, this is not absolutely necessary if ultrasound monitoring of the needle during the biopsy is optimal and if the macroscopic appearance of the material shows that it contains minute tissue fragments.

Limitations and Complications

The increasingly widespread use of ultrasound-guided fine-needle biopsy certainly owes something to the fact that it is regarded as a low-complication method. A multicenter study by Wiersema et al.[16] showed that the complication rate was ≈2%, with the majority being minor complications. Complications often only involve biopsy-point bleeding that is clinically insignificant. Heavier bleeding is rare; it may occur rarely due to shearing of the mucosa by the needle and due to injury to adjacent vessels when restless and nervous patients are being examined.

The infection rate is also remarkably low, so that antibiotic prophylaxis is not usually necessary. Biopsy of pancreatic pseudocysts is an exception to this, in which it has been shown that antibiotic prophylaxis is preferable, as there is a relatively high risk of infection.[17] Pancreatitis has been reported as a complication, particularly when pancreatic biopsies are performed in patients with benign pancreatic diseases.[15]

Tumor cell seeding has always been a matter of debate and concern; however, there are as yet no "hard facts" providing evidence that this is a potential risk. Penetrating through malignant tissue to reach a suspicious lesion is in any case not recommended. An example of this might be a patient with gastric or esophageal cancer, with a suspicious lymph node adjacent to the primary tumor.

Despite the rapid technological advances being made with other imaging methods, endoscopic ultrasonography has strengthened its position as a diagnostic method, particularly since the development of the fine-needle biopsy technique. It is therefore all the more important to take advantage of the diagnostic advantages and low complication rate of EUS by standardizing the procedure and providing training programs, so that it becomes even more widely used in gastrointestinal practice.

References

1. Fukuda M, Nakano Y, Saito K, Hirata K, Terada S, Urushizaki I. Endoscopic ultrasonography in the diagnosis of pancreatic carcinoma. The use of a liquid-filled stomach method. Scand J Gastroenterol Suppl 1984;94:65–76.
2. DiMagno EP, Buxton JL, Regan PT, et al. Ultrasonic endoscope. Lancet 1980;1(8169):629–631.
3. Strohm WD, Phillip J, Hagenmüller F, Classen M. Ultrasonic tomography by means of an ultrasonic fiberendoscope. Endoscopy 1980;12(5):241–244.
4. Vilmann P, Jacobsen GK, Henriksen FW, Hancke S. Endoscopic ultrasonography with guided fine needle aspiration biopsy in pancreatic disease. Gastrointest Endosc 1992;38(2):172–173.
5. Vilmann P, Hancke S, Henriksen FW, Jacobsen GK. Endosonographically-guided fine needle aspiration biopsy of malignant lesions in the upper gastrointestinal tract. Endoscopy 1993;25(8):523–527.
6. Vilmann P, Hancke S, Henriksen FW, Jacobsen GK. Endoscopic ultrasonography-guided fine-needle aspiration biopsy of lesions in the upper gastrointestinal tract. Gastrointest Endosc 1995;41(3):230–235.
7. Vilmann P. Endoscopic ultrasonography with curved array transducer in diagnosis of cancer in and adjacent to the upper gastrointestinal tract: scanning and guided fine needle aspiration biopsy [dissertation]. Copenhagen: Munksgaard, 1998.
8. Giovannini M, Seitz JF, Monges G, Perrier H, Rabbia I. Fine-needle aspiration cytology guided by endoscopic ultrasonography: results in 141 patients. Endoscopy 1995;27(2):171–177.
9. Vilmann P. Endoscopic ultrasonography-guided fine-needle aspiration biopsy of lymph nodes. Gastrointest Endosc 1996;43(2 Pt 2):S24–S29.
10. Pedersen BH, Vilmann P, Folke K, et al. Endoscopic ultrasonography and real-time guided fine-needle aspiration biopsy of solid lesions of the mediastinum suspected of malignancy. Chest 1996;110(2):539–544.
11. Pedersen BH, Vilmann P, Milman N, Folke K, Hancke S. Endoscopic ultrasonography with guided fine needle aspiration biopsy of a mediastinal mass lesion. Acta Radiol 1995;36(3):326–328.
12. Larsen SS, Krasnik M, Vilmann P, et al. Endoscopic ultrasound guided biopsy of mediastinal lesions has a major impact on patient management. Thorax 2002;57(2):98–103.
13. Larsen SS, Vilmann P, Krasnik M, et al. Endoscopic ultrasound guided biopsy performed routinely in lung cancer staging spares futile thoracotomies: preliminary results from a randomised clinical trial. Lung Cancer 2005;49(3):377–385.
14. Larsen SS, Vilmann P, Krasnik M, et al. Endoscopic ultrasound guided biopsy versus mediastinoscopy for analysis of paratracheal and subcarinal lymph nodes in lung cancer staging. Lung Cancer 2005;48(1):85–92.
15. Vilmann P, Hancke S. A new biopsy handle instrument for endoscopic ultrasound-guided fine-needle aspiration biopsy. Gastrointest Endosc 1996;43(3):238–242.
16. Wiersema MJ, Vilmann P, Giovannini M, Chang KJ, Wiersema LM. Endosonography-guided fine-needle aspiration biopsy: diagnostic accuracy and complication assessment. Gastroenterology 1997;112(4):1087–1095.
17. Chang KJ, Katz KD, Durbin TE, et al. Endoscopic ultrasound-guided fine-needle aspiration. Gastrointest Endosc 1994;40(6):694–699.

II Diagnostic Imaging and Interventions

10 EUS-Guided Biopsy—Indications, Problems, Pitfalls, Troubleshooting, and Clinical Impact

C. Jenssen, K. Moeller, M. Sarbia, S. Wagner

Endoscopic ultrasound-guided needle biopsies (EUS-guided fine-needle aspiration, EUS-FNA; EUS-guided Tru-Cut biopsy, EUS-TCB) are reliable, safe, and effective techniques for obtaining samples for cytological or histological examinations, either as a primary procedure or in cases in which other biopsy techniques have failed. EUS-FNA and EUS-TCB have become cornerstone techniques in visceral medicine, pulmonary medicine, and oncology. EUS-guided needle biopsy (EUS-NB) has considerably increased the diagnostic potential of endoscopic ultrasound (EUS). Between May 1, 2008, and April 3, 2009, 58 of 185 (31.3%) original publications on EUS reported on EUS-NB.[1] The initial reports on EUS-FNA were published in gastroenterology journals in 1992.[2,3] EUS-NB has also in the meantime become a topic in the cytopathology literature, following an initial report in 1997.[4] Cytopathological diagnoses based on EUS-NB may have a major impact on therapeutic decision-making and on the individual prognoses for patients—avoiding major surgery, dispensing with invasive diagnostic interventions such as thoracoscopy, mediastinoscopy, and laparoscopy, and determining whether neoadjuvant treatment or nonsurgical therapy is needed. This is the reason why the endosonographer and cytopathologist share a common responsibility for the quality with which biopsy material is acquired and processed, as well as for the cytological and histological diagnosis. This chapter discusses the problems and pitfalls of EUS-NB from the clinical and cytopathological points of view and considers reasonable solutions for problems that arise.

Indications and Contraindications

EUS-NB is indicated for cytopathological diagnosis of mass lesions in the gastrointestinal tract and adjacent to it, and of lymph nodes in its vicinity, if sampling using less invasive methods (e.g., forceps biopsy) is not possible or has failed. EUS-NB can therefore be of considerable value in the primary diagnosis and staging of malignant diseases, as well as for differentiating benign diseases. For EUS-NB to be justified, there must be potential clinical implications of the resulting cytopathological diagnosis—for example, a change in diagnostic pathways, avoidance of invasive or surgical treatment, or a decision in favor of specific treatments (**Tables 10.1, 10.2, 10.3, 10.4**).[5–8] EUS-NB is contraindicated in all circumstances in which the risks of the procedure outweigh the expected benefits of the diagnostic information it can provide (**Table 10.5**).

Table 10.1 Pancreatic indications for EUS-guided needle biopsy

Nonresectable tumors
Cytological/histological diagnosis before initiation of chemotherapy
Proof of nonresectability (liver metastasis, mediastinal lymph-node metastasis, pleural and peritoneal carcinosis)
Resectable tumors
Suspicion of solid tumors other than ductal adenocarcinoma (e.g., neuroendocrine tumor, malignant lymphoma, pancreatic metastases)
Differentiation of cystic pancreatic lesions
Suspicion of ductal adenocarcinoma only in cases in which the surgical decision depends on cytological/histological diagnosis
Unclear findings
Cytological/histological proof of a benign diagnosis in case of a low pretest probability for a malignant tumor (e.g., focal pancreatitis, autoimmune pancreatitis)

Table 10.2 Other indications for EUS-guided needle biopsy in gastroenterology

Primary diagnosis
Method of first choice in hypoechoic subepithelial tumors: gastrointestinal stromal tumor (GIST), schwannoma, leiomyoma, neuroendocrine tumor, granular cell tumor, etc.
After failure, or if other biopsy methods are contraindicated, in diffuse infiltrating gastric cancer (linitis plastica), cholangiocarcinoma, hepatocellular carcinoma
Staging
Esophageal cancer: celiac lymph-node metastasis, liver metastasis, peritoneal carcinosis
Biliary and gastrointestinal cancer: liver metastasis, peritoneal and pleural carcinosis, adrenal metastasis, mediastinal lymph-node metastases
Follow-up
Diagnosis of extraluminal recurrence after surgery for rectal cancer or other gastrointestinal malignancies

Table 10.3 Indications for EUS-guided needle biopsy in pneumology (lung cancer, other mediastinal tumors, mediastinal lymph nodes)

Primary diagnosis
Suspicion of lung cancer: after failure of bronchoscopic biopsy (central, periesophageal tumors; lymph-node metastases; metastases in the left adrenal gland or the liver)
Staging
Mediastinal staging: proof of N2 or N3 metastasis (NSCLC) or any mediastinal lymph-node metastasis (SCLC); proof of pleural carcinosis
Infradiaphragmatic staging: proof of distant metastasis (adrenal gland, liver, infradiaphragmatic lymph node)
Follow-up
Diagnosis of recurrence after curative surgery for lung cancer
Diagnosis of ambiguous and benign mass lesions
Ambiguous mediastinal lymphadenopathy or solid mass lesions
Suspicion of sarcoidosis or tuberculosis

NSCLC, non–small cell cancer; SCLC, small cell lung cancer.

Table 10.4 Oncological and other indications for EUS-guided needle biopsy

Primary diagnosis
Retroperitoneal tumors (adrenal glands after exclusion of pheochromocytoma; mesenchymal tumors)
Suspicion of malignant lymphoma (mediastinal and infradiaphragmatic lymph nodes, splenic lesions)
Suspicion of inflammatory mass lesions (mediastinum, retroperitoneum, gastrointestinal wall)
Staging
Various cancers: liver metastasis, adrenal metastasis, splenic metastasis, mediastinal or infradiaphragmatic lymph-node metastases, peritoneal and pleural carcinosis
Follow-up
Diagnosis of recurrence after curative treatment for various malignancies

Table 10.5 Contraindications for EUS-guided fine-needle aspiration (EUS-FNA) and EUS-guided Tru-Cut biopsy (EUS-TCB)[7]

No informed consent
Lack of cooperation or insufficient sedation
Anticoagulation treatment or coagulopathy (international normalized ratio INR > 1.5; platelet count < 50000; heparin in therapeutic doses)
Inhibition of platelet aggregation by clopidogrel[9]
Failure of ultrasound needle control
EUS-NB of the liver, pancreatic head, or ampulla in cases of insufficient drainage of obstructed bile ducts
Cystic mediastinal lesions[a, b]
Interposition of vessels[a, c]
Results of EUS-NB are unlikely to have a significant clinical impact

[a] A relative contraindication; benefit has to be weighed against risk very carefully.
[b] Peri-interventional antibiotic treatment is mandatory.
EUS-NB, EUS-guided needle biopsy.
[c] Transaortic EUS-FNA of mediastinal lymph nodes and tumors,[10,11] of the pericardium and a left atrial mass,[12] and of intravascular tumors[13] without any major complications has been reported.

Positive results of EUS-FNA from:		Treatment decision (depending on particular tumor type)
Ascites, pleural effusion, liver metastasis, adrenal gland metastasis, nonregional lymph nodes	M	Decision against surgery
Regional lymph nodes	N	Neoadjuvant treatment (palliative treatment)
Suspected primary tumor	T	Treatment according to histological diagnosis

Fig. 10.1 An algorithm for EUS-NB in oncological staging. Sampling should start in lesions in which positive findings would confirm the presence of distant metastases, then proceed to possible lymph-node metastases, and conclude with the suspected primary tumor, if needed (inverse TNM system).

Planning the Procedure

Before EUS-guided biopsy is carried out, all of the endoscopic and imaging studies available—such as transabdominal ultrasound (TUS), computed tomography (CT), and magnetic resonance imaging (MRI)—should be reviewed in order to generate a "road map" of the procedure. The endoscopy suite and team should be adequately prepared. The indication for EUS-NB has to be verified, and contraindications and risk factors must be checked. We would suggest that a complete EUS examination should first be conducted, looking specifically for findings that would probably represent the most advanced stage of a malignant gastrointestinal process—for example, a celiac lymph node in a patient with suspected esophageal cancer, or a liver lesion, ascites, or a mediastinal lymph node in a patient with a suspected pancreatic mass lesion. If malignant disease has been confirmed or is suspected, the first EUS-NB procedure should always target the lesion that would prove to represent the most advanced stage in case of positive cytological or histological findings (**Fig. 10.1**)[7].

The aim of the complete EUS examination should also be to detect intervening vessels, ascites, or gastrointestinal wall infiltrations so that the optimal needle track can be chosen. The clinical consequences of possible needle-tract seeding should also be taken into account when planning an EUS-NB procedure. In cases of pancreatic head tumor, the transduodenal needle route is preferable rather than a transgastric approach, as the duodenal wall will later be resected during a Kausch–Whipple operation if the findings are positive.

Diagnostic Yield

The diagnostic yield of EUS-NB varies depending on the nature of the target lesion, the skill and experience of the endoscopist and cytopathologist, and on numerous technical and procedural variables. It can potentially be improved with additional techniques such as real-time elastography and contrast-enhanced EUS. In various studies, EUS-FNA of solid pancreatic masses provided adequate material for cytological examination in 86.8–98.5% of cases, and for histological assessment in 68.9–89.0% of cases. The diagnostic yield of EUS-FNA was 65%–100% for lymph nodes, 91–100% for solid liver lesions, 97.7–100.0% for biliary structures, and 82.0–91.8% for subepithelial tumors of the gastrointestinal tract (**Tables 10.6, 10.7, 10.8, 10.9**).

It is difficult to compare sensitivity and specificity data between different studies. In some studies, inadequate biopsies are excluded from the statistical analysis, while others treat these as false-negatives. In statistical analyses, some authors treat "suspicious for malignancy" and "atypical" cytological findings as negative findings (true or false negatives), while others regard suspicious and sometimes even atypical findings as true or false positives. Rating suspicious findings as true positives is based on observations from EUS-FNA studies of solid pancreatic mass lesions, in which 82–100% of cases of suspicious cytology proved to be malignant neoplasms during the follow-up.[18,29,73–75] Different gold standards have also been used for statistical evaluation of EUS-NB studies. Most studies have used a combination of surgical pathology, other histological findings, radiological studies, and clinical follow-up to confirm a malignant diagnosis. Only a few studies have correlated the findings of EUS-NB with surgical pathology in all or almost all cases.[65,76–80]

Another problem causing difficulties in comparing the results of EUS-NB studies is the absence of a consensus definition of "inadequate," "insufficient," and "nondiagnostic" biopsy findings. Mitsuhashi et al. assessed smears as satisfactory if unequivocally malignant cells were identified. For negative cases, at least 5–10 groups of ≥ 10 epithelial cells or pancreatic acini had to be present on each slide. When only blood or normal gastrointestinal epithelial cells were seen, the specimen was regarded inadequate.[21] Noh et al. defined smears with two or three clusters of benign or malignant pancreatic glandular cells as adequate. For diagnostic smears from EUS-FNA of lymph nodes, the same authors postulated the presence of abundant lymphocytes and tingible body macrophages.[81] In studies on EUS-FNA including large numbers of patients, the reported rates of inadequate smears vary very widely (0–35%) depending on the definition of adequacy and the type of target lesion (**Tables 10.6, 10.7, 10.8, 10.9**).

There are few published data on the ability of EUS-FNA to provide adequate material for cytological or histological assessment. Combining cytological and histological analyses of samples obtained by EUS-FNA may improve diagnostic accuracy slightly (**Table 10.10**). The effectiveness of EUC-TCB in providing core biopsies of solid pancreatic masses, lymph nodes, and various other solid lesions varies between 50% and 99% (**Table 10.11**).

Table 10.6 Rates of inadequate material sampling and sensitivity of EUS-guided fine-needle aspiration (EUS-FNA) in studies including large numbers of patients: pancreatic mass lesions

First author, year	Target lesions	EUS-FNAs (n)	On-site cytology	Inadequate material (%)	Sensitivity (%)
1) Solid or mostly solid pancreatic mass lesions					
Yusuf 2009[14]	Pancreatic lesions (mostly solid)	842 (540 22-G; 302 25-G)	+ (90%)	8.6 (22-gauge) 3.8 (25-gauge)	84 (22-gauge)[a] 92 (25-gauge)[a]
Ardengh 2007[15]	Pancreatic lesions (solid, cystic)	611 (405 solid, 206 cystic)	–	2.6	78.4[a] (solid < 3 cm: 82.4; solid ≥ 3 cm: 78.8; cystic: 72.2)[a]
Turner BG 2010[16]	Solid pancreatic mass lesions	560	+/– (in 43.8%)	8.8 (adenocarcinoma and neuroendocrine tumors: 2.3; only adenocarcinoma: 0.9; only neuroendocrine tumors: 17.5)	76[a] (adenocarcinoma: 77[a]; 93[d] neuroendocrine tumor 68[a]; 80[d])
Eloubeidi 2006[17]	Solid pancreatic mass lesions	547	+	No data	95
Volmar 2005[18]	Pancreatic mass lesions	489	+ (in 89.2%)	1.5	79.9
Varadarajulu 2005[19]	Pancreatic mass lesions	300	+	No data	89.5
Zhang 2010[20]	Solid pancreatic mass lesions	279	+	7.2	94.7[a]
Mitsuhashi 2006[21]	Pancreatic mass lesions	267	+	5.2	94.6
Raut 2003[22]	Pancreatic mass lesions	233	+	6.9	91[a]
Rocca 2007[23]	Pancreatic mass lesions	232	–	12	80[c]
Eloubeidi 2008[24]	Solid pancreatic mass lesions	224	+	No data	92.4
Fritscher-Ravens 2002[25]	Pancreatic mass lesions	207	–	3.4	85
Möller 2009[26]	Pancreatic mass lesions	192	–	1.1 (cytology or histology) 7.3 (cytology) 13.5 (histology)	82.9[a] (cytology: 68[a], 74.2[c]; histology: 60[a], 69.8[c])
Harewood 2002[27]	Pancreatic mass lesions	185	+	7.1	94[c]
Shin 2002[28]	Mostly pancreatic mass lesions	179	–	13.2	81.7[a]
Eloubeidi 2003[29]	Pancreatic mass lesions	158	+	2	84.3[c] (96.7)[d]
Will 2009[30]	Pancreatic mass lesions	153	–	0.7	83[c]
Wiersema 1997[31]	Pancreatic mass lesions	124	+/–[e]	3.2	86
Gress 2001[32]	Pancreatic mass lesions	101	+	7.8	93.4[c]
2) Cystic lesions of the pancreas					
Brugge 2004[33]	Cystic mass lesions of the pancreas	341	No data	No data	34.5[a, b]
Zhang 2010[20]	Cystic mass lesions of the pancreas	186	+	23.7	45.4[a]
Frossard 2003[34]	Cystic mass lesions of the pancreas	127	No data	23[f]	97[g]

Sensitivity is given for the diagnosis of a "malignant lesion," unless otherwise stated.
[a] Analysis of all cases ("intention to diagnose").
[b] Sensitivity for differentiating between mucinous and nonmucinous cysts.
[c] Analysis of all cases with adequate material.
[d] Sensitivity was calculated on the basis of regarding definitely malignant, suspicious, and atypical cases as positive for malignancy.
[e] On-site cytology in two of four centers.
[f] Cases of insufficient cellularity or contamination by cells from the gastrointestinal wall.
[g] Sensitivity for differentiation of cases in which surgery is indicated against cases in which surgery is not necessary.

Table 10.7 Rates of inadequate material sampling and sensitivity of EUS-guided fine-needle aspiration (EUS-FNA) in studies including large numbers of patients: lymph nodes

First author, year	Target lesions	EUS-FNAs (n)	On-site cytology	Inadequate material (%)	Sensitivity (%)
Zhang 2010[20]	Mediastinal and abdominal lymph nodes	249	+	5.6	95[a]
Eloubeidi 2008[24]	Mediastinal and abdominal lymph nodes	246	+	No data	92.6
Annema 2005[35]	Mediastinal lymph nodes	242	+	3	91
Stelow 2004[36]	Mediastinal and abdominal lymph nodes	217	+	16 (12% of patients)	No data
Wiersema 1997[31]	Mediastinal and abdominal lymph nodes	192	+/–[b]	4.2	92 (84–97)[c]
Kramer 2006[37]	Mediastinal and celiac lymph nodes	155	–	35	92[d] 72[a]
Fritscher-Ravens 2000[38]	Mediastinal lymph nodes	153	–	2	92
Eloubeidi 2005[39]	Mediastinal lymph nodes	117	No data	No data	92.5[e]
Yasuda 2006[40]	Mediastinal and abdominal lymph nodes	104	–	0[f]	Accuracy 98

Sensitivity is given for the diagnosis of a "malignant lesion," unless otherwise stated.
[a] Analysis of all cases ("intention to diagnose").
[b] On-site cytology in two of four centers.
[c] Variation among the four centers.
[d] Analysis of all cases with adequate material.
[e] Sensitivity was calculated on the basis of regarding definitely malignant, suspicious, and atypical cases as positive for malignancy.
[f] Material for cytological and/or histological diagnosis.

Table 10.8 Rates of inadequate material sampling and sensitivity of EUS-guided fine-needle aspiration (EUS-FNA) in studies including large numbers of patients: various lesions

First author, year	Target lesions	EUS-FNAs (n)	On-site cytology	Inadequate material (%)	Sensitivity (%)
Eloubeidi 2008[24]	Lymph nodes, solid and cystic pancreatic masses, mural lesions, biliary lesions, liver lesions, mediastinal masses, masses of adrenal glands, spleen and kidney	641	+	No data	91.7
Anand 2007[41]	Nonpancreatic mass lesions	246	+	22	92[a]
Jhala 2004[42]	Various (pancreatic mass lesions and lymph nodes)	209	+	4.0	96[b]
Gress 1997[43]	Various (pancreatic mass lesions, lymph nodes, perirectal lesions, subepithelial tumors)	208	+	9	89
Südhoff 2004[44]	Various	106	–	5.6	78[a]
Chhieng 2002[45]	Various	103	+	5.8	71[b] (46)[a]

Sensitivity is given for the diagnosis of a "malignant lesion," unless otherwise stated.
[a] Analysis of all cases with adequate material.
[b] Analysis of all cases ("intention to diagnose").

Table 10.9 Rates of inadequate material sampling and sensitivity of EUS-guided fine-needle aspiration (EUS-FNA) in studies including large numbers of patients: lesions in various anatomic sites

First author, year	Target lesions	EUS-FNAs (n)	On-site cytology	Inadequate material (%)	Sensitivity (%)
1) Adrenal gland					
DeWitt 2007[46]	Left adrenal gland	38	+	24	100
Eloubeidi 2004[47]	Left adrenal gland	31	+	0	No data
Jhala 2004[48]	Left adrenal gland	24	+	0	100
2) Liver					
tenBerge 2002[49]	Liver masses	167	No data	No data	No data[a]
DeWitt 2003[50]	Liver masses	77	+	9	82–94 (depending on the status of seven unclassified lesions)
Hollerbach 2003[51]	Liver masses	41	–	2.4	94[b]
3) Biliary lesions					
Meara 2006[52]	Lesions in the bile duct and gallbladder	46	+	2.2	87
Fritscher-Ravens 2004[53]	Suspected hilar cholangio-carcinoma	44	–	2.3	89
Byrne 2004[54]	Bile duct lesions	35	+	0	100
Rösch 2004[55]	Biliary strictures	28	–	No data	75
Eloubeidi 2004[56]	Suspected cholangiocarci-noma	25	+	0	86
DeWitt 2006[57]	Proximal biliary strictures	24	+	0	77
4) Spleen					
Fritscher-Ravens 2003[58]	Focal lesions of the spleen	12	–	8	No data
Eloubeidi 2006[59]	Focal lesions of the spleen	6	+	0	66.7
5) Idiopathic mediastinal mass lesions					
Devereaux 2002[60]	Idiopathic mediastinal mass lesions	49	+	6	100[c] 94[d]
Catalano 2002[61]	Idiopathic mediastinal mass lesions	26	+	0	84 (Accuracy)
6) Mural lesions in the gastrointestinal tract					
Hoda 2009[62]	Suspected GISTs in the upper GI tract	112	+	16.1	83.9[c, e, f] (accuracy of cytology) 61.6[c, e] (accuracy of immuno-histochemistry)
Wiersema 1997[31]	Gastrointestinal wall (subepi-thelial tumors excluded)	103	+/–[g]	17.5	61 (40–67)[h]
Vander Noot 2004[63]	Intramural and extramural lesions in the gastrointestinal tract	62	+	0	89[e] (96)[f]
Akahoshi 2007[64]	Hypoechoic subepithelial tumors	53	?	7.5	97[e]
Ando 2002[65]	GISTs in the stomach and esophagus	49	–	8.2[i]	66.7[e] (100)[i]
Chen 2005[66]	Intramural and extramural lesions in the gastrointestinal tract	42	+	No data	100
Eloubeidi 2008[24]	Mural lesions	40	+	No data	86.2
Sepe 2009[67]	Histologically confirmed GISTs	37	–/+ (19%)	21.6	78.4[c, e] (accuracy for spindle cell neoplasm)
Sasaki 2005[68]	Intramural and extramural lesions in the rectum and colon	22	–	4.5	100[d] 93.3[c]

Table 10.9 (continued)

First author, year	Target lesions	EUS-FNAs (n)	On-site cytology	Inadequate material (%)	Sensitivity (%)
7) Ascites					
DeWitt 2007[69]	Ascites	60	+	0	No data
Nguyen 2001[70]	Ascites	31	+	0	50
Kaushik 2006[71]	Ascites	25	−	0	94
8) Renal tumors					
DeWitt 2009[72]	Kidney tumors	13	+	8	83 (five of six cases with surgical pathology)

Sensitivity is given for the diagnosis of a "malignant lesion," unless otherwise stated.
[a] No data for sensitivity due to the study design (survey of EUS centers).
[b] Sensitivity for combined cytology and histology.
[c] Analysis of all cases ("intention to diagnose").
[d] Analysis of all cases with adequate material.
[e] Sensitivity/accuracy for neoplastic lesions.
[f] Sensitivity was calculated on the basis of regarding definitely malignant, suspicious, and atypical cases as positive for malignancy.
[g] On-site cytology in two of four centers.
[h] Variation among the four centers.
[i] Sensitivity for diagnosis of malignant GIST.

Table 10.10 Diagnostic yield and sensitivity of EUS-guided fine-needle aspiration (EUS-FNA) (22-gauge): cytology versus histology

First author, year, no. of cases	Adequate specimens (%)			Sensitivity (%)		
	Cytology	Histology	Combined	Cytology	Histology	Combined
Solid pancreatic tumors						
Möller 2009 n = 192[26]	92.7	86.5	98.9	68.1[a] 74.2[b]	60.0[a] 69.8[b]	82.9[a]
Takahashi 2005 n = 77[82]	100	89	100	82	44[a] 74[b]	84[a]
Iglesias-Garcia 2007 n = 62[83]	82.3	83.9	90.3	68.4[a] 76.5[b]	68.4[a] 92.9[b]	84.2[a] 100[b]
Lymph nodes and various solid mass lesions						
Südhoff 2004 n = 106[44]	95.4	82.1	No data	No data	No data	78[a]
Niehaus 2006 n = 51[84]	96	71	No data	80, 91, 95[c]	51	No data

[a] Analysis of all cases (intention to diagnose).
[b] Analysis only of cases with adequate material.
[c] Sensitivity of smears from core biopsies, 80%; of smears from material expelled from the needle, 91%; and of smears from material expelled from the needle by air pressure, 95%.

Table 10.11 Diagnostic yield and accuracy of EUS-guided Tru-Cut biopsy (EUS-TCB): histology (compared with cytology: EUS-guided fine-needle aspiration or touch imprint cytology)

First author, year, no. of cases	Adequate specimens (%) 22-gauge FNA (cytology)	19-gauge Tru-Cut (histology)	Diagnostic accuracy (%) Cytology	Histology	Combined
Thomas 2009 n = 247 (V: P, NP, GIW)[85]	Not performed	87	–	75 [a] P: 67.5 NP: 80 GIW: 88	–
Aithal 2007 n = 167 (V)[86]	No data	89	82	89	93
Wittmann 2006 n = 159 (V) (EUS-TCB in 60%)[87]	94	88	77	73	91
Shah 2008 n = 123 (P)[88]	100	86	88.9[a]	52.9[a]	96.1[a]
Vanderheyden 2008 n = 109 (V)[89]	Touch imprint cytology, EUS-FNA not performed	No data	82.6[a] (touch imprint)	92.7[a]	95.4[a]
Kipp 2009 n = 86 (V)[75]	96 (V) 84 (SMT)	93 (V) 89.5 (SMT)	Sensitivity 55 (V) 16 (SMT)	Sensitivity 62 (V) 79 (SMT)	Sensitivity 78 (V) 79 (SMT)
Berger 2009 n = 70 (Med)[90]	90 EUS-FNA or EUS-TCB: 99	94	93[b]	90[b]	98[b]
Storch 2006 n = 41 (V)[91]	No data	76	76	76	95
Storch 2008 n = 48 (Med)[92]	No data	No data	79	79	98
Ginés 2005 n = 39 (V)[93]	No data (n = 13)	92	No data	87[a]	97[a]
Polkowski 2009 n = 31 (SMT)[94]	Not performed	78	–	63[a]	–
Thomas 2009 n = 31 (GIW)[95]	Not performed	90	–	81[a] 90[b]	–
Saftoiu 2007 n = 30 (V)[96]	96.4	89.3	73.7[a, c]	68.4[a, c]	No data
Sakamoto 2009 n = 24 (P)[97]	100 (25-G) 79 (22-G)	50	25-G: 91.7[a, b] 22-G: 75[a]; 94.5[b]	46[a]; 92[b]	No data
Wahnschaffe 2009 n = 24 (V)[98]	No data (n = 13)	83	No data	79[a]	92[a]
Larghi 2004 n = 23 (P)[99]	Not performed	74	–	61[a] 87.5[b]	–
Levy 2003 n = 20 (V)[100]	No data	No data	60[a]	85[a]	90[a]
Varadarajulu 2004 n = 18 (V)[101]	100	83	89[a]	78[a]	94[a]

[a] Analysis of all cases (intention to diagnose).
[b] Analysis of all cases with adequate material.
[c] Analysis only of the 18 mediastinal mass lesions.
GIW, EUS-TCB of thickened gastrointestinal wall; Med, mediastinal EUS-TCB; NP, nonpancreatic EUS-TCB; P, pancreatic EUS-TCB; SMT, EUS-TCB of gastrointestinal submucosal tumors; V, EUS-TCB from various sites.

Table 10.12 Possible influences on diagnostic yield

Factors	Relevance	Problem
1) Target organ, target tissue		
Anatomic site	+	Problems in obtaining diagnostic material: pancreatic head (especially uncinate process) and neck, gastrointestinal wall lesions; interposition of vessels
Biological tissue characteristics	+	Problems in obtaining diagnostic material: benign lesions, well-differentiated ductal pancreatic adenocarcinoma
Type of neoplasia	++	Problems in obtaining diagnostic material: subepithelial gastrointestinal tumors, pancreatic cancer, cystic lesions
Vascularization of target lesion	+	Bloody contamination of aspirates
Size of lesion	+	Problems in obtaining diagnostic material: very small lesions, very large and necrotic mass lesions
2) Methodological aspects		
Type and diameter of needle	+	Influence on: diagnostic yield (cytology, histology), technical feasibility
Aspiration	+	Influence on: cellularity, yield of histological material, bloody contamination
Number of needle passes	++	Dependent on target organ, features of lesion, and needle type
3) Organization and structure		
Cooperation between endosonographer and cytopathologist	+	On-site cytology: possible improvement of diagnostic yield by 10–15%
Experience, training (endosonographer, cytopathologist)	++	Steep learning curve
Cytopathological methodology	+	Diagnostic improvement by immunohistochemistry and other auxiliary methods in special cases
Quality management	+	Reduction in inaccurate and uncertain diagnoses
4) Other factors		
Contamination: cells from the needle tract and pancreatic acinus cells	+	Differential-diagnostic problems, limitations of cytological evaluation
Contamination: blood	+	Obstructs assessment of smears

Influences on Diagnostic Yield

The diagnostic yield of EUS-NB is influenced by a wide variety of factors—the anatomic and structural characteristics of the target lesions, methodological aspects of the acquisition and processing of material, the level of experience and training of both the endosonographer and the cytopathologist, and the structure and organization of diagnostic centers (**Table 10.12**).

■ Technical Problems

There have been very few published reports on the number of cases in which EUS-NB was not technically possible—for example, due to technical problems, interposed vessels, the anatomic location, or failed needle penetration of very hard tissue. Voss et al. reported on 99 consecutive

EUS-FNAs of solid pancreatic lesions. EUS-FNA was not possible with a 22-gauge needle in nine cases. Biopsy was not carried out due to interposed vessels in four cases. Needle penetration into the tumor tissue was not possible in three cases. Anatomic problems (such as duodenal stenosis, duodenal mobility) prevented EUS-FNA in two further cases.[102] Very hard tumor tissue is a negative predictive factor for the success of EUS-FNA.[103] In a large series of 541 EUS-FNAs of solid pancreatic lesions, repeated endosonographic investigations turned out to be necessary. In seven of 24 patients who underwent repeated investigations, technical problems, interposed vessels, or ascites were the reason for failure of the first attempt at EUS-FNA.[104] The same investigators detected periduodenal venous collaterals in 22 of 338 patients (6.5%) undergoing EUS for pancreatobiliary disorders. Twenty-one of the patients had pancreatic cancer. Venous collaterals impeded transduodenal EUS-FNA in nine patients (41%). However, the investigators succeeded in carrying out transgastric EUS-FNA of the lesion or were alter-

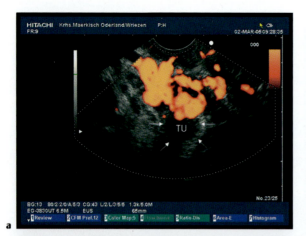

a

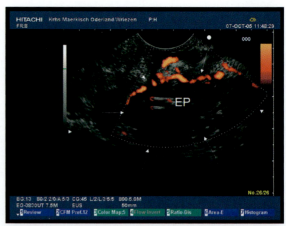

b

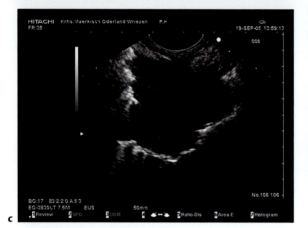

c

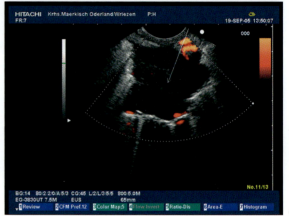

d

Fig. 10.2a–d Interposition of vessels in the needle tract.
a Peripancreatic portovenous collaterals in a patient with a small pancreatic tumor (TU, arrows).
b Small collaterals crossing the needle track in a patient with pancreatic cancer (the arrows mark the borders of the tumor). EP, endoprosthesis.

c A large mediastinal tumor adjacent to the esophagus before EUS-FNA.
d Color-coded duplex scanning shows vessels in the needle track.

natively able to sample liver metastases in six of these patients[105] (**Fig. 10.2**).

Mass lesions in the head and neck of the pancreas are difficult to sample, as the echoendoscope is in a "long" position. It may be difficult in this position to extend the needle from the accessory channel, and power transmission to the needle tip is impaired due to increased friction within the angulated needle shaft. A transduodenal approach to lesions in the pancreatic head using the large-caliber Tru-Cut and aspiration needles (19-gauge) is therefore not possible in most cases.[93,99,106] As a rule, it is always easier to position and move the needle if the echoendoscope is straightened. If the tumor is very hard or difficult to approach, it may be advantageous to use a 25-gauge needle with a pointed tip on the stylet. In technically challenging cases, we would suggest a controlled, step-by-step procedure: firstly, the gastrointestinal wall is penetrated. The thin wall of the duodenum and esophagus is not drawn aside by the needle, and penetration is there-

fore easy. Particularly in the upper third of the stomach, the more robust stomach wall tends to give way to the needle. We therefore prefer to thrust the needle forward through the gastric wall with a short, rapid, and powerful movement like a dart shot. After the gastrointestinal wall has been penetrated, the position of the echoendoscope and the angle of the needle are optimized to ensure contact between the transducer and the wall and to restore ultrasound control of the needle tip. The needle tip is now positioned in close contact with the surface of the target lesion. Very short, but rapid and powerful forward movements of the needle, repeatedly if necessary, will allow the penetration of the needle even into very hard tumor tissue.

Small lymph nodes that are embedded in loose connective tissue, as well as hard subepithelial tumors, may tend to evade the needle. In this situation as well, it is advisable to penetrate the gastrointestinal wall or its superficial layers in a first step. After the needle tip has been repositioned centrally on the capsule of the node or the surface of

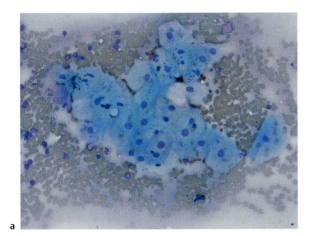

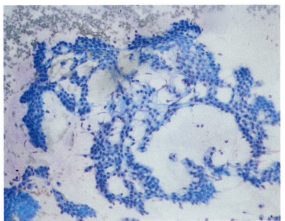

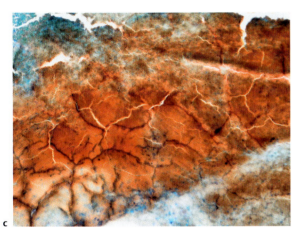

Fig. 10.3a–c Contamination of EUS-FNA specimens in some circumstances may lead to diagnostic confusion or may compromise the assessment of slides.
a Benign esophageal squamous cells.
b Benign gastric epithelia.
c Blood.

the tumor, it is possible to identify the optimal angle for advancing the needle into the lesion. Some groups have reported encouraging results in EUS-guided biopsy of very hard pancreatic and subepithelial tumors and of lymph nodes using an automated spring-loaded "power-shot" needle (Olympus NA-11 J-KB).[107]

■ Contamination

Contamination of cytological smears by epithelial cells or other cells from the needle tract is a common phenomenon in EUS-FNA. In one study, significant contamination of smears was noted in 23 of 72 cases (32%) and was reported to impede diagnostic interpretation.[108] In another study, normal duodenal or gastric epithelial cells and pancreatic acini were found in 52.4% of positive and suspicious cases and 93.8% of negative cases of EUS-FNA of pancreatic lesions, respectively.[21] Cellular contamination results in the aspirate being highly cellular, so that scarce malignant cells are overlooked (resulting in false-negative findings) or a neoplastic lesion is simulated (false-positive findings). Problems with differential diagnosis may arise

especially in cases of chronic pancreatitis, well-differentiated carcinoma (pancreas, lymph-node metastasis), cystic lesions of the pancreas, foregut duplication cysts, and mesenchymal tumors (**Fig. 10.3a, b**).[21,109–113] Pronounced bloody contamination as a result of inadvertent puncture of vessels near the target lesion, or when highly perfused lesions are being biopsied, also makes it difficult to assess aspirates (**Fig. 10.3c**).

Administration of acetylsalicylic acid (ASA), nonsteroidal anti-inflammatory drugs (NSAIDs), and low-molecular-weight heparin at prophylactic dosages has not been found to significantly increase the rate of blood contamination of EUS-FNA specimens from solid lesions. Bloody aspirates were seen in 5% of patients (one of 20) taking ASA, NSAIDs, or heparin and in 12.6% of control individuals (19 of 151).[114] Applying suction during EUS-FNA of lymph nodes led to poorer results in node aspiration by increasing the risk of a nondiagnostic bloody aspirate by factor of five.[115]

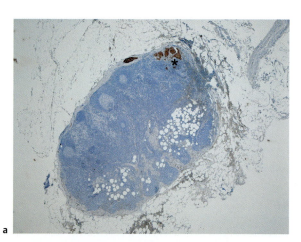

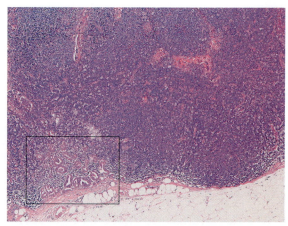

Fig. 10.4a, b Diminutive focal metastatic infiltrations on the edge of lymph nodes (markers), which are very difficult to sample with EUS-NB.

■ Features of the Target Lesion

Location of the Target Lesion

A large multicenter study by Wiersema et al.,[31] as well as three other studies,[20,24,116] showed that the rate of adequate specimens and the sensitivity were lower for lesions of the gastrointestinal tract wall in comparison with all other lesions. In solid pancreatic tumors, a location in the pancreatic head and accessibility of the lesion only from the descending duodenum are negative predictive factors for the diagnostic efficiency of EUS-FNA and EUS-TCB.[97,103] The actual location in the upper gastrointestinal tract may influence the yield of EUS-FNA for hypoechoic subepithelial tumors. In two studies, the diagnostic yield was found to be significantly higher for gastrointestinal stromal tumors (GISTs) located in the stomach in comparison with duodenal or esophageal GISTs.[67,117]

Size of the Target Lesion

In pancreatic tumors and lymph nodes, the diagnostic yield and accuracy of EUS-FNA were comparable when lesions had a diameter of up to 25 mm or larger than 25 mm.[42] Due to tumor necrosis in very large pancreatic masses, the negative predictive value of EUS-FNA may be unsatisfactory.[15] In another study, however, the sensitivity of EUS-FNA was significantly lower in lesions less than 10 mm in size in comparison with lesions with a diameter of 10 mm or more.[118] With regard to subepithelial tumors in the gastrointestinal tract, the diagnostic yield of EUS-FNA was lower for tumors < 20 mm in comparison with larger lesions.[64,117] In one study, EUS-FNA of very large subepithelial tumors (> 10 cm) proved to be unsuccessful in all cases.[67]

Focal Infiltration

Focal malignant infiltration of lymph nodes represents an obvious limitation of EUS-NB. Eloubeidi et al. used endoscopic ultrasound to examine 102 patients with esophageal cancer, searching for celiac lymph-node metastases. In patients with detectable celiac lymph nodes, the accuracy of EUS-FNA was 98%. In 14 patients in whom celiac lymph nodes were not endosonographically detectable, postoperative pathological investigation revealed the presence of 89 celiac lymph nodes with a median diameter of 5 mm (1–15 mm), 44% of which were malignant. The median diameter of metastatic infiltration in the EUS-negative celiac lymph-node metastases was only 4 mm.[119] Micrometastases in lymph nodes may be missed on EUS-NB (**Fig. 10.4**).

Histological Type

EUS-FNA of tumors with a high density of tumor cells (such as neuroendocrine tumors and malignant lymphomas) normally produces diagnostic samples with high cellularity. By contrast, EUS-NB of ductal adenocarcinoma of the pancreas yields much less cellular material, due to marked desmoplasia and surrounding inflammation.[21,112] In solid pancreatic and biliary mass lesions, the diagnostic yield and sensitivity of EUS-FNA are significantly impaired by the presence of chronic pancreatitis and marked acute inflammation.[19,25,30,52,120,121] In patients who ultimately have a benign condition diagnosed (chronic pancreatitis), the rate of nondiagnostic EUS-FNA of focal pancreatic mass lesions is significantly higher than in patients with a final diagnosis of ductal adenocarcinoma.[43,73] Significantly more needle passes are needed in order to diagnose well-differentiated pancreatic adenocarcinoma in comparison with pancreatic adenocarcinoma with moderate or poor differentiation.[122] Obtaining diagnostic material from cystic pancreatic tumors poses a challenge for the endosonographer. Aspirating the cyst contents yields extremely hypocellular samples, but biopsying small solid parts of cystic lesions or of the cyst wall involves technical difficulties. With the exception of one study,[34] therefore, the sensitivity of cytopathology alone for differentiating between mucinous and serous cystic lesions of the pancreas is reported to be unsatisfactory (27–60%) (**Table 10.6**; see also Chapter 18). The high cohesiveness of tumor cells limits the effectiveness of EUS-NB for assessing subepithelial spindle cell neoplasms in the gastrointestinal wall.[31,123]

■ Technical and Procedural Variables

Number of Needle Passes

The number of needle passes needed to obtain diagnostic material varies depending on the site, size, and type of lesion, and can potentially be optimized by immediate cytological assessment of the adequacy of specimens.[6,7,124,125] A systematic study of 109 patients in whom a 95% sensitivity rate for diagnosing malignancy was achieved showed that for lymph nodes and liver lesions, the number of needle passes needed for diagnosis (1.43 ± 0.66) was significantly lower than for solid mass lesions in the head of the pancreas (3.59 ± 2.29) or body/tail of the pancreas (3.10 ± 1.93). Cytological diagnosis of well-differentiated ductal adenocarcinoma of the pancreas required significantly more needle passes than diagnosis of moderate or poorly differentiated adenocarcinoma. A limitation to five needle passes in solid pancreatic lesions would have reduced the proportion of definitive cytological diagnoses by 13%.[126] The results of this and other studies concerning on-site cytological evaluation show that correct diagnosis of solid pancreatic lesions may require five to seven passes. In the case of lymph nodes, tumors of the liver, and lesions of the adrenal gland, two to five passes are estimated to be sufficient.[42,115,116,126,127] Factors increasing the number of needle passes necessary for definitive cytopathological diagnosis of solid pancreatic tumors are: a large diameter,[42] tumors with cystic parts (necrosis),[122] and a setting of chronic pancreatitis.[19] Interestingly, in one recent study conducted by three centers in Germany, gross macroscopic assessment by the EUS examiner of the adequacy of specimens for cytological and histological examination appeared to be sufficient to guide the number of needle passes, resulting in limitation of the number of needle passes to only one or two in 92% of patients with solid pancreatic masses. Macroscopic assessment failed in only 7% of cases for cytology and 13.5% for histology.[26] Another very recent study similarly showed that in the absence of on-site cytology, only two or three passes were needed to achieve a good level of accuracy for EUS-FNA of solid pancreatic lesions.[16] Various other groups with no access

to an on-site cytology service have reported similar experience.[30,83] The number of back-and-forth motions of the needle within a lesion needed to obtain diagnostic material has not been specifically investigated. Making ≈ 10 movements inside the lesion (with rapid inward thrusts and slow withdrawal) appears to be appropriate.[6]

Suction

Applying suction to the needle may increase the cellular yield of the aspirate, but on the other hand it may also increase artifacts and contamination with blood.[115] One study reported no difference between suction and no suction with regard to quality and diagnostic accuracy.[128] In another recent controlled study, EUS-guided fine-needle sampling with suction of solid masses increased the sensitivity and negative predictive value without increasing the overall bloodiness of each sample in comparison with the nonsuction group.[129] An in vitro study of EUS-FNA of lymph nodes favored continuous suction using a 5–10 mL volume instead of intermittent suction using larger syringes (20 and 30 mL).[130] In practical terms, we would suggest performing one or two needle passes with continuous suction first, and adding further passes without suction if very bloody aspirates are obtained.

There are a few data suggesting that EUS-FNA with high suction (30–35 mL) may make it easier to aspirate tissue cores suitable for histological investigation. Using continuous negative pressure with a 30-mL syringe in EUS-FNA (22-gauge) of solid pancreatic tumors, Voss et al. were able to obtain small core particles in 81% of cases.[102] Larghi et al. in EUS-FNA (22-G) of various solid tumors applied continuous high negative pressure suction at 35 mL with a 60-mL balloon inflation syringe and were able to obtain tissue specimens for histological examination with only one needle pass in 26 of 27 cases (96%). In two cases, in which cytological smears obtained by five needle passes using 5 mL suction failed to allow a definitive diagnosis, histological and immunohistochemical examination of the tissue cores established a diagnosis of neoplasia (recurrent thymoma, schwannoma of the gastric wall) or a benign condition (chronic pancreatitis, normal adrenal tissue).[131] However, a recent randomized study comparing EUS-FNA with high suction and EUS-TCB in various solid mass lesions was not able to reproduce these promising findings. Histological core particles were obtained in only 10 of 36 cases with high-suction FNA (27.8%), in comparison with 42 of 44 cases with EUS-TCB (95.3%).[132]

Selection of Lymph Nodes for EUS-NB

The assessment of lymph-node metastases is a crucial factor in oncological staging. Several guidelines recommend neoadjuvant treatment in cases of nodal involvement—for instance, in esophageal and rectal cancer, and

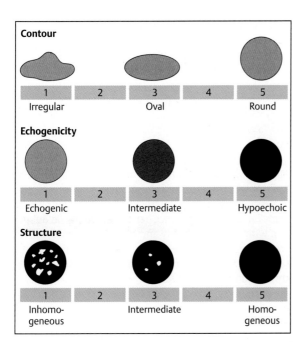

Fig. 10.5 Morphological scoring system for lymph nodes (adapted from D.O. Faigel).[140] Three lymph-node features are assessed using a visual analogue scale, resulting in a morphology score between 3 and 15. In 93% of lymph nodes with a morphological score of 3–6, the final diagnosis was benign. Approximately 50% of lymph nodes with an intermediate morphology score of 7–12, and 79% of lymph nodes with the highest morphology score (15) proved to be malignant. For esophageal cancer, lymph nodes with a diameter of >10 mm that were within 10 mm of the tumor, and which had a morphology score of 14 or 15, had a positive predictive value for malignancy of 87% when previous chemoradiotherapy was excluded.

only recently in gastric cancer. For non–small cell lung cancer (NSCLC) patients, metastasis to the contralateral mediastinal hilum (N3) is a negative prognostic marker, and surgery cannot be recommended in these patients. With ipsilateral mediastinal lymph-node metastases (N2), neoadjuvant treatment may be an option. Correct nodal staging and appropriate selection of lymph nodes for EUS-NB are therefore decisively important in most patients with suspected or proven malignancies.

Lymph-Node Size

Several pathological studies have shown that lymph-node size alone is not a reliable indicator for metastatic lymph-node infiltration in esophageal,[133] gastric,[134] colorectal,[135,136] or lung cancer.[137] In all of these types of cancer, metastatic lymph nodes are significantly larger than benign nodes. However, in patients with esophageal, gastric and colorectal cancer, more than 50% of metastatic lymph nodes are ≤5 mm in size.[133,135,137] In patients with non–small cell lung cancer without metastatic lymph-node involvement, 73% had at least one lymph node that was

≥10 mm in diameter. By contrast, 12% of patients with metastatic lymph-node involvement had no lymph nodes larger than 10 mm.[137] Despite the significant differences in diameter between metastatic and nonmetastatic lymph nodes, therefore, in gastrointestinal cancer and non–small cell lung cancer there is no definite correlation between metastatic involvement and the size of lymph nodes.

Sonomorphological Features

In addition to size, several other endosonographic criteria for malignant involvement of lymph nodes have been investigated. The standard EUS criteria typically used to assess malignant nodal involvement are based on a study of patients with esophageal cancer. In comparison with benign nodes, malignant lymph nodes are significantly more often hypoechoic, round or nearly round, and homogeneous, with a diameter ≥10 mm and smooth borders.[138,139] In addition, a short distance from the location of the primary tumor, an advanced primary tumor, the occurrence of groups of more than five lymph nodes, and the detection of lymph nodes at specific anatomical sites such as the celiac region, should raise a suspicion of malignant lymph-node infiltration.[119,140] Irregular nonshadowing, noncentral echogenic areas have been reported to correlate with coagulation necrosis and proved to be a very specific, although rather nonsensitive criterion for malignant infiltration of a mediastinal lymph node.[141] By contrast, benign lymph nodes are typically hyperechoic, heterogeneous, and small. They tend to have irregular borders, a triangular or flat shape, and a regular intranodal vasculature.[138–140,142]

However, the diagnostic selectivity of these ultrasound criteria is rather low. One study found all of the classic criteria of malignancy in only 25% of malignant nodes.[138] In rectal cancer, only 68% of malignant nodes were found to have three or more of four endosonographic features of malignancy. On the other hand, 48% of benign lymph nodes showed three echo features suggestive of malignancy.[143] For lung cancer, esophageal cancer, and pancreatobiliary cancer, 4–20% of lymph nodes that did not show any of the endosonographic features of malignancy proved to have malignant infiltration.[139,140,144,145] In patients with hilar cholangiocarcinoma, there were no significant differences in size or morphological appearance between benign and malignant lymph nodes.[146]

Assessing the size of the largest lymph node, the distance of the different lymph nodes from the primary tumor, and three morphological criteria (echogenicity, roundness, and homogeneity) on a five-point visual analogue scale, Faigel[140] was able to classify lymph nodes in only 25% of 238 cases with 80–90% certainty (**Figs. 10.5** and **10.6**). Using this morphological scoring system, the presence of at least one lymph node ≥10 mm with a distance of ≥10 mm from the primary tumor and with a morphology score of ≥14 (the prevalence of this pattern

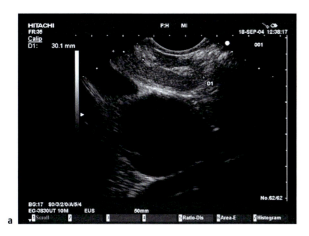 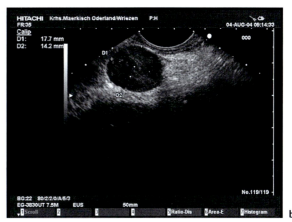

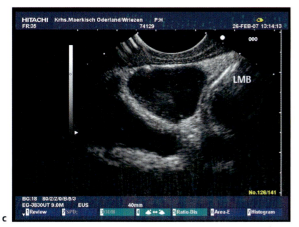 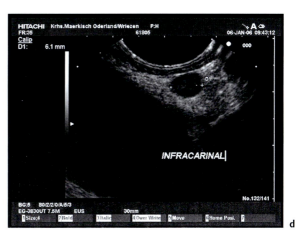

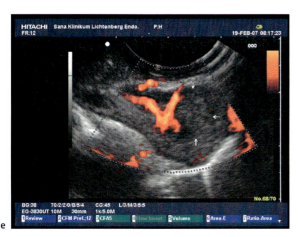 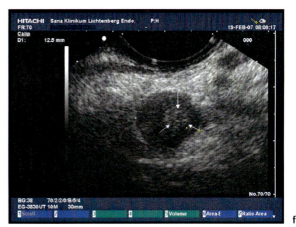

Fig. 10.6a–f Examples of lymph nodes with variable probabilities of malignant infiltration, based on the Faigel morphological score.[140]
a A typical benign, but large, subcarinal lymph node with distinct hilar structures (score 5).
b A typical malignant mediastinal lymph node in a patient with prostate cancer (score 13).
c A large subcarinal lymph node (score 14) in a patient without a known malignancy. EUS-FNA led to a diagnosis of sarcoidosis. LMB, left main bronchus.

d A small (6-mm) lymph node with typical malignant echo features (score 13) in a patient with non–small cell lung cancer. On the basis of the criteria used in computed tomography (CT), this lymph node would not be suspicious for malignancy. However, EUS-FNA confirmed malignant infiltration.
e, f Subcarinal and infradiaphragmatic lymph-node metastases in a patient with squamous cell cancer of the esophagus. The hyperechoic areas (arrows) are consistent with coagulation necrosis.

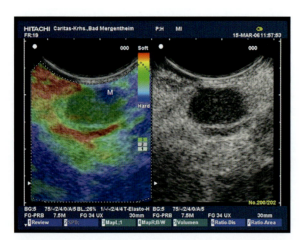

Fig. 10.7 A medium-sized hypoechoic mediastinal lymph node. Real-time elastography delineates a small area of hard tissue corresponding to metastatic infiltration (M). In this case, elastography may be helpful for targeting the needle.

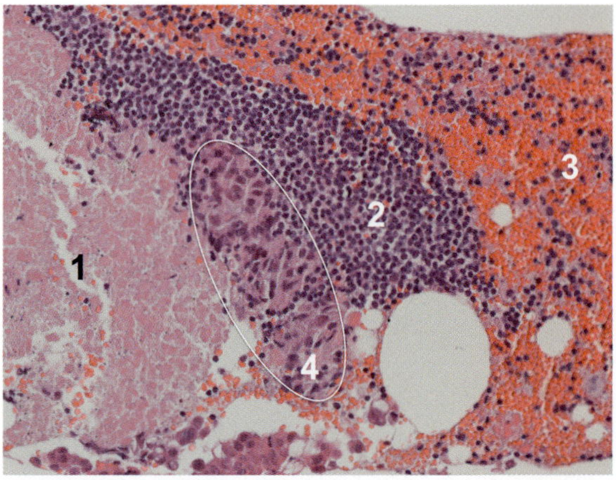

Fig. 10.8 Necrosis (1), normal lymph node tissue (2), red blood cell contamination (3), and malignant tumor cells (4, highlighted) in a specimen of mediastinal lymph-node tissue in a patient with non–small cell lung cancer (adenocarcinoma). (Hematoxylin–eosin, original magnification × 200.)

was 16% of cases) had a positive predictive value of 76%. On the other hand, a morphology score of ≤ 6 (occurring in 12% of cases) had a negative predictive value of 92%. However, 54% of the lymph nodes had an indeterminate morphological score of between 7 and 12.[140]

In view of the high background prevalence of inflammatory and reactive lymph nodes in the mediastinum, the reliability of endosonographic lymph-node features in this location appears to be much lower than for celiac nodes, for example.[140,147] In a northern European population with no malignant diagnoses, mediastinal lymph nodes were found in 62% of cases,[148] while in a North American population the rate was as high as 86% of cases.[149] On the other hand, abdominal lymph nodes were found in only 12% of northern European patients without malignancies—preferentially in the hepatoduodenal ligament in patients with current or previous acute pancreatitis. No celiac lymph nodes at all were detected in these patients.[148] In one study, the likelihood of a mediastinal lymph node being malignant was estimated to be 2.77 times lower in comparison with celiac, peripancreatic, perigastric, and perirectal lymph nodes.[147]

However, the classic[138,139] or modified[140,145] endosonographic lymph-node features may be helpful in selecting the most appropriate node for EUS-NB. Due to the limited accuracy of these predictive factors, EUS-NB even of small nodes with only an intermediate probability of malignancy should be performed in all cases in which proof of malignant involvement of a particular lymph node station would alter the management of the patient.[144] Hopefully, new ancillary endosonographic techniques (contrast-enhanced EUS, real-time elastography, EUS spectrum analysis) will not only improve differentiation between malignant and benign lymph nodes, but will also help identify

areas of malignant infiltration within a lymph node (**Fig. 10.7**).[150–156]

■ Targeting

Selecting the specific needle target within a tumor or lymph node may influence the diagnostic yield of EUS-FNA. In a metastatic lymph node, for example, preexisting lymphoid tissue may coexist with viable tumor cells and necrosis (**Fig. 10.8**).

For large, solid pancreatic tumors, the negative predictive value of EUS-FNA was found to be considerably lower in one large study in comparison with tumors with a diameter of less than 30 mm, presumably due to tumor necrosis.[15] In another study, the presence of intratumoral anechoic foci potentially representing necrotic areas was shown to be a significant predictive factor for the number of needle passes required to diagnose pancreatic cancer.[122] Particularly in larger tumors, therefore, the biopsy yield is likely to be higher if the needle is passed into the periphery of the lesion, rather than into its necrotic center or into areas with a "cystic" appearance.

In lymph nodes, metastatic infiltration selectively starts in the subcapsular sinus and only later occupies the entire parenchyma (**Fig. 10.4**). In one randomized controlled trial, however, selective sampling of the edge of the lymph nodes did not significantly improve the likelihood of a correct diagnosis in comparison with sampling the center of the lymph nodes.[115]

As a practical consequence of these data, the needle should be "fanned" throughout the lesion with multiple (rapid) forward and (slow) backward motions, gradually deflecting the scope tip or alternatively using the elevator.

In addition, ancillary endosonographic techniques such as contrast enhancement or elastography can be used to guide the needle in order to avoid puncture of necrotic areas.

■ Cytology or Histology? Needle Type and Needle Size

The 22-gauge needle is the standard needle for EUS-FNA. Thinner (25-gauge) as well as thicker (19-gauge) aspiration needles are less frequently used. The overwhelming majority of available studies have been conducted using 22-gauge needles and report on cytological examination of smears. Only a few centers have attempted to acquire histological material using aspiration needles (**Table 10.10**).[26,30,40,44,51,65,82–84,102,131,157] Histological diagnosis is reasonable in all cases in which diagnosis of a specific type of neoplasia is necessary, as well as in various benign diseases. Some neoplasms, such as malignant lymphomas, gastrointestinal mesenchymal tumors, rare pancreatic neoplasms, and well-differentiated adenocarcinomas, as well as some benign diseases (e.g., autoimmune pancreatitis) are difficult to diagnose solely on the basis of cytological examination. In the case of lymph-node metastases from an unknown primary lesion, it may be crucial to specify the malignant diagnosis using immunohistochemistry or gene expression profiling.

Aspiration Needles of Different Sizes

Various recent studies concur in suggesting that in terms of diagnostic yield in the cytological diagnosis of solid pancreatic lesions and various other types of lesion, the 25-gauge FNA needle is at least equivalent[14,158–160] or even superior[97,161] to the standard 22-gauge needle. A 25-gauge needle may be useful particularly for highly cellular and highly vascularized targets such as lymph nodes or neuroendocrine tumors, as well as in technically difficult cases (with excessive scope bending or angulation, or very hard lesions). With 22-gauge or 25-gauge aspiration needles, satisfactory cytological smears are obtained from solid pancreatic lesions in 87–100% of cases, from lymph nodes in 65–98%, and from various other lesions in 76–100% of cases (**Tables 10.6, 10.7, 10.8, 10.9**). However, most of these studies have focused on distinguishing between cancer and benign disease, rather than on the ability to diagnose a specific tumor entity. To achieve a specific diagnosis in benign as well as in malignant diseases, supplementary studies such as immunostaining, molecular studies, and flow cytometry may be necessary. In this setting, taking core biopsies using 22-gauge or 19-gauge needles may be advantageous. In one prospective study of technically successful EUS-NBs using the 25-gauge aspiration needle, histological diagnosis was feasible significantly less frequently in comparison with the 22-gauge

aspiration needle or the 19-gauge Tru-Cut needle.[97] Using 18-gauge or 19-gauge aspiration needles, it was possible to obtain core particles for histological analysis in 69–100% of cases.[40,106,157] Several groups have demonstrated that obtaining histological material is also feasible with the standard 22-gauge aspiration needle, with a comparable rate of 71–92% (**Fig. 10.9, Table 10.11**). In 131 consecutive EUS-FNA (22-gauge) procedures, mainly from lymph nodes, mediastinal tumors, the adrenal gland, and pancreatic lesions, our own group was able to obtain adequate material for histological assessment in 126 cases (96.2%). In four cases (3.1%), diagnosis was only possible on the basis of a histological examination of the core particles. In 18 cases (13.8%, with 11 benign diagnoses) only cytological diagnosis was possible. Immunohistochemical staining of paraffin-embedded material was necessary for specific tumor diagnosis in 10 cases (7.7%) (Wagner S, Jenssen C, Siebert C, 2007, unpublished data). Data from three centers in Germany have shown that in 166 of 192 cases (86.5%), it was possible to harvest adequate core specimens for histological assessment from solid pancreatic masses with a mean of 1.88 needle passes (22 G).[26]

One prospective, randomized, and controlled study compared the accuracy of EUS-FNA using the standard 22-gauge needle with that using the 19-gauge aspiration needle in patients with solid pancreatic and peripancreatic masses. The authors showed that the larger aspiration needle was advantageous for lesions in the pancreatic body and tail and for technically successful biopsies.[162]

19-Gauge Tru-Cut Needle

The yield of EUS-TCB has varied widely in several studies, in the range of 53–93% (**Fig. 10.10, Table 10.11**). In one large tertiary referral center, adequate samples were obtained in 215 of 247 patients (87%), and the overall sensitivity for diagnosing malignancy was 71%. The yield of EUS-TCB was independently predicted by the site of biopsy (transgastric procedures were better than transduodenal ones) and by the number of needle passes (more than two was better than two or fewer).[85] The use of EUS-TCB is limited by technical problems, especially in targeting pancreatic head lesions[85,87,97,100,106,163] and small lesions,[93] and by the higher costs of the technique in comparison with aspiration needles.

In a group of patients with various lesions and in patients with mediastinal lesions, Săftoiu et al. and Berger et al. showed that specific diagnosis of malignant tumors and granulomatous disease was achieved significantly more often using the 19-gauge Tru-Cut needle than with the 22-gauge aspiration needle. This was particularly important in cases of lung cancer, mediastinal lymph-node metastases, neuroendocrine tumors, malignant lymphoma, and mesenchymal tumors.[90,96] Case studies and small series have also demonstrated that EUS-TCB may be particularly valuable for diagnosing autoimmune pancreatitis,[164] unexplained thickening of the gastrointestinal

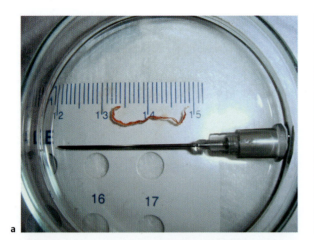

a

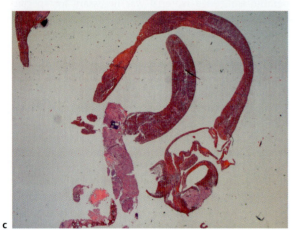

c

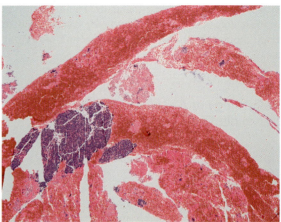

b

Fig. 10.9a–c The yield of EUS-FNA using aspiration needles (22-gauge, 19-gauge). In ≈ 80% of cases, it is possible to obtain small core particles suitable for histological assessment (**a** reproduced with permission from [124]).

a A core particle (EUS-FNA, 22-gauge needle).

b The specimen contains coagulated blood, fibrin, and small fragments of tumor tissue. Poorly differentiated cancer; material obtained from a lymph node using a 22-gauge needle. (Hematoxylin–eosin, original magnification × 40.)

c The core particles obtained using 19-gauge aspiration needles are slightly larger. Squamous cell cancer of the lung; material obtained from a celiac lymph node. (Hematoxylin–eosin, original magnification × 40.)

wall,[85,95] cystic pancreatic tumors,[127–129,165,188] gastrointestinal stromal tumors,[75,94,96,166] malignant lymphomas,[90,167] nonmalignant hepatic parenchymal disease,[168,169] and rare benign and malignant lesions that are difficult to diagnose.[170–173]

Aspiration Needles versus the 19-Gauge Tru-Cut Needle

In 24 patients with solid pancreatic masses, the overall accuracy rates for the 25-gauge aspiration needle, 22-gauge aspiration needle, and 19-gauge Tru-Cut needle were reported to be 91.7%, 75.0%, and 45.8%, respectively.[97] All other studies have shown that the diagnostic efficacy of EUS-TCB is comparable with that of EUS-FNA (**Table 10.11**).[86,87,90–92,96,100,101,106] Interesting laboratory simulations have shown that there is very high resistance to the advancement of 19-gauge needles (aspiration needles, Tru-Cut needles) through the instrumentation channels of echoendoscopes in an upward-angulated position. The maneuverability of the endoscope and ability to angulate the Albarrán lever were reduced when 19-gauge needles were used. Only the 22-gauge or 25-gauge FNA needles appeared to be suitable for insertion into the target

regions if tight angulation of the endoscope or of the Albarrán lever were necessary.[163]

■ Cytology and/or Histology

A combination of cytological analysis with histological and immunohistochemical assessment is capable of enhancing diagnostic accuracy (**Tables 10.9** and **10.10**). This applies to "dual sampling" (EUS-FNA and EUS-TCB in one session),[87,88,90,91,96] "sequential sampling" (firstly EUS-FNA or EUS-TCB and then the complementary method in a second examination, as required),[86,93,98,167] performing touch imprint cytology from tissue cores obtained with EUS-TCB,[89] and to the sampling of material by EUS-FNA for cytological smears as well as formalin-fixed core particles or cell blocks for histological analysis.[26,51,82,83,157,174–176] Particularly in cases in which there is a suspicion of metastasis from an unknown primary, pancreatic neoplasia other than ductal adenocarcinoma, malignant lymphoma, sarcoidosis, and gastrointestinal mesenchymal tumors, we would suggest complementing cytological smears with core biopsies or cell blocks, allowing for histological inves-

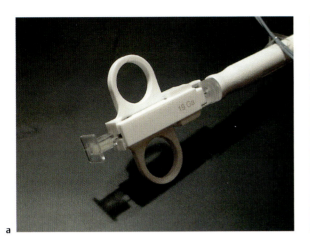

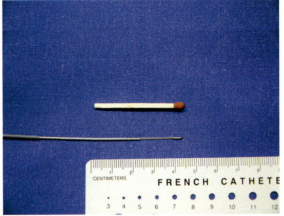

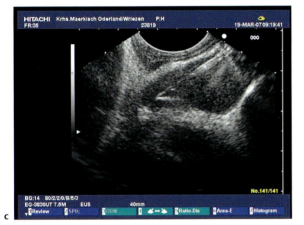

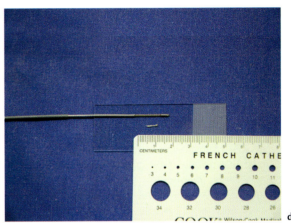

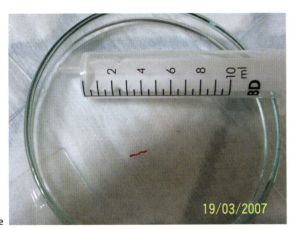

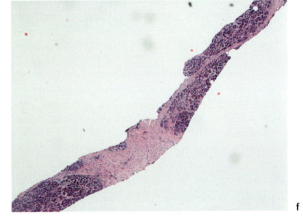

Fig. 10.10a–f 19-gauge Tru-Cut needle (Quickcore, Wilson-Cook).
a The handle of the device.
b The extended tip of the needle, with the tissue tray.
c The extended needle tip inside a subcarinal lymph node.
d The extended needle tip with a core particle from a solid lesion in the pancreatic head.
e A core particle obtained with a Tru-Cut biopsy from the lymph node.
f Microscopic assessment of the same particle, showing chronic fibrosing pancreatitis. (Hematoxylin–eosin, original magnification ×40.)

tigation, immunohistochemical staining, and other ancillary examinations. Depending on the size and site of the target lesion, as well as the individual risk assessment, this is possible either with EUS-guided aspiration using a 22-gauge or 19-gauge aspiration needle or by combining EUS-FNA (25-gauge, 22-gauge) and EUS-TCB (19-gauge) in selected cases.[7,124]

On-Site Cytology

Rapid on-site evaluation (ROSE) of the adequacy of specimens and preliminary cytological diagnosis is carried out in many centers in the United States, but this is not commonly done in Europe. The aim with ROSE is to provide immediate feedback regarding the quality and adequacy of the aspirates obtained with EUS-FNA in order to optimize the efficacy of the procedure. Selected smears are air-dried, immediately stained using a quick stain, and assessed for the adequacy of tissue sampling by a cytopathologist or a cytotechnician who is present in the endoscopy suite or in an adjacent room. Rapid on-site evaluation takes ≈ 5 minutes for each needle pass. EUS-FNA is continued until diagnostic material is obtained, avoiding an unnecessarily high number of needle passes. It has been claimed that on-site cytology thus potentially shortens the procedure, improves the yield of EUS-FNA, reduces the rate of inadequate aspirates, and lowers the costs of the procedure, as well as potentially decreasing potential complications and obviating the need for repeat diagnostic procedures.[6,126,177] In addition, real-time cytopathology reviewing allows an immediate preliminary diagnosis. The preliminary diagnoses resulting from ROSE are highly reliable; in three large studies, they differed from the definitive diagnoses in only 5.8%,[178] 8.4%,[179] and 11.5%[180] of cases, respectively. Depending on the preliminary diagnosis, it is also possible to allocate material for ancillary studies (microbiological culture, flow cytometry, cell-block techniques, immunochemistry, and molecular studies) if necessary.[181]

Although several experts advocate the use of on-site cytopathology, there are few data to support the claim that EUS centers should allocate resources for ROSE. Klapman et al. retrospectively compared the diagnostic yield of EUS-FNA samples between two academic hospitals that did and did not have facilities for performing rapid on-site cytological interpretation. The EUS-FNA procedures at both institutions were performed by the same endoscopist. Patients in the hospital with a cytopathologist were more likely to have a definitive diagnosis of malignancy and were less likely to have inadequate sampling or require a repeat procedure.[182] However, there have as yet been no prospective, randomized, and controlled trials to confirm that ROSE improves the sensitivity and/or effectiveness of EUS-FNA. Some retrospective comparative studies have reported that ROSE reduces the number of needle passes needed for diagnosis, improves the rate of conclusive diagnoses, and increases the total diagnostic yield of EUS-FNA by 10–15%.[16,182,183] In a large multicenter study, however, only the negative predictive value of EUS-FNA for extraintestinal mass lesions proved to be significantly better in two centers with on-site cytology in comparison with two other centers in which ROSE was not available. The sensitivity, specificity, accuracy, and positive predictive value of EUS-FNA of lymph nodes, extraintestinal mass lesions, and mural lesions in the gastrointestinal tract did not differ between centers with or without on-site cytology.[31]

ROSE also has several shortcomings. EUS has expanded from being available at only a few academic centers to community hospitals and outpatient endoscopy units. In Germany, for example, there are now some 800 centers providing EUS facilities, representing approximately 40% of all hospitals in the country.[1] The majority of these smaller centers are not capable of providing on-site cytology at the time of each EUS-FNA. Despite potentially reducing the number of needle passes needed, ROSE may slightly increase the costs of EUS-FNA and the procedure time required for it. In addition, an on-demand cytopathology service creates several challenges for the cytopathologist with regard to work flow, time management, resource allocation, and reimbursement of expenditure. Alternative options are therefore still being investigated—for example, telecytopathology for on-site cytology diagnoses, or assessment of the adequacy of specimens by cytotechnologists, EUS assistants, or endosonographers without the need for a cytopathologist to attend. The results of these studies have been inconsistent. For example, the ability of cytotechnologists or trained endosonographers to carry out on-site evaluation of the adequacy of smears obtained with EUS-FNA is a matter of controversy. In one study, three experienced endosonographers who had completed formal cytology training with the cytopathologist were found to have a poorer ability to interpret the adequacy of specimens in comparison with cytotechnologists.[184] In a recent study, by contrast, ROSE conducted by the endosonographer himself proved to be as effective as ROSE by a cytopathologist.[185] In solid pancreatic masses, gross visual assessment of smears by trained EUS assistants or by cytotechnologists was shown not to be as reliable as ROSE.[186] On the other hand, another study showed that assessment of the gross appearances of FNA specimens reliably predicts the adequacy of the samples.[187] For specific types of lesion (e.g., cystic pancreatic lesions), the gross visual appearance of the aspirated material may also provide valuable additional information toward a specific diagnosis.[187,188] One retrospective study recently suggested that telecytopathology may be an appropriate substitute for ROSE, showing that it was statistically equivalent in accuracy to rapid on-site cytopathological examinations of EUS-FNA specimens from pancreatic lesions.[189]

Experience, Training, and Dialogue

The skill and experience of both the EUS examiner and the cytopathologist play a key role in the diagnostic yield of EUS-NB. A large multicenter study showed that the accuracy of EUS-FNA of lymph nodes, extraintestinal mass lesions, and mural lesions of the gastrointestinal tract improved with time and growing experience. In the period from January 1994 to February 1995 (92%, n = 226) accuracy was significantly higher than in the initial period from January 1991 to December 1993 (80%, n = 193).[31]

On the basis of the published learning curve for a single endosonographer with limited experience (with 130 independent EUS examinations) in EUS-FNA of pancreatic lesions, it appears that at least 30 EUS-FNA procedures are required before the sensitivity for diagnosing pancreatic adenocarcinoma reaches 80%, and that 50 procedures are needed to constantly achieve a sensitivity of ≈ 90%.[190] However, the learning curve also needs to continue after this initial experience. Approximately 150 EUS-FNAs of pancreatic lesions proved to be necessary to gain comprehensive expertise in EUS-FNA of the pancreas, not only with regard to a reliably high accuracy, but also in terms of safety and efficiency.[191]

Another study impressively emphasized the invaluable significance of hands-on training. Mentoring was provided by an endosonographer with 12 years' experience in endoscopic ultrasound (more than 10,000 EUS examinations and more than 2500 EUS-FNAs). A very brief training period substantially improved the performance of three endosonographers with very limited experience in EUS-FNA (only 20 procedures in a 17-month period, with no supervision).[192] These data provide support for the American Society for Gastrointestinal Endoscopy (ASGE) recommendation that at least 150 supervised procedures, including 50 EUS-FNAs (25 pancreatic and 25 nonpancreatic) have to be performed in order to achieve comprehensive competence in all aspects of EUS.[193]

The diagnostic success of EUS-FNA depends of course not only on the endosonographer's experience, but also on the cytopathologist's expertise. In comparison with CT-guided and TUS-guided biopsies, the material obtained with EUS-NB has several special features—for example, contamination by gastrointestinal epithelia from the needle track.[113,124] This may cause difficulties for general pathologists and cytopathologists who have no experience in EUS-FNA. The problems can be overcome through training courses and dialogue. One recent study showed that following a short but intensive training session, experienced general pathologists who had little experience with EUS-FNA followed a steep learning curve, resulting in markedly improved reproducibility of their cytological diagnoses from EUS-FNA of mediastinal lymph nodes.[194] In a gastroenterological tertiary referral center, the percentage of nondiagnostic specimens from EUS-FNA similarly decreased significantly from 27% to 6% after a 1-month joint training period in EUS-FNA cytology for cytopathologists and endosonographers.[81] Experience at a large academic EUS center clearly demonstrates that the usual learning curves for EUS examiners and cytopathologists in EUS-FNA depend on the tissues that are targeted and are much steeper for lymph nodes than for pancreatic lesions. In a high-volume center in the United States, an acceptable rate of less than 10% for nondiagnostic (inadequate, atypical, or suspicious) findings and false findings (false-negative and false-positive cases) was achieved after 48 EUS-FNAs of mediastinal lymph nodes had been carried out, in comparison with 171 (nondiagnostic) and 186 (misdiagnosed) pancreatic EUS-FNAs.[195]

Whatever approaches to EUS-NB a specific center prefers, continuous and direct dialogue between the endosonographic examiner and the cytopathologist is the cornerstone of diagnostic success. The major prognostic and therapeutic impact of cytopathological diagnoses resulting from EUS-FNA or EUS-TCB requires a sense of shared responsibility.[7,124,125,181,196]

Handling, Preparation, and Processing of EUS-NB Specimens

The aspirate is initially expressed from the needle by slowly advancing the stylet. Once the stylet has been completely advanced onto the tip of the needle, a 2–10-mL air-filled syringe should be used to express further material. After the last needle pass has been completed, the final step should be to flush the needle with saline to expel all remaining material from it. There are several promising approaches to preparing the material obtained with EUS-FNA, and each of them has its own advantages and drawbacks. To obtain the maximum diagnostic information, complementary use of different preparations is worthwhile. For cytological analysis, smears (air-dried or alcohol-fixed) or liquid-based preparations can be used alternatively. For histological and immunohistochemical examinations of paraffin-embedded sections, small core particles and cell blocks can be used. Aspirates from different lesions should be carefully separated from each other. Unambiguous marking of each sample or smear is mandatory.[181]

Cytological Smears

Cytological smears can be prepared by the endoscopist, by a trained endoscopy nurse, by a cytotechnologist, or by a cytopathologist. The smearing technique requires appropriate training, and is described in detail in Chapter 11. Properly produced smears are decisive for establishing an unequivocal diagnosis. Appropriate fixation of cytology specimens is crucial to the preservation of the cellular

Table 10.13 Advantages and disadvantages of different fixation methods

Criteria	Air-dried smears	Wet-fixed smears	Liquid-based preparations
Rapid staining and on-site examination	+++	–	–
Dependence on smear technique	+++	++	–
Artifacts	Cellular and nuclear spreading, exaggeration of pleomorphism, condensation of chromatin	Shrinkage and rounding of cells	Optimal preservation of cells, some shrinkage, but significant changes in cellular architecture (e.g., disaggregation of cell clusters)
Extracellular background	Heavy, extracellular substances highlighted	Modest	Clean, almost complete disappearance of extracellular substances (e.g., mucins)
Cytoplasmic details	Well demonstrated	Poorly differentiated; good cytoplasmic transparency; visible keratinization	Preserved
Nuclear details and chromatin quality	Limited delineation	Highlighted	Enhanced nuclear features, prominent nucleoli
Stromal components	Well differentiated	Poorly demonstrated	Poorly demonstrated
Partially necrotic tissue	Poor definition of cell details	Good definition of intact single cells	Good definition of intact single cells

components. Depending on the planned staining technique, two types of smear can be prepared: air-dried or alcohol-fixed.[181] The specific fixation method used determines subsequent staining and also modifies the cells in various ways. Fixation and staining consequently highlight different cytological details (**Table 10.13**). Air-dried smears are typically stained using a Romanowsky stain—for example, May–Grünwald–Giemsa (MGG) or Diff-Quick (Chapter 11). Air-dried smears allow rapid staining (Diff-Quick or Hemacolor), followed by on-site assessment of smears. Immunocytochemistry in particular is possible using air-dried material. Other stains, such as the periodic acid–Schiff (PAS) reaction, Alcian blue, Ziehl–Neelsen, or Gram can be used, depending on the diagnostic needs in each specific case. If a smear is air-dried, it should not be placed in an alcohol fixative and must not be exposed to formalin or formalin fumes, which alter the cells and interfere with the staining reactions. Romanowsky stains are commonly used to examine blood smears and bone-marrow aspirates, and are therefore also suitable for evaluating lymph-node aspirates. Alcohol fixation preserves nuclear features well and is typically followed by Papanicolaou (Pap) or hematoxylin–eosin (H&E) staining. It is important to prevent air-drying before alcoholic fixation.

Liquid-Based Monolayer Preparations

Preparations such as Autocyte, ThinPrep, and Pap-Spin are interesting alternatives for processing samples obtained by EUS-FNA. The sample is placed in a specific transport and fixative medium. In an automated process, slices are prepared with a uniformly monolayer cell dispersion. The theoretical advantages of these preparations are that they do not depend on an individual smear technique; they eliminate mucus, erythrocytes, and protein precipitates from the sample; and there is highly consistent cell preservation, with an increase in diagnostic material with high cellularity on the slide and optimal assessment of single cells. In addition, ancillary studies (immunocytochemistry, DNA analysis) are possible using these monolayer preparations.[181] However, interpretive difficulties may arise as a result of disaggregation of cell clusters, loss of characteristic extracellular features (e.g., mucin in mucinous pancreatic neoplasms), and alteration of some cytological features. There is as yet only limited experience with liquid-based preparations of material obtained by EUS-FNA. Two nonrandomized studies have shown that liquid-based preparations are less sensitive in comparison with conventional smears after EUS-FNA of pancreatic lesions and lymph nodes.[197,198]

Cell Blocks

Cell blocks can be prepared from aspirated fluids (cyst contents, ascites, pleural fluid), from the needle rinse, and from part of the material collected in the proprietary fixative used for liquid-based preparations. They can be useful adjuncts to smears for establishing a more definitive cytopathologic diagnosis.[176] The effectiveness of cell blocks lies in the availability of diagnostic material for further histological examination, histochemistry, and immunohistochemistry for better typing of malignancies, and for identifying the infectious cause with microbiologic stains. A wide range of histological fixatives has been used for cell-blocks—primarily, neutrally buffered formaldehyde solution, Bouin solution, picric acid fixative, Carnoy fixative, and ethanol. Following a series of centrifugations, the resulting pellet undergoes routine formalin fixation, paraffin embedding, and sectioning for standard hematoxylin–eosin staining and a variety of other stains and immunohistochemical studies.[181] Sufficient material for cell-block preparation can be obtained in more than half of EUS-FNA procedures.[36,42] The overwhelming majority of studies have reported an increase in diagnostic information, particularly in cases of neuroendocrine and mesenchymal tumors, cystic lesions, and lymphoma.[21,28,34,41–43,45,62,74,112,174] Additional passes for cell blocks are highly recommended for lesions that may require ancillary studies, whenever core particles are not obtained by EUS-FNA.

Histology and Immunohistochemistry

Core particles that are sufficient for traditional histological techniques are obtained by EUS-TCB in 80–90% of cases (**Table 10.11**). However, depending on the specific method used to handle the samples, this can also be done with EUS-FNA using 22-gauge and 19-gauge needles (**Table 10.10**). After the material has been expelled from the aspiration needle onto slides, a gross visual inspection of the slides is carried out, looking for small tissue particles and cylinders of coagulated blood. These particles and cylinders are withdrawn from the slides using a small needle and placed in a formalin solution. The remaining material is smeared onto the slides and air-dried or fixed with alcohol. In our experience, these cylinders consist not only of blood and fibrin clots, but very often also contain small tissue fragments that can be processed for traditional histological assessment and ancillary studies (**Fig. 10.9**).

Molecular Studies and Flow Cytometry

Several studies have shown that molecular analyses are feasible with samples obtained using EUS-FNA.[199] Material for molecular studies has to be protected from potential RNA degradation by immediate cooling and incubation with a specific medium containing ribonuclease inhibitors. For flow-cytometric analysis, material from approximately three additional needle passes is collected into either heparinized, phosphate-buffered saline or a tissue culture transport medium containing calf serum, such as Hanks solution or Roswell Park Memorial Institute (RPMI) medium. Flow cytometry of EUS-FNA specimens has been shown to improve the diagnosis of non-Hodgkin lymphoma significantly.[44,59,200–203]

Microbiology

Case studies have shown that EUS-FNA is useful for obtaining samples suitable for fungal and bacterial cultures.[204,205]

Reliability of Diagnoses and Diagnostic Pitfalls

There are several possible reasons for misdiagnoses in the cytopathological interpretation of material obtained with EUS-NB: sampling error, inadequate sample processing, errors in interpretation by the cytopathologists, and insufficient dialogue between the clinician, endosonographer, and cytopathologist (**Table 10.14**). There are few published data relevant for assessing the scale of difficulties and errors occurring in cytopathological interpretation of material obtained with EUS-FNA.

■ Reproducibility of Cytopathological Diagnoses

Only two studies have analyzed the reproducibility of cytopathological diagnoses of specimens from EUS-FNA, both documenting good to excellent diagnostic agreement between experienced cytopathologists in assessing EUS-guided fine-needle aspiration samples from mediastinal lymph nodes and mass lesions. In one study, the kappa value for diagnostic agreement between two experienced cytopathologists was 0.88.[76] Another study compared the level of diagnostic agreement regarding materials obtained with EUS-FNA and endobronchial ultrasound–guided transbronchial needle aspiration (EBUS-TBNA) between pathologists with different levels of experience before and after an educational session. There was excellent reproducibility between the two observers, who were both highly experienced in assessing mediastinal fine-needle aspirates ($\kappa = 0.89$ and 0.87). The reproducibility of diagnoses made by experienced pathologists with little experience in EUS-FNA and EBUS-TBNA improved markedly following a training session.[194]

Three studies showed a very high level of agreement between preliminary on-site cytopathological diagnoses and final diagnoses. The on-site diagnosis and final diagnoses differed in only 51 of 656 cases (8.4%),[179] 80 of 1368 cases (5.8%),[178] and 52 of 485 cases (11.5%).[180] Scant cellularity or nondiagnostic material on the slides interpreted on site were the most frequent reasons for discrepancies, accounting for 21 of 51 (41%)[179] and 38 of 80 (47.5%)[178] cases, respectively, of disagreement between preliminary and final diagnoses. Cytopathological interpretation was difficult or discrepant in only 72 of 1934 cases (3.7%) and was ultimately possible using ancillary studies or intradepartmental/extradepartmental consultations in 40 (56%) of the 72 difficult cases.[178,179] The level of agreement between preliminary on-site diagnosis and final cytological interpretation was significantly better for malignant than for nonmalignant diseases (98.8% vs. 67.2%). Upgrading of preliminary diagnoses occurred more often than downgrading.[180]

Table 10.14 Possible influences on the diagnostic yield of EUS-guided needle biopsy

Factors	Relevance	Problem
1) Target organ / target tissue		
Anatomic site	+	Problems in obtaining diagnostic material: pancreatic head (especially uncinate process) and neck, gastrointestinal wall lesions; interposition of vessels
Biological tissue characteristics	+	Problems in obtaining diagnostic material: benign lesions, well-differentiated ductal pancreatic adenocarcinoma
Type of neoplasia	++	Problems in obtaining diagnostic material: subepithelial gastro-intestinal tumors, pancreatic cancer, cystic lesions
Vascularization of target lesion	+	Bloody contamination of aspirates
Size of lesion	+	Problems in obtaining diagnostic material: very small lesions, very large and necrotic mass lesions
2) Methodological aspects		
Type and diameter of needle	+	Influence on: diagnostic yield (cytology, histology), technical feasibility
Aspiration	+	Influence on: cellularity, yield of histological material, bloody contamination
Number of needle passes	++	Dependent on target organ and tumor type
3) Organization and structure		
Cooperation between endosonographer and cytopathologist	+	On-site cytology: possible improvement of diagnostic yield by 10–15%
Experience, training (endosonographer, cytopathologist)	++	Steep learning curve
Cytopathological methodology	+	Diagnostic improvement by immunohistochemistry and other auxiliary methods in special cases
Quality management	+	Reduction in inaccurate and uncertain diagnoses
4) Other factors		
Contamination: cells from needle track and pancreatic acinus cells	+	Differential-diagnostic problems, limitations of cytological evaluation
Contamination: blood	+	Obstructs assessment of smears

■ False-Negative and False-Positive Diagnoses

The frequency of false-negative diagnoses varies and mainly depends on the type of target lesion involved. In cases with adequate material, it has been estimated at 8–9% for EUS-FNA of lymph nodes, 0–25% for EUS-FNA of biliary strictures, and 4–25% for EUS-FNA of solid pancreatic lesions (**Tables 10.6, 10.7, 10.8, 10.9**). In patients with chronic pancreatitis, the sensitivity of EUS-FNA for diagnosing pancreatic cancer is still low, and in several studies has been reported to be only in the range of 44–74% (see Chapter 16).[19,25,82,120,121] On the basis of these data, it should be borne in mind that there is still a significant risk of malignancy with negative findings in EUS-NB, particularly in solid pancreatic and biliary lesions.

The specificity and positive predictive value of cancer diagnosis with EUS-FNA have been estimated at 100% in the overwhelming majority of studies. A thorough review of studies on EUS-FNA conducted in 2008 was able to identify only 10 studies (with a total of 1750 cases) and

one case study reporting on a total of 27 false-positive diagnoses using EUS-FNA.[7] In the majority of these cases, benign pancreatic conditions (such as chronic pancreatitis, intrapancreatic splenic heterotopia, and mucinous cystic adenoma) were misdiagnosed as ductal adenocarcinomas or neuroendocrine pancreatic tumors (**Figs. 10.11** and **10.12**).[17,18,41,63,76,77,102,119,206,207]

A recent study of a group of 377 patients in whom the EUS-FNA results were positive or suspicious for malignancy, and who underwent surgery without neoadjuvant therapy, identified 20 false-positive cases (5.3%) when only "positive" cytopathological interpretations were regarded as indicative of malignancy, and 27 false-positive cases (7.2%) when "suspicious" findings were also taken into account. Half of the cases of disagreement resulted from malignant cell contamination during EUS-FNA of lymph nodes in cases of luminal cancer (mostly esophageal). The other 50% of retrospectively inconsistent cases were attributed to interpretive errors by the cytopathologists.[208] The same group identified malignant cells in gastrointestinal luminal fluid not only in 48% of patients with luminal cancer, but also in 10% of patients with ex-

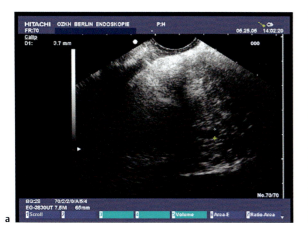
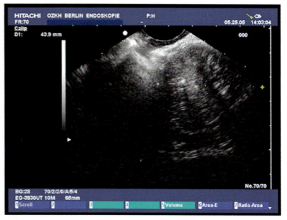

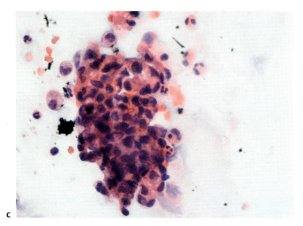
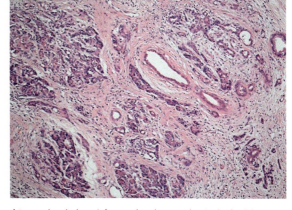

Fig. 10.11a–d A false-positive diagnosis of pancreatic cancer in a patient with chronic pancreatitis.
a, b The enlarged head of the pancreas.
c EUS-FNA, showing clusters of atypical epithelial cells. The diagnosis was "suspicious for malignancy." (Hematoxylin–eosin, original magnification × 400.)

d Surgical pathology (after a Whipple procedure). The final diagnosis was chronic sclerosing pancreatitis; there was no evidence of cancer. (Hematoxylin–eosin, original magnification × 400.)

traluminal (pancreatic) cancer undergoing EUS-FNA.[209] This shows that technical aspects of EUS-FNA—such as inadvertent aspiration of contaminated luminal fluid or traversing an area of mucosal high-grade dysplasia or malignant infiltration of the gastrointestinal wall—may be possible reasons for false-positive EUS-FNA findings.[210]

■ Difficult Differential Diagnoses and Diagnostic Pitfalls

The risk of misdiagnosis is greatest when the differential diagnosis includes entities with very similar cytological morphologies (cellular mimicry) and when a specific diagnosis is not expected—for example, in patients with very rare neoplasms.[113,125,196]

Pancreatic Adenocarcinoma, Focal Chronic Pancreatitis, Benign Pancreatic Glandular Epithelium

The cytopathological criteria for *ductal adenocarcinoma* of the pancreas are well established and include increased cellularity with predominance of one cell type, three-dimensional (overlapping) cell groups, loss of regular nuclear arrangement ("drunken honeycomb"), pleomorphic single cells, anisonucleosis, increased nuclear–cytoplasmic ratio, coarse and clumped chromatin, irregular nuclear contours, macronucleoli, coagulation necrosis, and atypical mitoses.[112,113] The use of various methods of processing the aspirates (air drying, immediate alcohol fixation, various stains) has a substantial influence on the individual diagnostic weight assigned to these features. Ductal adenocarcinoma is difficult to distinguish from *focal chronic pancreatitis* due to concomitant desmoplastic reaction and inflammation. Reactive inflammatory epithelial alterations may mimic well-differentiated cancer (see

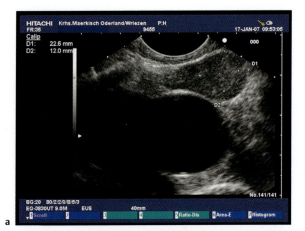

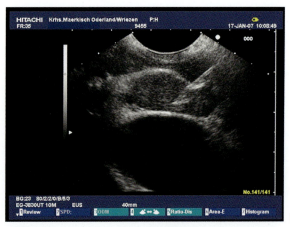

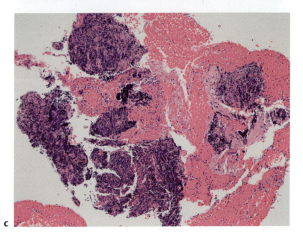

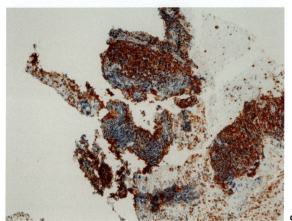

Fig. 10.12a–d A suspicious subcarinal lymph node in a patient with idiopathic mediastinal lymphadenopathy.
a EUS: intermediate likelihood of malignancy.
b EUS-FNA.
c Cytopathological suspicion of small cell lung cancer. (Hematoxylin–eosin, original magnification × 100).

d Immunohistochemistry (original magnification × 100): positive staining with leukocyte common antigen, CD45 (LCA), negative staining with monoclonal antibodies for cytokeratins AE1/AE3, thyroid transcription factor-1 (TTF-1), chromogranin A, and synaptophysin (not shown). The final diagnosis was artificially modified lymphatic tissue.

Fig. 10.11) (Chapter 16).[19,25,73,120,207] In addition, due to the close proximity to the lesion and contamination with glandular cells from the gastric or duodenal mucosa (see **Fig. 10.3b**), increased cellularity is a typical feature of FNA samples obtained under EUS guidance.[112]

It is very difficult to differentiate between focal *autoimmune pancreatitis* and solid pancreatic neoplasias using transabdominal ultrasound, computed tomography, and EUS-FNA.[164,211–214] Some recent studies have suggested that EUS-TCB may be a safe and accurate diagnostic procedure in patients with suspected autoimmune pancreatitis.[164]

A large number of complementary cytopathological and molecular techniques aimed at improving the unsatisfactory ability to distinguish between pancreatic adenocarcinoma, focal chronic pancreatitis, and intraductal papillary mucinous neoplasms in the pancreas have recently been described. These ancillary methods include immunochemical stains for biomarker profiles and proliferation

markers (e.g., monoclonal carcinoembryonic antigen, CA 19-9, B72.3, B7-H4, p53, Smad4, mesothelin, clusterin-beta, survivin, NQO1, mucin profiles, and Ki-67),[109,215–218] as well as molecular tests (DNA arrays for detecting microsatellite instability or K-*ras* point mutations and expression profiling of tumor-associated genes).[82,219–224] For example, three studies have demonstrated that specific mucin expression profiles may facilitate cytomorphological diagnosis of pancreatic ductal adenocarcinoma and pancreatic mucinous neoplasms in EUS-FNA specimens.[225–227] In addition, an immunohistochemical panel of mucin antibodies (MUC1, MUC2, MUCAC5, MUC6), as well as other biomarkers, have proved to be highly suitable for cytomorphologic differentiation between pancreatic neoplasms, reactive ductal atypia, and inadvertently sampled gastroduodenal mucosa.[109,218,226] K-*ras* mutations are not observed in samples of chronic pancreatitis obtained at EUS-FNA, but are present in some 70% of cases of pancreatic cancer.[82,219] When K-*ras* point mutation analysis was added to cytological assessment, Takahashi et al. were able to improve the diagnostic accuracy of EUS-FNA for suspected pancreatic cancer from 82% to 94%.[82] Similar results were obtained in a French multicenter study in which the authors demonstrated that in EUS-FNA of solid pancreatic masses, a combination of inflammation and fibrosis with wild-type K-*ras* is strongly suggestive of a benign condition (mass-forming pancreatitis).[219]

In a study in which cases of pancreatic cancer in which EUS-FNA cytology was not diagnostic, another investigation showed that overexpression of telomerase is a helpful marker of malignancy. Overall, in 98% of all pancreatic adenocarcinomas sampled by EUS-FNA, either diagnostic cytological findings (75% of cases) were obtained or telomerase overexpression was detectable (79% of cases).[223] Similarly, broad-panel microsatellite loss and K-*ras* point mutation analysis was reliably performed on EUS-FNA samples from pancreatic masses and improved the reliability of differentiation between malignancies and benign lesions (chronic pancreatitis, autoimmune pancreatitis).[221]

Cystic Lesions of the Pancreas

Differential diagnosis of cystic pancreatic lesions is challenging. The diagnosis should be based on a combination of the patient's history, clinical data, endosonographic morphology, cytomorphological features, and biochemical analysis of cyst fluid (Chapters 16 and 18).[34,112,113,228]

Cytology. Aspirates of cystic pancreatic lesions obtained with EUS-FNA have the drawback that in a high percentage of cases they contain gastrointestinal contaminants from the needle track (see **Fig. 10.3b**). Neoplastic low-grade glandular epithelium of mucinous pancreatic neoplasms and its mucinous contents are sometimes virtually indistinguishable from these contaminants. Goblet cells, which are normal constituents of the duodenal mucosa and intestinal metaplasia in the gastric mucosa, may also be present in the epithelium of mucinous neoplasms. Consequently, contamination of the EUS-FNA needle with epithelial cells and mucinous contents of the stomach or duodenum may lead to misinterpretation of bland pseudocysts or serous cystic adenoma. Conversely, aspirates from neoplastic mucinous lesions often lack both mucin and mucinous epithelium. An absence of mucin and mucinous epithelial cells on aspiration cytology therefore does not exclude a mucinous pancreatic neoplasm.[111,229–232] To provide a template for assessing mucin and epithelial contamination on pancreatic EUS-FNA specimens, Nagle et al. described specific cytomorphological and immunocytochemical baseline characteristics of duodenal and gastric mucosa and mucins. In both gastric and duodenal mucosa, the tumor marker B72.3 stained goblet cells with a strong, coarsely granular pattern and stained epithelial cells focally in a finely granular, punctate, perinuclear distribu-

tion; mucin also stained strongly in all cases.[109] In another very recent study, a lack of carcinoembryonic antigen (CEA) expression was more reliable than B72.3 for identifying both gastric and duodenal contamination.[233]

As a consequence of sampling difficulties, the differential diagnosis and grading of cystic pancreatic lesions on EUS fine-needle aspirates is challenging (**Figs. 10.13** and **10.14**).[230,232]

Papillary structures, which are diagnostic of *intraductal papillary mucinous neoplasms* (IPMNs), are not common in fine-needle aspirates from low-grade IPMNs. However, in cases in which there is a markedly dilated pancreatic duct, with or without a side branch cyst, the presence of thick "colloidlike" mucin is consistent with an IPMN. There are some cytological features that can predict the histological grade. Tight epithelial clusters of cells with a high nuclear–cytoplasmic ratio and an inflammatory smear background support the presence of a neoplasm with at least moderate dysplasia. Epithelial cells with pale nuclei and parachromatin clearing, as well as the presence of necrosis, are suspicious for (pre)malignant IPMNs.[230,234] *Mucinous cystic neoplasms* (MCNs) are histologically defined by an ovarian stroma, which is unfortunately not verifiable on cytological smears (**Figs. 10.13** and **10.14**).[232] Cytological features of MCNs are honeycombed sheets and clusters of mucin-containing cells. In addition, MCNs have abundant mucin in their background.[232] However, *duplication cysts* closely mimic low-grade MCN, which can lead to false-positive diagnoses.[235] EUS-FNA specimens from *serous cystadenomas* (SCAs) only very rarely contain glycogenated serous epithelial cells, which are the typical feature of these benign pancreatic cystic lesion.[111,229–232] One recent study suggested that recognizing hemosiderin-laden macrophages in a clean, nonmucinous background may serve as a clue to diagnosing a highly vascularized SCA.[229] Correct prospective diagnosis of benign *lymphoepithelial cysts* of the pancreas may be hindered by their very infrequent occurrence and some cytological pitfalls. Characteristic features are an often creamy or foamy aspirate, abundant anucleate squamous cells, a few benign-appearing nucleated squamous cells, amorphous keratinous debris, cholesterol crystals, and occasionally lymphocytes and multinucleate giant cells.[236,237] The cytological features of *pancreatic pseudocysts* (PCs) are frequently nonspecific. In one study, a definitive cytopathological diagnosis of pseudocyst was possible in only 10% of cases. The majority of smears (75%) from PCs revealed neutrophils and/or histiocytes. Yellow-pigmented material was identified in 31% of the aspirates from PCs, but was not observed in neoplastic mucinous cysts. Special stains for mucin (Alcian blue, mucicarmine) did not distinguish pseudocysts from neoplastic mucinous cysts.[238]

Due to these problems, the sensitivity of EUS-FNA cytology for diagnosing cystic pancreatic lesions is considerably lower than for solid pancreatic lesions. Although the sensitivity of EUS-FNA for identifying mucinous cystic

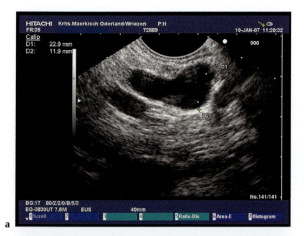

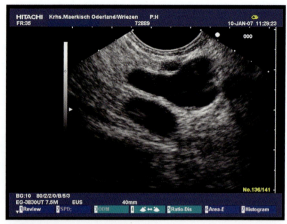

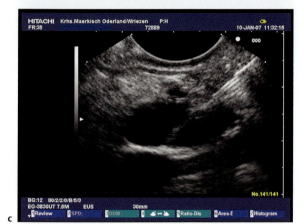

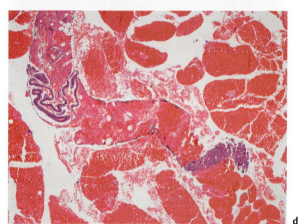

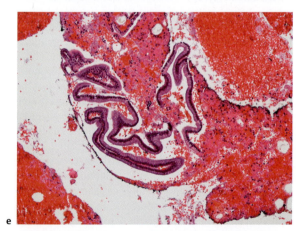

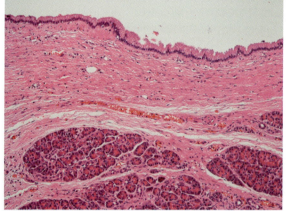

Fig. 10.13a–f A 64-year-old woman with an incidental ultrasound finding of a hypoechoic lesion in the pancreatic body.
a, b EUS: several small cysts without any solid components.
c EUS-FNA (22-G): there are clear cyst contents with low viscosity, CEA 450 ng/mL, very hypocellular smears.
d, e Histology (hematoxylin-eosin, original magnification ×40 and ×100). There are small core particles containing a large amount of blood, but also monolayered mucinous epithelia without any atypia, normal pancreatic tissue, and small amounts of connective tissue. The preoperative diagnosis was a benign mucinous cystic neoplasm (MCN).
f Surgical pathology confirmed the diagnosis, showing a multilocular mucinous cystadenoma with typical ovarianlike stroma and focal mucinous hyperplasia (PanIN 1a).

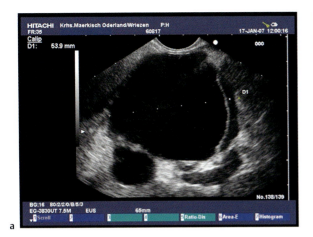

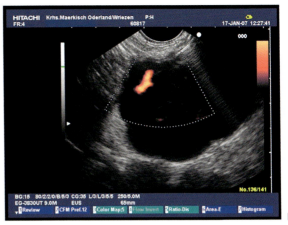

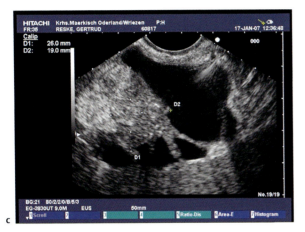

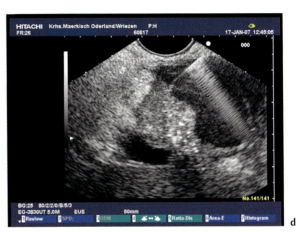

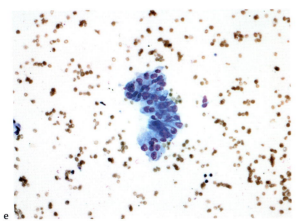

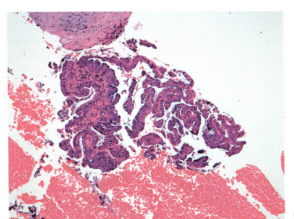

Fig. 10.14a–h A 65-year-old woman suffering from nonspecific abdominal symptoms. Computed tomography identified a cystic tumor in the splenic hilum.

a EUS: a large cystic lesion in the tail of the pancreas.

b EUS-FNA (22-gauge), with aspiration of viscous fluid (the color-coded area represents cyst contents flowing into the needle). The carcinoembryonic antigen (CEA) level was well above detection limits.

c, d Following aspiration of cyst contents, solid parts of the lesion were detected and sampled using EUS-FNA (22-G).

e Cytology: a cluster of atypical columnar epithelium (May–Grünwald–Giemsa, original magnification × 100).

f, g Histology (**f**: hematoxylin–eosin, original magnification × 100) and histochemistry (**g**: periodic acid–Schiff, original magnification × 100) show a mucinous papillary tumor with partially PAS-positive cytoplasm. There is no cytopathological proof of malignancy, but the excessively high CEA level is predictive of a malignant mucinous cystic neoplasm.

Fig. 10.14 g, h ▷

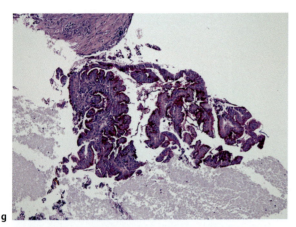
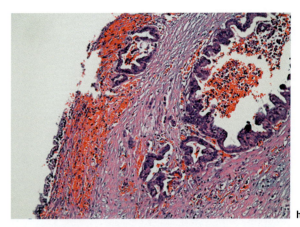

Fig. 10.14 g, h (continued)

h Surgical pathology: mucinous cystadenocarcinoma.

pancreatic lesions was as high as 97% in a recent study,[34] some studies have reported a sensitivity of only 10–59%.[33,231,238–240] However, when biochemical analyses of cyst fluid, histology, immunohistochemistry, and mucin stains are added to cytology alone, the diagnostic accuracy increases to 80–90%.[33,228,241]

Fluid markers. Despite considerable overlap, CEA has the greatest diagnostic value among fluid markers for distinguishing between nonmucinous and mucinous cystic lesions. However, studies vary regarding the threshold value that best discriminates between definitely benign and (potentially) malignant lesions (Chapter 16, **Table 16.7**). The cooperative pancreatic cyst study found that a cut-off value of 192 ng/mL had an accuracy of 79% for differentiating mucinous from nonmucinous cystic lesions. The accuracy of CEA was significantly greater than the accuracy of EUS morphology (51%), cytology (59%), or any combination of tests.[33] In intraductal papillary mucinous neoplasms, a CEA level below 200 ng/mL and a CA 72-4 level below 40 U/mL had excellent predictive values for excluding malignant IPMN.[242] Higher cut-off levels—for example, 400 ng/mL—have a higher positive predictive value, but lower sensitivity for diagnosing mucinous neoplasia. A very high CEA level (> 6000 ng/mL) is predictive of malignancy.[241] The cyst-fluid levels of pancreatic enzymes may help differentiate pseudocysts from other cystic lesions without ductal communication.[34,243] Prostaglandin E_2 levels may help differentiate IPMNs from MCNs and may be useful to predict the dysplastic grade of IPMNs.[244]

Mucin stain and apomucin phenotype. In one study, the presence of mucin in samples from cystic pancreatic lesions proved to be a stronger predictor of mucinous cystic neoplasms of the pancreas than a CEA level of more than 300 ng/mL[245] (**Fig. 10.13**).

The expression patterns of mucin antigens may provide useful information for assessing the invasive potential of a cystic mucinous tumor. In a recent study, pancreatic tissues with noninvasive IPMNs, irrespective of the degree of atypia, were positive for MUC5AC and negative for MUC1. Conversely, lesions with invasive behavior expressed MUC1.[246] The mucin expression profile may also help distinguish between the rare benign mucinous nonneoplastic cysts, which originate from acinar duct mucinous metaplasia, and mucinous pancreatic neoplasms.[247] A combination of mucin profile, CD10, and CK20 can be used for differential diagnosis of MCN and branch duct IPMN.[248]

DNA mutational analysis. Molecular-genetic studies of cyst-fluid DNA, using loss of heterozygosity analysis, have recently shown that K-*ras* tumor suppressor gene mutations occur more frequently in malignant lesions than in benign lesions.[224,234,249,250] However, other studies have not reported that DNA mutational analysis is of any value in addition to the established practice of testing cyst-fluid CEA and cytomorphology.[251]

EUS-TCB and EUS-guided brushing. The results of limited series and case studies suggest that EUS-TCB of the cyst wall can provide histological samples[165] and that cytological brushing using a 19-gauge aspiration needle for access (the Echo Brush)[252] can provide sufficient material to identify the type of cystic pancreatic neoplasia and detect malignant transformation.

Comprehensive view of clinical data and history, EUS morphology, fluid markers, and cytopathology. Due to the significant differences in natural history and prognosis between the various types of cystic pancreatic lesion, the final pretherapeutic diagnosis determines the indication for and the extent of pancreatic surgery, and ultimately affects the individual outcome for the patient. Despite recent developments, the preoperative diagnosis of pancreatic cystic lesions is still clearly difficult, and EUS-NB alone is unlikely to provide the high level of diagnostic accuracy necessary to allow a nonsurgical approach to asymptomatic cystic lesions in which there is no risk of malignant transformation. The decision on whether to proceed with nonsurgical management should not be based on a negative or nondiagnostic EUS-FNA alone, since according to one recent study, 67% of negative specimens and 92% of nondiagnostic specimens were associated with malignant or premalignant pathology.[239] Information about the patient's clinical data (sex, age, race, history of pancreatitis) and about morphological features on EUS and radiological studies (size, pancreatic duct dilation, wall thickness, ductal communication, mural protuberances and solid components), as well as information about the gastrointestinal wall structures traversed by the FNA needle (stomach, duodenum) is therefore decisively important for integrated cytopathological and clinical diagnosis of cystic pancreatic lesions. Exceptionally high cyst fluid CEA levels,[242,243,253–255] malignant cytology,[256,257] morphological features such as size, thickened wall, and intracystic solid growth,[253,254] and some patient-related factors (age, male gender, white race, weight loss, and other symptoms)[253,256,258] may help better predict cyst malignancy and the need for surgical treatment.

Rare Pancreatic Neoplasms (Neuroendocrine Tumor, Acinar Cell Cancer, Solid Pseudopapillary Tumor, Metastases, Lymphoma)

A reliable differential diagnosis between ductal pancreatic adenocarcinoma and the variety of other rare solid pancreatic neoplasms, including pancreatic metastases, provides the basis for appropriate treatment decisions.[16,228,259,260] The treatment options and prognosis differ widely between these tumors. *Solid pseudopapillary tumors* (SPTs) only very rarely have a malignant clinical course. By contrast, *acinar cell cancer* (ACC) has a particularly poor outcome. The aggressive potential *of neuroendocrine tumors of the pancreas* (P-NETs) varies. *Pancreatic metastases*—for example, from renal cell cancer, breast cancer, lung cancer, colorectal cancer, and malignant melanoma—account for 2–11% of solid pancreatic masses. The 5-year survival rate for patients with isolated pancreatic metastases from renal cell cancer and colorectal cancer who undergo radical surgery is much more favorable than that in patients with pancreatic cancer and pancreatic metastases from malignant melanoma or lung cancer. Remarkably, for solitary pancreatic metastases from renal cell cancer or colorectal cancer undergoing surgery, the 5-year survival may be more than 70%.[261,262] Nonsurgical diagnosis of *pancreatic lymphoma* typically results in a decision to carry out chemotherapy or chemoradiotherapy.

Four case series including 51 patients, as well as several case studies, have shown that EUS-FNA has the potential to diagnose pancreatic metastases from epithelial and mesenchymal tumors[263–266] as well as primary pancreatic lymphomas.[201]

Typical cytomorphological criteria in samples obtained with EUS-NB have been described for P-NETs, SPTs, and ACCs. There is considerable overlap among the cellular features ("cellular mimicry") between these different types of rare pancreatic solid tumor (**Table 10.15**).[77,112,113,259,263–272]

Immunochemical staining—with pancytokeratin, synaptophysin, chromogranin, vimentin, neuron-specific enolase (NSE), specific peptide hormones, or light chains—and molecular genetic techniques allow reliable differential diagnosis of these tumors (**Figs. 10.15** and **10.16**; see also **Fig. 18.6**).[77,112,113,259,263–272,274]

We have observed a case of P-NET in which a primary diagnosis of extramedullary plasmocytoma was corrected only by immunohistochemical verification of synaptophysin and chromogranin in the tumor cells (see **Fig. 18.18a–j**). Some of these tumors are also characterized by association with specific age groups or gender (SPT, ACC), typical endosonographic or radiological features (hypervascularization: P-NET, lymphoma, metastases), and specific symptoms or patient histories (functioning P-NETs, metastases, ACC). These data are helpful for assigning the scanty material obtained from EUS-FNA to selected immunochemical staining (**Table 10.15**). Determining the grade of malignancy of a P-NET is challenging. Proliferation markers (Ki-67) and DNA analysis (microsatellite loss) are potential predictive factors for aggressive biological behavior in P-NETs.[273–275]

Gastrointestinal Wall Lesions

Whereas cystic and hyperechoic subepithelial lesions in almost all cases are benign, the large and very heterogeneous group of hypoechoic subepithelial tumors poses a number of differential-diagnostic problems for the examiner. In our own patients, 247 of 346 (71.4%) nonvascular subepithelial lesions showed low echogenicity.[276] In addition to definitely benign tumors (leiomyomas, glomus tumors, granular cell tumors, schwannomas, pancreatic heterotopia, and inflammatory fibroid polyps), potentially malignant lesions such as gastrointestinal stromal tumors (GISTs), neuroendocrine tumors, leiomyosarcomas, malignant lymphomas, and submucosal metastases also typically appear as hypoechoic subepithelial lesions. The overwhelming majority of hypoechoic subepithelial tumors have a mesenchymal histogenesis (GISTs, leiomyomas, or schwannomas), and approximately three-quarters of these are GISTs.[123,277] Correct cytopathological diagnosis of hypoechoic subepithelial tumors in the gastrointestinal wall is therefore essential, as these lesions differ widely in their biological behavior and prognosis and therefore require different management strategies.

However, there are several problems in diagnosing this group of tumors using EUS-NB. Due to the high level of cellular cohesion present in most mesenchymal tumors, the yield of EUS-NB in mesenchymal subepithelial tumors is low in comparison with the results for lymph nodes and solid pancreatic tumors. The results of eight studies including a total of 523 patients showed an overall

Table 10.15 Differential diagnosis of rare solid pancreatic neoplasms (EUS and EUS-guided needle biopsy; data from[77,112,113,259,263–275])

P-NET	EUS morphology
	Often small, solid, hypoechoic, smooth outline, hypervascularized; sometimes capsulated
	Rarely cystic appearance
	Cytomorphology
	Distinctive cytomorphological variance
	Hypercellular aspirates
	Poorly cohesive population of monomorphic, small and medium-sized cells
	Moderate amount of cytoplasm with granules and vacuoles
	Pseudorosettes, sometimes acinar structures
	Bland, round to oval nuclei with smooth membrane and finely granular, sometimes coarse chromatin ("salt and pepper," "plasmacytoid appearance")
	Risk assessment
	Nuclear polymorphism, multinucleation, nucleoli
	Ki-67 > 2%
	Microsatellite loss (fractional allelic loss > 0.2)
	Immunochemistry
	Well-differentiated tumors: chromogranin, synaptophysin, NSE, PGP 9.5, CD56, peptide hormones, E-cadherin (membranous pattern), CK 10, CK 19
	Poorly differentiated tumors: NSE, PGP 9.5, CD56, synaptophysin, p53, often negative for chromogranin and peptide hormones

Tumor type	Potentially overlapping cytomorphological features	Criteria for differential diagnosis
SPT versus P-NET		**SPTs:**
	Highly cellular aspirates	*History:* almost exclusively young women
	Small, loose aggregates of small monomorphic cells, numerous single cells with small, round or oval nuclei	*EUS morphology:* large tumors with variable solid and cystic components
	Finely granular chromatin, small nucleoli, narrow cytoplasmic fringe, pseudorosettes, acini	*Cytomorphology:* branching papillae with fibrovascular stroma, nuclear dentations, PAS-positive nuclear inclusions
	CD56 +, NSE+, synaptophysin+	*Immunochemistry:* positive to vimentin, CD10, β-catenin, NSE; negative to chromogranin, cytokeratins, peptide hormones
ACC versus P-NET		**ACCs:**
	Hypercellular smears	*History:* predominantly older male patients, polyarthralgia, hyperlipasemia, multifocal necroses of fatty tissue
	Loosely cohesive cell clusters and single cells with finely vacuolized cytoplasm	*EUS morphology:* often very large tumors containing necroses and cystic areas
	Prominent nucleoli, irregularities of cellular membrane	*Cytomorphology:* larger, somewhat polygonal cells, acinar formations, coarsely clumped chromatin
		Immunochemistry: negative for neuroendocrine markers; positive for enzyme markers (trypsin, chymotrypsin, lipase)
Lymphoma and multiple myeloma versus P-NET		**Lymphoma, multiple myeloma:**
	Hypercellular aspirates	*Cytomorphology:* lack of cellular cohesion, scanty cytoplasm; coarse and clumpy peripheral chromatin pattern; irregular nuclear membrane
	Small monomorphic single cells	*Immunochemistry:* negative for neuroendocrine and epithelial markers; positive for lymphoid markers, plasma cell markers (CD138, light chains), leukocyte common antigen (LCA, CD45) in lymphoma
	Cellular mimicry of P-NET	

Additional difficult differential diagnoses
P-NET versus metastases of small cell cancer and of amelanotic melanoma
Clear cell P-NET versus metastasis of clear cell renal cancer
Helpful for discrimination: history of malignancy, multilocular metastases, immunohistochemistry (malignant melanoma: S-100, Melan-A, HMB-45; small cell lung cancer: TTF-1, cytokeratins, chromogranin, synaptophysin; renal cell cancer: CD10, vimentin)

ACC, acinar cell cancer; EUS, endoscopic ultrasonography; NSE, neuron-specific enolase; P-NET, neuroendocrine tumor of the pancreas; SPT, solid pseudopapillary tumor.

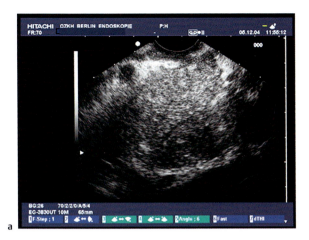

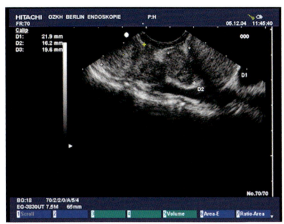

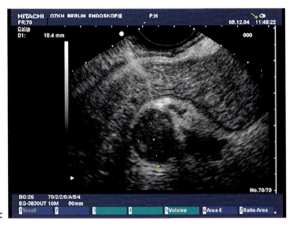

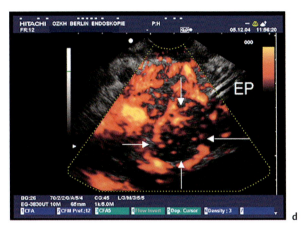

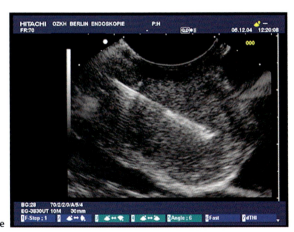

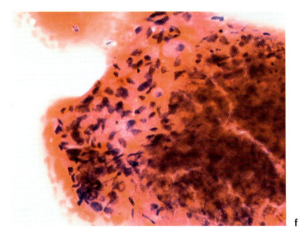

Fig. 10.15a–i A male patient with jaundice and double-duct sign on endoscopic retrograde pancreatography who was undergoing drainage of the biliary tract with a plastic endoprosthesis.

a–c EUS shows an enlarged pancreatic head without a clearly delineated mass lesion (**a**), and multiple suspicious lymph nodes in the mediastinum (**b**) and paraduodenal region (**c**).

d Contrast-enhanced EUS (SonoVue) shows a hypovascularized area in the enlarged pancreatic head (arrows).

e EUS-FNA of that part of the pancreatic head.

f–i Cytological (**f, h**: hematoxylin–eosin, original magnification ×100–×400) and histological (**i**: hematoxylin–eosin, x 100) confirmation of non–small cell cancer. Immunohistochemistry excluded a neuroendocrine tumor of the pancreas (not shown). The final diagnosis was acinar cell cancer.

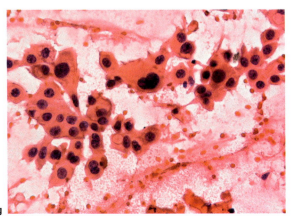

Fig. 10.15 h, i ▷

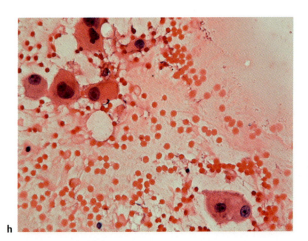
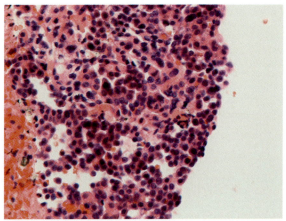

Fig. 10.15 h, i (continued)

diagnostic yield of 73% with EUS-FNA in subepithelial tumors (see Chapter 14, **Table 14.11**; **Table 10.9**). Even when EUS-NB of a subepithelial tumor is successful, differential cytological diagnosis between GISTs, other subepithelial mesenchymal tumors, and some types of epithelial tumor, is clearly difficult owing to overlapping between their cytomorphological features. Most gastrointestinal mesenchymal neoplasms are spindle cell lesions. Cytological features alone only rarely allow definitive discrimination between GISTs, leiomyoma, schwannomas, and other very rare mesenchymal neoplasms that have a spindle cell appearance. Smears from GISTs are more likely than leiomyomas to show occasional intact single cells with numerous stripped nuclei and cell groups with high cellularity.[113] When one is examining spindle cell fragments on smears and in cell blocks, concerns may also arise regarding their possible origin from the needle track through the deep muscle layer of the gastrointestinal wall. There are also difficulties in the differential cytological diagnosis of subepithelial tumors that have epithelioid cell pattern. Gastric glomus tumors, granular cell tumors, ≈ 25% of GISTs and leiomyomas, and occasional cases of schwannomas may have an epithelioid appearance and resemble epithelial neoplasms, particularly subepithelial neuroendocrine neoplasms and subepithelial metastases (**Fig. 10.17**).[113,277]

Two case studies have reported subepithelial metastases from ovarian cancer in the gastric wall, which appeared to be mesenchymal tumors arising from the muscularis propria on EUS. Correct diagnosis was possible with EUS-FNA using immunostaining (**Fig. 10.18**).[278,279]

Immunohistochemical analysis of a cell block or of core particles is therefore indispensable when diagnosing hypoechoic subepithelial tumors of the gastrointestinal tract using EUS-NB. It has been shown that phenotypic discrimination between the various types of mesenchymal subepithelial tumor is possible using a limited battery of immunostains (CD117, CD34, desmin or smooth-muscle actin, S-100 protein) on material obtained with EUS-FNA

or EUS-TCB (**Fig. 10.19**; see also Chapter 14, **Figs. 14.47** and **14.48**).[277]

There are also some rare and potentially difficult differential diagnoses, however. For example, 4–26% of GISTs are negative for c-*kit* (CD117), but may show focal immunoreactivity against smooth-muscle actin. These c-*kit*– negative GISTs are more likely to have epithelioid cell morphology (see Chapter 14). Other diagnostic pitfalls may be rare cases of subepithelially growing malignant melanomas, cancer metastases, clear cell sarcomas, Kaposi sarcomas, desmoid-type fibromatoses, solitary fibrous tumors, inflammatory fibroid polyps, and neuroendocrine tumors, which may be composed of epithelioid or spindle cells and are immunoreactive with some of the antibodies used to characterize GISTs, leiomyomas, and schwannomas. The differential diagnoses can be managed by careful interpretation of the hematoxylin–eosin sections and of the complete immunohistochemical panel, and by using antibodies to epithelial markers or specific antigens, to chromogranin, to β-catenin, to DOG1, and to PDGFR-α, in selected cases.[277] In addition to immunostaining, molecular analysis of mutations in the c-*kit* and PDGFR-α genes is possible in cell blocks or core particles obtained with EUS-NB and can be helpful when there is a difficult differential diagnosis.[280]

In addition to phenotypic differentiation between subepithelial mesenchymal tumors, the pretherapeutic diagnosis of these tumors should include information about possible malignancy. In GISTs, there are only a few cytological characteristics that suggest malignancy, such as dominant single cells or (very rarely) pleomorphic or hyperchromatic nuclei. However, cytological assessment of fine-needle aspirates is not sufficient to assess the biological behavior of GISTs.[113] In addition to the size of the tumor, the mitotic index characterizes the biological risk of GISTs. Core particles obtained with EUS-FNA and EUS-TCB are too small to be used to reliably assess the number of mitoses per 50 high-powered fields.[94] However, the

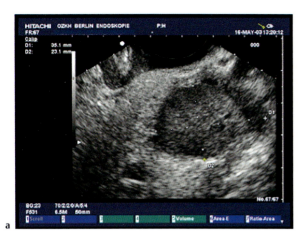

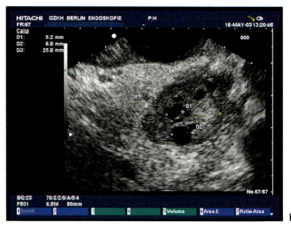

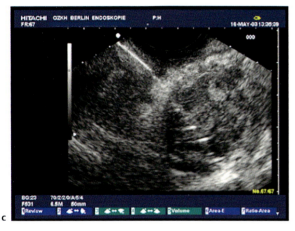

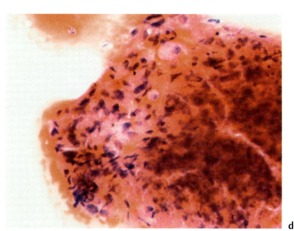

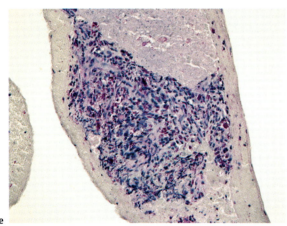

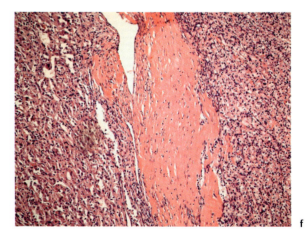

Fig. 10.16a–f A woman with a history of surgery for renal cell cancer 15 years previously.
a, b EUS shows a hypoechoic mass lesion in the head of the pancreas, with some small cystic areas.
c EUS-FNA (22-G).
d Cytology (hematoxylin–eosin, original magnification × 400): neoplastic cells with clear cytoplasm.

e Histology of the core particle (periodic acid–Schiff, original magnification × 200): a malignant tumor with PAS-positive tumor cells.
f Surgical pathology (hematoxylin–eosin, original magnification × 100): pancreatic metastasis from a clear cell renal cell cancer.

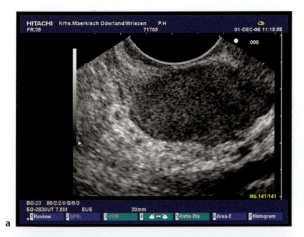

a

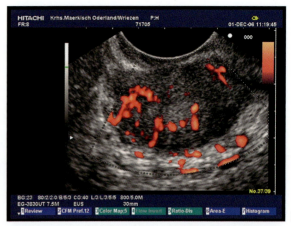

b

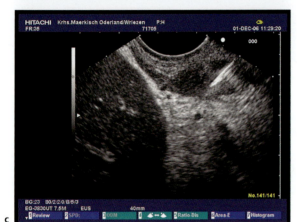

c

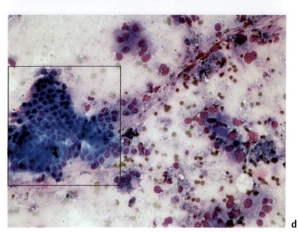

d

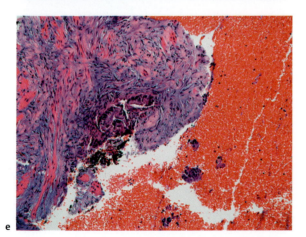

e

Fig. 10.17a–e A hypoechoic tumor in the body of the pancreas was detected in a 74-year-old female patient suffering from weight loss. EUS-FNA led to a diagnosis of ductal adenocarcinoma.

a, b EUS also shows a hypoechoic and hypervascularized tumor in the deep wall layers of the gastric antrum, with no association with any pancreatic structures.

c EUS-FNA (22-G).

d Cytology (May–Grünwald–Giemsa, original magnification × 200) revealed clusters of epithelial cells from the gastric wall (highlighted) and clusters of malignant cells (adenocarcinoma).

e Histology (hematoxylin–eosin, original magnification × 100): adenocarcinoma, with a pronounced desmoplastic reaction. Positive immunohistochemical staining with antibodies to CA19.9 but not to DPC4 (Smad4) made it possible to diagnose a gastric wall metastasis from the pancreatic cancer (not shown).

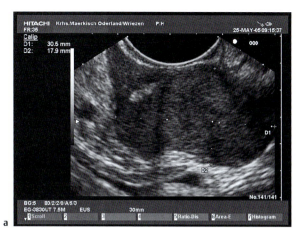

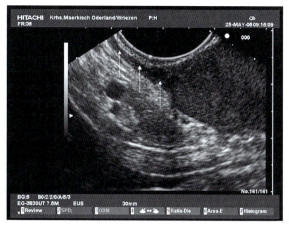

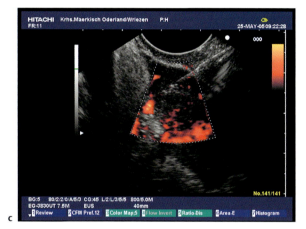

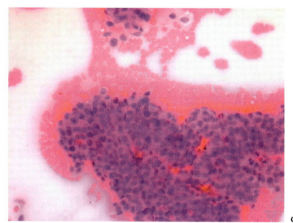

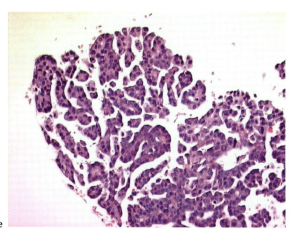

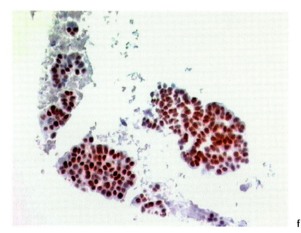

Fig. 10.18a–f A 39-year-old woman presented with weight loss, pleural effusions, and ascites of unknown origin. Esophagogastroduodenoscopy showed a distinct impression on the posterior wall of the gastric antrum.

a, b EUS depicts a large hypoechoic tumor in the gastric wall, apparently arising from the deep muscle layer (arrows).

c EUS-FNA (22-G).

d, e Cytology (**d**: May–Grünwald–Giemsa, original magnification × 200) and histology (**e**: hematoxylin–eosin, original magnification × 200) both show a malignant tumor with micropapillary cell clusters.

f The strong reaction of the tumor cell nuclei to Wilms tumor antigen (WT1) and negative staining to CD34 and CD117 (not shown) established a diagnosis of gastric wall metastasis from an ovarian cancer, which was later confirmed on computed tomography peritoneoscopy later. (Reproduced with permission from [278].)

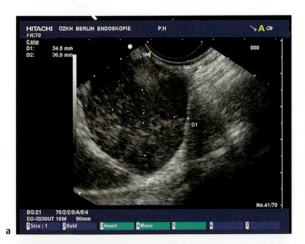

a

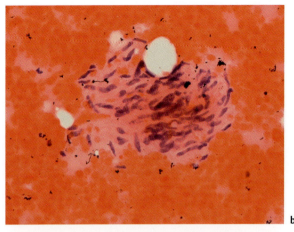

b

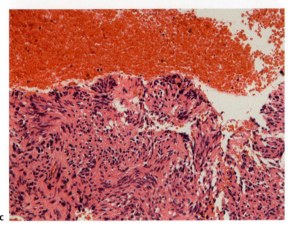

c

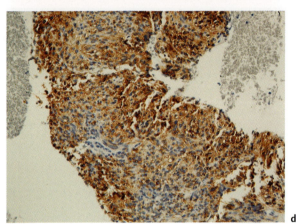

d

Fig. 10.19a–d A woman with an impression on the body of the stomach.

a EUS shows a hypoechoic tumor (35 × 37 mm) in the gastric wall, arising from the deep muscle layer. The patient decided against surgery, and EUS-FNA (22-gauge) was carried out. MP, muscularis propria; SM, submucosa.

b Cytology (hematoxylin–eosin, original magnification × 200), showing spindle cells with flat, elongated nuclei, indicating a mesenchymal tumor.

c Histology (hematoxylin-eosin, original magnification × 100), showing a typical fascicular cellular architecture, diagnostic of spindle cell mesenchymal neoplasia.

d Immunohistochemistry (c-kit, original magnification × 100): positive staining for CD117 established a diagnosis of gastrointestinal stromal tumor (GIST), and the patient then agreed to undergo surgical treatment (laparoscopic wedge resection) for the potentially malignant tumor.

presence of any mitosis in EUS-NB specimens of GISTs is highly suggestive of a high-risk GIST, and in two studies, the accuracy of a MIB-1 (Ki-67) index > 5% (or > 3%) in diagnosing a "malignant" GIST was high (see Chapter 14, **Figs. 14.47e** and **14.48e**).[65,80] Two very recent studies have shown that EUS-TCB is not superior to EUS-FNA in GISTs, due to the high rate of technical failure of the Tru-Cut needle.[94,166]

Lymph Nodes

There are two main indications for EUS-NB of lymph nodes: staging of malignant tumors (especially lung cancer, esophageal cancer, and pancreatobiliary cancer) and diagnosing lymph-node enlargement of unknown origin. One

of the major pitfalls is overinterpreting a lesion as positive for metastatic malignancy as a result of contamination with dysplastic or malignant cells when the needle passes through the primary tumor or dysplastic mucosa—for example, in Barrett's esophagus (**Fig. 10.20**).[36,210]

In patients with luminal cancer, contamination of gastrointestinal fluids and consequently of the needle with cells from the primary tumor may lead to false-positive lymph-node staging.[208,209] Repeat staging of lymph nodes after neoadjuvant chemoradiotherapy may be compromised by the presence of myxoid and hyaline changes, as well as necrotic material, in smears obtained with EUS-FNA. However, EUS-FNA has been found to be more accurate and to have higher positive predictive value than positron-emission tomography (PET) or CT for confirming

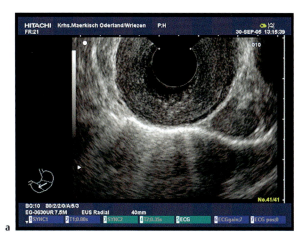

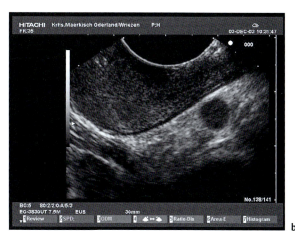

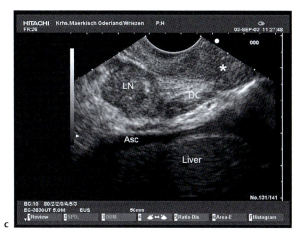

Fig. 10.20a–c Examples of lymph nodes in which EUS-FNA would only be possible by traversing the primary tumor with the needle. A positive result of a lymph-node biopsy would change the management, but on the other hand, there is a high risk of tumor cell contamination of the needle, resulting in a false-positive diagnosis of lymph-node metastasis and potential tumor cell seeding.
a Gastric cancer (T2) and a suspicious lymph node in the vicinity of the tumor (N1?).
b Cancer of the esophagogastric junction (T2) with probable lymph-node metastasis.
c Cancer of the esophagogastric junction (T3, asterisk) with probable metastasis to a celiac lymph node (LN). DC, diaphragmatic crus; Asc, ascites.

persistent malignant infiltration of mediastinal lymph nodes after neoadjuvant treatment.[112,281,282]

The major problem with lymph-node staging is sampling error. Despite careful aspiration using a fanning technique and a sufficient number of needle passes, focal malignant infiltration and micrometastases (see **Fig. 10.8**) may be missed. Two studies have investigated overexpression of telomerase and of markers specific for the primary tumor (CEA, CK19, LunX, PDEF, MUC1, KS1/4) in material obtained by EUS-FNA using reverse transcriptase polymerase chain reaction (PCR) as an indirect proof of micrometastatic involvement of mediastinal lymph nodes. Wallace et al. demonstrated overexpression of these markers in approximately 19% of cytology-negative lymph nodes and interpreted these findings as proof of micrometastases of lung cancer.[199,283] Using gene promoter hypermethylation, Pellisé et al. were able to increase the sensitivity of EUS-FNA for detecting lymph-node metastases from esophageal and other gastrointestinal cancers from 76% (with cytology alone) to 90% (with cytology and molecular assay).[284]

In EUS-NB of idiopathic lymph-node enlargement in patients with no history of malignant disease, the differential diagnosis is very broad, including nonspecific reactive lymphadenopathy, lymph-node silicosis, granulomatous disease (sarcoidosis, mycobacteriosis, fungal disease), metastases from a hitherto unknown primary tumor, and malignant lymphoma.[36,38,40,44,90,92,167,172,175,200,202,285–296] It is therefore essential in these cases to obtain sufficient material suitable for ancillary methods, including flow cytometry, molecular diagnosis, cytogenetics, and microbiological culture. We were able to diagnose tuberculosis in an EUS-FNA sample from an enlarged celiac lymph node using PCR in one patient (**Fig. 10.21**).

A frequent finding in EUS-FNA of enlarged mediastinal lymph nodes is granulomatous inflammation of the sarcoidosis type. In a retrospective study conducted by our own group, sarcoidosis-type granulomas were diagnosed using EUS-FNA in 18 of 120 patients (15%) with idiopathic mediastinal or abdominal lymphadenopathy (**Fig. 10.22**).

Despite the highly variable endosonographic features of lymph-node sarcoidosis (**Fig. 10.23**), cytopathological diagnosis of sarcoidosis using EUS-FNA has been shown to be very reliable[175,285–288,295] (**Figs. 10.24** and **10.25**).

If EUS-FNA provides cytological proof of lymph-node metastasis in a patient with no history of malignant disease, then immunochemical staining—for example, cytokeratin markers, tumor-specific antigens such as carci-

II Diagnostic Imaging and Interventions

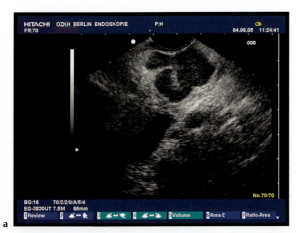

a

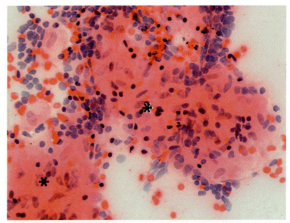

b

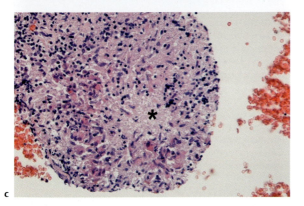

c

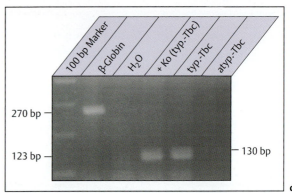

d

Fig. 10.21a–d A woman with abdominal symptoms and weight loss. Computed tomography showed a large lymph node (25 mm) at the celiac trunk.
a EUS shows a large suspicious lymph node. EUS-FNA (22-gauge) was performed.
b Cytology (hematoxylin–eosin, original magnification × 200), showed smears with a large amount of lymphocytes and some epithelioid cells (asterisks).
c Histology (hematoxylin–eosin, original magnification × 100), revealing an epithelioid cell granuloma with central necrosis (asterisk).

d Molecular genetics: confirmation of mycobacterial DNA by polymerase chain reaction. From left to right, the gel electrophoresis tracks show 1, the DNA size standard; 2, verification of amplifiable DNA in the sample from the patient (control gene: β-globulin); 3, negative control (H_2O); 4, positive control (*Mycobacterium tuberculosis*); 5, a sample from the patient, showing DNA from *M. tuberculosis*; and 6, a sample from the patient with no DNA from an atypical mycobacterium.

noembryonic antigen (CEA), prostate-specific antigen (PSA), vimentin, mucins, thyroid transcription factor-1 (TTF-1), estrogen receptor, progesterone receptor, S100 protein, Wilms tumor 1 (WT-1), HepPar, HMB 45, Melan-A, uroplakin—can in many cases allow conclusions to be drawn regarding the type and anatomic location of the primary tumor involved (**Figs. 10.26, 10.27, 10.28**).

Even for specialized cytopathologists, subtyping of malignant lymphomas on cytological smears is difficult and unreliable. Several studies have reported successful use of ancillary methods such as flow cytometry and immunochemical staining for specific lymphocyte markers in materials obtained with EUS-FNA[36,40,44,59,167,200–203] (**Fig. 10.29**). Ideal logistical arrangements and cooperation with specialized laboratories are obviously necessary here. On-site cytology is almost ideal for selective use of ancillary methods. If on-site cytology is not available, specific endosonographic features (e.g., large, very hypoechoic, round lymph nodes, bulky lesions, vascularization) can be used to guide the allocation of additional samples for flow cytometry and immunostaining.

Adrenal Glands/Retroperitoneal Tumors

When a mass lesion is detected in the adrenal glands in a patient with a history of malignant disease, particularly lung cancer, it is highly suspicious for—but by no means represents conclusive evidence of—adrenal metastasis. An adrenal gland mass is found in 5–16% of patients with lung cancer. However, several studies have shown that only 25–82% of adrenal mass lesions histologically match proven adrenal metastases. In incidentally discovered lesions of the adrenal gland in patients without cancer,

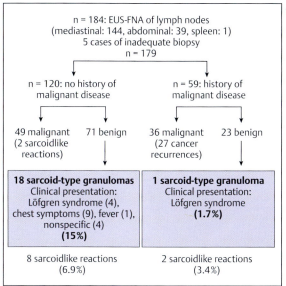

◁ **Fig. 10.22** The frequency of sarcoid-type granuloma in EUS-FNA samples from mediastinal and abdominal lymph nodes in patients with and without a history of malignant disease (Jenssen C, Siebert C, Wiegand A, Bartho S, Zels K, Wagner S, 2009, unpublished data).

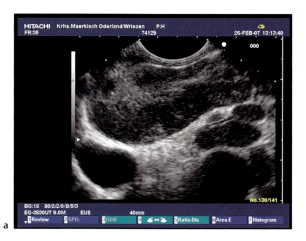

a

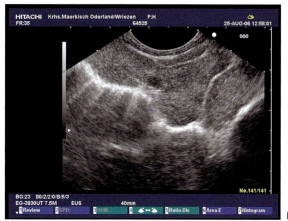

b

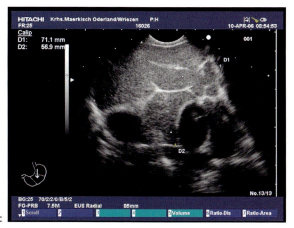

c

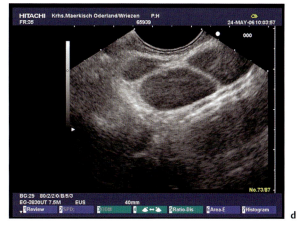

d

Fig. 10.23a–d Mediastinal lymph nodes with varying echo features in four different patients in whom EUS-FNA demonstrated sarcoidlike granulomatous inflammation.

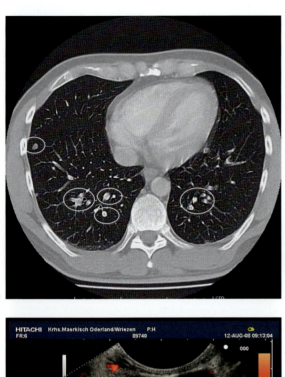

a

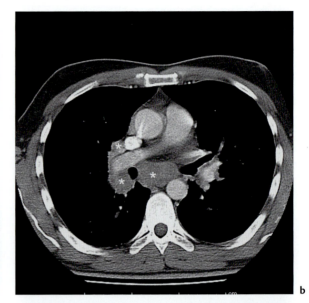

b

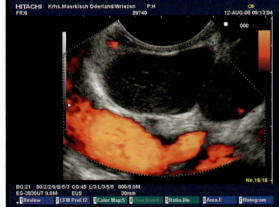

c

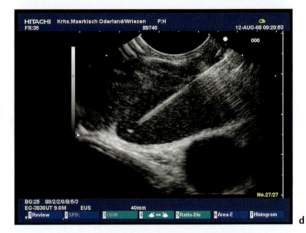

d

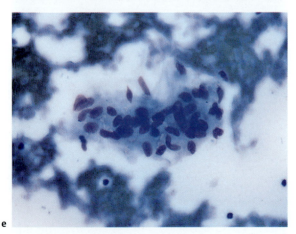

e

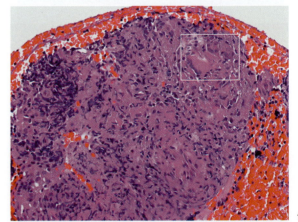

f

Fig. 10.24a–f A 38-year-old patient who presented with weight loss, intermittent fever, night sweats, and fatigue.

a, b Chest computed tomography, showing large mediastinal lymph nodes (asterisks) and small nodules in the lung parenchyma (highlighted). The radiologist's diagnosis was suspected malignant lymphoma.

c EUS shows very large, homogeneous, hypoechoic, and hypovascular (suspicious) lymph nodes.

d EUS-FNA with a 19-gauge aspiration needle was carried out due to suspected malignant lymphoma.

e Cytology (May–Grünwald–Giemsa, original magnification × 400), showing an epithelioid cell group.

f Histology (hematoxylin–eosin, original magnification × 200): a typical noncaseating epithelioid cell granuloma with a multinucleate giant cell (highlighted; sarcoidlike granuloma). The clinical diagnosis was sarcoidosis (stage II).

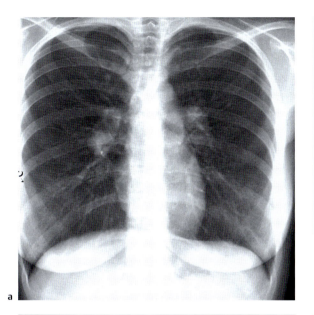

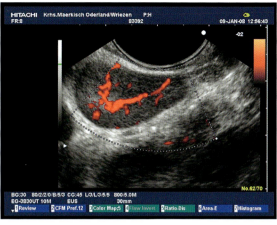

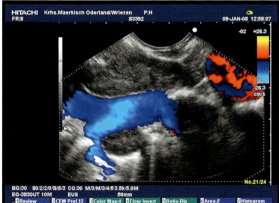

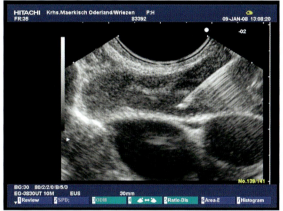

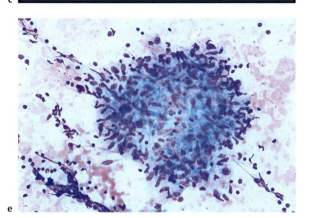

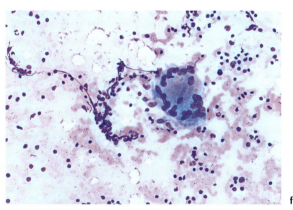

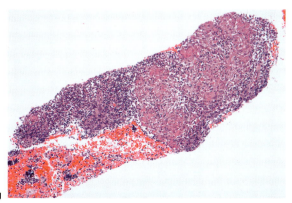

Fig. 10.25a–g A 28-year-old female patient had purple-colored, painful subcutaneous nodules on the lower legs (erythema nodosum), arthralgia (knee, ankle joints), and fever (**b–g** reproduced with permission from [124]).

a–c Bihilar lymphadenopathy (**a**: radiography; **b, c**: EUS). There is regular delineation of the vascular hilum of the large hypoechoic mediastinal lymph nodes, suggesting benign lymphadenopathy (**c**).
d EUS-FNA (22-gauge).

e, f Cytology (Pappenheim, original magnification ×200) shows clusters of epithelioid cells (**e**) and a multinucleate giant cell (**f**).

g Histology (hematoxylin–eosin, original magnification ×100) shows a typical noncaseating epithelioid cell granuloma (sarcoidlike granuloma). The clinical diagnosis was Löfgren syndrome.

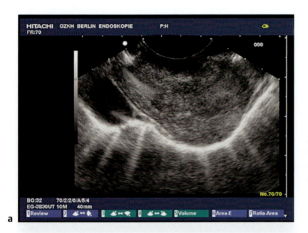

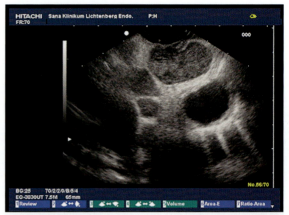

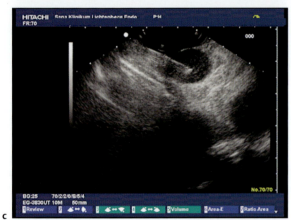

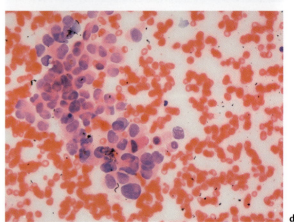

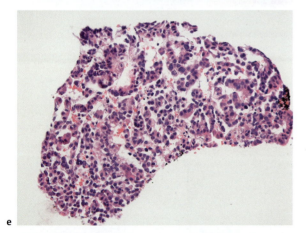

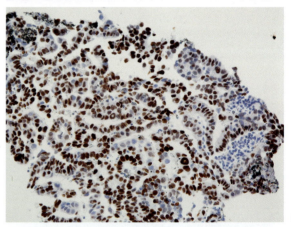

Fig. 10.26a–f A patient presented with vomiting due to pyloric stenosis.

a, b EUS shows a secondary finding of a large mediastinal mass lesion adjacent to the esophagus, with multiple enlarged subcarinal lymph nodes.

c EUS-FNA (22-G).

d Cytology (hematoxylin–eosin, original magnification × 400), showing malignant tumor cells (non–small cell cancer).

e Histology (hematoxylin–eosin, original magnification × 40): adenocarcinoma.

f Immunohistochemistry (original magnification × 40): there is strong expression of thyroid transcription factor-1 (TTF-1), which in this clinical context has a high specificity for lung cancer.

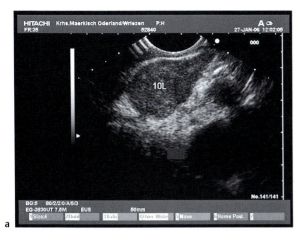
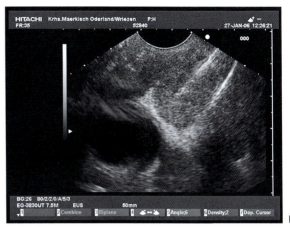

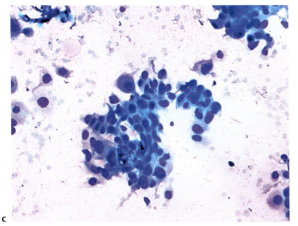
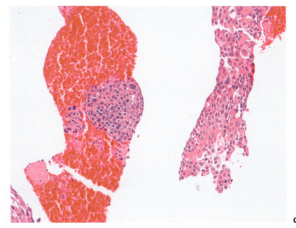

Fig. 10.27a–d A man with a histological diagnosis (bronchoscopic biopsy) of squamous cell cancer of the right upper lobe.
a, b EUS shows an enlarged lymphoma at the subcarinal station (7) and both main bronchi (10 L, R). EUS-FNA was carried out at a contralateral mediastinal lymph node (10 L).

c, d The cytological findings (May–Grünwald–Giemsa, original magnification × 200) and histological findings (hematoxylin–eosin, original magnification × 100) were consistent in diagnosing lymph-node metastasis (N3) from a non–small cell lung cancer (squamous cell cancer). This finding precludes surgical treatment.

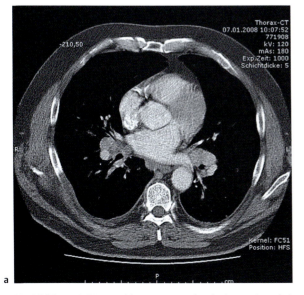
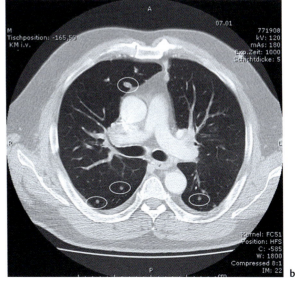

Fig. 10.28a–g A 54-year-old man presented with chest pain and shortness of breath.
a, b Chest computed tomography, showing mediastinal lymphadenopathy and small parenchymal nodules (highlighted).

Fig. 10.28 c–g ▷

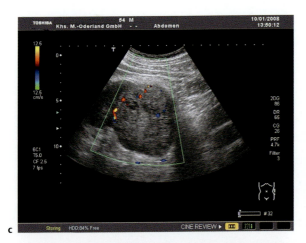

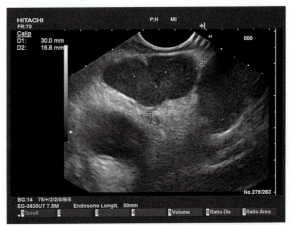

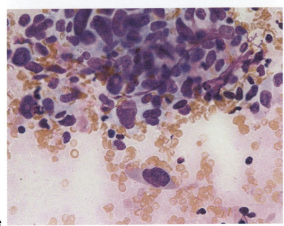

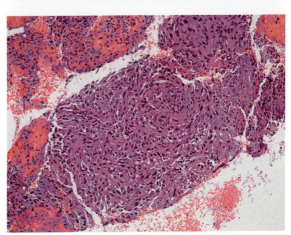

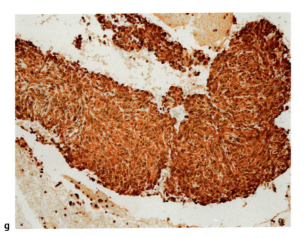

Fig. 10.28c–g (continued)   **c** Transabdominal ultrasound shows a large, hypoechoic tumor in the left kidney.

d EUS shows a large, hypoechoic, and homogeneous mediastinal lymphoma. EUS-FNA (22-gauge) was carried out.

e, f Cytology (**e**: May–Grünwald–Giemsa, original magnification ×200) and histology (**f**: hematoxylin–eosin, original magnification ×100): a malignant tumor, with partially spindle-shaped tumor cells.

g Immunohistochemistry (original magnification ×100): positive staining with vimentin and monoclonal antibodies for cytokeratins AE1/AE3 (not shown), negative for uroplakin (not shown). The final diagnosis was mediastinal metastasis from a sarcomatoid renal cell cancer.

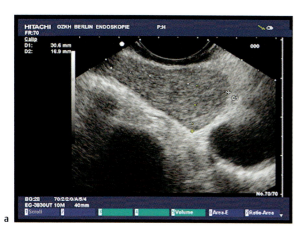

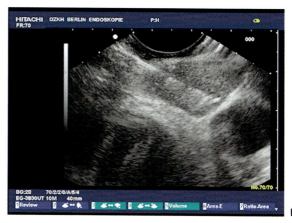

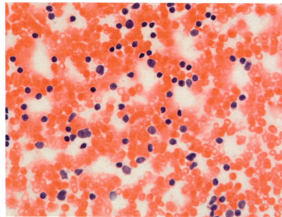

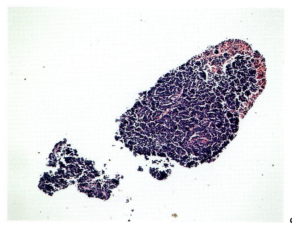

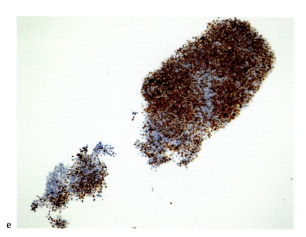

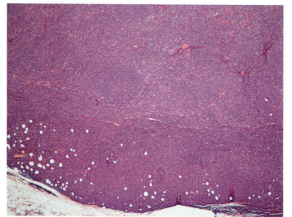

Fig. 10.29a–f A man presented with idiopathic leg vein thrombosis and dyspnea. Chest computed tomography was performed to exclude a pulmonary embolism, but showed multiple mediastinal lymphoma.

a, b EUS and EUS-FNA (22-gauge) of an enlarged subcarinal lymph node.

c Cytology (hematoxylin–eosin, original magnification × 200), showing lymphocytes with nuclear atypia.

d Histology (hematoxylin–eosin, original magnification × 20), showing a dense lymphatic infiltrate.

e Immunohistochemistry (original magnification × 20): nuclear expression of cyclin D1 (a brown-staining product), which is highly specific for mantle cell lymphoma.

f Histological examination of an excised peripheral lymph node confirmed this diagnosis (hematoxylin–eosin, original magnification × 20).

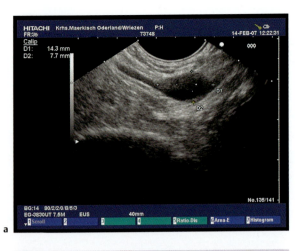

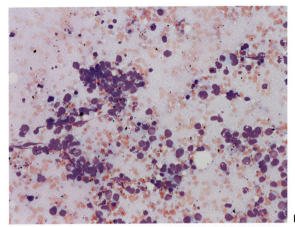

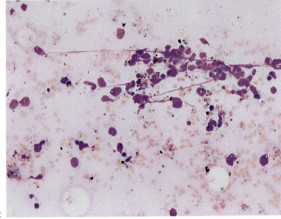

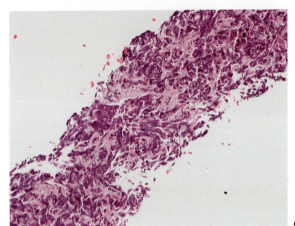

Fig. 10.30a–d A man in whom peripheral lung cancer was suspected on radiography. A bronchoscopy was nondiagnostic.
a EUS shows a small hypoechoic mass lesion (7 × 14 mm) in the left adrenal gland. EUS-FNA (22-gauge) was performed.

b, c Cytology (May–Grünwald–Giemsa, original magnification × 200) shows small cell cancer, with typical nuclear streaks.
d Histology (hematoxylin–eosin, original magnification × 200) confirmed an adrenal gland metastasis from small cell lung cancer.

the risk of malignancy is very low (1–2%) but is related to the size of the adrenal gland mass.[297] EUS-NB is a safe and very successful method for taking samples from the left adrenal gland,[46–48,298] and is also possible in enlarged right adrenal glands.[299,300] It is difficult to distinguish between adrenal hyperplasia, adrenocortical adenoma, and adrenal cancer using material obtained with EUS-FNA.[48] On the other hand, distinguishing between adrenal tissue (hyperplasia, adenoma) and extrinsic tissue (metastases, lymphoma, multiple myeloma, mesenchymal tumors) is comparatively straightforward in EUS-FNA samples. Pheochromocytoma can be diagnosed easily. It should be noted that biopsies of pheochromocytoma are associated with a considerable risk of hypertensive crisis.[297] To facilitate specific diagnoses by immunostaining, the aim in EUS-NB of adrenal glands should be to obtain core particles or cell blocks (**Figs. 10.30** and **10.31**).

EUS-NB with immunostaining is also a valuable tool for diagnosing nonadrenal and nonpancreatic retroperitoneal mass lesions, such as paragangliomas and mesenchymal neoplasms (**Fig. 10.32**).[13,41,301]

Various Other Organs

There have been reports, mainly in small case series, on results with EUS-NB in patients with mass lesions in the liver[49,51,302–307] (**Figs. 10.33** and **10.34**), diffuse parenchymal liver disease,[168,169] and lesions in the bile ducts,[52,53,56,57,308] spleen,[58,59,202,309] kidneys,[72] and mediastinal space[41,60,61,110,310,311] (**Fig. 10.35**)—particularly in patients with very small lesions in whom percutaneous or endoscopic sampling methods are associated with high risk, or in whom the lesions are inaccessible ("hidden lesions"). In these cases, it is essential to obtain material for ancillary diagnostic methods.

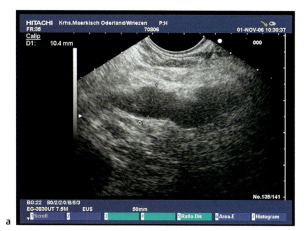

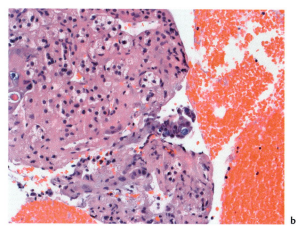

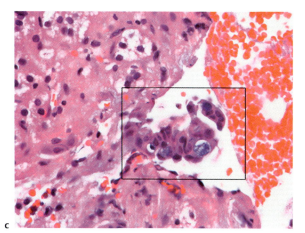

Fig. 10.31a–c a EUS, showing diffuse enlargement of the left adrenal gland in a patient with pancreatic cancer.
b, c Histology (hematoxylin–eosin, original magnification × 200 and × 400): the core particle obtained with EUS-FNA (22-gauge) shows adrenal gland tissue with focal metastatic infiltration (highlighted) by moderately differentiated adenocarcinoma.

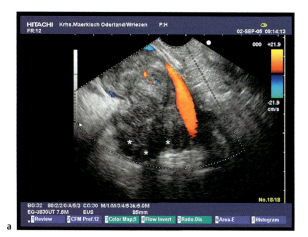

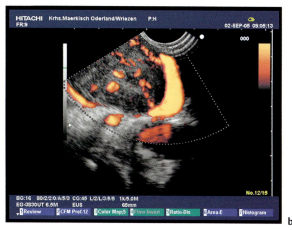

Fig. 10.32a–h In a 69-year-old woman suffering from abdominal pain and vomiting, transabdominal ultrasound and computed tomography revealed a right retroperitoneal mass, possibly arising from the right adrenal gland. (Reproduced with permission from [13].)

a, b EUS (with the transducer positioned in the second part of the duodenum) shows a large, hypoechoic, highly vascularized tumor growing inside the lumen of the inferior vena cava and infiltrating its wall and the surrounding retroperitoneal space (asterisks).

Fig. 10.32 c–h ▷

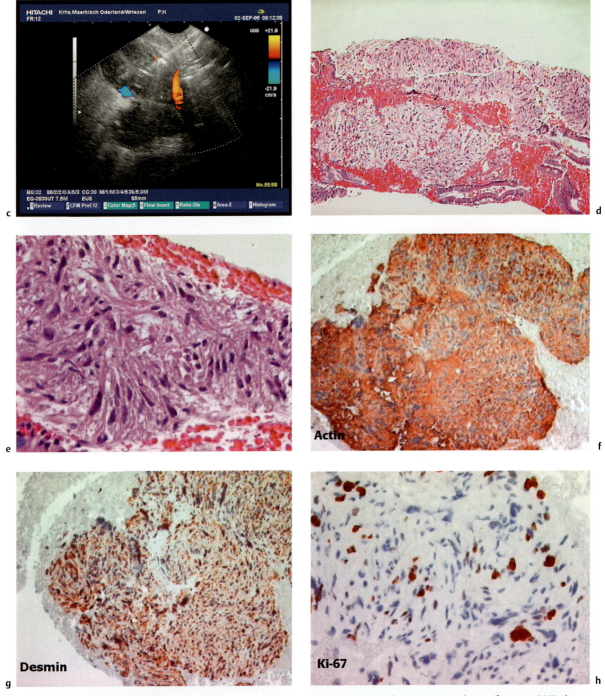

Fig. 10.32c–h (continued)   **c** EUS-FNA (22-gauge).
d, e Histology (hematoxylin–eosin, original magnification × 200 and × 400) shows that the lesion is a mesenchymal tumor consisting of tortuous fascicles of spindle cells. There are oval and elongated, slightly polymorphic nuclei, with eosinophilic, fibrillary cytoplasm.

f–h Immunohistochemistry (original magnification × 200): the tumor cells stain with smooth-muscle actin (**f**) and desmin (**g**). Approximately 20% of the tumor cells are reactive to the proliferation marker Ki-67. The final diagnosis of leiomyosarcoma of the inferior vena cava was confirmed by surgical pathology (not shown).

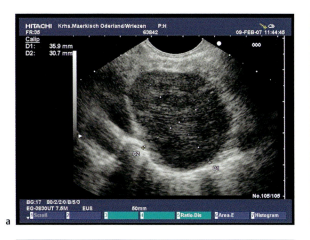

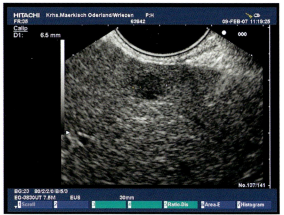

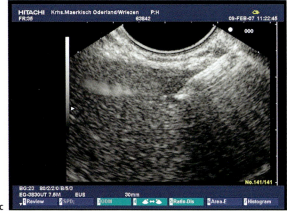

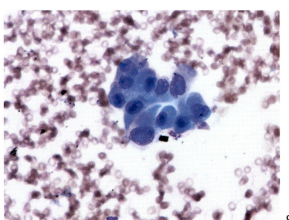

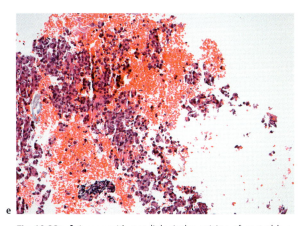

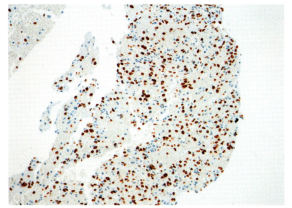

Fig. 10.33a–f A man with a radiological suspicion of central lung cancer. Bronchoscopy was nondiagnostic.
a, b EUS shows a primary lung tumor adjacent to the esophagus (**a**) and a small hypoechoic lesion (6.5 mm) in the left liver lobe (**b**).
c EUS-FNA (22-gauge) of the small liver lesion.
d, e Cytology (**d**: May–Grünwald–Giemsa, original magnification ×400) and histology (**e**: hematoxylin–eosin, original magnification ×100) show that the lesion was a hepatic metastasis from an adenocarcinoma.
f Immunohistochemistry (original magnification ×100): positive staining for thyroid transcription factor-1 (TTF-1) is highly compatible with a pulmonary origin (non–small cell lung cancer).

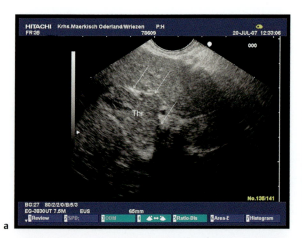

a

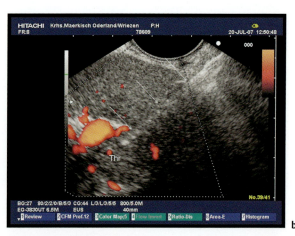

b

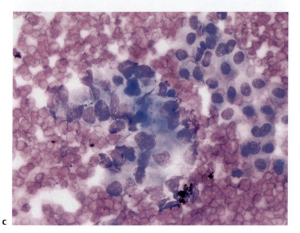

c

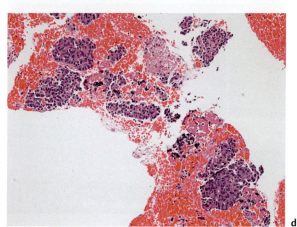

d

Fig. 10.34a–d A 64-year-old man with no history of liver disease presented with variceal bleeding. Contrast-enhanced transabdominal ultrasound showed a thrombosis of the left main branch of the portal vein, extending to the central intrahepatic part, and a small hypervascularized lesion in the left liver lobe.

a EUS: thrombosis in the left main branch of the portal vein (Thr, arrows).

b EUS-FNA (22-gauge) of the portal thrombus (the needle track is indicated by the arrows).

c Cytology (May–Grünwald–Giemsa, original magnification ×400) shows red blood cells and a group of epithelial tumor cells with large, hyperchromatic nuclei and prominent nucleoli.

d Histology (hematoxylin–eosin, original magnification ×100) shows a moderately differentiated adenocarcinoma, suggestive of hepatocellular carcinoma.

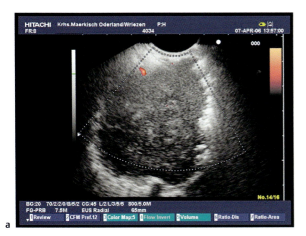

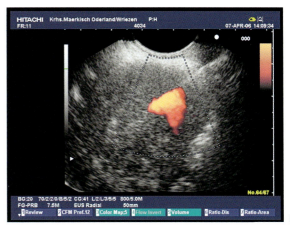

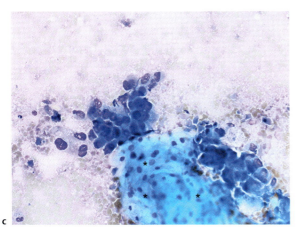

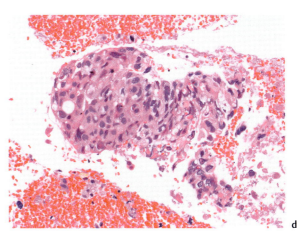

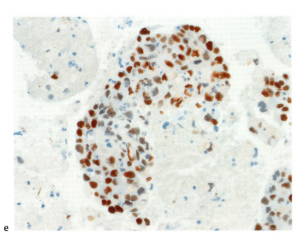

Fig. 10.35a–e A man with a suspected central lung cancer. The tumor was not accessible by bronchoscopic biopsy.
a EUS shows a large hypoechoic tumor adjacent to the esophagus.
b EUS-FNA (22-gauge).
c, d Cytology (**c**: May-Grünwald-Giemsa, original magnification ×200) and histology (**d**: hematoxylin-eosin, original magnification ×200) led to a diagnosis of adenocarcinoma. The smears are contaminated by esophageal squamous epithelia (asterisks).
e Immunohistochemistry (original magnification ×200): positive staining of tumor cells with thyroid transcription factor-1 (TTF-1) is typical of non–small cell lung cancer.

Quality Assessment and Benchmarking

In contrast to the situation in clinical studies, it is difficult to assess the diagnostic quality of EUS-NB samples in everyday clinical practice. The ideal benchmark for EUS-NB performance would be reliable positive and negative predictive values for diagnosing malignancy—requiring data from surgical pathology or from long-term follow-up studies. These data are not fully available in clinical routine work, as many patients undergo neoadjuvant treatment, are lost to follow-up, or are unfit for surgical treatment or decline it. There are consequently no currently accepted criteria for quality assessment in EUS-NB. Prospectively estimated complication rates[24,312] and surrogate parameters such as the reproducibility of cytopathological diagnoses,[194] the rate of nondiagnostic biopsies (e.g., due to technical failure or unsatisfactory specimens), the rate of inconclusive cytopathological diagnoses (e.g., "atypical," "suspicious for malignancy"),[195] and the yield of malignant diagnoses in EUS-FNA of solid pancreatic masses[313] appear to be suitable and simple tools for monitoring and benchmarking EUS-NB performance.

Clinical Impact of EUS-NB

■ Focal Pancreatic Lesions

In up to 50% of patients with focal pancreatic lesions, the final diagnosis is not ductal adenocarcinoma.[228] It is extremely important to identify patients with focal inflammatory masses (e.g., autoimmune pancreatitis), metastases, lymphoma, and neoplasias with low malignant potential or none. In most cases, diagnosing a distinct pancreatic mass lesion other than ductal adenocarcinoma will significantly alter the patient management and prognosis—for example, by indicating an organ-preserving surgical approach[260] or nonsurgical treatment. The patient's history and clinical symptoms and the morphological features of the lesion may help identify patients in whom there is a suspicion of pancreatic tumors other than adenocarcinoma. Typically, ductal adenocarcinoma of the pancreas is a hypovascular tumor. However, inflammatory lesions, microcystic adenomas, neuroendocrine tumors, metastases from renal cell cancer, and other rare pancreatic neoplasias, have been shown to be isovascular or hypervascular on contrast-enhanced (endoscopic) ultrasound. It should be noted that pancreatic necrosis also presents as an avascular or hypovascular hypoechoic mass lesion (**Figs. 10.15 d, 10.36, 10.37**).[314] In patients who are found to have isovascular or hypervascular lesions on contrast-enhanced EUS or other contrast-enhanced imaging studies, we would recommend performing a needle biopsy (US-guided or EUS-guided) in order to obtain smears and core particles allowing immunochemical differentiation. On the other hand, if there is a hypovascular pancreatic mass lesion, EUS-NB is only required before chemotherapy if there are definite criteria of nonresectability on EUS or radiological imaging, or if EUS-NB of possible liver metastases, malignant ascites or pleural fluid, or mediastinal lymph-node metastases, for example, might confirm advanced disease (**Fig. 10.38**).

In one study, the results of EUS-FNA contraindicated surgical treatment for pancreatic cancer in 13.5% of patients, as they confirmed the presence of hepatic metastases or mediastinal lymph-node metastases that had not been identified on CT.[315] In two other studies, EUS-FNA diagnosed mediastinal lymph-node metastases in 5–7% of pancreatic cancer patients[290,316] (**Figs. 10.39** and **10.40**).

In these cases, a cytopathological diagnosis of cancer may avoid the morbidity and costs of a noncurative and unnecessary operation.[17] EUS-FNA confirmation of malignant ascites or liver metastases in patients with pancreatic cancer is associated with very poor survival (median survival < 3 months) and may help guide treatment decisions—for example, in palliative treatment for obstructive jaundice.[317] In the near future, typifying unresectable solid pancreatic malignancies and using molecular profiling to predict responsiveness to chemotherapeutic agents (e.g., gemcitabine) or targeted therapies (hedgehog signaling pathway inhibitors) may help establish optimized individual treatment strategies.[318–321]

■ Esophageal and Other Gastrointestinal Cancers

In patients with esophageal cancer, the presence of lymph-node metastases may have a major impact on treatment decisions and on the prognosis. EUS has been shown to be superior to computed tomography for detecting celiac lymph nodes.[322,323] EUS-FNA substantially improves the sensitivity and specificity of EUS in evaluating nodal metastases (**Fig. 10.41**).[322,324]

Cytopathological confirmation of malignancy in celiac lymph nodes aspirated under EUS guidance is predictive of a poorer prognosis in patients with esophageal cancer and can have a major impact on treatment decisions for these patients.[5,119,325] Introducing EUS and EUS-FNA into the staging approach for esophageal cancer used in one study prompted appropriate use of preoperative neoadjuvant therapy in patients with advanced disease. EUS-FNA was associated with a significantly reduced risk of recurrence (hazard ratio 0.63) and mortality (HR 0.66).[326] Detecting or excluding subcarinal or proximal mediastinal lymph-node metastases using EUS-FNA also has a significant impact on surgical decision-making in patients with esophageal carcinoma (in relation to transthoracic versus transhiatal

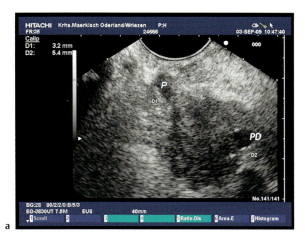
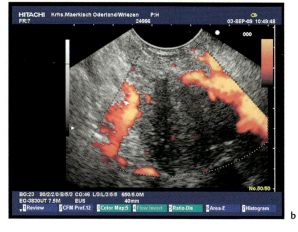

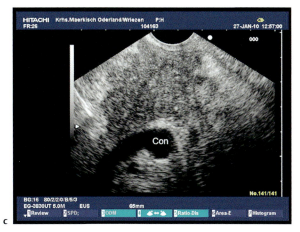
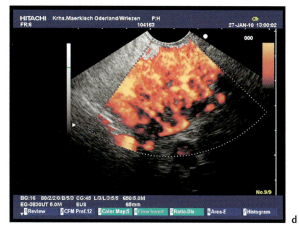

Fig. 10.36a–d Contrast-enhanced EUS (in power angio mode) after an intravenous injection of the contrast-enhancing agent SonoVue. **a, b** Hypoechoic tumor of the pancreatic head. Following injection of 1.25 mL SonoVue, the tumor has a hypovascular appearance in comparison with the surrounding pancreatic parenchyma (PD, pancreatic duct). The final diagnosis was ductal adenocarcinoma.

c, d Hypoechoic tumor of the pancreatic head. The color power angio mode after injection of 1.25 mL SonoVue (**d**) shows pronounced hypervascularity. The final diagnosis was autoimmune pancreatitis. Con, confluence of the portal vein.

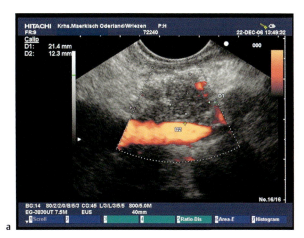
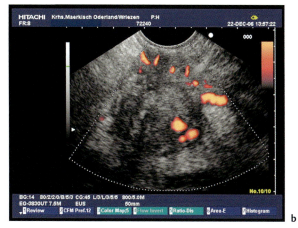

Fig. 10.37a–j EUS in a patient with acute pancreatitis.
a, b Two hypoechoic lesions were detected (**a**: body of the pancreas, **b**: tail of the pancreas).
c, d On the contrast-enhanced color power Doppler study, both lesions were hypovascular.
e, f EUS-FNA of the two lesions.

g, i The cytological (**g**) and histological (**i**) diagnosis of the small lesion in the pancreatic body was adenocarcinoma.
h, j The large lesion in the tail of the pancreas was found to be a necrosis (**g, h**: May–Grünwald–Giemsa, original magnification × 400; **i, j**: hematoxylin–eosin, original magnification × 100).

Fig. 10.37 c–j ▷

II Diagnostic Imaging and Interventions

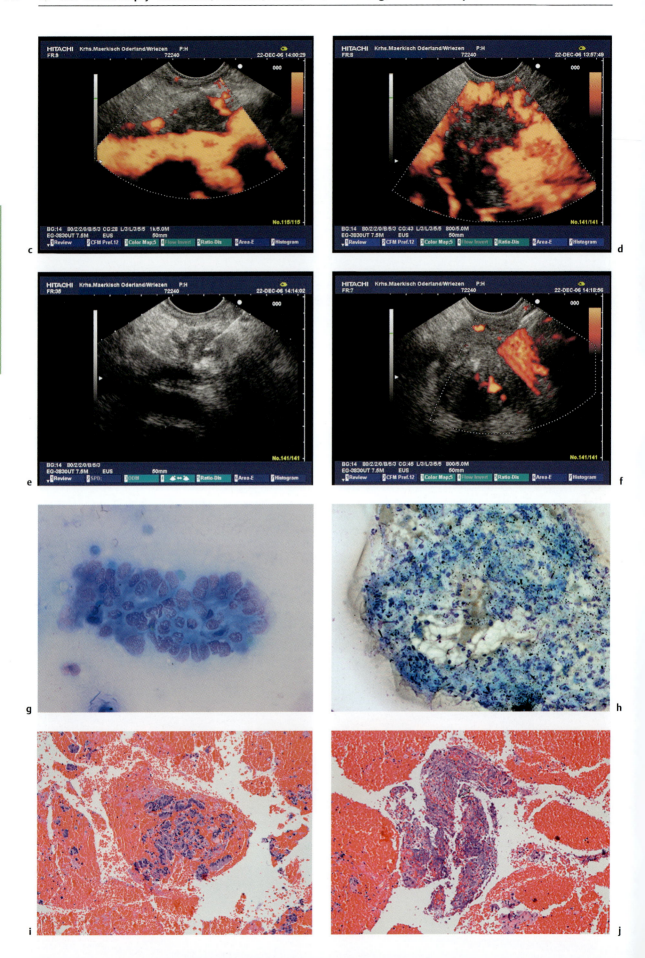

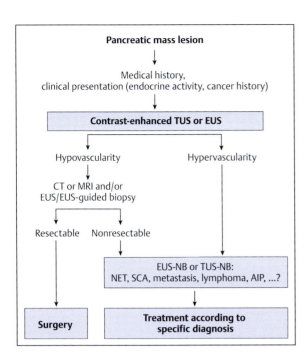

Fig. 10.38 The diagnostic algorithm for solid pancreatic lesions using EUS, contrast-enhanced (endoscopic) ultrasound, and needle biopsy, guided by endoscopic or transabdominal ultrasound (adapted from [7]). AIP, autoimmune pancreatitis; CT, computed tomography; EUS-NB, endoscopic ultrasound-guided needle biopsy; MRI, magnetic resonance imaging; NET, neuroendocrine tumor; SCA, serous cystic adenoma; TUS, transabdominal ultrasound; TUS-NB, transabdominal ultrasound–guided needle biopsy.

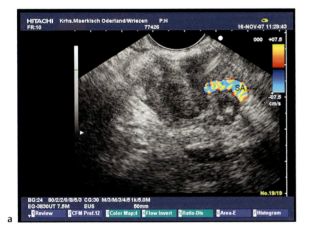

a

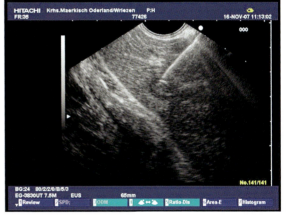

b

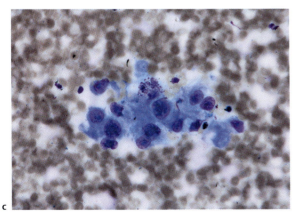

c

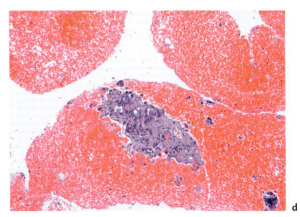

d

Fig. 10.39a–d A 47-year-old man who was suffering from back pain (**a**, **b** reproduced with permission from [125]).

a EUS shows a large hypoechoic mass lesion in the pancreatic tail (SA, splenic artery) and a small hypoechoic liver lesion.

b EUS-FNA (22-G) of the small liver lesion suspected to be a metastasis.

c, d Cytology (**c**: May–Grünwald–Giemsa, original magnification × 400) and histology (**d**: hematoxylin–eosin, original magnification × 100) of the liver lesion confirmed that the lesion was a metastasis from a moderately differentiated (pancreatic) adenocarcinoma. EUS-FNA of the primary pancreatic tumor was done in the same session and showed the same type of tumor (not shown).

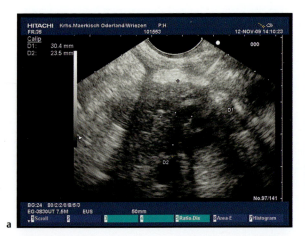

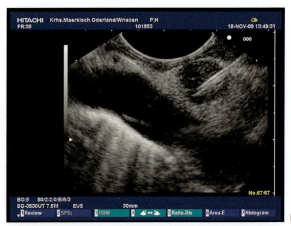

a

b

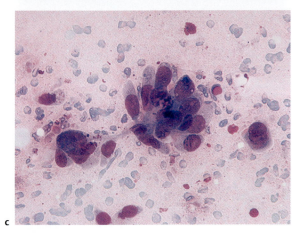

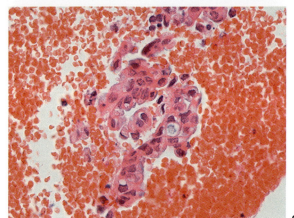

c

d

Fig. 10.40a–d A 51-year-old man who presented with acute pancreatitis and obstructive jaundice.
a, b EUS showed a pancreatic head mass (**a**) and an unexpected finding of a small (8 × 11 mm) hypoechoic mediastinal lymph node. EUS-FNA (22-gauge) of the lymph node was carried out (**b**) to confirm a distant metastasis.

c, d Cytology (**c**: May–Grünwald–Giemsa, original magnification × 400) and histology (**d**: hematoxylin–eosin, original magnification × 400) confirmed the mediastinal metastasis from pancreatic cancer.

esophagectomy).[327] In the course of EUS staging of cancer of the esophagus and esophagogastric junction, EUS and EUS-FNA also allowed detection and cytopathological diagnosis of unsuspected small left hepatic lobe metastases in a small group of patients, helping to avoid unnecessary surgery.[306] In patients with an endoscopic diagnosis of early Barrett's neoplasia, EUS-FNA may detect and confirm lymph-node metastases. In one study, this changed the course of management toward a surgical approach in 20% of patients who were initially referred for endoscopic resection.[328] One very interesting recent study showed that EUS and EUS-FNA had a significant influence on management decisions in a panel of three gastroenterologists, three medical oncologists, three radiation oncologists, and four thoracic surgeons in relation to 50 consecutive patients with esophageal cancer. EUS and EUS-FNA changed the patient management most for patients with stage IIA, IIB, or III disease—mostly from primary surgery to multimodal treatment. EUS and EUS-FNA not only had a strong

influence on management, but the results also increased the consensus among specialists regarding management recommendations.[329] EUS with EUS-NB is therefore strongly recommended during staging procedures in patients with esophageal cancer who are eligible for surgical treatment. However, a survey in the United States regarding the use of EUS-FNA for esophageal cancer staging in clinical practice showed that most thoracic surgeons' positive view of EUS-FNA as the most accurate locoregional staging modality in esophageal cancer was not fully reflected in utilization patterns, due to the poor quality of EUS services in some centers. In addition, the implications of celiac lymph-node involvement in patients with distal esophageal cancer confirmed by EUS-FNA was a matter of controversy in this study.[330]

In one study, EUS and EUS-guided FNA were shown to be helpful in identifying residual malignant infiltration in the lymph nodes after preoperative chemoradiotherapy. This proved to be helpful for identifying patients capable of

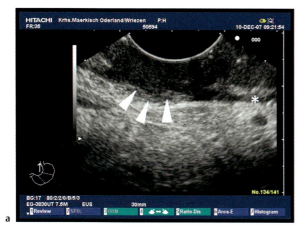
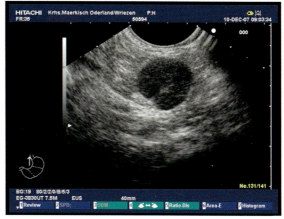
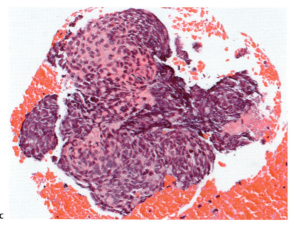
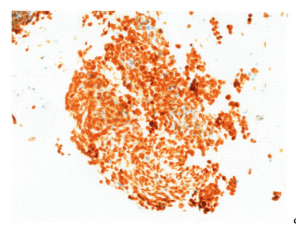

Fig. 10.41a–d A 68-year-old woman with poorly differentiated squamous cell cancer of the esophagus. (Reproduced with permission from [125.])

a EUS shows hypoechoic infiltration of all of the wall layers of the esophagus (arrows) beyond the outer borders of the muscularis propria (asterisk, T3).

b EUS-FNA (22-G) of a round, hypoechoic lymph node at the celiac trunk.

c Histology (hematoxylin–eosin, original magnification × 100): undifferentiated non–small cell cancer.

d Immunohistochemistry (original magnification × 100): positive staining with the transcription marker p63 and with cytokeratin 5/6 (not shown) is highly specific for celiac metastasis from a squamous cell cancer.

benefiting maximally from surgery.[331] However, another study did not confirm these results. PET-CT was more accurate than EUS-FNA in predicting nodal status and complete response after neoadjuvant therapy in patients with esophageal cancer.[332] The role of EUS-FNA in restaging patients with esophageal cancer after neoadjuvant treatment has therefore not yet been adequately defined.

In various types of gastrointestinal malignancy, EUS-NB may also be helpful in preventing unnecessary surgery by providing cytopathological confirmation of "occult" (CT-negative) hepatic metastases,[8,306,307,333] "occult" ascites,[69–71,317] or nodal metastases.[8,146,284,334–336] The staging-related clinical impact of EUS-FNA in one study ranged from 11.0% to 12.5% in patients with esophageal, gastric, and pancreatic cancer.[8] In another recent study, EUS-FNA changed the management plan in 34 of 234 patients (15%) with gastric cancer.[336] EUS-FNA is also of considerable value in decision-making regarding palliative treatment,

by making it possible to diagnose extraluminal recurrences of esophageal, gastric, and rectal cancer[303,337–340] (**Figs. 10.42** and **10.43**) and in detecting secondary malignancies—for example, in the lung (**Fig. 10.44**).[340]

■ Lung Cancer

In patients with suspected lung cancer, flexible bronchoscopy and image-guided transthoracic needle biopsy are the techniques most commonly used to obtain a tissue diagnosis. However, many tumors are not visible at bronchoscopy and also may not be sampled using transthoracic needle biopsy, for anatomic reasons. In patients with tumors adjacent to the esophagus, EUS-FNA and EBUS-TBNA can help establish a cytopathological diagnosis (**Figs. 10.26** and **10.34**).[76,341,342]

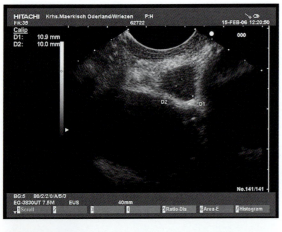

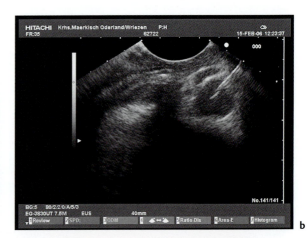

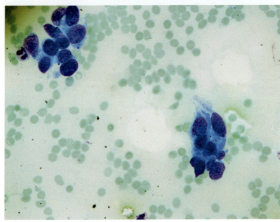

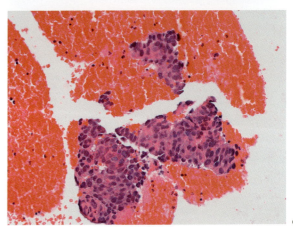

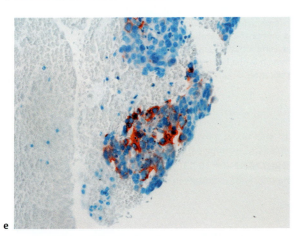

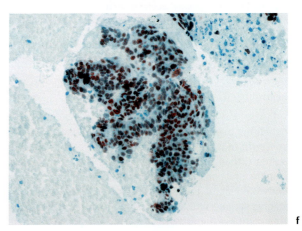

Fig. 10.42a–f A 75-year-old female patient who presented with coughing and dyspnea. Computed tomography demonstrated small pulmonary nodules. The patient had undergone surgery for rectal cancer 8 years previously.
a, b EUS-FNA of small (10-mm) subcarinal lymph nodes.
c, d Cytology (**c**: May–Grünwald–Giemsa, original magnification × 200) and histology (**d**: hematoxylin–eosin, original magnification × 200): metastasis from an adenocarcinoma.

e, f Immunohistochemistry (original magnification × 200): positive staining for cytokeratin 20 (**e**) and for CDX2 (**f**), but not for thyroid transcription factor-1 (TTF-1, not shown) confirmed a late metastasis from the patient's earlier rectal cancer.

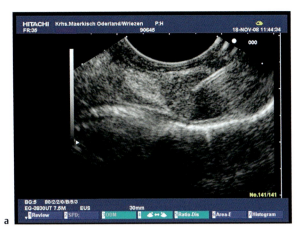

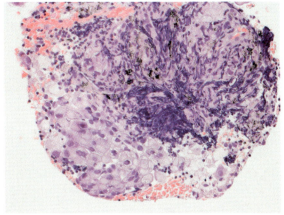

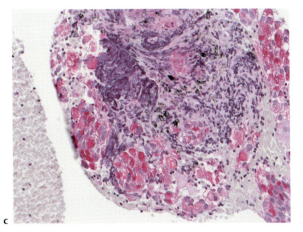

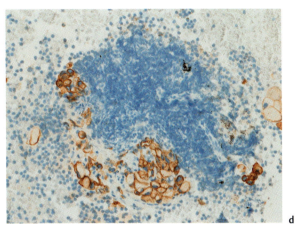

Fig. 10.43a–d A man who presented with weight loss 18 months after gastrectomy for signet-ring cell cancer of the stomach (pT2 N2 (10/50) cM0 pL0 V0 R0). (Reproduced with permission from [7].)
a EUS-FNA (22-gauge) of a small periesophageal lymph node.
b Histology (hematoxylin–eosin, original magnification × 200): the specimen contains lymphatic cells, histiocytes, anthracotic pigment, and large tumor cells with foamy cytoplasm and polymorphic nuclei.

c Histochemistry (periodic acid–Schiff, original magnification × 200): the cytoplasm in the tumor cells is PAS-positive.
d Immunohistochemistry (original magnification × 200): positive staining for cytokeratin 7 (CK7). Positive PAS staining and the cytokeratin type are evidence of a nodal recurrence of signet-ring cell cancer of the stomach.

Correct staging in patients with lung cancer is mandatory to allow them to be assigned to treatment strategies appropriately. Surgery cannot be recommended in patients with small cell lung cancer (SCLC), or in those with non–small cell cancer (NSCLC), with the following stages in the most recent TNM classification:[343] T4 (N0, N1: stage IIIA; N2, N3: stage IIIB) and/or N2/N3 (stage IIIA/IIIB) and/or M1 (stage IV). These patients with advanced or disseminated lung cancer are preferably treated with chemotherapy and radiotherapy (**Figs. 10.27, 10.30, 10.33, 10.44**). Neoadjuvant treatment is considered particularly in patients with stage IIIA N2 disease. Only NSCLC patients with localized disease are directly referred for surgery with curative intent.[344]

More than 150 studies have been published on EUS-FNA in the diagnosis and staging of lung cancer.[345] Two large meta-analyses reported pooled sensitivity and specificity rates of 88% and 96%[346] and 83% and 97%,[347] respectively,

for diagnosing mediastinal lymph-node metastases. EUS-FNA has been reported in several studies to have superior sensitivity and specificity for mediastinal lymph-node metastases in comparison with both CT and PET.[345] EUS and EUS-FNA are able to confirm the presence of mediastinal lymph-node metastases in up to 25% of lung cancer patients in whom CT had not demonstrated any enlarged mediastinal nodes.[348,349] However, in comparison with patients with enlarged mediastinal lymph nodes on CT, the sensitivity of EUS-FNA and EBUS-TBNA is lower in CT-negative patients.[346,350]

Several studies have been published reporting the major impact of EUS-FNA and EBUS-TBNA on clinical management in lung cancer patients. In one randomized study, routine use of EUS-FNA in the staging of lung cancer reduced the number of unnecessary thoracotomies from 25% to 9% in comparison with a conventional staging strategy including EUS-FNA only in CT-positive patients.[351] If

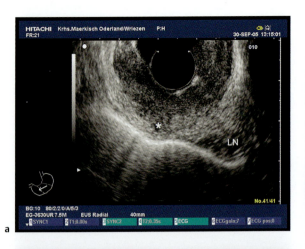

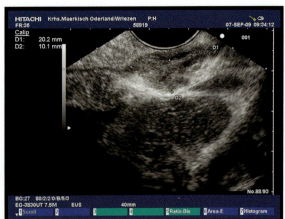

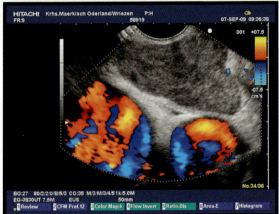

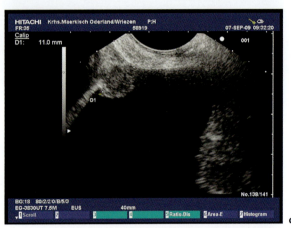

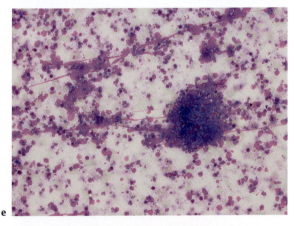

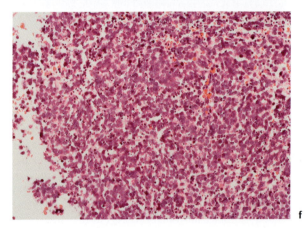

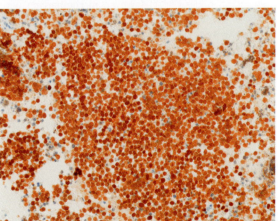

Fig. 10.44a–g Four years after neoadjuvant chemoradiotherapy and surgical treatment for signet-ring cell cancer of the proximal stomach (pT3 N1 cM0 pL1 V0 R0), a male patient presented with dysphagia and shortness of breath.

a The preoperative staging EUS. LN, lymph node.

b–d EUS 4 years later. There is a hypoechoic mass at the surgical esophagojejunal anastomosis (**b**), as well as large mediastinal lymph nodes (**c**) and pleural infiltration and effusion (**d**).

e–g Cytology (**e**: May–Grünwald–Giemsa, original magnification ×400), histology (**f**: hematoxylin–eosin, original magnification ×200), and immunohistochemistry (**g**: TTF-1, original magnification ×200). Therefore, EUS-FNA (22-G) of the anastomotic tumor (and of the mediastinal lymph nodes and pleural nodules) shows evidence of a small cell cancer of the lung.

Table 10.16 Yield of EUS-guided fine-needle aspiration (EUS-FNA) and endobronchial ultrasound-guided transbronchial needle aspiration (EBUS-TBNA) in comparison with surgical staging in patients with lung cancer (data from [347,350,360–362])

Diagnostic technique	Cervical (video-assisted) mediastinoscopy	Video-assisted thoracoscopy (VATS)	EUS-FNA	EBUS-TBNA
Sensitivity (pooled data)[a]	78% (19 studies, 6505 patients)[363]	75% (8 studies, 669 patients)[361]	83% (18 studies, 1201 patients)[346] 88% (32 studies, 2680 patients)[347]	93% (11 studies, 1299 patients)[350] 85–100% (14 studies)[362]
Complication rates	≈ 2%, mortality 0.08%	≈ 2%, no mortality	0–2.3% (0.8%), only minor, no mortality	0.15%, no mortality
Accessible mediastinal LN stations (in brackets: difficult or limited access)	1 L/R, 2 L/R, 4 L/R, 7, (8)[b], (10 L/R)	Right: 3 R, 4 R, 7, 8–10 R, (11–14 R) Left: 5–7, 8–10 L, (11–14 L)	2 L, (2 R), 3 p, 4 L, (4 R), (5), (6)[c], 7, 8, 9, (10LR)	1 L/R, 2 L/R, 3, 4 L/R, 7, (10–11 L/R), (12 L/R)
No access to mediastinal LN stations	3, 5, 6, 9, 11–14	Right: contralateral (L) stations, 5, 6 Left: contralateral (R) stations, 3, 4 L	3a, 11–14	5, 6, 8, 9, 13–14
Accessible predilection sites for distant metastases	No access	No access	Left adrenal gland, (right adrenal gland), left liver lobe, (right liver lobe), infra-diaphragmatic lymph nodes	No access

[a] Data from most recent meta-analyses or reviews.
[b] Access possible using video mediastinoscopy.
[c] Possible only by transaortic EUS-FNA, which was shown to be a relatively safe technique.[10,11]

EUS-FNA is used in addition to mediastinoscopy, significantly more patients with nodal metastases or tumor infiltration in neighboring structures may be identified than with each procedure alone.[76,352,353] In a prospective multicenter trial, Annema et al. demonstrated that in 107 consecutive patients with potentially resectable non–small cell lung cancer, one in six thoracotomies could haven been avoided by carrying out EUS-FNA in addition to mediastinoscopy.[76] A large study showed that in patients with suspected (n = 142) or proven (n = 100) lung cancer and enlarged mediastinal lymph nodes on CT, EUS-FNA avoided 70% of surgical procedures (mediastinoscopy, thoracoscopy, thoracotomy) that would otherwise have been scheduled, as it demonstrated mediastinal nodal metastases or T4 disease in NSCLC patients (61%) or provided cytopathological proof of SCLC (8%) or a benign diagnosis (1%).[35] In another recent study including 152 patients with proven or suspected lung cancer, patients were only sent to mediastinoscopy and/or thoracoscopy if EUS-FNA did not detect nodal disease. In this setting, EUS-FNA avoided the need for surgical staging in 39% of the patients.[353] Including EUS-FNA in staging procedures is also cost-effective in patients with lung cancer; in one study, it reduced the costs of staging by 40%.[354] However, in view of the limited sensitivity of EUS-FNA in patients who do not have enlarged lymph nodes on chest CTs or several lymph node stations, it is clear that EUS-FNA alone is not capable of replacing mediastinoscopy in the staging of lung cancer patients. In a recent study including 120 patients, the false-negative rate of mediastinal EUS-FNA was 25.3%. The sensitivity was limited in right-sided tumors, in patients with normal-sized lymph nodes on CT, and in lymph-node station 4.[355] These studies indicate that in a setting in which EBUS-TBNA is not available, EUS-FNA should be used to supplement rather than replace mediastinoscopy in the mediastinal staging of patients with lung cancer. However, the diagnostic yield and sensitivity of EBUS-TBNA has been found to be similar to that of cervical mediastinoscopy. According to data presented in two recent studies, surgical restaging of the mediastinum may not be mandatory in patients who have negative results on EBUS-TBNA.[356,357]

Virtually all mediastinal lymph-node stations can be examined and sampled using a combination of EUS-FNA and EBUS-TBNA (**Table 10.16**). This is the basis for the strategy of "complete endosonographic staging" of lung cancer, which can almost completely avoid the need for surgical staging of the disease.[358,359] The negative predictive value of combined nonsurgical staging in 150 patients with suspected and proven lung cancer was as high as 97% in one study.[359] This approach also appears to be highly cost-effective in patients with node-positive findings on CT.[360]

In addition to demonstrating and sampling ipsilateral and subcarinal (N2) or contralateral (N3) mediastinal lymph-node metastases, EUS-FNA is able to access relevant predilection spots for distant metastases (such as the adrenal glands, infradiaphragmatic lymph-node stations, liver, and pancreas) (**Figs. 10.30, 10.33**; see also **Figs. 10.45, 10.46, 10.47**).

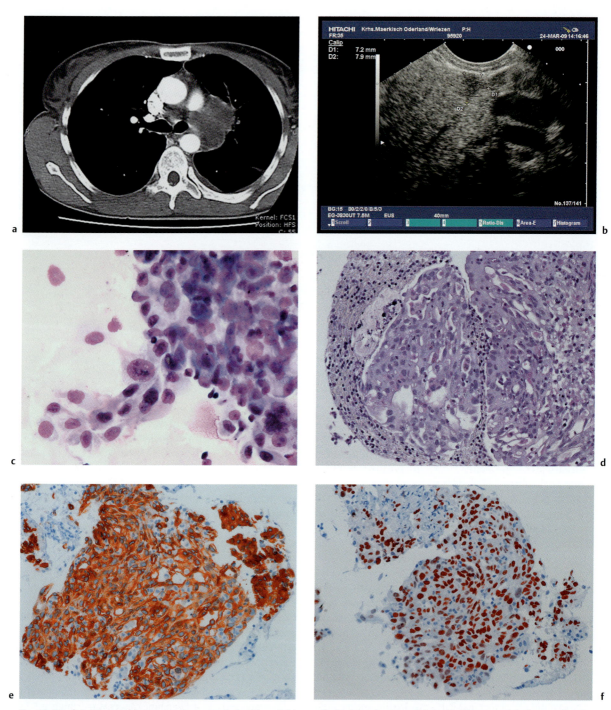

Fig. 10.45a–f A 41-year-old woman who presented with weight loss, coughing, and dyspnea.
a The chest computed tomogram shows a large tumor in the left hilum.
b Staging endosonography revealed multiple small hypoechoic mediastinal lymph nodes (not shown) and two small hypoechoic pancreatic mass lesions. EUS-FNA (22-gauge) of the most advanced lesion (suspected pancreatic metastasis) was performed.

c–f Cytology (**c**: May–Grünwald–Giemsa, original magnification × 400), histology (**d**: periodic acid–Schiff, original magnification × 200; negative staining) and immunohistochemistry (**e**: CK7, original magnification × 200; **f**: TTF-1, original magnification × 200) confirmed pancreatic metastasis from a non–small cell lung cancer (adenocarcinoma).

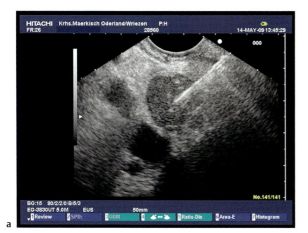

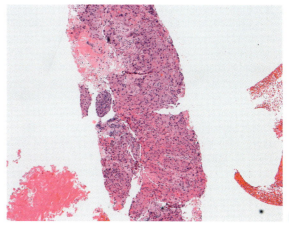

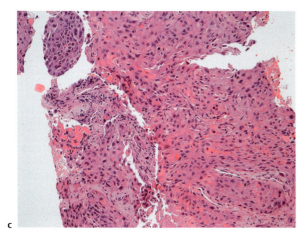

Fig. 10.46a–c A 50-year-old man who presented with obstructive jaundice caused by a hilar liver tumor (not shown). Endoscopic retrograde cholangiopancreatography was not possible due to a previous partial gastrectomy and Roux-en-Y anastomosis. Computed tomography of the chest showed a large tumor in the left mediastinal hilum (not shown).

a EUS-FNA of a large celiac lymph node (19-gauge) before EUS-guided cholangiodrainage.

b, c Histology (hematoxylin–eosin, original magnification × 100, × 200) shows a nonregional nodal metastasis from a squamous cell cancer in the lung.

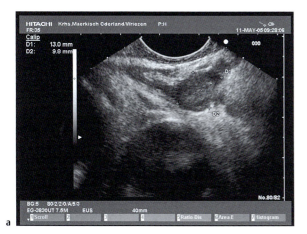

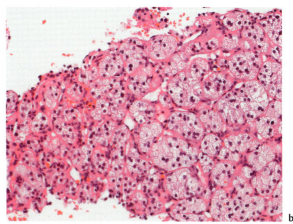

Fig. 10.47a, b Staging EUS in a patient with non–small cell cancer of the lung.

a EUS shows a small hypoechoic lesion (10 × 13 mm) in the central left adrenal gland.

b Histology (hematoxylin–eosin, original magnification × 200) shows that the core particle obtained with EUS-FNA (22-gauge) contains adrenal gland tissue with enlarged, ballooned cells and no nuclear atypia. A panel of laboratory tests did not show any endocrine activity. The final diagnosis was nonfunctional adrenal gland adenoma.

In a study of patients with enlarged adrenal glands at CT, EUS identified malignant infiltration of the left adrenal gland in 42% of the patients.[47] In patients with lung cancer, various studies have shown that in ≈ 50% of patients enlarged adrenal glands are caused by benign disease (adrenal hyperplasia, adenoma) (**Fig. 10.47**).[297] The adrenal glands are a very frequent location for distant metastases in lung cancer (**Fig. 10.30**). In one clinical tumor registry in Germany, the adrenal glands were involved in 25.7% of patients with stage IV disease. In 84.3% of patients with adrenal metastases, metastatic disease was also found in other locations.[364] One recent study showed that in patients with proven or suspected lung cancer, EUS-FNA of an enlarged left adrenal gland altered the staging results in 70% of cases—downstaging the disease in almost all of the patients. Treatment decisions were thus altered in almost half of the patient population. On the basis of the results of adrenal EUS-FNA, potentially curative surgery was planned in 25% of patients and unnecessary surgery was avoided in 5%.[298]

It has recently become possible to identify somatic mutations of the epidermal growth factor receptor (EGFR) in material obtained with EUS-FNA from lymph nodes or from the primary tumor in patients with non–small cell lung cancer. This may make it possible to predict the response to tyrosine kinase inhibitors in these patients and tailor the treatment accordingly.[199]

In conclusion, the inclusion of EUS-FNA and EBUS-TBNA in the guidelines for staging of lung cancer patients is strongly supported by the evidence emerging from recent research.[365]

Summary

EUS-FNA and EUS-TCB are minimally invasive and effective methods for sampling malignant and benign lesions in the pancreas, biliary system, gastrointestinal tract wall, and lymph nodes in the vicinity of the gastrointestinal tract. Both methods of EUS-guided biopsy play a key role in the primary diagnosis and staging of malignant gastrointestinal tumors. The preprocedural work-up includes evaluation of the appropriate indication, obtaining informed consent, checking coagulation status and risk factors, planning a case-specific diagnostic algorithm, and optimal preparation of the equipment for collecting, handling, and processing the specimens. The biopsy itself, as well as the processing of the cytological and histological material obtained, must be performed in an optimal fashion in order to ensure valid diagnoses. The yield of EUS-NB depends on the nature of the target lesion and a variety of technical and procedural variables. Contrast-enhanced EUS and EUS elastography are auxiliary methods which may allow further improvement of the diagnostic accuracy of EUS-guided biopsies. Immediate examination of aspi-

rates for adequacy during EUS-FNA may reduce the number of inadequate samples taken, and it also reduces the number of needle passes required. Alternatively, the aim in EUS-NB should be to obtain both cytological and histological material by means of EUS-FNA using 22-gauge needles, or through a combination of EUS-FNA and EUS-TCB.

Intensive training of both the endosonographic examiner and the cytopathologist, as well as continuous communication between them, are of vital importance for high-quality diagnostic EUS-NB with minimal sampling error and avoidance of diagnostic pitfalls.[7,124,125,181,196] The results of EUS-NB have a major impact on treatment decisions and on the prognosis, particularly in patients with pancreatic mass lesions, esophageal cancer, and lung cancer.

References

1. Jenssen C. Diagnostic endosonography—state of the art 2009. [Article in German] Endosk Heute 2009;22(2): 89–104.
2. Vilmann P, Jacobsen GK, Henriksen FW, Hancke S. Endoscopic ultrasonography with guided fine needle aspiration biopsy in pancreatic disease. Gastrointest Endosc 1992; 38(2):172–173.
3. Wiersema MJ, Hawes RH, Tao LC, et al. Endoscopic ultrasonography as an adjunct to fine needle aspiration cytology of the upper and lower gastrointestinal tract. Gastrointest Endosc 1992;38(1):35–39.
4. Erickson RA, Sayage-Rabie L, Avots-Avotins A. Clinical utility of endoscopic ultrasound-guided fine needle aspiration. Acta Cytol 1997;41(6):1647–1653.
5. Chang KJ, Soetikno RM, Bastas D, Tu C, Nguyen PT. Impact of endoscopic ultrasound combined with fine-needle aspiration biopsy in the management of esophageal cancer. Endoscopy 2003;35(11):962–966.
6. Erickson RA. EUS-guided FNA. Gastrointest Endosc 2004; 60(2):267–279.
7. Jenssen C, Dietrich CF. Endoscopic ultrasound-guided fine-needle aspiration biopsy and trucut biopsy in gastroenterology - An overview. Best Pract Res Clin Gastroenterol 2009;23(5):743–759.
8. Mortensen MB, Pless T, Durup J, Ainsworth AP, Plagborg GJ, Hovendal C. Clinical impact of endoscopic ultrasound-guided fine needle aspiration biopsy in patients with upper gastrointestinal tract malignancies. A prospective study. Endoscopy 2001;33(6):478–483.
9. Veitch AM, Baglin TP, Gershlick AH, Harnden SM, Tighe R, Cairns S; British Society of Gastroenterology; British Committee for Standards in Haematology; British Cardiovascular Intervention Society. Guidelines for the management of anticoagulant and antiplatelet therapy in patients undergoing endoscopic procedures. Gut 2008;57(9):1322–1329.
10. von Bartheld MB, Rabe KF, Annema JT. Transaortic EUS-guided FNA in the diagnosis of lung tumors and lymph nodes. Gastrointest Endosc 2009;69(2):345–349.
11. Wallace MB, Woodward TA, Raimondo M, Al-Haddad M, Odell JA. Transaortic fine-needle aspiration of centrally located lung cancer under endoscopic ultrasound guidance: the final frontier. Ann Thorac Surg 2007;84(3): 1019–1021.

12. Fritscher-Ravens A, Ganbari A, Mosse CA, Swain P, Koehler P, Patel K. Transesophageal endoscopic ultrasound-guided access to the heart. Endoscopy 2007;39(5):385–389.

13. Jenssen C, Siebert C, Bartho S. [Leiomyosarcoma of the inferior vena cava. Diagnosis using endoscopic ultrasound-guided fine-needle aspiration biopsy]. Dtsch Med Wochenschr 2008;133(15):769–772.

14. Yusuf TE, Ho S, Pavey DA, Michael H, Gress FG. Retrospective analysis of the utility of endoscopic ultrasound-guided fine-needle aspiration (EUS-FNA) in pancreatic masses, using a 22-gauge or 25-gauge needle system: a multicenter experience. Endoscopy 2009;41(5):445–448.

15. Ardengh JC, Lopes CV, de Lima LF, et al. Diagnosis of pancreatic tumors by endoscopic ultrasound-guided fine-needle aspiration. World J Gastroenterol 2007;13(22):3112–3116.

16. Turner BG, Cizginer S, Agarwal D, Yang J, Pitman MB, Brugge WR. Diagnosis of pancreatic neoplasia with EUS and FNA: a report of accuracy. Gastrointest Endosc 2010;71(1):91–98.

17. Eloubeidi MA, Varadarajulu S, Desai S, et al. A prospective evaluation of an algorithm incorporating routine preoperative endoscopic ultrasound-guided fine needle aspiration in suspected pancreatic cancer. J Gastrointest Surg 2007;11(7):813–819.

18. Volmar KE, Vollmer RT, Jowell PS, Nelson RC, Xie HB. Pancreatic FNA in 1000 cases: a comparison of imaging modalities. Gastrointest Endosc 2005;61(7):854–861.

19. Varadarajulu S, Tamhane A, Eloubeidi MA. Yield of EUS-guided FNA of pancreatic masses in the presence or the absence of chronic pancreatitis. Gastrointest Endosc 2005;62(5):728–736.

20. Zhang S, Defrias DV, Alasadi R, Nayar R. Endoscopic ultrasound-guided fine needle aspiration (EUS-FNA): experience of an academic centre in the USA. Cytopathology 2010;21(1):35–43.

21. Mitsuhashi T, Ghafari S, Chang CY, Gu M. Endoscopic ultrasound-guided fine needle aspiration of the pancreas: cytomorphological evaluation with emphasis on adequacy assessment, diagnostic criteria and contamination from the gastrointestinal tract. Cytopathology 2006;17(1):34–41.

22. Raut CP, Grau AM, Staerkel GA, et al. Diagnostic accuracy of endoscopic ultrasound-guided fine-needle aspiration in patients with presumed pancreatic cancer. J Gastrointest Surg 2003;7(1):118–126, discussion 127–128.

23. Rocca R, De Angelis C, Daperno M, et al. Endoscopic ultrasound-fine needle aspiration (EUS-FNA) for pancreatic lesions: effectiveness in clinical practice. Dig Liver Dis 2007;39(8):768–774.

24. Eloubeidi MA, Tamhane A. Prospective assessment of diagnostic utility and complications of endoscopic ultrasound-guided fine needle aspiration. Results from a newly developed academic endoscopic ultrasound program. Dig Dis 2008;26(4):356–363.

25. Fritscher-Ravens A, Brand L, Knöfel WT, et al. Comparison of endoscopic ultrasound-guided fine needle aspiration for focal pancreatic lesions in patients with normal parenchyma and chronic pancreatitis. Am J Gastroenterol 2002;97(11):2768–2775.

26. Möller K, Papanikolaou IS, Toermer T, et al. EUS-guided FNA of solid pancreatic masses: high yield of 2 passes with combined histologic-cytologic analysis. Gastrointest Endosc 2009;70(1):60–69.

27. Harewood GC, Wiersema MJ. Endosonography-guided fine needle aspiration biopsy in the evaluation of pancreatic masses. Am J Gastroenterol 2002;97(6):1386–1391.

28. Shin HJ, Lahoti S, Sneige N. Endoscopic ultrasound-guided fine-needle aspiration in 179 cases: the M. D. Anderson Cancer Center experience. Cancer 2002;96(3):174–180.

29. Eloubeidi MA, Chen VK, Eltoum IA, et al. Endoscopic ultrasound-guided fine needle aspiration biopsy of patients with suspected pancreatic cancer: diagnostic accuracy and acute and 30-day complications. Am J Gastroenterol 2003;98(12):2663–2668.

30. Will U, Mueller A, Topalidis T, Meyer F. Value of endoscopic ultrasonography-guided fine needle aspiration (FNA) in the diagnosis of neoplastic tumor(-like) pancreatic lesions in daily clinical practice. Ultraschall Med 2010;31(2):169–174.

31. Wiersema MJ, Vilmann P, Giovannini M, Chang KJ, Wiersema LM. Endosonography-guided fine-needle aspiration biopsy: diagnostic accuracy and complication assessment. Gastroenterology 1997;112(4):1087–1095.

32. Gress F, Gottlieb K, Sherman S, Lehman G. Endoscopic ultrasonography-guided fine-needle aspiration biopsy of suspected pancreatic cancer. Ann Intern Med 2001;134(6):459–464.

33. Brugge WR, Lewandrowski K, Lee-Lewandrowski E, et al. Diagnosis of pancreatic cystic neoplasms: a report of the cooperative pancreatic cyst study. Gastroenterology 2004;126(5):1330–1336.

34. Frossard JL, Amouyal P, Amouyal G, et al. Performance of endosonography-guided fine needle aspiration and biopsy in the diagnosis of pancreatic cystic lesions. Am J Gastroenterol 2003;98(7):1516–1524.

35. Annema JT, Versteegh MI, Veseliç M, Voigt P, Rabe KF. Endoscopic ultrasound-guided fine-needle aspiration in the diagnosis and staging of lung cancer and its impact on surgical staging. J Clin Oncol 2005;23(33):8357–8361.

36. Stelow EB, Lai R, Bardales RH, et al. Endoscopic ultrasound-guided fine-needle aspiration of lymph nodes: the Hennepin County Medical Center experience. Diagn Cytopathol 2004;30(5):301–306.

37. Kramer H, Sanders J, Post WJ, Groen HJ, Suurmeijer AJ. Analysis of cytological specimens from mediastinal lesions obtained by endoscopic ultrasound-guided fine-needle aspiration. Cancer 2006;108(4):206–211.

38. Fritscher-Ravens A, Sriram PV, Bobrowski C, et al. Mediastinal lymphadenopathy in patients with or without previous malignancy: EUS-FNA-based differential cytodiagnosis in 153 patients. Am J Gastroenterol 2000;95(9):2278–2284.

39. Eloubeidi MA, Cerfolio RJ, Chen VK, Desmond R, Syed S, Ojha B. Endoscopic ultrasound-guided fine needle aspiration of mediastinal lymph node in patients with suspected lung cancer after positron emission tomography and computed tomography scans. Ann Thorac Surg 2005;79(1):263–268.

40. Yasuda I, Tsurumi H, Omar S, et al. Endoscopic ultrasound-guided fine-needle aspiration biopsy for lymphadenopathy of unknown origin. Endoscopy 2006;38(9):919–924.

41. Anand D, Barroeta JE, Gupta PK, Kochman M, Baloch ZW. Endoscopic ultrasound guided fine needle aspiration of non-pancreatic lesions: an institutional experience. J Clin Pathol 2007;60(11):1254–1262.

42. Jhala NC, Jhala D, Eltoum I, et al. Endoscopic ultrasound-guided fine-needle aspiration biopsy: a powerful tool to obtain samples from small lesions. Cancer 2004;102(4):239–246.

43. Gress FG, Hawes RH, Savides TJ, Ikenberry SO, Lehman GA. Endoscopic ultrasound-guided fine-needle aspiration biopsy using linear array and radial scanning endosonography. Gastrointest Endosc 1997;45(3):243–250.

44. Südhoff T, Hollerbach S, Wilhelms I, et al. [Clinical utility of EUS-FNA in upper gastrointestinal and mediastinal disease]. Dtsch Med Wochenschr 2004;129(42):2227–2232.

45. Chhieng DC, Jhala D, Jhala N, et al. Endoscopic ultrasound-guided fine-needle aspiration biopsy: a study of 103 cases. Cancer 2002;96(4):232–239.

46. DeWitt J, Alsatie M, LeBlanc J, McHenry L, Sherman S. Endoscopic ultrasound-guided fine-needle aspiration of left adrenal gland masses. Endoscopy 2007;39(1):65–71.

47. Eloubeidi MA, Seewald S, Tamhane A, et al. EUS-guided FNA of the left adrenal gland in patients with thoracic or GI malignancies. Gastrointest Endosc 2004;59(6):627–633.

48. Jhala NC, Jhala D, Eloubeidi MA, et al. Endoscopic ultrasound-guided fine-needle aspiration biopsy of the adrenal glands: analysis of 24 patients. Cancer 2004;102(5):308–314.

49. tenBerge J, Hoffman BJ, Hawes RH, et al. EUS-guided fine needle aspiration of the liver: indications, yield, and safety based on an international survey of 167 cases. Gastrointest Endosc 2002;55(7):859–862.

50. DeWitt J, LeBlanc J, McHenry L, et al. Endoscopic ultrasound-guided fine needle aspiration cytology of solid liver lesions: a large single-center experience. Am J Gastroenterol 2003;98(9):1976–1981.

51. Hollerbach S, Willert J, Topalidis T, Reiser M, Schmiegel W. Endoscopic ultrasound-guided fine-needle aspiration biopsy of liver lesions: histological and cytological assessment. Endoscopy 2003;35(9):743–749.

52. Meara RS, Jhala D, Eloubeidi MA, et al. Endoscopic ultrasound-guided FNA biopsy of bile duct and gallbladder: analysis of 53 cases. Cytopathology 2006;17(1):42–49.

53. Fritscher-Ravens A, Broering DC, Knoefel WT, et al. EUS-guided fine-needle aspiration of suspected hilar cholangiocarcinoma in potentially operable patients with negative brush cytology. Am J Gastroenterol 2004;99(1):45–51.

54. Byrne MF, Gerke H, Mitchell RM, et al. Yield of endoscopic ultrasound-guided fine-needle aspiration of bile duct lesions. Endoscopy 2004;36(8):715–719.

55. Rösch T, Hofrichter K, Frimberger E, et al. ERCP or EUS for tissue diagnosis of biliary strictures? A prospective comparative study. Gastrointest Endosc 2004;60(3):390–396.

56. Eloubeidi MA, Chen VK, Jhala NC, et al. Endoscopic ultrasound-guided fine needle aspiration biopsy of suspected cholangiocarcinoma. Clin Gastroenterol Hepatol 2004;2(3):209–213.

57. DeWitt J, Misra VL, Leblanc JK, McHenry L, Sherman S. EUS-guided FNA of proximal biliary strictures after negative ERCP brush cytology results. Gastrointest Endosc 2006;64(3):325–333.

58. Fritscher-Ravens A, Mylonaki M, Pantes A, Topalidis T, Thonke F, Swain P. Endoscopic ultrasound-guided biopsy for the diagnosis of focal lesions of the spleen. Am J Gastroenterol 2003;98(5):1022–1027.

59. Eloubeidi MA, Varadarajulu S, Eltoum I, Jhala D, Chhieng DC, Jhala NC. Transgastric endoscopic ultrasound-guided fine-needle aspiration biopsy and flow cytometry of suspected lymphoma of the spleen. Endoscopy 2006; 38(6):617–620.

60. Devereaux BM, Leblanc JK, Yousif E, et al. Clinical utility of EUS-guided fine-needle aspiration of mediastinal masses in the absence of known pulmonary malignancy. Gastrointest Endosc 2002;56(3):397–401.

61. Catalano MF, Rosenblatt ML, Chak A, Sivak MV Jr, Scheiman J, Gress F. Endoscopic ultrasound-guided fine needle aspiration in the diagnosis of mediastinal masses of unknown origin. Am J Gastroenterol 2002;97(10):2559–2565.

62. Hoda KM, Rodriguez SA, Faigel DO. EUS-guided sampling of suspected GI stromal tumors. Gastrointest Endosc 2009;69(7):1218–1223.

63. Vander Noot MR III, Eloubeidi MA, Chen VK, et al. Diagnosis of gastrointestinal tract lesions by endoscopic ultrasound-guided fine-needle aspiration biopsy. Cancer 2004;102(3):157–163.

64. Akahoshi K, Sumida Y, Matsui N, et al. Preoperative diagnosis of gastrointestinal stromal tumor by endoscopic ultrasound-guided fine needle aspiration. World J Gastroenterol 2007;13(14):2077–2082.

65. Ando N, Goto H, Niwa Y, et al. The diagnosis of GI stromal tumors with EUS-guided fine needle aspiration with immunohistochemical analysis. Gastrointest Endosc 2002;55(1):37–43.

66. Chen VK, Eloubeidi MA. Endoscopic ultrasound-guided fine-needle aspiration of intramural and extraintestinal mass lesions: diagnostic accuracy, complication assessment, and impact on management. Endoscopy 2005;37(10):984–989.

67. Sepe PS, Moparty B, Pitman MB, Saltzman JR, Brugge WR. EUS-guided FNA for the diagnosis of GI stromal cell tumors: sensitivity and cytologic yield. Gastrointest Endosc 2009;70(2):254–261.

68. Sasaki Y, Niwa Y, Hirooka Y, et al. The use of endoscopic ultrasound-guided fine-needle aspiration for investigation of submucosal and extrinsic masses of the colon and rectum. Endoscopy 2005;37(2):154–160.

69. DeWitt J, LeBlanc J, McHenry L, McGreevy K, Sherman S. Endoscopic ultrasound-guided fine-needle aspiration of ascites. Clin Gastroenterol Hepatol 2007;5(5):609–615.

70. Nguyen PT, Chang KJ. EUS in the detection of ascites and EUS-guided paracentesis. Gastrointest Endosc 2001;54(3):336–339.

71. Kaushik N, Khalid A, Brody D, McGrath K. EUS-guided paracentesis for the diagnosis of malignant ascites. Gastrointest Endosc 2006;64(6):908–913.

72. DeWitt J, Gress FG, Levy MJ, et al. EUS-guided FNA aspiration of kidney masses: a multicenter U.S. experience. Gastrointest Endosc 2009;70(3):573–578.

73. Catalano MF, Ahmed U, Chauhan S, et al. EUS-guided FNA of pancreatic mass lesions: significance of suspicious or atypical histopathology. (abstract) Gastrointest Endosc 2005;61(5):AB272.

74. Eloubeidi MA, Jhala D, Chhieng DC, et al. Yield of endoscopic ultrasound-guided fine-needle aspiration biopsy in patients with suspected pancreatic carcinoma. Cancer 2003;99(5):285–292.

75. Kipp BR, Pereira TC, Souza PC, Gleeson FC, Levy MJ, Clayton AC. Comparison of EUS-guided FNA and Trucut biopsy for diagnosing and staging abdominal and mediastinal neoplasms. Diagn Cytopathol 2009;37(8):549–556.

76. Annema JT, Versteegh MI, Veselic M, et al. Endoscopic ultrasound added to mediastinoscopy for preoperative staging of patients with lung cancer. JAMA 2005;294(8):931–936.

77. Ardengh JC, de Paulo GA, Ferrari AP. EUS-guided FNA in the diagnosis of pancreatic neuroendocrine tumors before surgery. Gastrointest Endosc 2004;60(3):378–384.

78. Caddy G, Conron M, Wright G, Desmond P, Hart D, Chen RY. The accuracy of EUS-FNA in assessing mediastinal lymphadenopathy and staging patients with NSCLC. Eur Respir J 2005;25(3):410–415.

79. Fritscher-Ravens A, Bohuslavizki KH, Brandt L, et al. Mediastinal lymph node involvement in potentially resectable lung cancer: comparison of CT, positron emission tomog-

raphy, and endoscopic ultrasonography with and without fine-needle aspiration. Chest 2003;123(2):442–451.

80. Okubo K, Yamao K, Nakamura T, et al. Endoscopic ultrasound-guided fine-needle aspiration biopsy for the diagnosis of gastrointestinal stromal tumors in the stomach. J Gastroenterol 2004;39(8):747–753.

81. Noh KW, Raimondo M, Woodward TA, et al. Eliminating the "non-diagnostic" EUS-FNA specimen: effect of a quality improvement program on cytologic interpretation. (abstract) Gastrointest Endosc 2005;61(5):AB295.

82. Takahashi K, Yamao K, Okubo K, et al. Differential diagnosis of pancreatic cancer and focal pancreatitis by using EUS-guided FNA. Gastrointest Endosc 2005;61(1):76–79.

83. Iglesias-Garcia J, Dominguez-Munoz E, Lozano-Leon A, et al. Impact of endoscopic ultrasound-guided fine needle biopsy for diagnosis of pancreatic masses. World J Gastroenterol 2007;13(2):289–293.

84. Niehaus J, Burmester E, Rode M, et al. EUS-FNA: a prospective study for the evaluation of the histological and cytological material. (abstract) Gastrointest Endosc 2006;63(5):AB275.

85. Thomas T, Kaye PV, Ragunath K, Aithal G. Efficacy, safety, and predictive factors for a positive yield of EUS-guided Trucut biopsy: a large tertiary referral center experience. Am J Gastroenterol 2009;104(3):584–591.

86. Aithal GP, Anagnostopoulos GK, Tam W, et al. EUS-guided tissue sampling: comparison of "dual sampling" (Trucut biopsy plus FNA) with "sequential sampling" (Trucut biopsy and then FNA as required). Endoscopy 2007;39(8):725–730.

87. Wittmann J, Kocjan G, Sgouros SN, Deheragoda M, Pereira SP. Endoscopic ultrasound-guided tissue sampling by combined fine needle aspiration and trucut needle biopsy: a prospective study. Cytopathology 2006;17(1):27–33.

88. Shah SM, Ribeiro A, Levi J, et al. EUS-guided fine needle aspiration with and without trucut biopsy of pancreatic masses. JOP 2008;9(4):422–430.

89. Vanderheyden AD, Proctor KA, Rizk MK, Silva RG Jr, Jensen CS, Gerke H. The value of touch imprint cytology in EUS-guided Trucut biopsy. Gastrointest Endosc 2008;68(1):44–50.

90. Berger LP, Scheffer RC, Weusten BL, et al. The additional value of EUS-guided Tru-cut biopsy to EUS-guided FNA in patients with mediastinal lesions. Gastrointest Endosc 2009;69(6):1045–1051.

91. Storch I, Jorda M, Thurer R, et al. Advantage of EUS Trucut biopsy combined with fine-needle aspiration without immediate on-site cytopathologic examination. Gastrointest Endosc 2006;64(4):505–511.

92. Storch I, Shah M, Thurer R, Donna E, Ribeiro A. Endoscopic ultrasound-guided fine-needle aspiration and Trucut biopsy in thoracic lesions: when tissue is the issue. Surg Endosc 2008;22(1):86–90.

93. Ginès A, Wiersema MJ, Clain JE, Pochron NL, Rajan E, Levy MJ. Prospective study of a Trucut needle for performing EUS-guided biopsy with EUS-guided FNA rescue. Gastrointest Endosc 2005;62(4):597–601.

94. Polkowski M, Gerke W, Jarosz D, et al. Diagnostic yield and safety of endoscopic ultrasound-guided trucut [corrected] biopsy in patients with gastric submucosal tumors: a prospective study. Endoscopy 2009;41(4):329–334.

95. Thomas T, Kaye PV, Ragunath K, Aithal GP. Endoscopic-ultrasound-guided mural trucut biopsy in the investigation of unexplained thickening of esophagogastric wall. Endoscopy 2009;41(4):335–339.

96. Săftoiu A, Vilmann P, Guldhammer Skov B, Georgescu CV. Endoscopic ultrasound (EUS)-guided Trucut biopsy adds significant information to EUS-guided fine-needle aspiration in selected patients: a prospective study. Scand J Gastroenterol 2007;42(1):117–125.

97. Sakamoto H, Kitano M, Komaki T, et al. Prospective comparative study of the EUS guided 25-gauge FNA needle with the 19-gauge Trucut needle and 22-gauge FNA needle in patients with solid pancreatic masses. J Gastroenterol Hepatol 2009;24(3):384–390.

98. Wahnschaffe U, Ullrich R, Mayerle J, Lerch MM, Zeitz M, Faiss S. EUS-guided Trucut needle biopsies as first-line diagnostic method for patients with intestinal or extraintestinal mass lesions. Surg Endosc 2009;23(10):2351–2355.

99. Larghi A, Verna EC, Stavropoulos SN, Rotterdam H, Lightdale CJ, Stevens PD. EUS-guided trucut needle biopsies in patients with solid pancreatic masses: a prospective study. Gastrointest Endosc 2004;59(2):185–190.

100. Levy MJ, Jondal ML, Clain J, Wiersema MJ. Preliminary experience with an EUS-guided trucut biopsy needle compared with EUS-guided FNA. Gastrointest Endosc 2003;57(1):101–106.

101. Varadarajulu S, Fraig M, Schmulewitz N, et al. Comparison of EUS-guided 19-gauge Trucut needle biopsy with EUS-guided fine-needle aspiration. Endoscopy 2004;36(5):397–401.

102. Voss M, Hammel P, Molas G, et al. Value of endoscopic ultrasound guided fine needle aspiration biopsy in the diagnosis of solid pancreatic masses. Gut 2000;46(2):244–249.

103. Catalano MF, Fazel A, Quadri A, et al. Factors that influence accuracy of tissue sampling in pancreatic mass lesions: an EUS-FNA study. (abstract) Gastrointest Endosc 2002;55(5):AB246.

104. Eloubeidi MA, Varadarajulu S, Desai S, Wilcox CM. Value of repeat endoscopic ultrasound-guided fine needle aspiration for suspected pancreatic cancer. J Gastroenterol Hepatol 2008;23(4):567–570.

105. Eloubeidi MA, Iseman DT, Chen VK, Vickers SM, Wilcox CM. Prevalence and significance of periduodenal venous collaterals in patients evaluated for pancreaticobiliary disorders by endosonography. Endoscopy 2003;35(12):1015–1019.

106. Itoi T, Itokawa F, Sofuni A, et al. Puncture of solid pancreatic tumors guided by endoscopic ultrasonography: a pilot study series comparing Trucut and 19-gauge and 22-gauge aspiration needles. Endoscopy 2005;37(4):362–366.

107. Binmoeller KF, Jabusch HC, Seifert H, Soehendra N. Endosonography-guided fine-needle biopsy of indurated pancreatic lesions using an automated biopsy device. Endoscopy 1997;29(5):384–388.

108. Meyer S, Bittinger F, Keth A, Von Mach MA, Kann PH. [Endosonographically controlled transluminal fine needle aspiration biopsy: diagnostic quality by cytologic and histopathologic classification]. Dtsch Med Wochenschr 2003;128(30):1585–1591.

109. Nagle JA, Wilbur DC, Pitman MB. Cytomorphology of gastric and duodenal epithelium and reactivity to B72.3: a baseline for comparison to pancreatic lesions aspirated by EUS-FNAB. Diagn Cytopathol 2005;33(6):381–386.

110. Fazel A, Moezardalan K, Varadarajulu S, Draganov P, Eloubeidi MA. The utility and the safety of EUS-guided FNA in the evaluation of duplication cysts. Gastrointest Endosc 2005;62(4):575–580.

111. Huang P, Staerkel G, Sneige N, Gong Y. Fine-needle aspiration of pancreatic serous cystadenoma: cytologic features and diagnostic pitfalls. Cancer 2006;108(4):239–249.

112. Jhala NC, Jhala DN, Chhieng DC, Eloubeidi MA, Eltoum IA. Endoscopic ultrasound-guided fine-needle aspiration. A cytopathologist's perspective. Am J Clin Pathol 2003;120(3):351–367.

113. Stelow EB, Bardales RH, Stanley MW. Pitfalls in endoscopic ultrasound-guided fine-needle aspiration and how to avoid them. Adv Anat Pathol 2005;12(2):62–73.

114. Kien-Fong Vu C, Chang F, Doig L, Meenan J. A prospective control study of the safety and cellular yield of EUS-guided FNA or Trucut biopsy in patients taking aspirin, nonsteroidal anti-inflammatory drugs, or prophylactic low molecular weight heparin. Gastrointest Endosc 2006;63(6):808–813.

115. Wallace MB, Kennedy T, Durkalski V, et al. Randomized controlled trial of EUS-guided fine needle aspiration techniques for the detection of malignant lymphadenopathy. Gastrointest Endosc 2001;54(4):441–447.

116. Pellisé Urquiza M, Fernández-Esparrach G, Solé M, et al. Endoscopic ultrasound-guided fine needle aspiration: predictive factors of accurate diagnosis and cost-minimization analysis of on-site pathologist. Gastroenterol Hepatol 2007;30(6):319–324.

117. Hamerski C, Shergill A, DeLusong M, et al. Yield of endoscopic ultrasound guided fine needle aspiration (EUS-FNA) in diagnosing submucosal lesions of the upper GI tract. (abstract) Gastrointest Endosc 2008;67(5):AB222.

118. Giovannini M, Seitz JF, Monges G, Perrier H, Rabbia I. Fine-needle aspiration cytology guided by endoscopic ultrasonography: results in 141 patients. Endoscopy 1995;27(2):171–177.

119. Eloubeidi MA, Wallace MB, Reed CE, et al. The utility of EUS and EUS-guided fine needle aspiration in detecting celiac lymph node metastasis in patients with esophageal cancer: a single-center experience. Gastrointest Endosc 2001;54(6):714–719.

120. Ardengh JC, Lopes CV, Campos AD, Pereira de Lima LF, Venco F, Módena JL. Endoscopic ultrasound and fine needle aspiration in chronic pancreatitis: differential diagnosis between pseudotumoral masses and pancreatic cancer. JOP 2007;8(4):413–421.

121. Krishna NB, Mehra M, Reddy AV, Agarwal B. EUS/EUS-FNA for suspected pancreatic cancer: influence of chronic pancreatitis and clinical presentation with or without obstructive jaundice on performance characteristics. Gastrointest Endosc 2009;70(1):70–79.

122. Cheng TY, Wang HP, Jan IS, Chen JH, Lin JT. Presence of intratumoral anechoic foci predicts an increased number of endoscopic ultrasound-guided fine-needle aspiration passes required for the diagnosis of pancreatic adenocarcinoma. J Gastroenterol Hepatol 2007;22(3):315–319.

123. Polkowski M. Endoscopic ultrasound and endoscopic ultrasound-guided fine-needle biopsy for the diagnosis of malignant submucosal tumors. Endoscopy 2005;37(7):635–645.

124. Jenssen C, Möller K, Wagner S, Sarbia M. [Endoscopic ultrasound-guided biopsy: diagnostic yield, pitfalls, quality management part 1: optimizing specimen collection and diagnostic efficiency]. Z Gastroenterol 2008;46(6):590–600.

125. Jenssen C, Möller K, Wagner S, Sarbia M. [Endoscopic ultrasound-guided biopsy: diagnostic yield, pitfalls, quality management part 2: opportunities of differential diagnosis, pitfalls, and problem solutions]. Z Gastroenterol 2008;46(9):897–908.

126. Erickson RA, Sayage-Rabie L, Beissner RS. Factors predicting the number of EUS-guided fine-needle passes for diagnosis of pancreatic malignancies. Gastrointest Endosc 2000;51(2):184–190.

127. LeBlanc JK, Ciaccia D, Al-Assi MT, et al. Optimal number of EUS-guided fine needle passes needed to obtain a correct diagnosis. Gastrointest Endosc 2004;59(1):475–481.

128. Storch IM, Sussman DA, Jorda M, Ribeir A. Evaluation of fine needle aspiration vs. fine needle capillary sampling on specimen quality and diagnostic accuracy in endoscopic ultrasound-guided biopsy. Acta Cytol 2007;51(6):837–842.

129. Puri R, Vilmann P, Săftoiu A, et al. Randomized controlled trial of endoscopic ultrasound-guided fine-needle sampling with or without suction for better cytological diagnosis. Scand J Gastroenterol 2009;44(4):499–504.

130. Bhutani MS, Suryaprasad S, Moezzi J, Seabrook D. Improved technique for performing endoscopic ultrasound guided fine needle aspiration of lymph nodes. Endoscopy 1999;31(7):550–553.

131. Larghi A, Noffsinger A, Dye CE, Hart J, Waxman I. EUS-guided fine needle tissue acquisition by using high negative pressure suction for the evaluation of solid masses: a pilot study. Gastrointest Endosc 2005;62(5):768–774.

132. Gerke H, Rizk MK, Vanderheyden AD, Jensen CS. Randomized study comparing endoscopic ultrasound-guided Trucut biopsy and fine needle aspiration with high suction. Cytopathology 2010;21(1):44–51.

133. Schröder W, Baldus SE, Mönig SP, Beckurts TK, Dienes HP, Hölscher AH. Lymph node staging of esophageal squamous cell carcinoma in patients with and without neoadjuvant radiochemotherapy: histomorphologic analysis. World J Surg 2002;26(5):584–587.

134. Mönig SP, Zirbes TK, Schröder W, et al. Staging of gastric cancer: correlation of lymph node size and metastatic infiltration. AJR Am J Roentgenol 1999;173(2):365–367.

135. Kotanagi H, Fukuoka T, Shibata Y, et al. The size of regional lymph nodes does not correlate with the presence or absence of metastasis in lymph nodes in rectal cancer. J Surg Oncol 1993;54(4):252–254.

136. Mönig SP, Baldus SE, Zirbes TK, et al. Lymph node size and metastatic infiltration in colon cancer. Ann Surg Oncol 1999;6(6):579–581.

137. Prenzel KL, Mönig SP, Sinning JM, et al. Lymph node size and metastatic infiltration in non-small cell lung cancer. Chest 2003;123(2):463–467.

138. Bhutani MS, Hawes RH, Hoffman BJ. A comparison of the accuracy of echo features during endoscopic ultrasound (EUS) and EUS-guided fine-needle aspiration for diagnosis of malignant lymph node invasion. Gastrointest Endosc 1997;45(6):474–479.

139. Catalano MF, Sivak MV Jr, Rice T, Gragg LA, Van Dam J. Endosonographic features predictive of lymph node metastasis. Gastrointest Endosc 1994;40(4):442–446.

140. Faigel DO. EUS in patients with benign and malignant lymphadenopathy. Gastrointest Endosc 2001;53(6): 593–598.

141. Bhutani MS, Saftoiu A, Chaya C, et al. Irregular echogenic foci representing coagulation necrosis: a useful but perhaps under-recognized EUS echo feature of malignant lymph node invasion. J Gastrointestin Liver Dis 2009;18(2):181–184.

142. Hall JD, Kahaleh M, White GE, Talreja J, Northup PG, Shami VM. Presence of lymph node vasculature: a new EUS criterion for benign nodes? Dig Dis Sci 2009;54(1):118–121.

143. Gleeson FC, Clain JE, Papachristou GI, et al. Prospective assessment of EUS criteria for lymphadenopathy associated with rectal cancer. Gastrointest Endosc 2009;69(4):896–903.

144. Schmulewitz N, Wildi SM, Varadarajulu S, et al. Accuracy of EUS criteria and primary tumor site for identification of mediastinal lymph node metastasis from non-small-cell lung cancer. Gastrointest Endosc 2004;59(2):205–212.
145. Gill KR, Ghabril MS, Jamil LH, et al. Endosonographic features predictive of malignancy in mediastinal lymph nodes in patients with lung cancer. Gastrointest Endosc 2010;72(2):265–271.
146. Gleeson FC, Rajan E, Levy MJ, et al. EUS-guided FNA of regional lymph nodes in patients with unresectable hilar cholangiocarcinoma. Gastrointest Endosc 2008;67(3):438–443.
147. Chen VK, Eloubeidi MA. Endoscopic ultrasound-guided fine needle aspiration is superior to lymph node echofeatures: a prospective evaluation of mediastinal and peri-intestinal lymphadenopathy. Am J Gastroenterol 2004;99(4):628–633.
148. Kalaitzakis E, Sadik R, Doig L, Meenan J. Defining the lymph node burden in a Northern European population without malignancy: the potential effect of geography in determining a need for FNA? Dis Esophagus 2009; 22(5):409–417.
149. Wiersema MJ, Hassig WM, Hawes RH, Wonn MJ. Mediastinal lymph node detection with endosonography. Gastrointest Endosc 1993;39(6):788–793.
150. Das A, Nguyen CC, Li F, Li B. Digital image analysis of EUS images accurately differentiates pancreatic cancer from chronic pancreatitis and normal tissue. Gastrointest Endosc 2008;67(6):861–867.
151. Giovannini M, Thomas B, Erwan B, et al. Endoscopic ultrasound elastography for evaluation of lymph nodes and pancreatic masses: a multicenter study. World J Gastroenterol 2009;15(13):1587–1593.
152. Hocke M, Menges M, Topalidis T, Dietrich CF, Stallmach A. Contrast-enhanced endoscopic ultrasound in discrimination between benign and malignant mediastinal and abdominal lymph nodes. J Cancer Res Clin Oncol 2008;134(4):473–480.
153. Janssen J, Dietrich CF, Will U, Greiner L. Endosonographic elastography in the diagnosis of mediastinal lymph nodes. Endoscopy 2007;39(11):952–957.
154. Kanamori A, Hirooka Y, Itoh A, et al. Usefulness of contrast-enhanced endoscopic ultrasonography in the differentiation between malignant and benign lymphadenopathy. Am J Gastroenterol 2006;101(1):45–51.
155. Kumon RE, Pollack MJ, Faulx AL, et al. In vivo characterization of pancreatic and lymph node tissue by using EUS spectrum analysis: a validation study. Gastrointest Endosc 2010;71(1):53–63.
156. Săftoiu A, Vilmann P, Hassan H, Gorunescu F. Analysis of endoscopic ultrasound elastography used for characterisation and differentiation of benign and malignant lymph nodes. Ultraschall Med 2006;27(6):535–542.
157. Binmoeller KF, Thul R, Rathod V, et al. Endoscopic ultrasound-guided, 18-gauge, fine needle aspiration biopsy of the pancreas using a 2.8 mm channel convex array echoendoscope. Gastrointest Endosc 1998;47(2):121–127.
158. Imazu H, Uchiyama Y, Kakutani H, Ikeda K, Sumiyama K, Kaise M, et al A prospective comparison of EUS-guided FNA using 25-gauge and 22-gauge needles. Gastroenterol Res Pract 2009;2009:546390.
159. Lee JH, Stewart J, Ross WA, Anandasabapathy S, Xiao L, Staerkel G. Blinded prospective comparison of the performance of 22-gauge and 25-gauge needles in endoscopic ultrasound-guided fine needle aspiration of the pancreas and peri-pancreatic lesions. Dig Dis Sci 2009;54(10):2274–2281.
160. Siddiqui UD, Rossi F, Rosenthal LS, Padda MS, Murali-Dharan V, Aslanian HR. EUS-guided FNA of solid pancreatic masses: a prospective, randomized trial comparing 22-gauge and 25-gauge needles. Gastrointest Endosc 2009;70(6):1093–1097.
161. Nguyen TTH, Lee CE, Whang CS. A comparison of the diagnostic yield and specimen adequacy between 22 and 25 gauge needles for endoscopic ultrasound-guided needle aspiration (EUS-FNA) of solid pancreatic lesions (SPL): Is bigger better? (abstract) Gastrointest Endosc 2008; 67(5):AB100.
162. Song TJ, Kim JH, Lee SS, Eum JB, Moon SH, Park do H, et al The prospective randomized, controlled trial of endoscopic ultrasound-guided fine-needle aspiration using 22G and 19G aspiration needles for solid pancreatic or peripancreatic masses. Am J Gastroenterol 2010;105(8):1739–1745.
163. Itoi T, Itokawa F, Kurihara T, et al. Experimental endoscopy: objective evaluation of EUS needles. Gastrointest Endosc 2009;69(3 Pt 1):509–516.
164. Mizuno N, Bhatia V, Hosoda W, et al. Histological diagnosis of autoimmune pancreatitis using EUS-guided trucut biopsy: a comparison study with EUS-FNA. J Gastroenterol 2009;44(7):742–750.
165. Levy MJ, Smyrk TC, Reddy RP, et al. Endoscopic ultrasound-guided trucut biopsy of the cyst wall for diagnosing cystic pancreatic tumors. Clin Gastroenterol Hepatol 2005; 3(10):974–979.
166. Fernández-Esparrach G, Sendino O, Solé M, et al. Endoscopic ultrasound-guided fine-needle aspiration and trucut biopsy in the diagnosis of gastric stromal tumors: a randomized crossover study. Endoscopy 2010;42(4):292–299.
167. Eloubeidi MA, Mehra M, Bean SM. EUS-guided 19-gauge trucut needle biopsy for diagnosis of lymphoma missed by EUS-guided FNA. Gastrointest Endosc 2007;65(6):937–939.
168. Dewitt J, McGreevy K, Cummings O, et al. Initial experience with EUS-guided Tru-cut biopsy of benign liver disease. Gastrointest Endosc 2009;69(3 Pt 1):535–542.
169. Gleeson FC, Clayton AC, Zhang L, et al. Adequacy of endoscopic ultrasound core needle biopsy specimen of nonmalignant hepatic parenchymal disease. Clin Gastroenterol Hepatol 2008;6(12):1437–1440.
170. Gleeson F, Clarke E, Kelly S, et al. Diagnosis by EUS trucut biopsy of extrapulmonary tuberculosis in a patient with Crohn's disease treated with infliximab. Gastrointest Endosc 2005;61(3):489–492.
171. Larghi A, Rodriguez-Wulff E, Noffsinger A, Dye CE. Recurrent malignant thymoma diagnosed by EUS-guided Trucut biopsy. Gastrointest Endosc 2006;63(6):859–860.
172. Rhee KH, Lee SS, Huh JR. Endoscopic ultrasonography-guided trucut biopsy for the preoperative diagnosis of peripancreatic Castleman's disease: a case report. World J Gastroenterol 2008;14(13):2115–2117.
173. Silva RG, Dahmoush L, Gerke H. Pancreatic metastasis of an ovarian malignant mixed Mullerian tumor identified by EUS-guided fine needle aspiration and Trucut needle biopsy. JOP 2006;7(1):66–69.
174. Imaoka H, Yamao K, Bhatia V, et al. Rare pancreatic neoplasms: the utility of endoscopic ultrasound-guided fine-needle aspiration-a large single center study. J Gastroenterol 2009;44(2):146–153.
175. Iwashita T, Yasuda I, Doi S, et al. The yield of endoscopic ultrasound-guided fine needle aspiration for histological diagnosis in patients suspected of stage I sarcoidosis. Endoscopy 2008;40(5):400–405.

176. Noda Y, Fujita N, Kobayashi G, et al. Diagnostic efficacy of the cell block method in comparison with smear cytology of tissue samples obtained by endoscopic ultrasound-guided fine-needle aspiration. J Gastroenterol 2010; 45(8): 868–875.

177. Emery SC, Savides TJ, Behling CA. Utility of immediate evaluation of endoscopic ultrasound-guided transesophageal fine needle aspiration of mediastinal lymph nodes. Acta Cytol 2004;48(5):630–634.

178. Woon C, Bardales RH, Stanley MW, Stelow EB. Rapid assessment of fine needle aspiration and the final diagnosis—how often and why the diagnoses are changed. Cytojournal 2006;3:25.

179. Eloubeidi MA, Tamhane A, Jhala N, et al. Agreement between rapid onsite and final cytologic interpretations of EUS-guided FNA specimens: implications for the endosonographer and patient management. Am J Gastroenterol 2006;101(12):2841–2847.

180. Jhala NC, Eltoum IA, Eloubeidi MA, et al. Providing on-site diagnosis of malignancy on endoscopic-ultrasound-guided fine-needle aspirates: should it be done? Ann Diagn Pathol 2007;11(3):176–181.

181. Logroño R, Waxman I. Interactive role of the cytopathologist in EUS-guided fine needle aspiration: an efficient approach. Gastrointest Endosc 2001;54(4):485–490.

182. Klapman JB, Logrono R, Dye CE, Waxman I. Clinical impact of on-site cytopathology interpretation on endoscopic ultrasound-guided fine needle aspiration. Am J Gastroenterol 2003;98(6):1289–1294.

183. Cleveland P, Gill KR, Coe SG, et al. An evaluation of risk factors for inadequate cytology in EUS-guided FNA of pancreatic tumors and lymph nodes. Gastrointest Endosc 2010; 71(7):1194–1199.

184. Savoy AD, Raimondo M, Woodward TA, et al. Can endosonographers evaluate on-site cytologic adequacy? A comparison with cytotechnologists. Gastrointest Endosc 2007;65(7):953–957.

185. Hikichi T, Irisawa A, Bhutani MS, et al. Endoscopic ultrasound-guided fine-needle aspiration of solid pancreatic masses with rapid on-site cytological evaluation by endosonographers without attendance of cytopathologists. J Gastroenterol 2009;44(4):322–328.

186. Nguyen YP, Maple JT, Zhang Q, et al. Reliability of gross visual assessment of specimen adequacy during EUS-guided FNA of pancreatic masses. Gastrointest Endosc 2009;69(7): 1264–1270.

187. Mayall F, Cormack A, Slater S, McAnulty K. The utility of assessing the gross appearances of FNA specimens. Cytopathology 2010;21(6):395–397.

188. Zhu LC, Grieco V. Diagnostic value of unusual gross appearance of aspirated material from endoscopic ultrasound-guided fine needle aspiration of pancreatic and peripancreatic cystic lesions. Acta Cytol 2008;52(5):535–540.

189. Kim B, Chhieng DC, Crowe DR, et al. Dynamic telecytopathology of on site rapid cytology diagnoses for pancreatic carcinoma. Cytojournal 2006;3:27.

190. Mertz H, Gautam S. The learning curve for EUS-guided FNA of pancreatic cancer. Gastrointest Endosc 2004;59(1): 33–37.

191. Eloubeidi MA, Tamhane A. EUS-guided FNA of solid pancreatic masses: a learning curve with 300 consecutive procedures. Gastrointest Endosc 2005;61(6):700–708.

192. Harewood GC, Wiersema LM, Halling AC, Keeney GL, Salamao DR, Wiersema MJ. Influence of EUS training and pathology interpretation on accuracy of EUS-guided fine needle aspiration of pancreatic masses. Gastrointest Endosc 2002;55(6):669–673.

193. Eisen GM, Dominitz JA, Faigel DO, et al; American Society for Gastrointestinal Endoscopy. Guidelines for credentialing and granting privileges for endoscopic ultrasound. Gastrointest Endosc 2001;54(6):811–814.

194. Skov BG, Baandrup U, Jakobsen GK, et al. Cytopathologic diagnoses of fine-needle aspirations from endoscopic ultrasound of the mediastinum: reproducibility of the diagnoses and representativeness of aspirates from lymph nodes. Cancer 2007;111(4):234–241.

195. Eltoum IA, Chhieng DC, Jhala D, et al. Cumulative sum procedure in evaluation of EUS-guided FNA cytology: the learning curve and diagnostic performance beyond sensitivity and specificity. Cytopathology 2007;18(3):143–150.

196. Kulesza P, Eltoum IA. Endoscopic ultrasound-guided fine-needle aspiration: sampling, pitfalls, and quality management. Clin Gastroenterol Hepatol 2007;5(11):1248–1254.

197. de Luna R, Eloubeidi MA, Sheffield MV, et al. Comparison of ThinPrep and conventional preparations in pancreatic fine-needle aspiration biopsy. Diagn Cytopathol 2004; 30(2):71–76.

198. LeBlanc JK, Emerson RE, DeWitt J, et al. A prospective study comparing rapid assessment of smears and ThinPrep for endoscopic ultrasound-guided fine-needle aspirates. Endoscopy 2010;42(5):389–394.

199. Wallace MB. Micrometastasis, molecular markers, and their future role with EUS-guided FNA. Gastrointest Endosc 2009; 69(2, Suppl): S152–S154.

200. Al-Haddad M, Savabi MS, Sherman S, et al. Role of endoscopic ultrasound-guided fine-needle aspiration with flow cytometry to diagnose lymphoma: a single center experience. J Gastroenterol Hepatol 2009;24(12):1826–1833.

201. Khashab M, Mokadem M, DeWitt J, et al. Endoscopic ultrasound-guided fine-needle aspiration with or without flow cytometry for the diagnosis of primary pancreatic lymphoma - a case series. Endoscopy 2010;42(3):228–231.

202. Pugh JL, Jhala NC, Eloubeidi MA, et al. Diagnosis of deep-seated lymphoma and leukemia by endoscopic ultrasound-guided fine-needle aspiration biopsy. Am J Clin Pathol 2006;125(5):703–709.

203. Wiersema MJ, Gatzimos K, Nisi R, Wiersema LM. Staging of non-Hodgkin's gastric lymphoma with endosonography-guided fine-needle aspiration biopsy and flow cytometry. Gastrointest Endosc 1996;44(6):734–736.

204. Chaya CT, Schnadig V, Gupta P, Logrono R, Bhutani MS. Endoscopic ultrasound-guided fine-needle aspiration for diagnosis of an infectious mediastinal mass and/or lymphadenopathy. Endoscopy 2006;38(Suppl 2):E99–E101.

205. Fritscher-Ravens A, Schirrow L, Pothmann W, Knöfel WT, Swain P, Soehendra N. Critical care transesophageal endosonography and guided fine-needle aspiration for diagnosis and management of posterior mediastinitis. Crit Care Med 2003;31(1):126–132.

206. Fritscher-Ravens A, Sriram PV, Schröder S, Topalidis T, Bohnacker S, Soehendra N. Stromal tumor as a pitfall in EUS-guided fine-needle aspiration cytology. Gastrointest Endosc 2000;51(6):746–749.

207. Schwartz DA, Unni KK, Levy MJ, Clain JE, Wiersema MJ. The rate of false-positive results with EUS-guided fine-needle aspiration. Gastrointest Endosc 2002;56(6): 868–872.

208. Gleeson FC, Kipp BR, Caudill JL, et al. False positive endoscopic ultrasound fine needle aspiration cytology: incidence and risk factors. Gut 2010;59(5):586–593.

209. Levy MJ, Gleeson FC, Campion MB, et al. Prospective cytological assessment of gastrointestinal luminal fluid acquired during EUS: a potential source of false-positive FNA and needle tract seeding. Am J Gastroenterol 2010;105(6): 1311–1318.

210. Harbaum L, Pomjanski N, Hinterleitner TA, Böcking A, Langner C. False-positive mediastinal lymph node cytology due to translesional endoscopic ultrasound-guided fine-needle aspiration in a patient with Barrett's early cancer. Endoscopy 2009;41(Suppl 2):E150–E151.

211. De Lisi S, Buscarini E, Arcidiacono PG, et al. Endoscopic ultrasonography findings in autoimmune pancreatitis: be aware of the ambiguous features and look for the pivotal ones. JOP 2010;11(1):78–84.

212. Deshpande V, Mino-Kenudson M, Brugge WR, et al. Endoscopic ultrasound guided fine needle aspiration biopsy of autoimmune pancreatitis: diagnostic criteria and pitfalls. Am J Surg Pathol 2005;29(11):1464–1471.

213. Farrell JJ, Garber J, Sahani D, Brugge WR. EUS findings in patients with autoimmune pancreatitis. Gastrointest Endosc 2004;60(6):927–936.

214. Hoki N, Mizuno N, Sawaki A, et al. Diagnosis of autoimmune pancreatitis using endoscopic ultrasonography. J Gastroenterol 2009;44(2):154–159.

215. Agarwal B, Ludwig OJ, Collins BT, Cortese C. Immunostaining as an adjunct to cytology for diagnosis of pancreatic adenocarcinoma. Clin Gastroenterol Hepatol 2008; 6(12):1425–1431.

216. Awadallah NS, Dehn D, Shah RJ, et al. NQO1 expression in pancreatic cancer and its potential use as a biomarker. Appl Immunohistochem Mol Morphol 2008;16(1):24–31.

217. Awadallah NS, Shroyer KR, Langer DA, et al. Detection of B7-H4 and p53 in pancreatic cancer: potential role as a cytological diagnostic adjunct. Pancreas 2008;36(2):200–206.

218. Jhala N, Jhala D, Vickers SM, et al. Biomarkers in diagnosis of pancreatic carcinoma in fine-needle aspirates. Am J Clin Pathol 2006;126(4):572–579.

219. Bournet B, Souque A, Senesse P, et al. Endoscopic ultrasound-guided fine-needle aspiration biopsy coupled with KRAS mutation assay to distinguish pancreatic cancer from pseudotumoral chronic pancreatitis. Endoscopy 2009; 41(6): 552–557.

220. Itoi T, Takei K, Sofuni A, et al. Immunohistochemical analysis of p53 and MIB-1 in tissue specimens obtained from endoscopic ultrasonography-guided fine needle aspiration biopsy for the diagnosis of solid pancreatic masses. Oncol Rep 2005;13(2):229–234.

221. Khalid A, Nodit L, Zahid M, et al. Endoscopic ultrasound fine needle aspirate DNA analysis to differentiate malignant and benign pancreatic masses. Am J Gastroenterol 2006; 101(11):2493–2500.

222. Laurell H, Bouisson M, Berthelemy P, et al. Identification of biomarkers of human pancreatic adenocarcinomas by expression profiling and validation with gene expression analysis in endoscopic ultrasound-guided fine needle aspiration samples. World J Gastroenterol 2006;12(21): 3344–3351.

223. Mishra G, Zhao Y, Sweeney J, et al. Determination of qualitative telomerase activity as an adjunct to the diagnosis of pancreatic adenocarcinoma by EUS-guided fine-needle aspiration. Gastrointest Endosc 2006;63(4):648–654.

224. Schoedel KE, Finkelstein SD, Ohori NP. K-Ras and microsatellite marker analysis of fine-needle aspirates from intraductal papillary mucinous neoplasms of the pancreas. Diagn Cytopathol 2006;34(9):605–608.

225. Chhieng DC, Benson E, Eltoum I, et al. MUC1 and MUC2 expression in pancreatic ductal carcinoma obtained by fine-needle aspiration. Cancer 2003;99(6):365–371.

226. Giorgadze TA, Peterman H, Baloch ZW, et al. Diagnostic utility of mucin profile in fine-needle aspiration specimens of the pancreas: an immunohistochemical study with surgical pathology correlation. Cancer 2006;108(3):186–197.

227. Wang Y, Gao J, Li Z, Jin Z, Gong Y, Man X. Diagnostic value of mucins (MUC1, MUC2 and MUC5AC) expression profile in endoscopic ultrasound-guided fine-needle aspiration specimens of the pancreas. Int J Cancer 2007; 121(12): 2716–2722.

228. Dietrich CF, Jenssen C, Allescher HD, Hocke M, Barreiros AP, Ignee A. [Differential diagnosis of pancreatic lesions using endoscopic ultrasound]. Z Gastroenterol 2008;46(6): 601–617.

229. Belsley NA, Pitman MB, Lauwers GY, Brugge WR, Deshpande V. Serous cystadenoma of the pancreas: limitations and pitfalls of endoscopic ultrasound-guided fine-needle aspiration biopsy. Cancer 2008;114(2):102–110.

230. Michaels PJ, Brachtel EF, Bounds BC, Brugge WR, Pitman MB. Intraductal papillary mucinous neoplasm of the pancreas: cytologic features predict histologic grade. Cancer 2006;108(3):163–173.

231. Repák R, Rejchrt S, Bártová J, Malírová E, Tycová V, Bures J. Endoscopic ultrasonography (EUS) and EUS-guided fine-needle aspiration with cyst fluid analysis in pancreatic cystic neoplasms. Hepatogastroenterology 2009;56(91-92):629–635.

232. Stelow EB, Shami VM, Abbott TE, et al. The use of fine needle aspiration cytology for the distinction of pancreatic mucinous neoplasia. Am J Clin Pathol 2008;129(1):67–74.

233. Toll AD, Bibbo M. Identification of gastrointestinal contamination in endoscopic ultrasound-guided pancreatic fine needle aspiration. Acta Cytol 2010;54(3):245–248.

234. Emerson RE, Randolph ML, Cramer HM. Endoscopic ultrasound-guided fine-needle aspiration cytology diagnosis of intraductal papillary mucinous neoplasm of the pancreas is highly predictive of pancreatic neoplasia. Diagn Cytopathol 2006;34(7):457–462.

235. Wang B, Hunter WJ, Bin-Sagheer S, Bewtra C. Rare potential pitfall in endoscopic ultrasound-guided fine needle aspiration biopsy in gastric duplication cyst: a case report. Acta Cytol 2009;53(2):219–222.

236. Jian B, Kimbrell HZ, Sepulveda A, Yu G. Lymphoepithelial cysts of the pancreas: endosonography-guided fine needle aspiration. Diagn Cytopathol 2008;36(9):662–665.

237. Nasr J, Sanders M, Fasanella K, Khalid A, McGrath K. Lymphoepithelial cysts of the pancreas: an EUS case series. Gastrointest Endosc 2008;68(1):170–173.

238. Gonzalez Obeso E, Murphy E, Brugge W, Deshpande V. Pseudocyst of the pancreas: the role of cytology and special stains for mucin. Cancer Cytopathol 2009;117(2):101–107.

239. Maker AV, Lee LS, Raut CP, Clancy TE, Swanson RS. Cytology from pancreatic cysts has marginal utility in surgical decision-making. Ann Surg Oncol 2008;15(11):3187–3192.

240. Sedlack R, Affi A, Vazquez-Sequeiros E, Norton ID, Clain JE, Wiersema MJ. Utility of EUS in the evaluation of cystic pancreatic lesions. Gastrointest Endosc 2002;56(4): 543–547.

241. van der Waaij LA, van Dullemen HM, Porte RJ. Cyst fluid analysis in the differential diagnosis of pancreatic cystic lesions: a pooled analysis. Gastrointest Endosc 2005; 62(3):383–389.

242. Maire F, Voitot H, Aubert A, et al. Intraductal papillary mucinous neoplasms of the pancreas: performance of pancreatic fluid analysis for positive diagnosis and the prediction of malignancy. Am J Gastroenterol 2008;103(11):2871–2877.

243. Linder JD, Geenen JE, Catalano MF. Cyst fluid analysis obtained by EUS-guided FNA in the evaluation of discrete cystic neoplasms of the pancreas: a prospective single-center experience. Gastrointest Endosc 2006;64(5):697–702.

244. Schmidt CM, Yip-Schneider MT, Ralstin MC, et al. PGE(2) in pancreatic cyst fluid helps differentiate IPMN from MCN and predict IPMN dysplasia. J Gastrointest Surg 2008;12(2):243–249.

245. Shami VM, Sundaram V, Stelow EB, et al. The level of carcinoembryonic antigen and the presence of mucin as predictors of cystic pancreatic mucinous neoplasia. Pancreas 2007;34(4):466–469.

246. Ito H, Endo T, Oka T, et al. Mucin expression profile is related to biological and clinical characteristics of intraductal papillary-mucinous tumors of the pancreas. Pancreas 2005;30(4):e96–e102.

247. Cao W, Adley BP, Liao J, et al. Mucinous nonneoplastic cyst of the pancreas: apomucin phenotype distinguishes this entity from intraductal papillary mucinous neoplasm. Hum Pathol 2010;41(4):513–521.

248. Nishigami T, Onodera M, Torii I, et al. Comparison between mucinous cystic neoplasm and intraductal papillary mucinous neoplasm of the branch duct type of the pancreas with respect to expression of CD10 and cytokeratin 20. Pancreas 2009;38(5):558–564.

249. Khalid A, Zahid M, Finkelstein SD, et al. Pancreatic cyst fluid DNA analysis in evaluating pancreatic cysts: a report of the PANDA study. Gastrointest Endosc 2009;69(6):1095–1102.

250. Shen J, Brugge WR, Dimaio CJ, Pitman MB. Molecular analysis of pancreatic cyst fluid: a comparative analysis with current practice of diagnosis. Cancer Cytopathol 2009;117(3):217–227.

251. Sreenarasimhaiah J, Lara LF, Jazrawi SF, Barnett CC, Tang SJ. A comparative analysis of pancreas cyst fluid CEA and histology with DNA mutational analysis in the detection of mucin producing or malignant cysts. JOP 2009;10(2):163–168.

252. Al-Haddad M, Gill KR, Raimondo M, et al. Safety and efficacy of cytology brushings versus standard fine-needle aspiration in evaluating cystic pancreatic lesions: a controlled study. Endoscopy 2010;42(2):127–132.

253. Buscaglia JM, Giday SA, Kantsevoy SV, et al. Patient- and cyst-related factors for improved prediction of malignancy within cystic lesions of the pancreas. Pancreatology 2009;9(5):631–638.

254. Leung KK, Ross WA, Evans D, et al. Pancreatic cystic neoplasm: the role of cyst morphology, cyst fluid analysis, and expectant management. Ann Surg Oncol 2009;16(10):2818–2824.

255. Pitman MB, Deshpande V. Endoscopic ultrasound-guided fine needle aspiration cytology of the pancreas: a morphological and multimodal approach to the diagnosis of solid and cystic mass lesions. Cytopathology 2007;18(6):331–347.

256. Huang ES, Turner BG, Fernandez-Del-Castillo C, Brugge WR, Hur C. Pancreatic cystic lesions: clinical predictors of malignancy in patients undergoing surgery. Aliment Pharmacol Ther 2010;31(2):285–294.

257. Schmidt CM, White PB, Waters JA, et al. Intraductal papillary mucinous neoplasms: predictors of malignant and invasive pathology. Ann Surg 2007;246(4):644–651, discussion 651–654.

258. Lee CJ, Scheiman J, Anderson MA, et al. Risk of malignancy in resected cystic tumors of the pancreas < or = 3 cm in size: is it safe to observe asymptomatic patients? A multi-institutional report. J Gastrointest Surg 2008;12(2):234–242.

259. Chang F, Chandra A, Culora G, Mahadeva U, Meenan J, Herbert A. Cytologic diagnosis of pancreatic endocrine tumors by endoscopic ultrasound-guided fine-needle aspiration: a review. Diagn Cytopathol 2006;34(9):649–658.

260. Fritscher-Ravens A, Izbicki JR, Sriram PV, et al. Endosonography-guided, fine-needle aspiration cytology extending the indication for organ-preserving pancreatic surgery. Am J Gastroenterol 2000;95(9):2255–2260.

261. Masetti M, Zanini N, Martuzzi F, et al. Analysis of prognostic factors in metastatic tumors of the pancreas: a single-center experience and review of the literature. Pancreas 2010;39(2):135–143.

262. Tanis PJ, van der Gaag NA, Busch OR, van Gulik TM, Gouma DJ. Systematic review of pancreatic surgery for metastatic renal cell carcinoma. Br J Surg 2009;96(6):579–592.

263. DeWitt J, Jowell P, Leblanc J, et al. EUS-guided FNA of pancreatic metastases: a multicenter experience. Gastrointest Endosc 2005;61(6):689–696.

264. Fritscher-Ravens A, Sriram PV, Krause C, et al. Detection of pancreatic metastases by EUS-guided fine-needle aspiration. Gastrointest Endosc 2001;53(1):65–70.

265. Mesa H, Stelow EB, Stanley MW, Mallery S, Lai R, Bardales RH. Diagnosis of nonprimary pancreatic neoplasms by endoscopic ultrasound-guided fine-needle aspiration. Diagn Cytopathol 2004;31(5):313–318.

266. Varghese L, Ngae MY, Wilson AP, Crowder CD, Gulbahce HE, Pambuccian SE. Diagnosis of metastatic pancreatic mesenchymal tumors by endoscopic ultrasound-guided fine-needle aspiration. Diagn Cytopathol 2009;37(11):792–802.

267. Bardales RH, Centeno B, Mallery JS, et al. Endoscopic ultrasound-guided fine-needle aspiration cytology diagnosis of solid-pseudopapillary tumor of the pancreas: a rare neoplasm of elusive origin but characteristic cytomorphologic features. Am J Clin Pathol 2004;121(5):654–662.

268. Burford H, Baloch Z, Liu X, Jhala D, Siegal GP, Jhala N. E-cadherin/beta-catenin and CD10: a limited immunohistochemical panel to distinguish pancreatic endocrine neoplasm from solid pseudopapillary neoplasm of the pancreas on endoscopic ultrasound-guided fine-needle aspirates of the pancreas. Am J Clin Pathol 2009;132(6):831–839.

269. Jani N, DeWitt J, Eloubeidi M, et al. Endoscopic ultrasound-guided fine-needle aspiration for diagnosis of solid pseudopapillary tumors of the pancreas: a multicenter experience. Endoscopy 2008;40(3):200–203.

270. Salla C, Konstantinou P, Chatzipantelis P. CK19 and CD10 expression in pancreatic neuroendocrine tumors diagnosed by endoscopic ultrasound-guided fine-needle aspiration cytology. Cancer Cytopathol 2009;117(6):516–521.

271. Stelow EB, Woon C, Pambuccian SE, et al. Fine-needle aspiration cytology of pancreatic somatostatinoma: the importance of immunohistochemistry for the cytologic diagnosis of pancreatic endocrine neoplasms. Diagn Cytopathol 2005;33(2):100–105.

272. Stelow EB, Bardales RH, Shami VM, et al. Cytology of pancreatic acinar cell carcinoma. Diagn Cytopathol 2006;34(5):367–372.

273. Chatzipantelis P, Konstantinou P, Kaklamanos M, Apostolou G, Salla C. The role of cytomorphology and proliferative activity in predicting biologic behavior of pancreatic neuroendocrine tumors: a study by endoscopic ultrasound-guided fine-needle aspiration cytology. Cancer Cytopathol 2009;117(3):211–216.

274. Fasanella KE, McGrath KM, Sanders M, Brody D, Domsic R, Khalid A. Pancreatic endocrine tumor EUS-guided FNA DNA microsatellite loss and mortality. Gastrointest Endosc 2009;69(6):1074–1080.

275. Nodit L, McGrath KM, Zahid M, et al. Endoscopic ultrasound-guided fine needle aspirate microsatellite loss analysis and pancreatic endocrine tumor outcome. Clin Gastroenterol Hepatol 2006;4(12):1474–1478.

276. Jenssen C, Dietrich CF. Endoscopic ultrasound of gastrointestinal subepithelial lesions. Ultraschall Med 2008;29(3):236–256, quiz 257–264.

277. Stelow EB, Murad FM, Debol SM, et al. A limited immunocytochemical panel for the distinction of subepithelial gastrointestinal mesenchymal neoplasms sampled by endoscopic ultrasound-guided fine-needle aspiration. Am J Clin Pathol 2008;129(2):219–225.

278. Jenssen C, Schick B, Wagner S. Primary diagnosis of serous papillary-ovarian carcinoma by EUS-guided fine-needle aspiration biopsy of a submucosal gastric tumor: a case report. [Article in German] Endosk Heute 2006;19(1):32–35.

279. Sangha S, Gergeos F, Freter R, Paiva LL, Jacobson BC. Diagnosis of ovarian cancer metastatic to the stomach by EUS-guided FNA. Gastrointest Endosc 2003;58(6):933–935.

280. Gomes AL, Bardales RH, Milanezi F, Reis RM, Schmitt F. Molecular analysis of c-Kit and PDGFRA in GISTs diagnosed by EUS. Am J Clin Pathol 2007;127(1):89–96.

281. Annema JT, Veseliç M, Versteegh MI, Willems LN, Rabe KF. Mediastinal restaging: EUS-FNA offers a new perspective. Lung Cancer 2003;42(3):311–318.

282. Varadarajulu S, Eloubeidi M. Can endoscopic ultrasonography-guided fine-needle aspiration predict response to chemoradiation in non-small cell lung cancer? A pilot study. Respiration 2006;73(2):213–220.

283. Al-Haddad M, Wallace MB. EUS-FNA and biomarkers for the staging of non-small cell lung cancer. Endoscopy 2006;38(Suppl 1):S114–S117.

284. Pellisé M, Castells A, Ginès A, et al. Detection of lymph node micrometastases by gene promoter hypermethylation in samples obtained by endosonography- guided fine-needle aspiration biopsy. Clin Cancer Res 2004;10(13):4444–4449.

285. Annema JT, Veseliç M, Rabe KF. Endoscopic ultrasound-guided fine-needle aspiration for the diagnosis of sarcoidosis. Eur Respir J 2005;25(3):405–409.

286. Fritscher-Ravens A, Sriram PV, Topalidis T, et al. Diagnosing sarcoidosis using endosonography-guided fine-needle aspiration. Chest 2000;118(4):928–935.

287. Michael H, Ho S, Pollack B, Gupta M, Gress F. Diagnosis of intra-abdominal and mediastinal sarcoidosis with EUS-guided FNA. Gastrointest Endosc 2008;67(1):28–34.

288. Mishra G, Sahai AV, Penman ID, et al. Endoscopic ultrasonography with fine-needle aspiration: an accurate and simple diagnostic modality for sarcoidosis. Endoscopy 1999; 31(5):377–382.

289. Wildi SM, Judson MA, Fraig M, et al. Is endosonography guided fine needle aspiration (EUS-FNA) for sarcoidosis as good as we think? Thorax 2004;59(9):794–799.

290. Hahn M, Faigel DO. Frequency of mediastinal lymph node metastases in patients undergoing EUS evaluation of pancreaticobiliary masses. Gastrointest Endosc 2001;54(3):331–335.

291. Krishna NB, Gardner L, Collins BT, Agarwal B. Periportal lymphadenopathy in patients without identifiable pancreatobiliary or hepatic malignancy. Clin Gastroenterol Hepatol 2006;4(11):1373–1377.

292. Catalano MF, Nayar R, Gress F, et al. EUS-guided fine needle aspiration in mediastinal lymphadenopathy of unknown etiology. Gastrointest Endosc 2002;55(7):863–869.

293. Nakahara O, Yamao K, Bhatia V, et al. Usefulness of endoscopic ultrasound-guided fine needle aspiration (EUS-FNA) for undiagnosed intra-abdominal lymphadenopathy. J Gastroenterol 2009;44(6):562–567.

294. Khashab MA, Emerson RE, DeWitt JM. Endoscopic ultrasound-guided fine-needle aspiration for the diagnosis of anaplastic pancreatic carcinoma: a single-center experience. Pancreas 2010;39(1):88–91.

295. von Bartheld MB, Veseliç-Charvat M, Rabe KF, Annema JT. Endoscopic ultrasound-guided fine-needle aspiration for the diagnosis of sarcoidosis. Endoscopy 2010;42(3):213–217.

296. Puri R, Vilmann P, Sud R, et al. Endoscopic ultrasound-guided fine-needle aspiration cytology in the evaluation of suspected tuberculosis in patients with isolated mediastinal lymphadenopathy. Endoscopy 2010;42(6):462–467.

297. Jenssen C, Dietrich CF. [Ultrasound and endoscopic ultrasound of the adrenal glands]. Ultraschall Med 2010;31(3):228–247, quiz 248–250.

298. Bodtger U, Vilmann P, Clementsen P, Galvis E, Bach K, Skov BG. Clinical impact of endoscopic ultrasound-fine needle aspiration of left adrenal masses in established or suspected lung cancer. J Thorac Oncol 2009;4(12):1485–1489.

299. DeWitt JM. Endoscopic ultrasound-guided fine-needle aspiration of right adrenal masses: report of 2 cases. J Ultrasound Med 2008;27(2):261–267.

300. Eloubeidi MA, Morgan DE, Cerfolio RJ, Eltoum IA. Transduodenal EUS-guided FNA of the right adrenal gland. Gastrointest Endosc 2008;67(3):522–527.

301. Catalano MF, Sial S, Chak A, et al. EUS-guided fine needle aspiration of idiopathic abdominal masses. Gastrointest Endosc 2002;55(7):854–858.

302. Crowe DR, Eloubeidi MA, Chhieng DC, Jhala NC, Jhala D, Eltoum IA. Fine-needle aspiration biopsy of hepatic lesions: computerized tomographic-guided versus endoscopic ultrasound-guided FNA. Cancer 2006;108(3):180–185.

303. DeWitt J, Ghorai S, Kahi C, et al. EUS-FNA of recurrent postoperative extraluminal and metastatic malignancy. Gastrointest Endosc 2003;58(4):542–548.

304. Hollerbach S, Reiser M, Topalidis T, König M, Schmiegel W. Diagnosis of hepatocellular carcinoma (HCC) in a high-risk patient by using transgastric EUS-guided fine-needle biopsy (FUS-FNA). Z Gastroenterol 2003;41(10):995–998.

305. Lai R, Stephens V, Bardales R. Diagnosis and staging of hepatocellular carcinoma by EUS-FNA of a portal vein thrombus. Gastrointest Endosc 2004;59(4):574–577.

306. McGrath K, Brody D, Luketich J, Khalid A. Detection of unsuspected left hepatic lobe metastases during EUS staging of cancer of the esophagus and cardia. Am J Gastroenterol 2006;101(8):1742–1746.

307. Singh P, Mukhopadhyay P, Bhatt B, et al. Endoscopic ultrasound versus CT scan for detection of the metastases to the liver: results of a prospective comparative study. J Clin Gastroenterol 2009;43(4):367–373.

308. Fritscher-Ravens A, Broering DC, Sriram PV, et al. EUS-guided fine-needle aspiration cytodiagnosis of hilar chol-

angiocarcinoma: a case series. Gastrointest Endosc 2000;52(4): 534–540.

309. Iwashita T, Yasuda I, Tsurumi H, et al. Endoscopic ultrasound-guided fine needle aspiration biopsy for splenic tumor: a case series. Endoscopy 2009;41(2):179–182.

310. Eloubeidi MA, Cohn M, Cerfolio RJ, et al. Endoscopic ultrasound-guided fine-needle aspiration in the diagnosis of foregut duplication cysts: the value of demonstrating detached ciliary tufts in cyst fluid. Cancer 2004;102(4): 253–258.

311. Fritscher-Ravens A, Petrasch S, Reinacher-Schick A, Graeven U, König M, Schmiegel W. Diagnostic value of endoscopic ultrasonography-guided fine-needle aspiration cytology of mediastinal masses in patients with intrapulmonary lesions and nondiagnostic bronchoscopy. Respiration 1999;66(2):150–155.

312. Eloubeidi MA, Tamhane A, Varadarajulu S, Wilcox CM. Frequency of major complications after EUS-guided FNA of solid pancreatic masses: a prospective evaluation. Gastrointest Endosc 2006;63(4):622–629.

313. Savides TJ, Donohue M, Hunt G, et al. EUS-guided FNA diagnostic yield of malignancy in solid pancreatic masses: a benchmark for quality performance measurement. Gastrointest Endosc 2007;66(2):277–282.

314. Rickes S, Rauh P, Uhle C, Ensberg D, Mönkemüller K, Malfertheiner P. Contrast-enhanced sonography in pancreatic diseases. Eur J Radiol 2007;64(2):183–188.

315. Ardengh JC, Malheiros CA, Pereira V, Coelho DE, Coelho JF, Rahal F. Endoscopic ultrasound-guided fine-needle aspiration using helical computerized tomography for TN staging and vascular injury in operable pancreatic carcinoma. JOP 2009;10(3):310–317.

316. Agarwal B, Gogia S, Eloubeidi MA, Correa AM, Ho L, Collins BT. Malignant mediastinal lymphadenopathy detected by staging EUS in patients with pancreaticobiliary cancer. Gastrointest Endosc 2005;61(7):849–853.

317. DeWitt J, Yu M, Al-Haddad MA, Sherman S, McHenry L, Leblanc JK. Survival in patients with pancreatic cancer after the diagnosis of malignant ascites or liver metastases by EUS-FNA. Gastrointest Endosc 2010;71(2):260–265.

318. Ashida R, Nakata B, Shigekawa M, et al. Gemcitabine sensitivity-related mRNA expression in endoscopic ultrasound-guided fine-needle aspiration biopsy of unresectable pancreatic cancer. J Exp Clin Cancer Res 2009;28:83.

319. Itoi T, Sofuni A, Fukushima N, et al. Ribonucleotide reductase subunit M2 mRNA expression in pretreatment biopsies obtained from unresectable pancreatic carcinomas. J Gastroenterol 2007;42(5):389–394.

320. Ulla JL, Martinez MA, Paz-Esquete J, Garcia-Arroyo R, Dominguez-Comesaña E, Vazquez-Astray E. Types of Pancreatic Cancer in EUS-FNA and Chemotherapy. Am J Ther 2009 Dec 16 [Epub ahead of print] .

321. Steg A, Vickers SM, Eloubeidi M, et al. Hedgehog pathway expression in heterogeneous pancreatic adenocarcinoma: implications for the molecular analysis of clinically available biopsies. Diagn Mol Pathol 2007;16(4):229–237.

322. Puli SR, Reddy JB, Bechtold ML, Antillon MR, Ibdah JA. Accuracy of endoscopic ultrasound in the diagnosis of distal and celiac axis lymph node metastasis in esophageal cancer: a meta-analysis and systematic review. Dig Dis Sci 2008;53(9):2405–2414.

323. van Vliet EP, Heijenbrok-Kal MH, Hunink MG, Kuipers EJ, Siersema PD. Staging investigations for oesophageal cancer: a meta-analysis. Br J Cancer 2008;98(3):547–557.

324. Puli SR, Reddy JB, Bechtold ML, Antillon D, Ibdah JA, Antillon MR. Staging accuracy of esophageal cancer by endoscopic ultrasound: a meta-analysis and systematic review. World J Gastroenterol 2008;14(10):1479–1490.

325. Eloubeidi MA, Wallace MB, Hoffman BJ, et al. Predictors of survival for esophageal cancer patients with and without celiac axis lymphadenopathy: impact of staging endosonography. Ann Thorac Surg 2001;72(1):212–219, discussion 219–220.

326. Harewood GC, Kumar KS. Assessment of clinical impact of endoscopic ultrasound on esophageal cancer. J Gastroenterol Hepatol 2004;19(4):433–439.

327. Marsman WA, Brink MA, Bergman JJ, et al. Potential impact of EUS-FNA staging of proximal lymph nodes in patients with distal esophageal carcinoma. Endoscopy 2006;38(8): 825–829.

328. Shami VM, Villaverde A, Stearns L, et al. Clinical impact of conventional endosonography and endoscopic ultrasound-guided fine-needle aspiration in the assessment of patients with Barrett's esophagus and high-grade dysplasia or intramucosal carcinoma who have been referred for endoscopic ablation therapy. Endoscopy 2006;38(2):157–161.

329. Ginès A, Cassivi SD, Martenson JA Jr, et al. Impact of endoscopic ultrasonography and physician specialty on the management of patients with esophagus cancer. Dis Esophagus 2008;21(3):241–250.

330. Maple JT, Peifer KJ, Edmundowicz SA, et al. The impact of endoscopic ultrasonography with fine needle aspiration (EUS-FNA) on esophageal cancer staging: a survey of thoracic surgeons and gastroenterologists. Dis Esophagus 2008;21(6):480–487.

331. Agarwal B, Swisher S, Ajani J, et al. Endoscopic ultrasound after preoperative chemoradiation can help identify patients who benefit maximally after surgical esophageal resection. Am J Gastroenterol 2004;99(7):1258–1266.

332. Cerfolio RJ, Bryant AS, Ohja B, Bartolucci AA, Eloubeidi MA. The accuracy of endoscopic ultrasonography with fine-needle aspiration, integrated positron emission tomography with computed tomography, and computed tomography in restaging patients with esophageal cancer after neoadjuvant chemoradiotherapy. J Thorac Cardiovasc Surg 2005;129(6):1232–1241.

333. Prasad P, Schmulewitz N, Patel A, et al. Detection of occult liver metastases during EUS for staging of malignancies. Gastrointest Endosc 2004;59(1):49–53.

334. Kramer H, Koëter GH, Sleijfer DT, van Putten JW, Groen HJ. Endoscopic ultrasound-guided fine-needle aspiration in patients with mediastinal abnormalities and previous extrathoracic malignancy. Eur J Cancer 2004;40(4):559–562.

335. Giovannini M, Monges G, Seitz JF, et al. Distant lymph node metastases in esophageal cancer: impact of endoscopic ultrasound-guided biopsy. Endoscopy 1999;31(7): 536–540.

336. Hassan H, Vilmann P, Sharma V. Impact of EUS-guided FNA on management of gastric carcinoma. Gastrointest Endosc 2010;71(3):500–504.

337. Giovannini M, Bernardini D, Seitz JF, et al. Value of endoscopic ultrasonography for assessment of patients presenting elevated tumor marker levels after surgery for colorectal cancers. Endoscopy 1998;30(5):469–476.

338. Hünerbein M, Totkas S, Moesta KT, Ulmer C, Handke T, Schlag PM. The role of transrectal ultrasound-guided biopsy in the postoperative follow-up of patients with rectal cancer. Surgery 2001;129(2):164–169.

339. Hünerbein M, Totkas S, Balanou P, Handke T, Schlag PM. EUS-guided fine needle biopsy: minimally invasive access to metastatic or recurrent cancer. Eur J Ultrasound 1999;10(2-3):151–157.

340. Peric R, Schuurbiers OC, Veseliç M, Rabe KF, van der Heijden HF, Annema JT. Transesophageal endoscopic ultrasound-guided fine-needle aspiration for the mediastinal staging of extrathoracic tumors: a new perspective. Ann Oncol 2010;21(7):1468–1471.

341. Hernandez A, Kahaleh M, Olazagasti J, et al. EUS-FNA as the initial diagnostic modality in centrally located primary lung cancers. J Clin Gastroenterol 2007;41(7):657–660.

342. Varadarajulu S, Hoffman BJ, Hawes RH, Eloubeidi MA. EUS-guided FNA of lung masses adjacent to or abutting the esophagus after unrevealing CT-guided biopsy or bronchoscopy. Gastrointest Endosc 2004;60(2):293–297.

343. Rami-Porta R, Crowley JJ, Goldstraw P. The revised TNM staging system for lung cancer. Ann Thorac Cardiovasc Surg 2009;15(1):4–9.

344. D'Addario G, Felip E; ESMO Guidelines Working Group. Non-small-cell lung cancer: ESMO clinical recommendations for diagnosis, treatment and follow-up. Ann Oncol 2008;19(Suppl 2):ii39–ii40.

345. Vilmann P, Annema J, Clementsen P. Endosonography in bronchopulmonary disease. Best Pract Res Clin Gastroenterol 2009;23(5):711–728.

346. Micames CG, McCrory DC, Pavey DA, Jowell PS, Gress FG. Endoscopic ultrasound-guided fine-needle aspiration for non-small cell lung cancer staging: A systematic review and metaanalysis. Chest 2007;131(2):539–548.

347. Puli SR, Batapati Krishna Reddy J, Bechtold ML, et al. Endoscopic ultrasound: its accuracy in evaluating mediastinal lymphadenopathy? A meta-analysis and systematic review. World J Gastroenterol 2008;14(19):3028–3037.

348. Wallace MB, Ravenel J, Block MI, et al. Endoscopic ultrasound in lung cancer patients with a normal mediastinum on computed tomography. Ann Thorac Surg 2004;77(5):1763–1768.

349. Fernández-Esparrach G, Ginès A, Belda J, et al. Transesophageal ultrasound-guided fine needle aspiration improves mediastinal staging in patients with non-small cell lung cancer and normal mediastinum on computed tomography. Lung Cancer 2006;54(1):35–40.

350. Gu P, Zhao YZ, Jiang LY, Zhang W, Xin Y, Han BH. Endobronchial ultrasound-guided transbronchial needle aspiration for staging of lung cancer: a systematic review and meta-analysis. Eur J Cancer 2009;45(8):1389–1396.

351. Larsen SS, Vilmann P, Krasnik M, et al. Endoscopic ultrasound guided biopsy performed routinely in lung cancer staging spares futile thoracotomies: preliminary results from a randomised clinical trial. Lung Cancer 2005;49(3):377–385.

352. Tournoy KG, De Ryck F, Vanwalleghem LR, et al. Endoscopic ultrasound reduces surgical mediastinal staging in lung cancer: a randomized trial. Am J Respir Crit Care Med 2008;177(5):531–535.

353. Talebian M, von Bartheld MB, Braun J, et al. EUS-FNA in the preoperative staging of non-small cell lung cancer. Lung Cancer 2010;69(1):60–65.

354. Kramer H, van Putten JW, Post WJ, et al. Oesophageal endoscopic ultrasound with fine needle aspiration improves and simplifies the staging of lung cancer. Thorax 2004;59(7):596–601.

355. Witte B, Neumeister W, Huertgen M. Does endoesophageal ultrasound-guided fine-needle aspiration replace mediastinoscopy in mediastinal staging of thoracic malignancies? Eur J Cardiothorac Surg 2008;33(6):1124–1128.

356. Szlubowski A, Herth FJ, Soja J, et al. Endobronchial ultrasound-guided needle aspiration in non-small-cell lung cancer restaging verified by the transcervical bilateral extended mediastinal lymphadenectomy—a prospective study. Eur J Cardiothorac Surg 2010;37(5):1180–1184.

357. Ømark Petersen H, Eckardt J, Hakami A, Olsen KE, Jørgensen OD. The value of mediastinal staging with endobronchial ultrasound-guided transbronchial needle aspiration in patients with lung cancer. Eur J Cardiothorac Surg 2009;36(3):465–468.

358. Vilmann P, Krasnik M, Larsen SS, Jacobsen GK, Clementsen P. Transesophageal endoscopic ultrasound-guided fine-needle aspiration (EUS-FNA) and endobronchial ultrasound-guided transbronchial needle aspiration (EBUS-TBNA) biopsy: a combined approach in the evaluation of mediastinal lesions. Endoscopy 2005;37(9):833–839.

359. Wallace MB, Pascual JM, Raimondo M, et al. Minimally invasive endoscopic staging of suspected lung cancer. JAMA 2008;299(5):540–546.

360. Harewood GC, Pascual J, Raimondo M, et al. Economic analysis of combined endoscopic and endobronchial ultrasound in the evaluation of patients with suspected non-small cell lung cancer. Lung Cancer 2010;67(3):366–371.

361. Schipper P, Schoolfield M. Minimally invasive staging of N2 disease: endobronchial ultrasound/transesophageal endoscopic ultrasound, mediastinoscopy, and thoracoscopy. Thorac Surg Clin 2008;18(4):363–379.

362. Varela-Lema L, Fernández-Villar A, Ruano-Ravina A. Effectiveness and safety of endobronchial ultrasound-transbronchial needle aspiration: a systematic review. Eur Respir J 2009;33(5):1156–1164.

363. Detterbeck FC, Jantz MA, Wallace M, Vansteenkiste J, Silvestri GA; American College of Chest Physicians. Invasive mediastinal staging of lung cancer: ACCP evidence-based clinical practice guidelines (2nd edition). Chest 2007;132(3, Suppl):202S–220S.

364. Nurnberg D, Jung A, Spengler J, Holle A. Nebennierentumor und Bronchialkarzinom—ist jeder Nebennierentumor eine Metastase? Ultraschall Med 2006;27(S1):V12_1.

365. Annema JT, van Meerbeck J, Rintoul RC, et al. Madiastinoscopy vs endosonography for mediastinal nodal staging of lung cancer: a randomized trial. JAMA 2010;304(20):2245–2252.

11 Tips and Tricks for Fine-Needle Puncture

T. Beyer, T. Topalidis

There is a very wide range of morphological equivalents for a pathological structure that is visualized on ultrasonography. Options include inflammatory conditions, benign or malignant tumors, and metastases. Cytological or histological confirmation of the diagnosis is often required in order to distinguish between the different possibilities. The hints and tips presented here are intended for cytological aspiration biopsy—better known as fine-needle aspiration biopsy (FNAB).

The advantages of the current microinvasive technique include:

- A high level of patient acceptance
- The high diagnostic yield
- A low risk of complications
- Low cost

These considerations have led to this valuable method being accepted throughout the world.

Definition of Fine-Needle Puncture

Various different terms are used for the fine-needle puncture technique (needle diameter < 1 mm) in everyday clinical practice:

- Fine-needle aspiration (FNA)
- Fine-needle aspiration biopsy (FNAB)
- Fine-needle aspiration cytology (FNAC)
- Fine-needle biopsy (FNB)
- Fine-needle cytology (FNC)

A variety of fine-needle systems are now commercially available, which can be used with endoscopic ultrasound (EUS) equipment for imaging-guided biopsy procedures. The main advantage of EUS-guided fine-needle puncture appears to be the ability to control the needle tip in real time during the puncture process. However, the results depend not only on the puncture process, but also on the processing of the resulting specimen and the quality of the cytologist.

Unfortunately, there is as yet no standard procedure for specimen processing. There is no consensus on whether it is necessary to use a fixation process for the specimens, or if so, whether fixation should be performed before or after smearing onto the microscopic slide. Nor is it clear which fixation method is best. However, we would like to discuss and clarify the following questions here:

- What fixation methods are available?
- How should the specimens be stained?
- Is it possible to create a standard for cytological diagnosis?

Cytological Examination

Nine steps are involved in a normal cytological examination process, according to Lopes Cardozo:[1]

- Indication for fine-needle aspiration
- Choice of the best way of obtaining the specimen
- Process of taking the specimen
- Preparation of the specimen
- Fixation process
- Staining process
- Preliminary analysis of the material
- Formulating a diagnosis on the basis of clinical information
- Matching the diagnosis to the patient's disease

All of these diagnostic steps are equally important in order to obtain an optimal result. Normally, steps 1–5 and 9 are performed by the clinical practitioner, whereas steps 6–8 are carried out by the cytologist. In our opinion, steps 2, 3, and 9 are the most difficult and require perfect teamwork between the clinical practitioner and the cytologist to ensure the best possible result.

It is important to mention two different ways of obtaining a cytological diagnosis at this point. On the one hand, there are central cytology laboratories with no direct connection to the clinical practitioner (as in the case of one of the present authors, T.T.); on the other hand, cytologically trained clinical practitioners (as in the case of the other author, T.B.) may have a direct link to a clinical department (such as pulmonology). The goal in both cases is to match the cytological specimens to the correct diagnosis. The cytologically trained clinical practitioner carries out a simultaneous preliminary analysis during the puncture process, which is advantageous as it reduces the number of specimen collections. This results in better patient comfort and increases the sensitivity of the method. On the other hand, the cytology specialist naturally has a wider knowledge of different diseases and can use immunocytology to obtain a clearer diagnosis.

Collection

It is important to obtain an optimal view of the lesion in question after an EUS examination of the patient. The most important consideration is to find the shortest possible route to the target, avoiding the surrounding blood vessels. One advantageous way of doing this is to use an assistant to control the needle movement into the lesion (in real-time puncture) while the examiner controls the echoendoscope to maintain optimal positioning. After the needle has entered the target, the stylet has to be removed. A syringe with a volume of 10 mL should then be attached at the end of the needle and used to produce suction (pressure below atmospheric level). While continuous suction through the syringe is being maintained, the needle should be passed through the lesion movement forward and backward in a fanlike pattern. After three to five needle passes, the suction should be released and the needle removed (**Fig. 11.1**).

Specimen Handling

After the puncture process has been performed, the fine-needle aspiration system should immediately be removed from the echoendoscope, and a new 10 mL syringe filled with 10 mL air should be placed at the end of the needle system. The collected specimen has to be spread onto slides by carefully emptying the air-filled syringe through the needle. During this process, the tip of the needle has to be held directly on the slide to ensure that only small portions of the specimen are released. Alternatively, the stylet can be carefully reintroduced into the needle and the resulting pressure can be used to eject the specimen (**Figs. 11.2** and **11.3**).

Immediately after this, the specimen should be smeared gently but quickly using another slide. The smaller the specimen drops, the thinner the specimen layer on the slide (**Figs. 11.4** and **11.5**). Too much pressure during the spreading process should be avoided, as it increases cell artifacts.

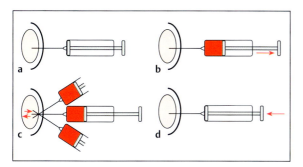

Fig. 11.1 a–d The fine-needle aspiration procedure.
a Introducing the needle into the lesion.
b Creating suction using a syringe.
c The fanlike pattern of needle passes (three to five passes).
d Releasing the suction and removing the needle.

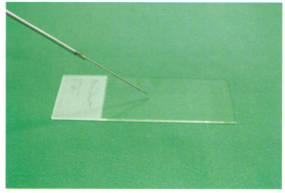

Fig. 11.2 Removal of the specimen from the needle (step 1). The Hancke–Vilmann fine-needle aspiration system is being used here.

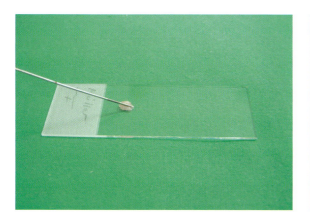

Fig. 11.3 Removal of the specimen from the needle (step 2). Releasing droplike portions onto the slide. It is important to prevent the resulting specimen from drying out by preparing no more than two or three slides and then immediately smearing them using another slide.

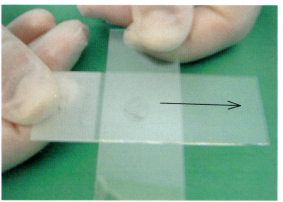

Fig. 11.4 Smearing technique (step 1). Another slide is laid crosswise over the first slide, and the specimen is smeared by moving the second slide with gentle pressure but fast movement (in the direction of the arrow).

Fixation

The fixation process is very important for the microscopic image, and fixation should be done immediately after the smearing of the specimen. The method of fixation used depends on the type and size of the specimen, as well as on the staining method chosen afterward. There are two different fixation methods (**Figs. 11.6, 11.7, 11.8**):

- Air-drying fixation
- Chemical fixation

Air-drying fixation allows later staining using May–Grün-wald–Giemsa solution (MGG), as well as immunocyto-chemical staining methods, and in the authors' opinion appears to be preferable to chemical fixation methods. Chemical fixation substances (alcohol, Delaunay solution, chemical spray fixation) allow later staining using Papanicolaou solution or hematoxylin-eosin solution. In this case, the fixation process has to be started immediately (< 5 seconds) after smearing. The specimen on the slide must still be moist during the fixation process, to avoid severe cell artifacts that could prevent proper examination by the cytologist. There should be a label on every slide

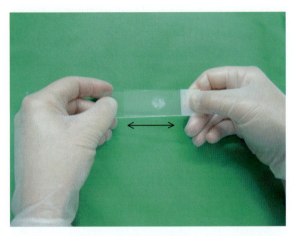

Fig. 11.5 Smearing technique (step 2). Another slide should be laid directly over the first slide. The two slides are moved against each other quickly, but with gentle pressure.

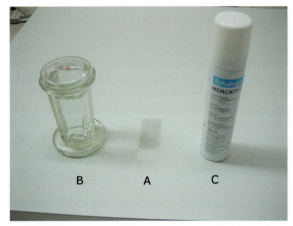

Fig. 11.6 a–c Three types of fixation.
a Air-drying fixation.
b Chemical liquid fixation (alcohol or Delaunay solution), with immersion of the loaded slides in a 95% alcohol solution for a period of 30 minutes.
c Chemical spray fixation.

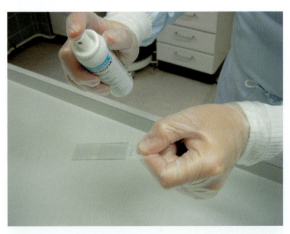

Fig. 11.7 Chemical spray fixation. This is best for subsequent staining using Papanicolaou solution or hematoxylin–eosin (HE) solution. Agreement from the cytologist is required before this is used. The loaded slide should be sprayed several times from a distance of 20–30 cm immediately after smearing. After spraying, the slides should be left in a horizontal position for 20 minutes.

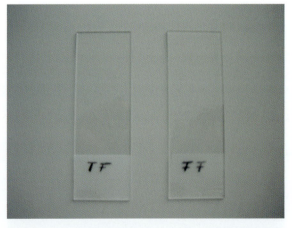

Fig. 11.8 Air-drying fixation or chemical fixation? Air-drying fixation is quick and therefore allows staining to be carried out at the bedside (with May–Grünwald–Giemsa staining or Pappenheim staining). It is also suitable for immunocytochemical examinations. Chemical fixation is necessary for Papanicolaou or hematoxylin–eosin staining and needs to be agreed on with the cytologist beforehand.

stating the type of fixation used and the name of the patient, to avoid mistakes and to ensure the optimal choice of staining method.

Staining

The air-drying method has proved to be the best way of allowing a quick "bedside" staining process such as Hemacolor (Merck Inc., Darmstadt, Germany) (**Figs. 11.9, 11.10, 11.11**).

Request Form, Clinical Data, Questions of Interest

It is essential for the cytologist to have important clinical facts from the patient's history in order to find the correct answer to the question being posed. Unfortunately, little information is often provided on the request form. It should be noted that data protection between the clinical physician and the cytologist is usually very strictly adhered to.

The following information is the minimum necessary to provide the best cytological results:
- Type of specimen
- Origin of specimen
- Important facts in the patient's history, for example:
  - Any previous carcinoma; if so, then an indication of the histological type and grading should be given
  - Known diagnosis
  - Important pathological data from the patient's laboratory results
- Question posed
- Needle track

On the other hand, the cytologist has to provide answers to the following questions:
- Is the material representative?
- What was the origin of the material?
- Is it an inflammatory process or a neoplasia?
- Is the neoplasia benign or malignant?
- In case of metastasis, what is the origin of the cancer?

Not all material contains the right cells for cytological analysis. In our own experience, the incidence of usable cells being present in all loaded slides is 89%[2] (**Fig. 11.12**).

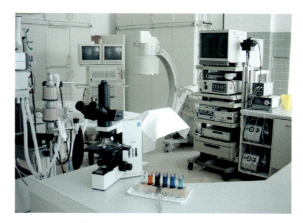

Fig. 11.9 Bedside cytology (clinical cytology). This allows fast preliminary evaluation of the specimen during the endoscopic investigation. If a sampling error occurs, up to two repeat punctures of the lesion should be performed.

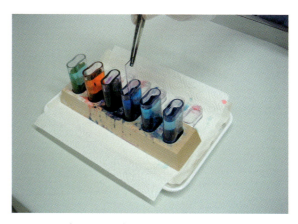

Fig. 11.10 A fast staining kit (Hemacolor; Merck no. 11661). Solution 1: the fixation solution (5 × 1 s). Solution 2: the red staining substance (3 × 1 s). Solution 3: the blue staining substance (6 × 1 s). Solution 4: buffer solution (2 × 1 s). Solution 5: buffer solution (2 × 1 s). Solution 6: buffer solution (2 × 1 s). The advantages of the staining kit are that it is a simple and fast method, one can check one's own results, and it is a time-saving technique.

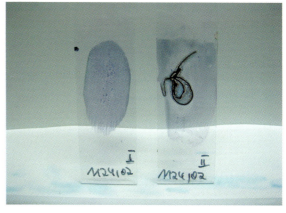

Fig. 11.11 Which is the ideal smear? I: An ideal smear—rich in cells (macroscopic small dark blue pixels, homogeneously dispersed).
II: An unusable smear, with large amounts of coagulated material and lumps.

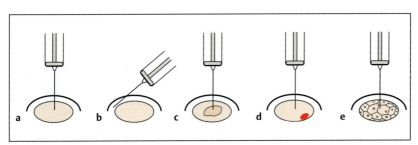

Fig. 11.12 a–e Sampling errors
a The best scenario: correct needle positioning and optimal fine-needle aspiration.
b Missing the target.
c Cystic, hemorrhagic, or necrotic material.
d Missing the cancer in a benign lesion.
e Low cell content in the lesion, or sclerotic lesion.

Causes of Errors in Fine-Needle Aspiration Biopsy

Sampling process: missing the target; not obtaining enough material from the target; material not representative.

Sample handling: smearing, fixing and staining process; cytologist's level of experience.

Capabilities and Limitations of Cytology

The primary aim in cytology is to distinguish between malignant and benign specimens. False-positive results are mainly due to mistakes by the cytologist, and may include:
- Granulomatous inflammations
- Cell artifacts caused by previous radiation or chemotherapy
- Benign tumors

False-negative results are often due to mistakes by the clinical physician, and may include:
- Target too small for a specimen to be obtained
- Necrotic material
- Lack of proficiency in the fine-needle aspiration technique

Limitations:
- Information about the infiltration of the lesion: invasion of the lymphatic system; invasion of different layers and/or vessels.
- Exclusion of malignancy using a single fine-needle aspiration with an inadequate specimen.

- Differentiation and classification of anaplastic or immature tumors and non-Hodgkin or Hodgkin lymphomas is nearly impossible using normal cell-staining methods. In these cases, immunocytochemical staining methods are required.

Standardized Documentation of Findings

The cytological documentation should contain:
- A description of the patient's history relevant to the specimen
- A description of the quality of the material (e.g., six air-dried, unstained slides with material)
- A description of the cells present
- A diagnosis, including the expected grade of malignancy:
  – Material not representative
  – Representative material with no signs of malignancy (negative)
  – Malignant cells not clearly ruled out (doubtful)
  – Malignant cells probable (suspicion)
  – Malignant cells visible (positive)

It should be noted that neither method (histology or cytology) is infallible. In all cases, the cytological diagnosis should be evaluated in conjunction with the patient's symptoms.

Example Findings

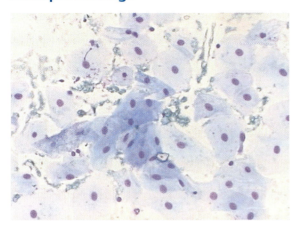

Fig. 11.13 Fine-needle aspiration cytology of a lymph node. There is no representative material, only squamous epithelium from the esophageal mucosa, with no lymphocytes or other diagnostically relevant cell material.

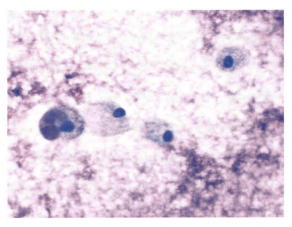

Fig. 11.14 Mediastinal tumor, 1. A bronchogenic cyst, with large amounts of amorphous eosinophilic background substance (mucus) and four typical macrophages. No tumor cells.

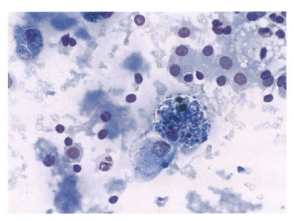

Fig. 11.15 Mediastinal tumor, 2. Thyrocytes, macrophages, and blue colloid. A combination of clinical findings, imaging, and cell findings suggested benign nodular goiter.

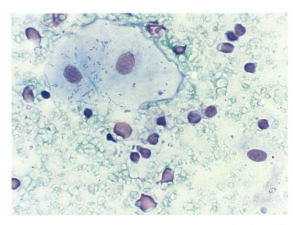

Fig. 11.16 Fine-needle aspiration cytology (station 7/mediastinal). Blood, two mature squamous cells from the esophagus, and loose mature lymphocytes are present, with no blast cells or epithelial tumor cells—suggesting benign lymph-node enlargement.

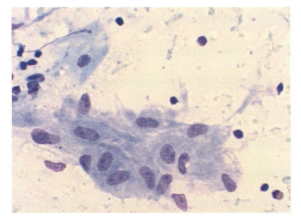

Fig. 11.17 Fine-needle aspiration cytology (station 4 L/mediastinal). There are a few small lymphocytes and a larger group of epithelioid cells, with no necrosis or epithelial tumor cells—suggesting noncaseating epithelioid granulomatosis.

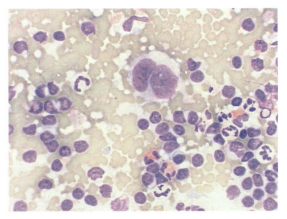

Fig. 11.18 Fine-needle aspiration cytology (station 4 R/mediastinal). Sanguineous smear with a plethora of small lymphocytes, a few eosinophilic granulocytes, and a typical Reed–Sternberg cell containing bilobar nuclei with prominent blue nucleoli—Hodgkin disease in a mediastinal lymph node.

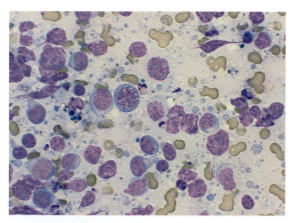

Fig. 11.19 Fine-needle aspiration cytology (station 4 L/mediastinal). Cell-rich smear with large numbers of enlarged lymphatic cells with prominent nucleoli and irregular (cleaved) or smooth (noncleaved) membranes. There are blue particles in the background (lymphoglandular bodies)—large cell non-Hodgkin lymphoma.

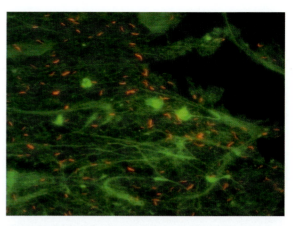

Fig. 11.20 Fine-needle aspiration cytology (station 4 R/mediastinal). Acridine orange staining, showing large amounts of red bacteria (*Mycobacterium tuberculosis*) against the dark background of the specimen—lymph-node tuberculosis.

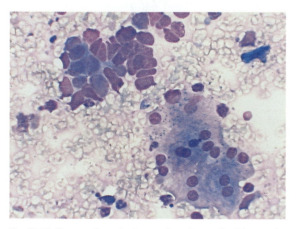

Fig. 11.21 Fine-needle aspiration cytology from a focal hepatic lesion. There is a cluster of hepatocytes and a larger group of tumor cells with bare nuclei, with no visible nucleoli, and typical molding—hepatic metastasis from a small cell anaplastic carcinoma (small cell lung cancer).

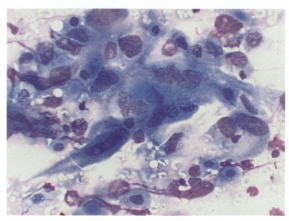

Fig. 11.22 Fine-needle aspiration cytology from a pulmonary mass in the right upper lobe. There are multiple atypical epithelial cells with dense blue cytoplasm, and the tumor cells have bizarre shapes (strap cells)—non–small cell lung cancer/moderate to well-differentiated squamous cell carcinoma.

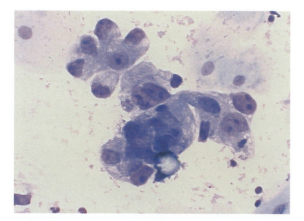

Fig. 11.23 Fine-needle aspiration cytology (station 4 L/mediastinal). There are a few small lymphocytes and mature squamous cells from the esophagus, as well as two atypical epithelial cell clusters from a differentiated adenoid carcinoma (rosette shape)—lymph-node metastasis from an adenocarcinoma.

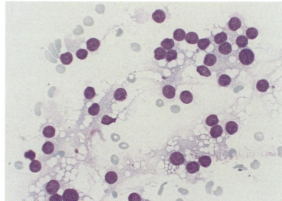

Fig. 11.24 Fine-needle aspiration cytology from the left adrenal gland. Typical cell groups from the adrenal area, with small, round nuclei and vacuolated cytoplasm. Anisonucleosis and intranuclear pseudoinclusions may be present. Some cells, stripped of their cytoplasm, appear as bare nuclei against a "bubbly" background—benign adrenal adenoma.

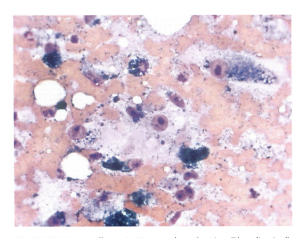

Fig. 11.25 Fine-needle aspiration cytology (station 7/mediastinal). Large numbers of tumorous components rich in melanin pigment are visible both in the cytoplasm and in the background. The sometimes gigantic nucleoli are a typical finding—lymph-node metastasis from a melanotic melanoma.

References

1. Lopes Cardozo P. In: Linke A, ed. Früherkennung des Krebses. Stuttgart: Schattauer; 1962.
2. Beyer T. Klinischer Stellenwert der endosonographisch gesteuerten transmuralen Feinnadelbiopsie für den Pneumologen. Dissertation, Medizinische Fakultät der Universität Leipzig. 2003.

12 Complications of Endoscopic Ultrasound: Risk Assessment and Prevention

C. Jenssen, M. Mayr, D. Nuernberg, S. Faiss

Endoscopic ultrasound (EUS) and EUS-guided interventions, including fine-needle aspiration biopsy (EUS-FNA) and Tru-Cut biopsy (EUS-TCB), have become an accepted part of the diagnosis, staging, and treatment of gastrointestinal diseases, as well as in benign and malignant pulmonary disorders. In the United States, 60% of gastroenterologists use EUS, and in four European countries ≈43% of gastroenterologists and visceral surgeons are reported to have access to EUS.[1,2] In Germany, EUS systems are now used not only in university and tertiary referral centers, but also in some 40% of the country's approximately 2000 hospitals.[3] Despite nearly 30 years' experience and a growing number of examinations and interventions, reliable and prospective data on the safety, risks, and complications of diagnostic and interventional EUS are limited.[4]

EUS-Specific Risk Factors

Endoscopic ultrasound systems differ from traditional forward-viewing and oblique-viewing endoscopes in the rigidity and stiffness of the tip of the scope, which holds the ultrasound transducer, and in that they have a somewhat larger diameter (12.4–14.6 mm) than gastroscopes (9.0–9.8 mm) or duodenoscopes (11.0–13.1 mm).[5] In addition, most echoendoscopes have a longer nonflexible segment just proximal to the transducer. The examination time in EUS is in most cases significantly longer than standard esophagogastroduodenoscopy. With the exception of the electronic radial-scanning echoendoscopes made by Pentax/Hitachi and Fujinon, all other echoendoscopes currently available are oblique-viewing instruments. Intubation and advancement of the echoendoscopes, especially in the esophagus, are therefore semi-blind maneuvers.

EUS-FNA and EUS-TCB differ from forceps biopsies in that all of the layers of the nonsterile gastrointestinal tract and sterile extraintestinal anatomical structures are penetrated in order to obtain access to the target organ or structure. The target lesions are often neighboring vascular structures and may have pathological vascularization themselves. For this reason, it is not possible to apply data from studies on the safety of upper gastrointestinal endoscopy to endoscopic ultrasound.

Complications of Diagnostic EUS

■ Perforation (Tables 12.1 and 12.2)

Esophageal perforation. In a survey of the members of the American Endosonography Club published in 2001, 86 members reported 16 cervical esophageal perforations among 43 852 upper gastrointestinal EUS procedures with radial echoendoscopes (0.03%).[6] Almost all of the patients in whom perforations occurred were elderly; seven of the 16 patients (44%) had a history of difficult intubation in previous endoscopic investigations. Large cervical osteophytes were identified in three cases.

Table 12.1 Possible risk factors for gastrointestinal perforation in endoscopic ultrasound investigations

Risk factor	References
Lack of operator experience	Das et al. 2001,[6] Jenssen et al. 2008,[10] Lachter 2007[14]
Esophagus	
Cancer of the esophagus and esophagogastric junction	Das et al. 2001,[6] Mortensen et al. 2005,[9] Rösch et al. 1993[7]
Dilation of esophageal stricture before EUS	Das et al. 2001,[6] Mortensen et al. 2005,[9] Rösch et al. 1993[7]
Advanced patient age	Das et al. 2001[6]
Difficult previous endoscopic intubation of the esophagus	Das et al. 2001[6]
Large cervical osteophytes	Das et al. 2001[6]
Duodenum	
Diverticula	Jenssen et al. 2008,[10] Lachter 2007[14]
Stenosis, pancreatic head tumor	Raut et al. 2003[11]
Longitudinal echoendoscope (long, rigid tip)	Lachter 2007[14]

In nine of the 16 patients with cervical esophageal perforation (56%), the procedure was being performed by an investigator with less than 1 year of experience in endoscopic ultrasonography. Two patients required surgery. In 13 of the 15 surviving patients (87%), the complication was managed successfully with conservative treatment. One patient died.[6]

Another early multicenter survey from Europe[7] reported 13 esophageal perforations in 37 915 radial EUS examinations (0.03%), accounting for 68% of all complications. The majority of these patients (77%) had undergone pre-EUS dilation of esophageal strictures to allow complete staging of esophageal cancer, including the celiac lymph-node station.[7] Only two studies prospectively investigated the frequency of esophageal perforations. In a single-center study in the Unites States, all patients who underwent EUS of the upper gastrointestinal tract by a single experienced endosonographer over a 7-year period were enrolled. Cervical esophageal perforations occurred in three of 4844 patients (0.06%). The curved-array echoendoscope was used in all three patients.[8] In a study from a department of surgical endoscopy in Denmark, complications of EUS in 3324 consecutive patients were investigated. Esophageal perforations occurred in five of 10 patients with complications (0.15% of all investigations, 0.94% of all patients with esophageal cancer). Balloon dilation had been carried out before the EUS examination in two cases. All five patients with esophageal perforation made a full recovery with conservative treatment (n = 4) or surgical treatment (n = 1).[9] From 2004 to 2006, we performed a survey in German centers performing endoscopic ultrasonography.[10] Thirty-two of the 67 centers that responded to the questionnaire reported keeping a prospective registry of complications. Esophageal perforation occurred in only eight of 85 084 reported diagnostic EUS procedures (0.009%). None of the perforations was related to previous dilation of esophageal strictures. Stenosing esophageal cancer was present in five cases.

Duodenal perforation. In the German survey, duodenal perforations were reported significantly more often than esophageal perforations, occurring in 19 additional cases (0.022%) (**Fig. 12.1**). In 10 of these 19 cases (47.4%) duodenal diverticula (n = 4), duodenal stenosis (n = 3), duodenal ulcer (n = 1), duodenal scarring (n = 1), or acute pancreatitis (n = 1) were reported to have potentially contributed to the perforation. Twenty-seven of the 28 perforations were managed surgically, and all the patients survived[10] (**Table 12.2**).

In a large series of 233 endoscopic ultrasound-guided fine-needle aspiration biopsies in patients with presumed pancreatic cancer, Raut and colleagues reported on two cases of duodenal perforation requiring surgical intervention (0.86%). There was no luminal narrowing of the duodenum in either case.[11] One case report has been published describing an iatrogenic duodenal perforation during endoscopic ultrasonography, which was managed success-

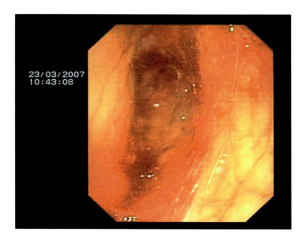

Fig. 12.1 Endoscopic view of a retroperitoneal perforation caused by a longitudinal scanning echoendoscope, diagnosed immediately at the time of EUS examination. The indication for the EUS examination was suspected bile duct stones in an 83-year-old woman. The patient recovered soon after the operation (image reproduced with permission from Jenssen et al.[10]).

Table 12.2 Frequency of perforations of the upper gastrointestinal tract by radial and longitudinal echoendoscopes in the German survey of EUS complications 2004–2006 (data from[10])

Perforation	Radial EUS (n = 47 417)	Longitudinal EUS (n = 37 667)	All diagnostic EUS examinations [a] (n = 85 084)
Esophageal	3 (0.087%)	5 (0.013%)	8 (0.009%)
Duodenal	8 (0.017%)	11 (0.029%)	19 (0.022%)[b]
Gastric	0	1 (0.003%)	1 (0.001%)
Total	11 (0.023%)	17 (0.045%)[c]	28 (0.033%)

[a] Without EUS-guided biopsies or EUS-guided therapeutic interventions.
[b] $P < 0.05$ in comparison with esophageal perforations.
[c] Not significant ($P > 0.05$) in comparison with radial echoendoscopes.

fully by endoscopic closure with hemoclips, followed by conservative treatment.[12] One duodenal perforation occurred in a series of 224 EUS-FNA procedures, representing one out of five severe complications (complication rate 2.2%).[13]

A national survey in Israel investigated the mortality rate associated with diagnostic EUS.[14] Thirteen of 18 reported cases of death related to EUS (seven in Israel and six from outside the country) resulted from duodenal tears, leading to retroperitoneal perforations. Two further cases occurred as a consequence of esophageal perforations. At least four of six cases of duodenal perforation reported in Israel involved patients with duodenal diverticula. Five of the eight fatal complications in Israel were associated with procedures conducted by examiners with experience of fewer than 300 EUS procedures.[14]

Table 12.3 Complications of diagnostic endoscopic ultrasound (EUS),[a] EUS-guided fine-needle aspiration biopsy (EUS-FNA), and EUS-guided therapeutic interventions (EUS-I) in 67 German centers, 2004–2006 (data from[10])

Complications	EUS[1] (n = 85 084)	EUS-FNA (n = 13 223)	EUS-I (n = 2297)	*Total* (n = 100 604)
Total	**29 (0.034%)**	**38 (0.29%)**	**37 (1.61%)**	**104 (0.10%)**
Major	29 (0.034%)	23 (0.17%)	36 (1.57%)	88 (0.087%)
Conservative treatment	2	15	13	31
Interventional treatment	0	4	6	10
Surgical treatment	27	4	17	47
Mortality	4 (0.005%)	0 (0.000%)	6 (0.3%)	10 (0.01%)
Minor (No treatment necessary)	0	15 (0.11%)	1 (0.04%)	16 (0.016%)

[a] Without EUS-guided biopsies or EUS-guided therapeutic interventions.

■ Aspiration

Endosonographic visualization of the gastrointestinal wall and of adjacent structures depends on appropriate acoustic coupling of the transducer to the gastrointestinal wall, either using a water-filled balloon at the tip of the echoendoscope or of the high-frequency ultrasound miniprobe or by filling the gastrointestinal lumen with water. As water-filling of the upper gastrointestinal tract is frequently used, the low frequency of reported cases of aspiration is somewhat surprising. There have only been three reported cases of aspiration of fluid contents from the upper gastrointestinal tract followed by aspiration pneumonia in endosonographic examinations.[14,15]

In the Danish prospective study, tracheal suction was needed in 15 of 293 patients (5.1%), and one patient aspirated during the procedure (0.3%). The "water-in-stomach" method was only used in nine patients (3.1%).[9]

■ Bacteremia

Few data are available concerning the frequency of bacteremia after diagnostic EUS without fine-needle aspiration biopsy. Janssen et al.[16] investigated 100 consecutive patients undergoing diagnostic EUS with a curvilinear echoendoscope by obtaining two pairs of blood cultures immediately before and 5 minutes after EUS. Significant bacteremia (*Streptococcus viridans* and *Propionibacterium* species; *S. mitis*) occurred in only two patients (2%), in both cases after an EUS investigation for staging of esophageal cancer (two of nine patients with esophageal cancer).[16] Levy et al.[17] noted transient bacteremia in one of 52 patients who underwent diagnostic EUS with a radial-scanning echoendoscope (1.9%). None of the three patients with bacteremia after diagnostic EUS in these two studies developed symptoms of infection.[16,17]

■ Hematogenous Tumor Cell Dissemination

Hematogenous tumor cell dissemination was documented in 11 of 45 patients (24%) after transrectal ultrasound (TRUS) staging of rectal cancer. In a further 17 patients (38%), circulating tumor cells were detected in peripheral blood samples before and after TRUS.[18] The clinical and prognostic significance of this observation is not clear at present, although data from the same group suggest that detection of circulating tumor cells in blood samples from patients with stage 2 colorectal cancer correlates with a poor outcome.[19]

Complications with EUS-Guided Biopsy

Patients who undergo EUS-guided biopsy—EUS-guided fine-needle aspiration (EUS-FNA) or EUS-guided Tru-Cut biopsy (EUS-TCB)—are more likely to experience complications or report symptoms following EUS in comparison with patients undergoing diagnostic EUS (**Tables 12.3** and **12.4**).[10,20,21] The major complications reported with EUS-guided biopsy are infections in cystic lesions, bleeding, and acute pancreatitis.[4,22]

■ Bacteremia and Infectious Complications

Bacteremia after EUS-FNA in the upper gastrointestinal tract appears to be a rare event. Its frequency has been investigated in three prospective studies including 202 patients.[16,17,23] In one study with 100 patients, all blood cultures obtained 30 minutes and 60 minutes after the procedure were negative, except in six patients in whom the culture was positive for coagulase-negative *Staphylococcus*, which the investigators regarded as a contaminant.[23] Among the 102 patients in the studies by Janssen

Table 12.4 Complications of diagnostic endoscopic ultrasound (EUS),[a] EUS-guided fine-needle aspiration biopsy (EUS-FNA) and EUS-guided therapeutic interventions (EUS-I): summary of large single-center and multicenter studies

First author (year)	Features of the study	Frequency of complications (%)		
		EUS[1]	EUS-FNA	EUS-I
1) Prospective, single-center				
Williams 1999[46]	333 EUS-FNAs	–	0.3	–
Mortensen 2005[9]	2518 EUSs, 670 EUS-FNAs, 136 EUS-Is	0.22	0.3	0.74
Bournet 2006[13]	3207 EUSs, 224 EUS-FNAs	0.093	2.2	–
Al-Haddad 2008[28]	483 EUS-FNAs	–	1.4	–
Eloubeidi 2008[149]	656 EUS-FNAs	–	1.1	–
Thomas 2009[140]	247 EUS-TCBs	–	2.4[b]	–
2) Retrospective, single-center				
O'Toole 2001[15]	322 EUS-FNAs	–	1.6	–
Carrara 2010[72]	1034 pancreatic EUS-FNAs	–	1.2	–
3) Retrospective, multicenter				
Rösch 1993[7]	42 105 EUSs	0.05	–	–
Wiersema 1997[44]	457 EUS-FNAs (four EUS centers)	–	1.1	–
Buscarini 2006[21]	11 539 EUSs, 787 EUS-FNAs, 21 EUS-Is (six EUS centers)	0.046	0.88	9.5
Jenssen 2008[10]	85 084 EUSs, 13 223 EUS-FNAs, 2297 EUS-Is (67 EUS centers)	0.034	0.29	1.61

[a] Without EUS-guided biopsies or EUS-guided therapeutic interventions.
[b] EUS-guided Tru-Cut biopsy (EUS-TCB), 19-G needle.

et al. and Levy et al. mentioned above, five patients had bacteremia after EUS-FNA (*Streptococcus viridans* in three cases; *Streptococcus* group F; Gram-negative bacillus). No signs or symptoms of infection developed in any of the patients.[16,17]

Large series reporting EUS-FNA in solid pancreatic masses have noted a 0.4–1.0% rate of febrile episodes.[24–26] One case of pyrexia and abdominal pain after EUS-FNA of a large pancreatic head mass, followed by extensive acute portal vein thrombosis, was reported.[27]

In addition to two cases of fever that resolved on antibiotics after EUS-FNA of lymph nodes, reported in larger studies,[28,29] there have been seven reports of serious infectious complications after EUS-FNA or EUS-TCB of mediastinal lymph nodes. After EUS-guided aspiration biopsy of a mediastinal lymph-node metastasis from hepatocellular carcinoma, a mediastinal abscess developed. The iatrogenic abscess was treated successfully with EUS-guided drainage and subsequent endoscopic closure of the resulting esophagomediastinal fistula.[30] Another mediastinal abscess requiring computed tomography–assisted drainage and subsequent thoracotomy developed following EUS-FNA of a mediastinal metastasis from a malignant teratoma.[31] Infectious mediastinitis also occurred as a consequence of transesophageal EUS-FNA of an enlarged necrotic lymph node[32] and of a small benign lymph node in the aortopulmonary window.[33] In one patient, EUS-FNA of a tuberculous subcarinal lymph node induced multiple symptomatic mediastinal–esophageal fistulas, which resolved in the course of tuberculostatic treatment.[34] Only

one case has so far been described of infective endocarditis (*Streptococcus salivarius*) due to EUS-FNA of a mediastinal lymph node in an oncologic patient.[35]

There have been five published reports of infection after EUS-FNA or EUS-TCB of a subepithelial tumor. In one case, EUS-FNA of an esophageal leiomyoma caused severe intramural infection, leading to an esophagectomy.[36] In another case, fever developed 2 hours after EUS-FNA of a large mesenchymal tumor of the esophagus, presumably due to left lobar pneumonia.[15] In the third case, a large duodenal gastrointestinal stromal tumor (GIST) became infected with *Enterobacter cloacae* following EUS-FNA. The resulting abscess resolved after endoscopic transduodenal drainage and antibiotic treatment.[37] Two cases of severe septic complications (streptococcus sepsis, gastric wall abscess) occurred in a series of 52 consecutive EUS-TCBs of gastric subepithelial tumors (3.9%).[38] In our own series of EUS-guided biopsies of hypoechoic subepithelial tumors in the stomach, using a 19-G aspiration needle, one septic infection and an extramural abscess (*Morganella morganii*) also developed in a patient with a large gastric GIST who was receiving 15 mg prednisolone per day (**Fig. 12.2**).

EUS-FNA of rectal, colonic, perirectal, and pericolic mass lesions appears to be a safe procedure. There have been only two reports of infectious complications following transrectal or transcolonic EUS-FNA of solid mass lesions.[39,40] In a prospective risk assessment of bacteremia in 100 patients undergoing EUS-FNA of rectal and perirectal lesions, six patients developed positive blood cultures.

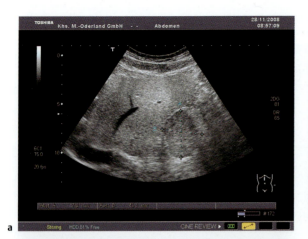

a

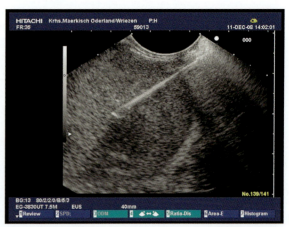

b

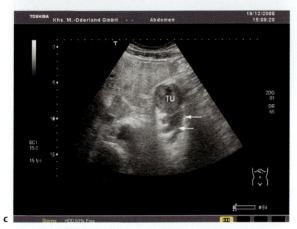

c

Fig. 12.2a–c Abscess 7 days after EUS-guided fine-needle aspiration (EUS-FNA), with a 19-G aspiration needle, of a large gastrointestinal stromal tumor (GIST) in the stomach.
a The transabdominal ultrasound image before EUS-FNA.
b EUS-FNA.
c The transabdominal ultrasound image 8 days after EUS-FNA, showing a hypoechoic mass (arrows) with irregular margins in the periphery of the tumor (Tu). The patient had fever and abdominal pain, and blood cultures were positive for *Morganella morganii*.

Four of these cases were considered to involve contaminants (coagulase-negative *Staphylococcus, Moraxella, Peptostreptococcus stomatis*). Two patients had true-positive blood cultures (*Bacteroides fragilis, Gemella morbillorum*). No immediate or delayed infectious complications occurred in any patients.[41] In two other investigations of the role of EUS-FNA in submucosal tumors and extrinsic masses of the colon and rectum, there were also no complications in 22 and 48 patients, respectively, who underwent transrectal or transcolonic EUS-FNA.[42,43]

EUS-FNA of cystic lesions in the retroperitoneal space or pancreas, and particularly in the mediastinum, appears to carry a significant risk of severe infectious complications. In a large multicenter study of EUS-FNA, two of 18 patients with EUS-FNA of a cystic pancreatic lesion without any preprocedural antibiotic prophylaxis developed cyst infections.[44] In spite of the substantially growing numbers of EUS-FNA procedures being carried out for cystic lesions in the pancreas, there have only been two reports of infection after EUS-FNA of cystic pancreatic lesions despite prophylactic antibiotics.[45,46]

EUS-FNA of bronchogenic and other mediastinal cysts may cause cyst infection, mediastinitis, and severe sepsis. Foregut duplication cysts account for 6–15% of primary

mediastinal masses.[47] It may be difficult to differentiate between esophageal bronchogenic cysts and subepithelial tumors or paraesophageal masses because of their hypoechoic and inhomogeneous mucoid contents.[48,49] One study showed that in 19 patients in whom a bronchogenic cyst was diagnosed with EUS, 13 cysts were anechoic, while the other six were hypoechoic, suggesting a solid mass lesion. Computed tomography or magnetic resonance imaging were diagnostic of a cyst in only four cases.[50] In another study, nine of 27 benign mediastinal cysts were misdiagnosed as solid masses on computed tomography.[51] There have been reports of eight cases of mediastinitis following EUS-FNA or EUS-TCB of mediastinal mass lesions, which were hypoechoic on EUS and had high computed tomography (CT) attenuation values, but proved to be bronchogenic cysts. As solid lesions were suspected, antibiotics had not been administered in five cases.[13,49,50,52,53] In three other cases, severe infection requiring surgical intervention occurred despite preinterventional and postinterventional intravenous antibiotic administration.[54] In one other case, asymptomatic contamination of a mediastinal foregut duplication cyst with *Candida albicans* developed despite preprocedural antibiotic prophylaxis.[55] On the other hand, no infectious complications were seen among 22 patients who underwent transesophageal EUS-FNA of suspected mediastinal cysts using peri-interventional antibiotic prophylaxis.[48]

EUS-FNA of ascites and pleural fluid also involves a risk of infection. Despite antibiotic prophylaxis with levofloxacin in one study, one of 25 patients with transgastric or transduodenal EUS-FNA of suspected malignant ascites developed bacterial peritonitis. Treatment with intravenous antibiotics was successful.[56] In another study, two of 60 patients (3%) developed self-limited fever following EUS-guided paracentesis.[57] A third study did not report any complications after EUS-FNA of ascites in 31 patients who did not receive prophylactic antibiotics.[58]

■ Bile Peritonitis and Cholangitis

Bile peritonitis is a severe complication that can develop due to inadvertent penetration or perforation of the common bile duct when EUS-FNA of a pancreatic mass is being performed in patients with biliary obstruction,[59] or after failure of an attempt at EUS-guided transduodenal cholangiography or bile-duct drainage.[10]

An attempt at EUS-guided gallbladder bile aspiration resulted in bile peritonitis in two of the first three patients who were enrolled in a study to identify patients with microlithiasis as a cause of idiopathic pancreatitis. These complications prompted the investigators to discontinue the study.[60] Inadvertent gallbladder puncture was a complication of transgastric EUS-guided drainage of an infected pancreatic pseudocyst. Thanks to immediate placement of a nasocystic drain in the gallbladder, only mild and localized bile peritonitis developed and surgery was avoided.[61] In an international survey of the indications, yield, and safety of EUS-FNA of liver lesions, one case of death due to septic cholangitis associated with EUS-FNA of a liver metastasis was reported. The background was an occluded biliary stent in a patient with biliary obstruction secondary to pancreatic cancer.[62]

As a consequence of mechanical irritation caused by the tip of the scope or by a water-filled balloon, endoscopic ultrasonography of the pancreas may cause proximal or distal biliary stent migration, possibly followed by cholangitis.[63]

■ Acute Pancreatitis

Hyperamylasemia is common after EUS-FNA of pancreatic lesions, occurring in 11 of 100 patients in one recent prospective study. However, only two patients developed mild acute pancreatitis.[64] Six large studies of EUS-FNA of pancreatic mass lesions have reported iatrogenic acute pancreatitis following EUS-FNA, with rates ranging from 0.4% to 2.0%.[15,20,26,46,64,65] A pooled analysis of 4909 EUS-

FNAs of solid pancreatic masses from 19 EUS centers in the United States identified 14 cases of iatrogenic postprocedural acute pancreatitis (0.29%).[66] The frequency of acute pancreatitis in individual centers ranged from 0% to 2.35%. Only two centers (413 cases of pancreatic EUS-FNA, two cases of acute pancreatitis) assessed complications of EUS-FNA in a prospective manner. Some of the centers with retrospective complication assessment did not report any cases of iatrogenic acute pancreatitis, suggesting that cases of acute pancreatitis may have been underreported for the retrospective cohort. Interestingly, the survey found that half of the patients who had acute pancreatitis after EUS-FNA had benign disease, suggesting that these patients may be at greater risk. Another possible risk factor for iatrogenic acute pancreatitis after EUS-FNA appears to be a history of acute recurrent pancreatitis.[66] This observation is in good accordance with experience with percutaneous pancreatic FNA. In the German survey, eight of nine patients (89%) with reported acute pancreatitis turned out to have benign disease after EUS-FNA of pancreatic mass lesions (**Table 12.2**).[10] In a large retrospective series of EUS-FNA in patients with pancreatic cystic lesions, acute pancreatitis occurred in six of 603 cases (1%).[45] In a prospective analysis of pancreatic EUS-FNA, pancreatitis did not occur in any of 134 patients with solid lesions, but in three of 114 (2.6%) patients with cystic lesions.[15] Two studies investigated the value of EUS-FNA and EUS-TCB in the diagnosis of chronic pancreatitis. Mild acute pancreatitis developed in two of 27 patients (7.4%) after EUS-FNA[67] and in one of 16 patients (6%) as a consequence of EUS-TCB.[68]

One very unusual complication was reported very recently: pancreatic ascites developed after EUS-FNA of a small pancreatic tail cyst, most probably due to elevated pancreatic duct pressure caused by an ampullary adenoma.[69]

■ Hemorrhage

Self-limiting mild intraluminal bleeding due to EUS-FNA has been reported to occur in as many as 4% of cases.[25] In a prospective study evaluating the risk of extraluminal hemorrhage caused by EUS-FNA, only three cases of mild extraluminal hemorrhage were observed among 227 patients (1.3%).[70] Extraluminal bleeding after EUS-FNA can be visualized with endoscopic ultrasound very well. The bleeding appears as an expanding hyperechoic or hypoechoic region adjacent to the sampled lesion (**Figs. 12.3, 12.4, 12.5, 12.6, 12.7, 12.8, 12.9, 12.10**).[70]

In the survey of German EUS centers mentioned above (13 223 EUS-FNAs; **Table 12.3**), bleeding was the most common complication of EUS-FNA (0.15% of cases). Mild and self-limiting bleeding after EUS-FNA occurred in 15 patients. Five patients suffered from severe hemorrhages requiring transfusion and in two cases surgical intervention.[10] One patient was treated with low-molecular-

II Diagnostic Imaging and Interventions

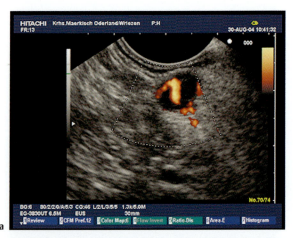

a

Fig. 12.3a, b Mild extraluminal hemorrhage (arrow) after endoscopic ultrasound-guided fine-needle aspiration (EUS-FNA) of a small neuroendocrine pancreatic tumor (X).
a Before EUS-FNA.

b

b Approximately 5 minutes after a second needle pass. The patient did not develop any symptoms.

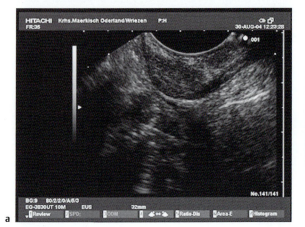

a

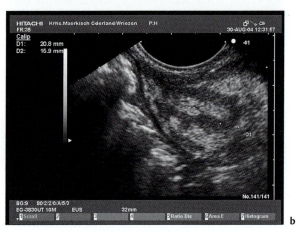

b

Fig. 12.4a, b A minute hematoma in the gastric wall after endoscopic ultrasound-guided fine-needle aspiration (EUS-FNA) of a small subepithelial tumor in a patient with cancer of the large intestine.
a Appearance before EUS-FNA.

b A small echogenic intramural hematoma after three needle passes. The EUS-FNA was nondiagnostic; pathological examination following surgical wedge resection revealed a pancreatic rest.

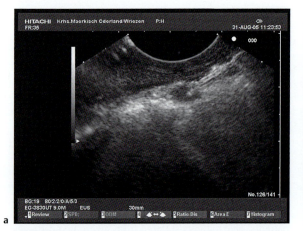

a

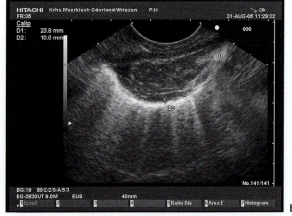

b

Fig. 12.5a, b Extraesophageal bleeding after endoscopic ultrasound-guided fine-needle aspiration (EUS-FNA) of a small mediastinal lymph node after neoadjuvant chemotherapy in a patient with non–small cell lung cancer.

a EUS-FNA.
b The hematoma appeared immediately after the first needle pass.

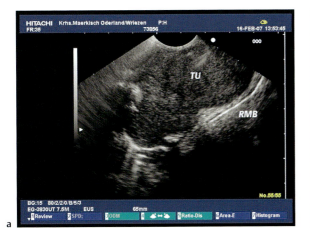

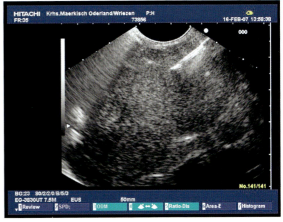

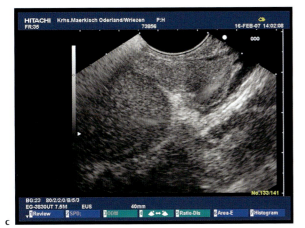

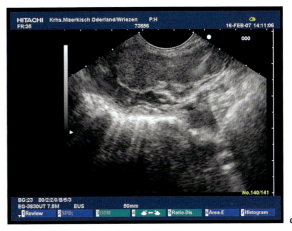

Fig. 12.6a–d An extraesophageal hematoma after endoscopic ultrasound-guided fine-needle aspiration (EUS-FNA) of a central small cell lung cancer.
a A large hypoechoic tumor (TU) adjacent to the right main bronchus (RMB).
b EUS-FNA (22-gauge).

c, d Bleeding is indicated by an expanding extraesophageal inhomogeneous mass above the tumor (**c**: 3 minutes after the first needle pass; **d**: 12 minutes after the first needle pass). The patient was treated with prophylactic antibiotics and did not develop any symptoms.

weight heparin (LWMH) immediately after the procedure and developed a large mediastinal hematoma and hematothorax. Seven units of packed red cells had to be transfused, and thoracoscopy was performed. Another patient needed transfusion of four units of packed red cells after EUS-FNA of pancreatic head carcinoma with portal hypertension. Patients with highly vascularized lesions—for example, subepithelial mesenchymal tumors (**Figs. 12.2, 12.4, 12.7**), neuroendocrine tumors (**Fig. 12.3**), and some metastases, as well as patients with cystic lesions (**Figs. 12.8, 12.9, 12.11**), may be at greater risk. In a retrospective study of EUS-FNA of pancreatic cystic lesions in 50 patients, Varadarajulu and Eloubeidi identified three cases of acute intracystic hemorrhage (6%).[71] Two patients experienced transient abdominal pain, and none of the three patients required blood transfusions. Intracystic bleeding was readily recognized during the investigation as an expanding hyperechoic area around the site of needle puncture within the targeted cyst (**Fig. 12.4**). It was not possible to identify any risk factors contributing to the bleeding events. None of the patients with acute intracystic hemorrhage had taken nonsteroidal anti-inflammatory drugs (NSAIDs), including aspirin, during the week before the procedure.[71] In a large Italian single-center study, bleeding was the most frequent complication of pancreatic EUS-FNA (0.96%, n = 1034), occurring in cystic lesions in seven of 10 cases.[72]

A prospective analysis compared the risk of bleeding after EUS-FNA or EUS-TCB in patients taking NSAIDs, acetylsalicylic acid (ASA), or prophylactic low-molecular-weight heparin (LWMH) with the risk in patients who were not treated. Two of six patients (33.3%) receiving prophylactic LWMH developed extraluminal bleeding, in comparison with none of 26 patients taking platelet inhibitors and seven of the 190 patients (3.7%) not receiving potentially risky medication. There appears to be no addi-

II Diagnostic Imaging and Interventions

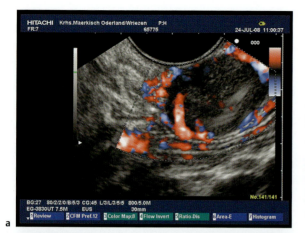

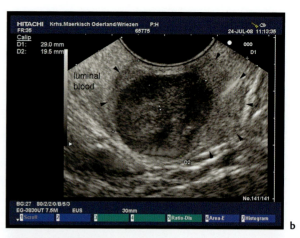

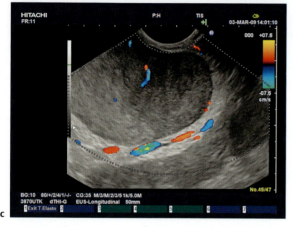

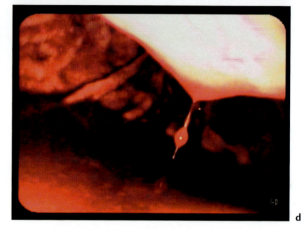

Fig. 12.7a–d Bleeding after endoscopic ultrasound-guided fine-needle aspiration (EUS-FNA), with a 19-gauge aspiration needle, of hypoechoic subepithelial tumors in the stomach.

a EUS image of a gastric leiomyoma, with numerous submucous vessels surrounding the tumor.

b Echogenic blood is seen within the submucosa surrounding the tumor (arrowheads) as well as in the gastric lumen.

c EUS image of a large gastrointestinal stromal tumor (GIST) in the stomach, with intermediate vascularity.

d Endoscopic image of intraluminal bleeding. The bleeding stopped spontaneously in both patients.

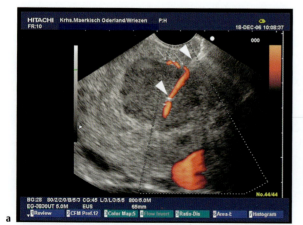

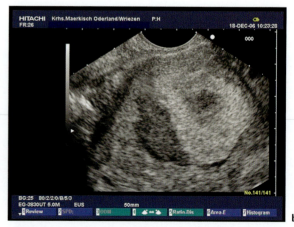

Fig. 12.8a, b Hemorrhage in the central necrotic cavity of a ductal adenocarcinoma of the pancreas after endoscopic ultrasound-guided fine-needle aspiration (EUS-FNA), with a 22-gauge aspiration needle.

a EUS-FNA of the "cystic" part of the tumor. The bleeding along the needle tip (arrowheads) is depicted using color-coded duplex EUS

(color-power angio mode; arrows: vessel in the periphery of the tumor).

b About 15 minutes after withdrawal of the needle, the "cystic" part of the tumor is filled with echogenic coagulum (images reproduced with permission from Adler et al.[4]).

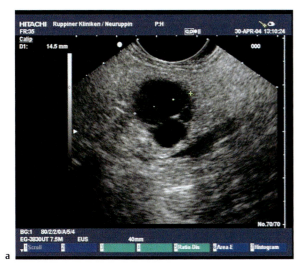

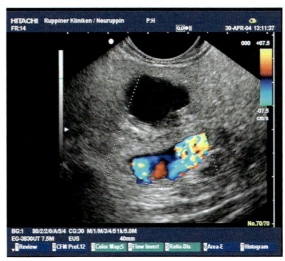

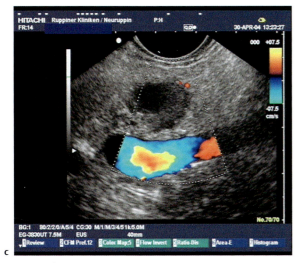

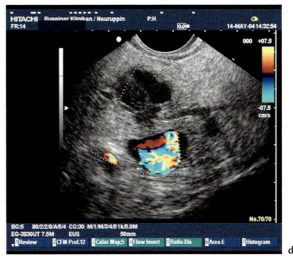

Fig. 12.9a–d Intraluminal cyst hemorrhage after endoscopic ultrasound-guided fine-needle aspiration (EUS-FNA) of a septated pancreatic cystic lesion.[152]

a, b The cystic lesion before EUS-FNA; the color Doppler does not show any vessels in the cyst wall.

c A hyperechogenic area is seen inside the cyst after EUS-FNA. The bleeding stopped spontaneously. At the time of puncture, the bleeding was immediately recognized with color-coded duplex ultrasound; it originated from a small septation inside the cyst.

d The appearance of the cyst 14 days after EUS-FNA. The patient did not develop any symptoms.

tional risk of bleeding related to EUS-FNA in patients taking aspirin or NSAIDs, but possibly in patients receiving prophylactic LMWH.[73] There are no data on the risk of EUS-guided biopsy in patients treated with clopidogrel. However, the results of a recent study showing that clopidogrel use, and in particular combined treatment with clopidogrel and ASA, greatly increased the risk of bleeding in patients undergoing transbronchial lung biopsy[74] suggest that the risk is presumably also increased with EUS-guided biopsy.

There have been several case reports on severe bleeding caused by EUS-guided biopsy—for example, with hemosuccus pancreaticus caused by EUS-FNA of cystic pancreatic lesions,[75] left adrenal gland hemorrhage,[76] retroper-

itoneal bleeding after EUS-FNA of a solid and cystic pancreatic lesion,[21,77] mesenteric bleeding,[78] and intramural bleeding following EUS-TCB of subepithelial tumors.[79,80] Two cases of fatal extraluminal bleeding after EUS-FNA of solid pancreatic lesions have been reported. One patient developed uncontrolled bleeding from a pseudoaneurysm and died. The FNA was performed using a radial-scanning echoendoscope.[81] The other patient developed massive gastrointestinal bleeding 6 hours after EUS-FNA of a pancreatic cancer. Autopsy revealed disseminated cancer, but no bleeding from the EUS puncture areas.[9]

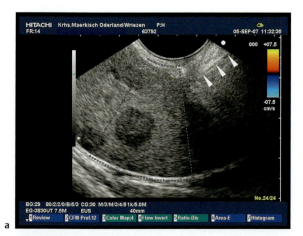

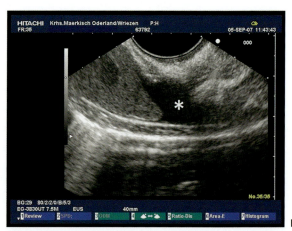

Fig. 12.10a, b
a Endoscopic ultrasound-guided fine-needle aspiration (EUS-FNA) (22-gauge) of a hypoechoic tumor in the spleen. The cytological and histological findings showed that the patient had noncaseating granulomatous splenitis of the sarcoidosis type. Arrowheads: needle.

b Ten minutes after the first of two needle passes, there is endosonographic proof of free fluid around the spleen (*), indicating intraperitoneal bleeding. There were no symptoms, and the hemoglobin level did not decrease (images reproduced with permission from Jenssen et al.[10]).

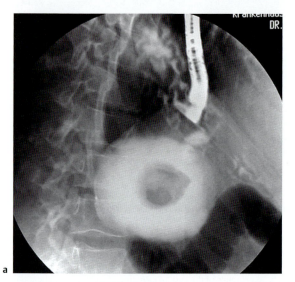

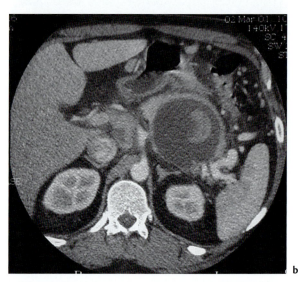

Fig. 12.11a, b Intraluminal bleeding after endoscopic ultrasound-guided pseudocystogastrostomy.
a The fluoroscopic image.
b The computed tomogram after termination of the procedure.

■ Abdominal and Thoracic Pain, Pneumothorax, and Pneumoperitoneum

Abdominal pain following EUS-FNA of pancreatic lesions and abdominal lymph nodes and thoracic pain after EUS-FNA of mediastinal lymph nodes and mediastinal mass lesions with no clinical, laboratory, or radiological findings suggestive of any specific complication have been described in several studies.[9,20,26] A case of massive pneumoperitoneum due to transduodenal EUS-FNA of a solid pancreatic lesion, which resolved without any intervention during antibiotic treatment, is of interest. In the absence of clinical and radiological evidence of bowel perforation, the authors explained the pneumoperitoneum as a result of insufflated air tracking into the peritoneal cavity through the EUS-FNA site. They suggest that some patients with abdominal pain after EUS-FNA may represent cases of unrecognized pneumoperitoneum. The authors therefore suggest that the evaluation of patients who report abdominal pain after EUS-FNA should include an upright plain abdominal radiograph.[82]

Pneumothorax as an adverse event after EUS-FNA has been reported in only a single case. One of three complications in a series of 159 EUS-FNA was pneumothorax after transesophageal biopsy of a mediastinal mass.[83]

■ Tumor Cell Seeding

Needle-tract seeding is a rare complication after percutaneous fine-needle biopsy of intra-abdominal tumors. Based on large retrospective series, its frequency is estimated to be as low as 0.003–0.009% of cases.[84–89] However, one prospective comparative study reported the incidence of needle-tract implantation of hepatocellular carcinoma and pancreatic carcinoma after ultrasound-guided percutaneous puncture to be ≈ 1.5%.[90]

The actual frequency of EUS-FNA–related needle-tract seeding is unknown, but four recent case reports have raised concern that the substantial increase in the numbers of EUS-FNA procedures being performed in the diagnosis of pancreatic masses and enlarged lymph nodes may lead to further cases of this harmful complication. In one case, a large gastric wall implantation metastasis with retroperitoneal invasion (50 × 30 mm) was diagnosed 16 months after potentially curative resection of a small (8 mm) T1N0M0 carcinoma of the pancreatic tail. The tumor had previously been sampled using transgastric EUS-FNA (with five needle passes).[91] In the second case, transgastric EUS-FNA (with one needle pass) of a melanoma metastasis to a perigastric lymph node was complicated by a large (30 mm) gastric implantation metastasis along the needle tract. It was detected and resected 6 months later in the course of surgical resection of the lymph-node metastasis after neoadjuvant chemotherapy had been administered.[92] Recently, a case of needle tract implantation metastasis of the esophageal wall after EUS-FNA of a large metastatic subcarinal lymph node metastasis of gastric cancer using a 19-G needle was reported. The esophageal implantation metastasis developed despite perioperative systemic chemotherapy and disappearance of the subcarinal metastatic lymph node, but fortunately resolved after 2 months of radiotherapy.[93] The potential risk of peritoneal carcinomatosis due to transgastric EUS-FNA of pancreatic malignancies was highlighted by a reported case of peritoneal dissemination of an intraductal papillary mucinous tumor (IPMT) of the pancreas following EUS-FNA of the tumor.[94] Nevertheless, the risk of peritoneal carcinomatosis appears to be significantly lower with EUS-FNA in comparison with percutaneous FNA under computed-tomographic or ultrasound guidance.[95]

Recent data have shown that vital tumor cells were present in the gastrointestinal luminal fluid in nearly half of patients with luminal cancers, as a result of tumor cell sloughing, as well as in 10% of patients with pancreatic cancer secondary to EUS-FNA.[96] However, the significance of this finding in relation to potential tumor cell dissemination during EUS-guided transmural biopsy is not at present clear.

EUS-Guided Therapeutic Interventions

EUS-guided celiac plexus block (EUS-CPB) and EUS-guided celiac plexus neurolysis (EUS-CPN) may lead to retroperitoneal abscess, which has only been reported in five cases (one case report and four cases in two large single-center series[97–99].) However, in one multicenter risk assessment in 41 patients undergoing EUS-CPB, no infectious complications were observed after the procedure; 46.3% of the patients were receiving proton-pump inhibitors (PPIs), and no antibiotic prophylaxis was administered in 58.5% of the procedures.[100] A very unusual complication of EUS-CPN is severe ischemic injury to end organs in the celiac trunk.[69] The pooled complication rate of 170 procedures from six studies was 1.6% (major complications: 0.5%). In a prospective study by O'Toole and Schmulewitz (189 procedures), the complication rate was 8.2% (major complications: 0.6%).[99]

The most common complications of EUS-guided drainage of pancreatic cysts and pancreatic necrosis, of the pancreatic duct, and of the bile ducts were pancreatitis, hemorrhage (**Fig. 12.11**), asymptomatic pneumoperitoneum (**Fig. 12.12**), perforation, and infection. Complication rates were reported to be in the wide range of 0–31% (**Tables 12.3** and **12.4**, see also **Table 16.8**, Chapter 16).

Newer EUS-guided therapeutic interventions include EUS-guided pancreatic cyst ablation and tumor injection therapy. In three studies in which 80–90% ethanol was injected into pancreatic neoplastic cysts, two cases of pancreatitis occurred in 64 patients (pooled complication rate: 3.1%).[101] In a small pilot study, 21 patients with locally advanced pancreatic cancer were given eight EUS-guided fine-needle injections of the antitumoral replication-sensitive adenovirus ONYX.015. Two patients developed sepsis before prophylactic antibiosis was started, and two patients suffered duodenal perforations.[102] EUS-guided ethanol ablation of pancreatic insulinomas may cause pancreatitis, ulceration of the gastroduodenal wall, and bleeding.[103–105]

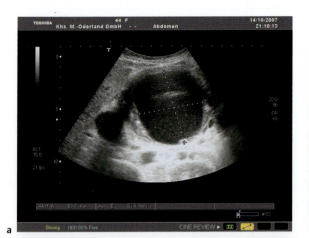

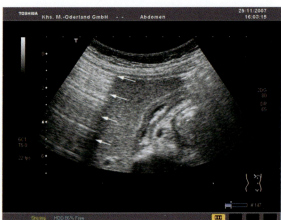

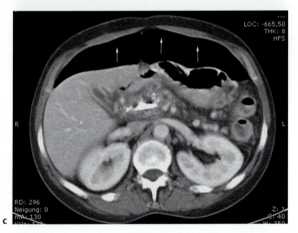

Fig. 12.12 a–c Pneumoperitoneum without peritonitis after endoscopic ultrasound-guided drainage of a pseudocyst in the pancreatic tail.

a Transabdominal ultrasound image of an infected pseudocyst in the pancreatic tail.

b, c After EUS-guided drainage of the pseudocyst, tenderness of the abdomen developed, but there were no signs of peritonitis. Transabdominal ultrasound (arrows in **b**) and computed tomography (**c**) showed large amounts of free air. The free air only disappeared 3 weeks later.

Prevention of EUS-Related Complications

Strategies aimed at minimizing the potential risk of EUS, EUS-guided biopsy, and EUS-guided therapeutic interventions include:

- Adequate education and training of examiners
- Deep familiarity with the results of previous investigations and of possible therapeutic implications
- Appropriate consideration of the patient's clinical condition and of the indications and contraindications of the investigation or procedure
- Careful consideration of a meaningful clinical strategy for investigating and treating each individual patient
- Optimization of the prerequisites and conditions for the planned investigation or procedure

■ Suggested Ways of Preventing Complications

- *Participation in supervised training programs in EUS, EUS-guided biopsy, and EUS-guided therapeutic interventions.* EUS and EUS-guided interventions are complex, technically demanding procedures in which the findings are difficult to interpret and which require advanced skills in diagnostic and therapeutic endoscopy, outstanding experience in diagnostic ultrasonography, and a fundamental understanding of the anatomy of the gastrointestinal tract and surrounding structures. The guidelines for credentialing and granting privileges for endoscopic ultrasound published by the American Society for Gastrointestinal Endoscopy recommend a minimum of 150 supervised EUS investigations, including 75 pancreatobiliary EUS investigations and 50 EUS-FNA procedures, to establish comprehensive competence in all aspects of EUS.[106] Specific guidelines for training in endoscopic ultrasonography should be implemented in the national gastroenterological societies' training programs.[107,108]
- *Diagnostic endoscopy of the upper or lower gastrointestinal tract should be conducted before EUS,* and the echoen-

doscope or high-frequency ultrasound miniprobe most suitable for the intended investigation or procedure should be selected.

- *EUS and in particular EUS-guided interventions should only be carried out in cooperative and adequately sedated patients.* The oxygen saturation, heart rate, and (whenever possible and necessary) blood pressure and electrocardiography should be monitored.
- *Water filling in the upper gastrointestinal tract should be restricted to the minimum amount needed,* and the endoscopy unit and team should be prepared to carry out nasopharyngeal suction.
- In EUS examinations of the pancreas, biliary duct, ampulla, and duodenum in patients with biliary stents, *the correct position of the stent should be checked before the examination is completed.*
- *When there is luminal narrowing—for instance, in patients with esophageal carcinoma—care needs to be taken when maneuvering the echoendoscope and one should consider carrying out the examination with a transendoscopic high-frequency ultrasound miniprobe. Dilation and passage of the stricture should only be performed in selected cases.* A malignant esophageal stricture restricts passage of the echoendoscope in approximately one-third of investigations for esophageal cancer staging and may limit complete evaluation of the tumor depth and lymph nodes at the celiac axis.[109] On the other hand, EUS is currently the most accurate modality available for locoregional staging of esophageal carcinoma.[110] In comparison with the limited diagnostic accuracy of computed tomography, EUS in combination with FNA is highly accurate for detecting and assessing lymph-node metastases at the celiac axis.[111] EUS in combination with EUS-FNA of suspicious celiac lymph nodes is essential for effective decision-making and may therefore potentially reduce the costs as well as the complications of managing patients with esophageal cancer, by preventing unnecessary thoracotomies.[112,113] In addition, EUS staging leads to appropriate administration of neoadjuvant therapy in patients with locally advanced disease and is associated with a recurrence-free survival advantage and an overall survival advantage in these patients.[114] This is why it is justified to carry out dilation before passage of a curvilinear echoendoscope through a malignant esophageal stricture in selected patients, to gain access to the celiac axis region to look for and aspirate celiac lymph nodes. Prospective studies of the role of dilation in patients with obstructing esophageal cancer undergoing EUS examinations by experienced endosonographers have not found any association between perforation and dilation.[115] However, in the case of high-grade strictures in one study, a substantial rate (24%) of esophageal perforation as a result of either wire-guided dilation, or as a direct consequence of the endosonographic staging procedure, was reported. On the other hand, 19 of 21 patients with a high-grade malignant stenosis were found to have stage III or IV

Table 12.5 Contraindications against EUS-FNA and EUS-TCB[125]

No informed consent
Lack of cooperation or insufficient sedation
Anticoagulation treatment or coagulopathy: International Normalized Ratio (INR) > 1.5; platelet count < 50 000; heparin in therapeutic doses
Inhibition of platelet aggregation with clopidogrel[151]
Failure of ultrasound needle control
EUS-guided biopsy of liver, pancreatic head, or ampulla in patients with insufficient drainage of obstructed bile ducts
Cystic mediastinal lesions [a,b]
Interposition of vessels[a]
Results of EUS-guided biopsy are unlikely to have significant clinical impact

[a] Relative contraindication; benefits have to be weighed up against risk very carefully. Transaortic EUS-FNA of mediastinal lymph nodes and tumors, of the pericardium and a left atrial mass, and of intravascular tumors have been reported without any major complications[153–156].

[b] Peri-interventional antibiotic treatment is mandatory.

disease on histopathological examination of the surgical specimen.[109] This is why we do not recommend dilation and complete endosonographic staging in patients with very tight malignant strictures. Dilation or bougienage should be limited to the minimal diameter needed for passage of the echoendoscope. Sequential dilation to a maximum of 16 mm has been reported in four studies with 160 patients, with no perforations.[115–118] One large multicenter study demonstrated the safety of through-the-scope balloon dilation before complete EUS staging of esophageal cancer. A perforation occurred in one of 71 cases.[119] Negotiating the echoendoscope through the tumor with the tip of the video scope closely following the path of the guide wire used for dilation under fluoroscopic guidance may help prevent perforation after dilation.[120] Dilation should be limited to patients in whom detection of celiac lymph-node metastases would change the course of treatment. Patients who are not suitable for surgery or neoadjuvant treatment schedules due to significant comorbidity or liver metastases (identified on ultrasonography or computed tomography) should be excluded from dilation. Using a tapered-tip, wire-guided, nonoptical radial echoendoscope[121,122] or through-the-scope high-frequency ultrasound miniprobes[123,124] allows complete staging of obstructing esophageal cancer in most cases, but does not allow cytological or histological confirmation of suspected celiac lymph-node metastases.

- *EUS-guided biopsy is contraindicated in all patients and in all conditions in which the risks of the procedure outweigh the expected benefits of the diagnostic information it can provide* (**Table 12.5**).[125]
- *Whenever possible, use color-coded duplex sonography (CCDS) or the color-power angio (CPA) mode before punc-*

ture to avoid vessels and highly vascularized structures in the needle trajectory.

- *Before EUS-guided biopsy of a large, solid-appearing mediastinal mass lesion, all appropriate methods should be used to exclude cystic lesions:*
  - Computed tomography (CT) or magnetic resonance imaging (MRI) before EUS-FNA.
  - CCDS, CPA and real-time EUS elastography to confirm that the structure really is solid, characterized by the detection of blood flow inside the lesion.
  - If there is any uncertainty regarding the solid character of the lesion, contrast-enhanced EUS should be used to confirm the flow signals.

- *EUS-guided biopsy of pancreatic masses should be restricted to those patients in whom definitive cytopathological diagnosis of the lesion is likely to alter the management significantly.* Knowing when to carry out EUS-FNA is as important as being able to perform the procedure itself.[22] In general, there is no indication for EUS-FNA of a pancreatic mass lesion that is typical of adenocarcinoma in patients who have no criteria of unresectability.[22,125] We suggest the following indications for EUS-FNA of pancreatic masses:[125]
  - *Unresectable mass:* documentation of malignancy and histological type before palliative (or neoadjuvant) chemotherapy or radiotherapy; proof of unresectability (liver metastases, mediastinal lymph node metastases, pleural or peritoneal carcinosis).
  - *Solid pancreatic mass lesions atypical for adenocarcinoma* (for example, suspected metastases, lymphoma, or neuroendocrine tumor): cytological or histological diagnosis in most cases will alter the course of therapy (avoiding surgical interventions, limited resections, chemotherapy, radiotherapy). More recent EUS techniques (CCDS, CPA, ultrasound contrast enhancement, ultrasound elastography) may help select resectable pancreatic masses that are atypical of pancreatic adenocarcinoma and should therefore be sampled.[126–139]
  - *Cystic pancreatic lesions:* differentiation between benign (pseudocyst, simple cyst, lymphoepithelial cyst) and (potentially) malignant cystic lesions (mucinous neoplasia).
  - If the patient is reluctant to undergo major pancreatic surgery without a definitive histological diagnosis, EUS-FNA appears to be the safest and most efficacious method of acquiring tissue.[22] In such cases, transgastric EUS-FNA of pancreatic mass lesions should be avoided in order to minimize the risk of implantation metastasis or intraperitoneal cancer dissemination.
  - *Unclear findings:* cytological/histological proof of a benign diagnosis if there is a low pretest probability of a malignant tumor (e.g., focal pancreatitis and autoimmune pancreatitis).

- *Tru-Cut needles should be used with caution in selected cases.*[4,125] Two large tertiary referral center experiences have shown that, in comparison with EUS-FNA, EUS-TCB

in the hands of very experienced investigators is not associated with an increased risk of complications. The complication rates of 0.6% and 2.4% with EUS-TCB were in the range of the adverse effects of EUS-FNA.[140,141] However, none of the studies conducted to date has addressed the issue of safety sufficiently and in comparison with EUS-FNA. On the other hand, there are several technical difficulties with this technique, especially in targeting pancreatic head lesions and small lymph nodes.[141–143] Subepithelial tumors, unexplained thickening of the gastrointestinal wall, suspected lymphoma, and suspected autoimmune pancreatitis are now beginning to emerge as special indications for EUS-TCB, as it provides an opportunity for histological versus cytological examination and because it has greater diagnostic efficacy and accuracy in comparison with EUS-FNA.[125]

- *Antibiotic prophylaxis should be administered in patients undergoing EUS-guided biopsy or EUS-guided drainage of cystic lesions (pancreas, peripancreatic, mediastinal). Antibiotic prophylaxis should also be considered in patients undergoing transrectal and transcolonic EUS-FNA.*[4] Antibiotic prophylaxis appears to reduce the incidence of clinically relevant infectious complications of EUS-FNA performed to sample cystic lesions of the pancreas. There are no data comparing EUS-FNA of cystic lesions with or without antibiotic prophylaxis in a prospective manner. However, in contrast to the high rate of cyst infections in older studies in which antibiotic prophylaxis was not provided, one large previous series (including 603 patients) using antibiotic prophylaxis reported only one infectious complication.[45] Some experts also recommend periprocedural antibiotic prophylaxis for EUS-FNA of the perirectal space,[144] for EUS-TCB of subepithelial tumors,[38] for EUS-FNA of ascites,[56] and for EUS-guided celiac plexus block in patients taking PPIs.[145] However, there are no valid data supporting routine use of antibiotics for these indications.[41,100] One experimental study demonstrated that flushing the gastrointestinal mucosa with 10 mL of a 5% povidone–iodine solution before EUS-FNA of cystic lesions substantially reduces, but does not eliminate, transmucosal transmission of bacteria. The authors therefore suggest combining systemic antibiotics and local 5% povidone–iodine when carrying out EUS-FNA of cystic lesions.[146]

- *Complications should be assessed in a prospective manner, and all complications that occur should be analyzed.* Prospective risk assessment is an essential prerequisite for the analysis and prevention of complications. Careful prospective studies show higher complication rates than retrospective studies. The American Society for Gastrointestinal Endoscopy recommends that specific quality indicators (in particular indications, sedation, immediate and delayed complications, procedure success) should be tracked routinely in all patients undergoing EUS.[147]

Summary: Morbidity and Mortality of EUS and EUS-FNA

Diagnostic EUS without EUS-guided intervention is a safe procedure. The complication rates are comparable to those in diagnostic endoscopy of the upper gastrointestinal tract (**Table 12.6**).[4] The most common complications are perforations of the esophagus and of the duodenum. Perforation may be made more likely by the specific mechanical and optical properties of echoendoscopes. To minimize the risk of perforation, examiners should be aware of the specific features of the echoendoscope used, as well as of the specific anatomical situation in the patient (e.g., esophageal stenosis, duodenal diverticula). Esophageal dilation before EUS staging of esophageal carcinoma should be avoided in very tight stenoses and in all cases in which the results of complete locoregional staging will probably not alter the course of management for the patient.

Most complications of EUS are associated with EUS-guided biopsy. The overall complication rate of EUS-FNA and EUS-TCB appears to be between 0.3% and 6.3%, and is comparable to that of colonoscopy with polypectomy (**Tables 12.4** and **12.6**). The mortality is close to zero.[9,10,13,15,21,22,26,28,44,62,72,81,83,140,141,148–150]

The major adverse effects are bleeding, acute pancreatitis, and infectious complications.[4,22,148] Cystic lesions are associated with an increased risk of infectious and bleeding complications in comparison with solid lesions.[44,71] Infection of pancreatic cystic lesions appears to have been substantially eliminated by prophylactic antibiotic use. The risk of bleeding is not increased in patients who are taking aspirin or NSAIDs, but in all probability in patients taking clopidogrel or receiving heparin in prophylactic and therapeutic doses. Treatment with clopidogrel

and heparin therefore should be discontinued in the case of planned EUS-guided biopsy or therapeutic intervention whenever possible.[151]

EUS-FNA of benign pancreatic lesions appears to be associated with a greater risk than EUS-FNA of pancreatic malignancies. Tumor cell seeding and peritoneal dissemination are very rarely reported serious events.

Complications occurring with EUS, EUS-guided biopsy, and EUS-guided therapeutic interventions should be assessed in a prospective manner in all endoscopy units.

Adequate education and training in EUS and EUS-guided biopsy and EUS-guided therapeutic intervention is the essential prerequisite for minimizing the risk and enhancing the efficacy of endosonographic examinations and interventions. Restricting EUS-guided biopsy only to patients in whom the cytological or histological results can be expected to change the course of management is the best way of preventing the complications of EUS-guided biopsy.

Table 12.6 Complication risk of diagnostic endoscopic ultrasound (EUS) and EUS-guided fine-needle aspiration biopsy (EUS-FNA) in comparison with other endoscopic examinations and interventions (pooled data from the literature)

Complications	Total (%)	Bleeding (%)	Perforation (%)
Diagnostic EGD	0.009–0.2	0.002–0.06	0.0009–0.04
Diagnostic colonoscopy	0.02–0.25	0–0.03	0.005–0.2
Colonoscopy and polypectomy	0.36–9.7	0.26–8.6	0.06–1.1
Diagnostic ERCP	1.38	0	0.11
Therapeutic ERCP	5.0–9.8	0.49–2.0	0.3–0.8
EUS	0.03–0.15	0	0.03–0.15
EUS-FNA and EUS-TCB	0.3–6.3	0.15–3.7	0–0.86

EGD, esophagogastroduodenoscopy; ERCP, endoscopic retrograde cholangiopancreatography; EUS, endoscopic ultrasonography; EUS-FNA, endoscopic ultrasound-guided fine-needle aspiration; EUS-TCB, endoscopic ultrasound-guided Tru-Cut biopsy.

References

1. Ahmad NA, Kochman ML, Ginsberg GG. Practice patterns and attitudes toward the role of endoscopic ultrasound in staging of gastrointestinal malignancies: a survey of physicians and surgeons. Am J Gastroenterol 2005;100(12): 2662–2668.
2. Kalaitzakis E, Panos M, Sadik R, Aabakken L, Koumi A, Meenan J. Clinicians' attitudes towards endoscopic ultrasound: a survey of four European countries. Scand J Gastroenterol 2009;44(1):100–107.
3. Jenssen C. Diagnostic endosonography – state of the art 2009 [Article in German] Endosk Heute 2009;22:89–104.
4. Adler DG, Jacobson BC, Davila RE, et al; ASGE. ASGE guideline: complications of EUS. Gastrointest Endosc 2005; 61(1): 8–12.
5. Tierney WM, Adler DG, Chand B, et al; ASGE Technology Committee. Echoendoscopes. Gastrointest Endosc 2007;66(3):435–442.
6. Das A, Sivak MV Jr, Chak A. Cervical esophageal perforation during EUS: a national survey. Gastrointest Endosc 2001;53(6):599–602.
7. Rösch T, Dittler HJ, Fockens P, Yasuda K, Lightdale C. Major complications of endoscopic ultrasonography: results of a survey of 42 105 cases. Gastrointest Endosc 1993;39:344.
8. Eloubeidi MA, Tamhane A, Lopes TL, Morgan DE, Cerfolio RJ. Cervical esophageal perforations at the time of endoscopic ultrasound: a prospective evaluation of frequency, outcomes, and patient management. Am J Gastroenterol 2009;104(1):53–56.
9. Mortensen MB, Fristrup C, Holm FS, et al. Prospective evaluation of patient tolerability, satisfaction with patient information, and complications in endoscopic ultrasonography. Endoscopy 2005;37(2):146–153.
10. Jenssen C, Faiss S, Nürnberg D. Complications of endoscopic ultrasound and endoscopic ultrasound-guided interventions - results of a survey among German centers. [Article in German] Z Gastroenterol 2008;46(10):1177–1184.
11. Raut CP, Grau AM, Staerkel GA, et al. Diagnostic accuracy of endoscopic ultrasound-guided fine-needle aspiration in patients with presumed pancreatic cancer. J Gastrointest Surg 2003;7(1):118–126, discussion 127–128.

II Diagnostic Imaging and Interventions

12. Sebastian S, Byrne AT, Torreggiani WC, Buckley M. Endoscopic closure of iatrogenic duodenal perforation during endoscopic ultrasound. Endoscopy 2004;36(3):245.

13. Bournet B, Migueres I, Delacroix M, et al. Early morbidity of endoscopic ultrasound: 13 years' experience at a referral center. Endoscopy 2006;38(4):349–354.

14. Lachter J. Fatal complications of endoscopic ultrasonography: a look at 18 cases. Endoscopy 2007;39(8):747–750.

15. O'Toole D, Palazzo L, Arotçarena R, et al. Assessment of complications of EUS-guided fine-needle aspiration. Gastrointest Endosc 2001;53(4):470–474.

16. Janssen J, König K, Knop-Hammad V, Johanns W, Greiner L. Frequency of bacteremia after linear EUS of the upper GI tract with and without FNA. Gastrointest Endosc 2004;59(3):339–344.

17. Levy MJ, Norton ID, Wiersema MJ, et al. Prospective risk assessment of bacteremia and other infectious complications in patients undergoing EUS-guided FNA. Gastrointest Endosc 2003;57(6):672–678.

18. Koch M, Antolovic D, Kienle P, et al. Increased detection rate and potential prognostic impact of disseminated tumor cells in patients undergoing endorectal ultrasound for rectal cancer. Int J Colorectal Dis 2007;22(4):359–365.

19. Koch M, Kienle P, Kastrati D, et al. Prognostic impact of hematogenous tumor cell dissemination in patients with stage II colorectal cancer. Int J Cancer 2006;118(12): 3072–3077.

20. Eloubeidi MA, Chen VK, Eltoum IA, et al. Endoscopic ultrasound-guided fine needle aspiration biopsy of patients with suspected pancreatic cancer: diagnostic accuracy and acute and 30-day complications. Am J Gastroenterol 2003;98(12):2663–2668.

21. Buscarini E, De Angelis C, Arcidiacono PG, et al. Multicentre retrospective study on endoscopic ultrasound complications. Dig Liver Dis 2006;38(10):762–767.

22. Erickson RA. EUS-guided FNA. Gastrointest Endosc 2004;60(2):267–279.

23. Barawi M, Gottlieb K, Cunha B, Portis M, Gress F. A prospective evaluation of the incidence of bacteremia associated with EUS-guided fine-needle aspiration. Gastrointest Endosc 2001;53(2):189–192.

24. Chang KJ, Nguyen P, Erickson RA, Durbin TE, Katz KD. The clinical utility of endoscopic ultrasound-guided fine-needle aspiration in the diagnosis and staging of pancreatic carcinoma. Gastrointest Endosc 1997;45(5):387–393.

25. Voss M, Hammel P, Molas G, et al. Value of endoscopic ultrasound guided fine needle aspiration biopsy in the diagnosis of solid pancreatic masses. Gut 2000;46(2): 244–249.

26. Eloubeidi MA, Tamhane A, Varadarajulu S, Wilcox CM. Frequency of major complications after EUS-guided FNA of solid pancreatic masses: a prospective evaluation. Gastrointest Endosc 2006;63(4):622–629.

27. Matsumoto K, Yamao K, Ohashi K, et al. Acute portal vein thrombosis after EUS-guided FNA of pancreatic cancer: case report. Gastrointest Endosc 2003;57(2):269–271.

28. Al-Haddad M, Wallace MB, Woodward TA, et al. The safety of fine-needle aspiration guided by endoscopic ultrasound: a prospective study. Endoscopy 2008;40(3):204–208.

29. Eloubeidi MA, Wallace MB, Reed CE, et al. The utility of EUS and EUS-guided fine needle aspiration in detecting celiac lymph node metastasis in patients with esophageal cancer: a single-center experience. Gastrointest Endosc 2001; 54(6):714–719.

30. Will U, Meyer F, Bosseckert H. Successful endoscopic management of iatrogenic mediastinal infection and subsequent esophagomediastinal fistula, following endosonographically guided fine-needle aspiration biopsy. Endoscopy 2005;37(1):88–90.

31. Pai KR, Page RD. Mediastinitis after EUS-guided FNA biopsy of a posterior mediastinal metastatic teratoma. Gastrointest Endosc 2005;62(6):980–981.

32. Aerts JG, Kloover J, Los J, van der Heijden O, Janssens A, Tournoy KG. EUS-FNA of enlarged necrotic lymph nodes may cause infectious mediastinitis. J Thorac Oncol 2008;3(10):1191–1193.

33. Savides TJ, Margolis D, Richman KM, Singh V. Gemella morbillorum mediastinitis and osteomyelitis following transesophageal endoscopic ultrasound-guided fine-needle aspiration of a posterior mediastinal lymph node. Endoscopy 2007;39(Suppl 1):E123–E124.

34. von Bartheld MB, van Kralingen KW, Veenendaal RA, Willems LN, Rabe KF, Annema JT. Mediastinal-esophageal fistulae after EUS-FNA of tuberculosis of the mediastinum. Gastrointest Endosc 2009;71(1):210–212.

35. van Fraeyenhove F, Lamot C, Vogelaers D, Van Belle S, Cesmeli E, Rottey S. A rare infectious complication after endoscopic ultrasound guided fine needle aspiration in an oncological patient and review of the literature. Acta Clin Belg 2009;64(2):147–149.

36. Grandval P, Picon M, Coste P, Giovannini M, Thomas P, Lafon J. Infection of submucosal tumor after endosonography-guided needle biopsy. [Article in German] Gastroenterol Clin Biol 1999;23(5):566–568.

37. DeWitt J, Al-Haddad M, Fogel E, et al. Endoscopic transduodenal drainage of an abscess arising after EUS-FNA of a duodenal GI stromal tumor. Gastrointest Endosc 2009;70(1):185–188.

38. Polkowski M, Gerke W, Jarosz D, et al. Diagnostic yield and safety of endoscopic ultrasound-guided trucut [corrected] biopsy in patients with gastric submucosal tumors: a prospective study. Endoscopy 2009;41(4):329–334.

39. Faias S, Kaplan R, Hawes RH, et al. Role of endoscopic ultrasound with guided fine needle aspiration (EUS-FNA) in the diagnosis of pelvic masses [abstract]. Gastrointest Endosc 2005;61:AB276.

40. Mezzi G, Arcidiacono PG, Carrara S, Freschi M, Boemo C, Testoni PA. Complication after endoscopic ultrasound-guided fine-needle aspiration (EUS-FNA) of rectal lesion. Endoscopy 2007;39(Suppl 1):E137.

41. Levy MJ, Norton ID, Clain JE, et al. Prospective study of bacteremia and complications With EUS FNA of rectal and perirectal lesions. Clin Gastroenterol Hepatol 2007;5(6): 684–689.

42. Sailer M, Bussen D, Fein M, et al. Endoscopic ultrasound-guided transrectal biopsies of pelvic tumors. J Gastrointest Surg 2002;6(3):342–346.

43. Sasaki Y, Niwa Y, Hirooka Y, et al. The use of endoscopic ultrasound-guided fine-needle aspiration for investigation of submucosal and extrinsic masses of the colon and rectum. Endoscopy 2005;37(2):154–160.

44. Wiersema MJ, Vilmann P, Giovannini M, Chang KJ, Wiersema LM. Endosonography-guided fine-needle aspiration biopsy: diagnostic accuracy and complication assessment. Gastroenterology 1997;112(4):1087–1095.

45. Lee LS, Saltzman JR, Bounds BC, Poneros JM, Brugge WR, Thompson CC. EUS-guided fine needle aspiration of pancreatic cysts: a retrospective analysis of complications and their predictors. Clin Gastroenterol Hepatol 2005;3(3): 231–236.

46. Williams DB, Sahai AV, Aabakken L, et al. Endoscopic ultrasound guided fine needle aspiration biopsy: a large single centre experience. Gut 1999;44(5):720–726.

47. Ribet ME, Copin MC, Gosselin B. Bronchogenic cysts of the mediastinum. J Thorac Cardiovasc Surg 1995;109(5): 1003–1010.

48. Fazel A, Moezardalan K, Varadarajulu S, Draganov P, Eloubeidi MA. The utility and the safety of EUS-guided FNA in the evaluation of duplication cysts. Gastrointest Endosc 2005;62(4):575–580.

49. Westerterp M, van den Berg JG, van Lanschot JJ, Fockens P. Intramural bronchogenic cysts mimicking solid tumors. Endoscopy 2004;36(12):1119–1122.

50. Wildi SM, Hoda RS, Fickling W, et al. Diagnosis of benign cysts of the mediastinum: the role and risks of EUS and FNA. Gastrointest Endosc 2003;58(3):362–368.

51. Eloubeidi MA, Cohn M, Cerfolio RJ, et al. Endoscopic ultrasound-guided fine-needle aspiration in the diagnosis of foregut duplication cysts: the value of demonstrating detached ciliary tufts in cyst fluid. Cancer 2004;102(4): 253–258.

52. Annema JT, Veseliç M, Versteegh MI, Rabe KF. Mediastinitis caused by EUS-FNA of a bronchogenic cyst. Endoscopy 2003;35(9):791–793.

53. Varadarajulu S, Fraig M, Schmulewitz N, et al. Comparison of EUS-guided 19-gauge Trucut needle biopsy with EUS-guided fine-needle aspiration. Endoscopy 2004;36(5): 397–401.

54. Diehl DL, Cheruvattath R, Facktor MA, Go BD. Infection after endoscopic ultrasound-guided aspiration of mediastinal cysts. Interact Cardiovasc Thorac Surg 2010;10(2): 338–340.

55. Ryan AG, Zamvar V, Roberts SA. Iatrogenic candidal infection of a mediastinal foregut cyst following endoscopic ultrasound-guided fine-needle aspiration. Endoscopy 2002;34(10):838–839.

56. Kaushik N, Khalid A, Brody D, McGrath K. EUS-guided paracentesis for the diagnosis of malignant ascites. Gastrointest Endosc 2006;64(6):908–913.

57. DeWitt J, LeBlanc J, McHenry L, McGreevy K, Sherman S. Endoscopic ultrasound-guided fine-needle aspiration of ascites. Clin Gastroenterol Hepatol 2007;5(5):609–615.

58. Nguyen PT, Chang KJ. EUS in the detection of ascites and EUS-guided paracentesis. Gastrointest Endosc 2001;54(3): 336–339.

59. Chen HY, Lee CH, Hsieh CH. Bile peritonitis after EUS-guided fine-needle aspiration. Gastrointest Endosc 2002;56(4): 594–596.

60. Jacobson BC, Waxman I, Parmar K, Kauffman JM, Clarke GA, Van Dam J. Endoscopic ultrasound-guided gallbladder bile aspiration in idiopathic pancreatitis carries a significant risk of bile peritonitis. Pancreatology 2002;2(1):26–29.

61. Hikichi T, Irisawa A, Takagi T, et al. A case of transgastric gallbladder puncture as a complication during endoscopic ultrasound-guided drainage of a pancreatic pseudocyst. Fukushima J Med Sci 2007;53(1):11–18.

62. tenBerge J, Hoffman BJ, Hawes RH, et al. EUS-guided fine needle aspiration of the liver: indications, yield, and safety based on an international survey of 167 cases. Gastrointest Endosc 2002;55(7):859–862.

63. Gaylord KM, Nawras A. Incidence of biliary stent migration as a direct complication of performing endoscopic ultrasound [abstract]. Gastrointest Endosc 2005;61:AB279.

64. Fernández-Esparrach G, Ginès A, García P, et al. Incidence and clinical significance of hyperamylasemia after endoscopic ultrasound-guided fine-needle aspiration (EUS-FNA) of pancreatic lesions: a prospective and controlled study. Endoscopy 2007;39(8):720–724.

65. Gress F, Michael H, Gelrud D, et al. EUS-guided fine-needle aspiration of the pancreas: evaluation of pancreatitis as a complication. Gastrointest Endosc 2002;56(6):864–867.

66. Eloubeidi MA, Gress FG, Savides TJ, et al. Acute pancreatitis after EUS-guided FNA of solid pancreatic masses: a pooled analysis from EUS centers in the United States. Gastrointest Endosc 2004;60(3):385–389.

67. Hollerbach S, Klamann A, Topalidis T, Schmiegel WH. Endoscopic ultrasonography (EUS) and fine-needle aspiration (FNA) cytology for diagnosis of chronic pancreatitis. Endoscopy 2001;33(10):824–831.

68. DeWitt J, McGreevy K, LeBlanc J, McHenry L, Cummings O, Sherman S. EUS-guided Trucut biopsy of suspected nonfocal chronic pancreatitis. Gastrointest Endosc 2005; 62(1):76–84.

69. Babich JP, Bonasera RJ, Klein J, Friedel DM. Pancreatic ascites: complication after endoscopic ultrasound-guided fine needle aspiration of a pancreatic cyst. Endoscopy 2009;41(Suppl 2):E211–E212.

70. Affi A, Vazquez-Sequeiros E, Norton ID, Clain JE, Wiersema MJ. Acute extraluminal hemorrhage associated with EUS-guided fine needle aspiration: frequency and clinical significance. Gastrointest Endosc 2001;53(2):221–225.

71. Varadarajulu S, Eloubeidi MA. Frequency and significance of acute intracystic hemorrhage during EUS-FNA of cystic lesions of the pancreas. Gastrointest Endosc 2004;60(4): 631–635.

72. Carrara S, Arcidiacono PG, Mezzi G, Petrone MC, Boemo C, Testoni PA. Pancreatic endoscopic ultrasound-guided fine needle aspiration: complication rate and clinical course in a single centre. Dig Liver Dis 2010;42(7):520–523.

73. Kien-Fong Vu C, Chang F, Doig L, Meenan J. A prospective control study of the safety and cellular yield of EUS-guided FNA or Trucut biopsy in patients taking aspirin, nonsteroidal anti-inflammatory drugs, or prophylactic low molecular weight heparin. Gastrointest Endosc 2006;63(6):808–813.

74. Ernst A, Eberhardt R, Wahidi M, Becker HD, Herth FJ. Effect of routine clopidogrel use on bleeding complications after transbronchial biopsy in humans. Chest 2006;129(3): 734–737.

75. Singh P, Gelrud A, Schmulewitz N, Chauhan S. Hemosuccus pancreaticus after EUS-FNA of pancreatic cyst (with video). Gastrointest Endosc 2008;67(3):543.

76. Haseganu LE, Diehl DL. Left adrenal gland hemorrhage as a complication of EUS-FNA. Gastrointest Endosc 2009;69(6): e51–e52.

77. Carrara S, Arcidiacono PG, Giussani A, Testoni PA. Acute hemorrhage with retroperitoneal hematoma after endoscopic ultrasound-guided fine-needle aspiration of an intraductal papillary mucinous neoplasm of the pancreas. Am J Gastroenterol 2009;104(6):1610–1611.

78. Siddiqui A, Burdick S, Yang K, Cryer B. Acute mesenteric hemorrhage associated with EUS-guided fine needle aspiration. J Clin Gastroenterol 2007;41(7):722–723.

79. Inoue H, Mizuno N, Sawaki A, et al. Life-threatening delayed-onset bleeding after endoscopic ultrasound-guided 19-gauge Trucut needle biopsy of a gastric stromal tumor. Endoscopy 2006;38(Suppl 2):E38.

80. Varadarajulu S, Fraig M, Schmulewitz N, et al. Comparison of EUS-guided 19-gauge Trucut needle biopsy with EUS-guided fine-needle aspiration. Endoscopy 2004;36(5): 397–401.

81. Gress FG, Hawes RH, Savides TJ, Ikenberry SO, Lehman GA. Endoscopic ultrasound-guided fine-needle aspiration biopsy using linear array and radial scanning endosonography. Gastrointest Endosc 1997;45(3):243–250.

82. Andrews AH, Horwhat JD. Massive pneumoperitoneum after EUS-FNA aspiration of the pancreas. Gastrointest Endosc 2006;63(6):876–877.

83. Larino-Noia J, Iglesias-Garcia J, Seijo-Rios S et al. Assessment of EUS and EUS-guided FNA complications in a large cohort of patients [abstract]. Endoscopy 2006;38. DOI:101055/s-2006-947785.

84. Buscarini L, Fornari F, Bolondi L, et al. Ultrasound-guided fine-needle biopsy of focal liver lesions: techniques, diagnostic accuracy and complications. A retrospective study on 2091 biopsies. J Hepatol 1990;11(3):344–348.

85. Fornari F, Civardi G, Cavanna L, et al; The Cooperative Italian Study Group. Complications of ultrasonically guided fine-needle abdominal biopsy. Results of a multicenter Italian study and review of the literature. Scand J Gastroenterol 1989;24(8):949–955.

86. Smith EH. The hazards of fine-needle aspiration biopsy. Ultrasound Med Biol 1984;10(5):629–634.

87. Smith EH. Complications of percutaneous abdominal fine-needle biopsy. Review. Radiology 1991;178(1): 253–258.

88. Weiss H, Düntsch U. Complications of fine needle puncture. DEGUM survey II. [Article in German] Ultraschall Med 1996;17(3):118–130.

89. Weiss H, Düntsch U, Weiss A. Risks of fine needle puncture—results of a survey in West Germany (German Society of Ultrasound in Medicine survey). [Article in German] Ultraschall Med 1988;9(3):121–127.

90. Kosugi C, Furuse J, Ishii H, et al. Needle tract implantation of hepatocellular carcinoma and pancreatic carcinoma after ultrasound-guided percutaneous puncture: clinical and pathologic characteristics and the treatment of needle tract implantation. World J Surg 2004;28(1):29–32.

91. Paquin SC, Gariépy G, Lepanto L, Bourdages R, Raymond G, Sahai AV. A first report of tumor seeding because of EUS-guided FNA of a pancreatic adenocarcinoma. Gastrointest Endosc 2005;61(4):610–611.

92. Shah JN, Fraker D, Guerry D, Feldman M, Kochman ML. Melanoma seeding of an EUS-guided fine needle track. Gastrointest Endosc 2004;59(7):923–924.

93. Doi S, Yasuda I, Iwashita T, et al. Needle tract implantation on the esophageal wall after EUS-guided FNA of metastatic mediastinal lymphadenopathy. Gastrointest Endosc 2008;67(6):988–990.

94. Hirooka Y, Goto H, Itoh A, et al. Case of intraductal papillary mucinous tumor in which endosonography-guided fine-needle aspiration biopsy caused dissemination. J Gastroenterol Hepatol 2003;18(11):1323–1324.

95. Micames C, Jowell PS, White R, et al. Lower frequency of peritoneal carcinomatosis in patients with pancreatic cancer diagnosed by EUS-guided FNA vs. percutaneous FNA. Gastrointest Endosc 2003;58(5):690–695.

96. Levy MJ, Gleeson FC, Campion MB, et al. Prospective cytological assessment of gastrointestinal luminal fluid acquired during EUS: a potential source of false-positive FNA and needle tract seeding. Am J Gastroenterol 2010;105(6): 1311–1318.

97. Mahajan RJ, Nowell W, Theerathorn P, Lipscomb A, Hart R, Adams L. Empyema after endoscopic ultrasound guided celiac plexus pain block (EUS-CPB) in chronic pancreatitis (CP): experience at an academic center [abstract]. Gastrointest Endosc 2002;55:AB 101.

98. Muscatiello N, Panella C, Pietrini L, Tonti P, Ierardi E. Complication of endoscopic ultrasound-guided celiac plexus neurolysis. Endoscopy 2006;38(8):858.

99. O'Toole TM, Schmulewitz N. Complication rates of EUS-guided celiac plexus blockade and neurolysis: results of a large case series. Endoscopy 2009;41(7):593–597.

100. George J, Grobmann CR, Jowell PS, Michael H, Pollack B, Gress F. Risk assessment of infectious complications in patients undergoing endoscopic ultrasound (EUS) guided celiac plexus block (CPB): a multicenter experience [abstract]. Gastrointest Endosc 2005;61:AB 279.

101. Ho KY, Brugge WR; EUS 2008 Working Group. EUS 2008 Working Group document: evaluation of EUS-guided pancreatic-cyst ablation. Gastrointest Endosc 2009; 69(2, Suppl): S22–S27.

102. Hecht JR, Bedford R, Abbruzzese JL, et al. A phase I/II trial of intratumoral endoscopic ultrasound injection of ONYX-015 with intravenous gemcitabine in unresectable pancreatic carcinoma. Clin Cancer Res 2003;9(2):555–561.

103. Deprez PH, Claessens A, Borbath I, Gigot JF, Maiter D. Successful endoscopic ultrasound-guided ethanol ablation of a sporadic insulinoma. Acta Gastroenterol Belg 2008;71(3): 333–337.

104. Jürgensen C, Schuppan D, Neser F, Ernstberger J, Junghans U, Stölzel U. EUS-guided alcohol ablation of an insulinoma. Gastrointest Endosc 2006;63(7):1059–1062.

105. Muscatiello N, Salcuni A, Macarini L, et al. Treatment of a pancreatic endocrine tumor by ethanol injection guided by endoscopic ultrasound. Endoscopy 2008;40(Suppl 2): E258–E259.

106. Eisen GM, Dominitz JA, Faigel DO, et al; American Society for Gastrointestinal Endoscopy. Guidelines for credentialing and granting privileges for endoscopic ultrasound. Gastrointest Endosc 2001;54(6):811–814.

107. Krakamp B, Janssen J, Menzel J, Schäfer A, Rünzi M; Arbeitsgemeinschaft fur endoskopischen Ultraschall in Nordrhein-Westfalen (AGEUS). Requirements and recommendations for performing endosonographies. [Article in German] Z Gastroenterol 2004;42(2):157–166.

108. Van Dam J, Brady PG, Freeman M, et al; American Society for Gastrointestinal Endoscopy. Guidelines for training in electronic ultrasound: guidelines for clinical application. From the ASGE. Gastrointest Endosc 1999;49(6):829–833.

109. Van Dam J, Rice TW, Catalano MF, Kirby T, Sivak MV Jr. High-grade malignant stricture is predictive of esophageal tumor stage. Risks of endosonographic evaluation. Cancer 1993;71(10):2910–2917.

110. Puli SR, Reddy JB, Bechtold ML, Antillon D, Ibdah JA, Antillon MR. Staging accuracy of esophageal cancer by endoscopic ultrasound: a meta-analysis and systematic review. World J Gastroenterol 2008;14(10):1479–1490.

111. Puli SR, Reddy JB, Bechtold ML, Antillon MR, Ibdah JA. Accuracy of endoscopic ultrasound in the diagnosis of distal and celiac axis lymph node metastasis in esophageal cancer: a meta-analysis and systematic review. Dig Dis Sci 2008;53(9):2405–2414.

112. Chang KJ, Soetikno RM, Bastas D, Tu C, Nguyen PT. Impact of endoscopic ultrasound combined with fine-needle aspiration biopsy in the management of esophageal cancer. Endoscopy 2003;35(11):962–966.

113. Lightdale CJ, Kulkarni KG. Role of endoscopic ultrasonography in the staging and follow-up of esophageal cancer. J Clin Oncol 2005;23(20):4483–4489.

114. Harewood GC, Kumar KS. Assessment of clinical impact of endoscopic ultrasound on esophageal cancer. J Gastroenterol Hepatol 2004;19(4):433–439.
115. Parmar KS, Zwischenberger JB, Reeves AL, Waxman I. Clinical impact of endoscopic ultrasound-guided fine needle aspiration of celiac axis lymph nodes (M1a disease) in esophageal cancer. Ann Thorac Surg 2002;73(3):916–920, discussion 920–921.
116. Kallimanis GE, Gupta PK, al-Kawas FH, et al. Endoscopic ultrasound for staging esophageal cancer, with or without dilation, is clinically important and safe. Gastrointest Endosc 1995;41(6):540–546.
117. Pfau PR, Ginsberg GG, Lew RJ, Faigel DO, Smith DB, Kochman ML. Esophageal dilation for endosonographic evaluation of malignant esophageal strictures is safe and effective. Am J Gastroenterol 2000;95(10):2813–2815.
118. Wallace MB, Hawes RH, Sahai AV, Van Velse A, Hoffman BJ. Dilation of malignant esophageal stenosis to allow EUS guided fine-needle aspiration: safety and effect on patient management. Gastrointest Endosc 2000;51(3):309–313.
119. Jacobson BC, Shami VM, Faigel DO, et al. Through-the-scope balloon dilation for endoscopic ultrasound staging of stenosing esophageal cancer. Dig Dis Sci 2007;52(3):817–822.
120. Chandrashekar MV, Richardson DL, Preston S, Karat D, Griffin SM. Perforation of a nonobstructing gastro-oesophageal carcinoma by oblique-viewing endoscopic ultrasound videoscope: a need for a safe technique. Endoscopy 2002;34(11):934.
121. Bowrey DJ, Clark GW, Roberts SA, et al. Endosonographic staging of 100 consecutive patients with esophageal carcinoma: introduction of the 8-mm esophagoprobe. Dis Esophagus 1999;12(4):258–263.
122. Mallery S, Van Dam J. Increased rate of complete EUS staging of patients with esophageal cancer using the nonoptical, wire-guided echoendoscope. Gastrointest Endosc 1999;50(1):53–57.
123. Hünerbein M, Ghadimi BM, Haensch W, Schlag PM. Transendoscopic ultrasound of esophageal and gastric cancer using miniaturized ultrasound catheter probes. Gastrointest Endosc 1998;48(4):371–375.
124. Menzel J, Hoepffner N, Nottberg H, Schulz C, Senninger N, Domschke W. Preoperative staging of esophageal carcinoma: miniprobe sonography versus conventional endoscopic ultrasound in a prospective histopathologically verified study. Endoscopy 1999;31(4):291–297.
125. Jenssen C, Dietrich CF. Endoscopic ultrasound-guided fine-needle aspiration biopsy and trucut biopsy in gastroenterology - An overview. Best Pract Res Clin Gastroenterol 2009;23(5):743–759.
126. Dietrich CF, Ignee A, Braden B, Barreiros AP, Ott M, Hocke M. Improved differentiation of pancreatic tumors using contrast-enhanced endoscopic ultrasound. Clin Gastroenterol Hepatol 2008;6(5):590–597, e1.
127. Dietrich CF, Jenssen C, Allescher HD, Hocke M, Barreiros AP, Ignee A. Differential diagnosis of pancreatic lesions using endoscopic ultrasound. [Article in German] Z Gastroenterol 2008;46(6):601–617.
128. Dietrich CF. Contrast-enhanced low mechanical index endoscopic ultrasound (CELMI-EUS). Endoscopy 2009;41(Suppl 2):E43–E44.
129. Dietrich CF, Hirche TO, Ott M, Ignee A. Real-time tissue elastography in the diagnosis of autoimmune pancreatitis. Endoscopy 2009;41(8):718–720.
130. Giovannini M, Thomas B, Erwan B, et al. Endoscopic ultrasound elastography for evaluation of lymph nodes and pancreatic masses: a multicenter study. World J Gastroenterol 2009;15(13):1587–1593.
131. Hirche TO, Ignee A, Barreiros AP, et al. Indications and limitations of endoscopic ultrasound elastography for evaluation of focal pancreatic lesions. Endoscopy 2008;40(11):910–917.
132. Hocke M, Schulze E, Gottschalk P, Topalidis T, Dietrich CF. Contrast-enhanced endoscopic ultrasound in discrimination between focal pancreatitis and pancreatic cancer. World J Gastroenterol 2006;12(2):246–250.
133. Hocke M, Ignee A, Topalidis T, Stallmach A, Dietrich CF. Contrast-enhanced endosonographic Doppler spectrum analysis is helpful in discrimination between focal chronic pancreatitis and pancreatic cancer. Pancreas 2007;35(3):286–288.
134. Hocke M, Schmidt C, Zimmer B, Topalidis T, Dietrich CF, Stallmach A. Contrast enhanced endosonography for improving differential diagnosis between chronic pancreatitis and pancreatic cancer. [Article in German] Dtsch Med Wochenschr 2008;133(38):1888–1892.
135. Iglesias-Garcia J, Larino-Noia J, Abdulkader I, Forteza J, Dominguez-Munoz JE. EUS elastography for the characterization of solid pancreatic masses. Gastrointest Endosc 2009;70(6):1101–1108.
136. Janssen J, Schlörer E, Greiner L. EUS elastography of the pancreas: feasibility and pattern description of the normal pancreas, chronic pancreatitis, and focal pancreatic lesions. Gastrointest Endosc 2007;65(7):971–978.
137. Kitano M, Sakamoto H, Matsui U, et al. A novel perfusion imaging technique of the pancreas: contrast-enhanced harmonic EUS (with video). Gastrointest Endosc 2008;67(1):141–150.
138. Sãftoiu A, Vilmann P, Gorunescu F, et al. Neural network analysis of dynamic sequences of EUS elastography used for the differential diagnosis of chronic pancreatitis and pancreatic cancer. Gastrointest Endosc 2008;68(6):1086–1094.
139. Sakamoto H, Kitano M, Suetomi Y, Maekawa K, Takeyama Y, Kudo M. Utility of contrast-enhanced endoscopic ultrasonography for diagnosis of small pancreatic carcinomas. Ultrasound Med Biol 2008;34(4):525–532.
140. Thomas T, Kaye PV, Ragunath K, Aithal G. Efficacy, safety, and predictive factors for a positive yield of EUS-guided Trucut biopsy: a large tertiary referral center experience. Am J Gastroenterol 2009;104(3):584–591.
141. Wittmann J, Kocjan G, Sgouros SN, Deheragoda M, Pereira SP. Endoscopic ultrasound-guided tissue sampling by combined fine needle aspiration and trucut needle biopsy: a prospective study. Cytopathology 2006;17(1):27–33.
142. Itoi T, Itokawa F, Sofuni A, et al. Puncture of solid pancreatic tumors guided by endoscopic ultrasonography: a pilot study series comparing Trucut and 19-gauge and 22-gauge aspiration needles. Endoscopy 2005;37(4):362–366.
143. Sakamoto H, Kitano M, Komaki T, et al. Prospective comparative study of the EUS guided 25-gauge FNA needle with the 19-gauge Trucut needle and 22-gauge FNA needle in patients with solid pancreatic masses. J Gastroenterol Hepatol 2009;24(3):384–390.
144. Schwartz DA, Harewood GC, Wiersema MJ. EUS for rectal disease. Gastrointest Endosc 2002;56(1):100–109.
145. Gress F, Schmitt C, Sherman S, Ciaccia D, Ikenberry S, Lehman G. Endoscopic ultrasound-guided celiac plexus block for managing abdominal pain associated with chronic pancreatitis: a prospective single center experience. Am J Gastroenterol 2001;96(2):409–416.

146. Sing J Jr, Erickson R, Fader R. An in vitro analysis of microbial transmission during EUS-guided FNA and the utility of sterilization agents. Gastrointest Endosc 2006;64(5): 774–779.

147. Jacobson BC, Chak A, Hoffman B, et al; ASGE/ACG Taskforce on Quality in Endoscopy. Quality indicators for endoscopic ultrasonography. Am J Gastroenterol 2006;101(4): 898–901.

148. Eloubeidi MA, Chen VK, Eltoum IA, et al. Endoscopic ultrasound-guided fine needle aspiration biopsy of patients with suspected pancreatic cancer: diagnostic accuracy and acute and 30-day complications. Am J Gastroenterol 2003;98(12):2663–2668.

149. Eloubeidi MA, Tamhane A. Prospective assessment of diagnostic utility and complications of endoscopic ultrasound-guided fine needle aspiration. Results from a newly developed academic endoscopic ultrasound program. Dig Dis 2008;26(4):356–363.

150. Mahnke D, Chen YK, Antillon MR, Brown WR, Mattison R, Shah RJ. A prospective study of complications of endoscopic retrograde cholangiopancreatography and endoscopic ultrasound in an ambulatory endoscopy center. Clin Gastroenterol Hepatol 2006;4(7):924–930.

151. Veitch AM, Baglin TP, Gershlick AH, Harnden SM, Tighe R, Cairns S; British Society of Gastroenterology; British Committee for Standards in Haematology; British Cardiovascular Intervention Society. Guidelines for the management of anticoagulant and antiplatelet therapy in patients undergoing endoscopic procedures. Gut 2008;57(9):1322–1329.

152. Nürnberg D, Jung A, Löschner C. Blutung in eine zystische Pankreasläsion während der EUS-gezielten Punktion. Ultraschall Med 2004;25:S81.

153. Bartheld MB, Rabe KF, Annema JT. Transaortic EUS-guided FNA in the diagnosis of lung tumors and lymph nodes. Gastrointest Endos. 2009;69:345–349..

154. Wallace MB, Woodward TA, Raimondo M, Al-Haddad M, Odell JA. Transaortic fine-needle aspiration of centrally located lung cancer under endoscopic ultrasound guidance: the final frontier. Ann Thorac Surg 2007;84: 1019–1021.

155. Fritscher-Ravens A, Ganbari A, Mosse CA, Swain P, Koehler P, Patel K. Transesophageal endoscopic ultrasound-guided access to the heart. Endoscopy 2007;39:385–389..

156. Jenssen C, Siebert C, Bartho S. [Leiomyosarcoma of the inferior vena cava. Diagnosis using endoscopic ultrasound-guided fine-needle aspiration biopsy.] Dtsch Med Wochenschr 2008;133:769–772.

III Gastrointestinal Tract

13 Esophagus, Stomach, Duodenum

C.F. Dietrich, S. Faiss

Endoscopic ultrasound (EUS) is an extremely valuable tool for the local staging of various types of gastrointestinal tumor. Initial enthusiastic reports on the technique's diagnostic value were later qualified, but EUS-guided fine-needle aspiration (EUS-FNA) has extended the method's range of applications.

Wall Layers in the Esophagus, Stomach, and Duodenum

The accuracy of EUS measurement of the thickness of the gastrointestinal wall depends on physiological peristalsis; a contracted segment can resemble a thickened intestinal wall. Published studies provide some reference values for the "normal" thickness of the gastrointestinal wall, but these tend to have a wide range due to the use of different examination techniques (e.g., more or less application pressure) and technical parameters (such as the frequency used and the accuracy of measurement), and in addition there is considerable interobserver variability. As in conventional transabdominal ultrasound of the bowel, EUS can delineate five layers in the wall of the esophagus, stomach, and duodenum (**Table 13.1**). In the esophagus, the muscularis propria can be divided into a hypoechoic inner layer (ring) and a hypoechoic outer layer (longitudinal). A hyperechoic connective-tissue layer can be detected between these two layers of muscle (**Fig. 13.1, Table 13.1**). Further differentiation of the mucosa is possible in some cases, but is of less clinical significance.

Although acoustic changes in the impedance cannot in principle be equated with the histological structure of the intestinal wall, the endosonographic image of the layers can provide orientation. Edema, cellular infiltration, cicatricial changes, and neoplastic masses can produce an endosonographic image of a thickened intestinal wall. Hypoechoic parts of the intestinal wall predominate when there are active inflammatory processes. However, echogenicity alone is not a sufficient marker of inflammatory activity. In addition, echogenicity may be biased by the frequency of the transducer used. Mucosal edema with

Table 13.1 Endoscopic ultrasound (EUS) layers in the normal esophageal, gastric, and duodenal wall

EUS morphology of the intestinal wall	Interpretation
Hyperechoic (echo-rich) inner layer	Physical entrance echo (transition between the lumen and the mucosa)
Hypoechoic (echo-poor) inner layer	Mucosa
Hyperechoic middle layer	Submucosa
Hypoechoic outer layer	Muscularis propria
Hyperechoic outer layer	Physical emission echo (serosa, adventitia/surroundings)

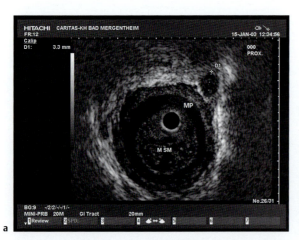

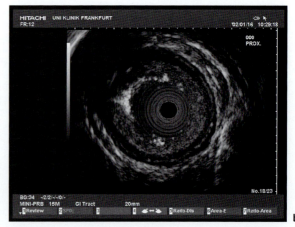

Fig. 13.1a, b The layers of the esophageal wall.
a Normal esophageal layers, showing the mucosa (M) and submucosa (SM; not clearly defined here), as well as the muscularis propria (MP). A small normal periesophageal lymph node is indicated between the markers.

b The inner (ring) muscular layer and outer (longitudinal) muscular layer are circumscribed.

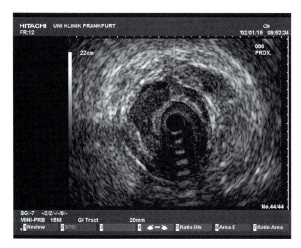

Fig. 13.2 Disrupted layers of the esophageal wall in a patient with a mucosal tear. This type of mucosal tear, as well as a conventional biopsy, can lead to intramural bleeding or edema, with considerable changes in the layers that prevent adequate endosonographic assessment.

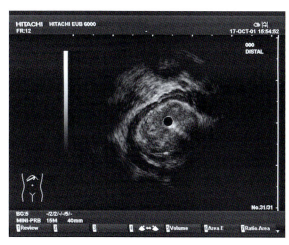

Fig. 13.3 Disrupted layers of the esophageal wall after radiotherapy. Due to a variety of changes, and particularly as a result of fusion of the anatomical layers, re-staging with EUS after radiotherapy is not reliably possible.

normal or slightly reduced peristalsis can lead to accentuated intestinal layers. By contrast, the typical layers of the intestinal wall can be disrupted by invasive processes (such as neoplasms and lymphomas) (**Figs. 13.2** and **13.3**).

Esophagus

■ Orientation

Thorough anatomical knowledge of the abdominal and thoracic region, familiarity with different imaging qualities (e.g., radial or linear EUS and the effects of the angle of the acoustic level relative to the tip of the EUS probe), a feeling for the position of the probe tip, and a strong three-dimensional spatial sense are necessary for correct anatomical classification of findings in the intestinal wall. In addition to having good endoscopic skills and familiarity with ultrasound, examiners have to go through an extensive learning process to be able to grasp the different and variable acoustic levels in EUS. Basically, the gastrointestinal tract and the adjacent organs can be examined at the horizontal, sagittal, frontal, and subsequently at mixed and variable levels. With the radial EUS scanners currently available, the acoustic level that is mapped is pivotable in a user-defined way. This means that different views from cranial and caudal can be obtained without moving the probe tip.

Older EUS devices (e.g., the Olympus UM-3 generation) only had two settings. However, these systems already had remarkable spatial resolution. In addition to anatomical knowledge and a basic understanding of the special imaging view provided by EUS devices, observing specific conventions during the course of an examination is useful for maintaining continuous anatomical orientation. In the ideal case, the EUS device can be passed through the gastrointestinal tract with only ultrasound and manual guidance, without endoscopic viewing. Rotating the stem of the EUS device produces comparable rotation of the EUS image, so that optional imaging positions can be achieved. In EUS, the esophagus is usually examined with the spine at the 6-o'clock position and the patient's left side at the 3-o'clock position. This approach facilitates comparison with other imaging modalities (such as computed tomography). However, other different approaches are also used.

■ Optimizing the Examination

Filling the organ with water and/or using a water-filled balloon at the tip of the EUS device can help provide a better view. Starting in the distal part of the esophagus, water filling can be carried out to improve the imaging quality. Filling the balloon slightly after inserting the scope can help prevent mucosal damage by smoothing the potentially traumatic tip of the device. Water filling of the lumen is contraindicated in the proximal part of the esophagus, due to the risk of aspiration.

■ Indications

EUS is indicated for staging malignant tumors in patients with no distant metastases, and for clarifying unclear findings. Endosonographic assessment of the esophageal wall is the method of choice and provides unrivaled resolution (**Fig. 13.1**).

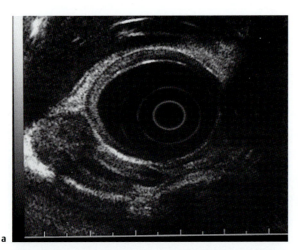 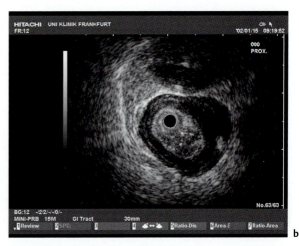

Fig. 13.4a, b A leiomyoma is visible in the outer muscular layer on radial EUS (**a**) and with the miniprobe (**b**).

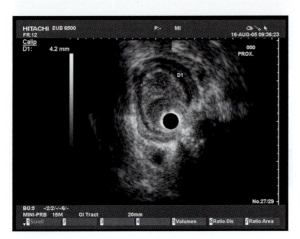

Fig. 13.5 Lipoma. EUS demonstration of a lipoma, achieved by assigning the submucosa as the underlying anatomic layer. The echogenicity depends on the size of the fat droplets and the EUS frequency used. Lipomas may be hypoechoic but are more often hyperechoic or mixed.

■ Benign Diseases

The value of EUS in histologically confirmed benign diseases of the esophagus is unclear. There have been no large prospective studies on the clinical impact of EUS in benign esophageal diseases. Depending on the presence of Barrett's epithelium, differences in the thickness of the esophageal wall can be measured endosonographically, but as these lie in a range of less than 1 mm they have not become clinically relevant. However, EUS is helpful for clarifying submucosal lesions and assessing impressions on the esophageal wall. EUS can distinguish between mesenchymal tumors, which are often encountered—e.g., leiomyoma (**Fig. 13.4**), fibroma, lipoma (**Fig. 13.5**), hemangioma, myxoma—and rare epithelial tumors (such as cysts and papillomas). The symptoms of the various lesions are not characteristic; the principal symptom is dysphagia. Before endoscopic resection of such tumors, vessels need to be excluded as the cause of mucosal or submucosal swelling to avoid fatal complications.

The success of treatment for esophageal varices is assessed endoscopically. Conventional EUS can provide adequate assessment of intraluminal and extramural varices that are not endoscopically visible, but the management implications of this are not clear (**Fig. 13.6**).

■ Malignant Tumors of the Esophagus

Malignant intratumoral and extramural tumor growth can normally be evaluated very well with EUS. However, tumor-related esophageal stenoses that prevent passage of the endoscope are problematic, since in these cases the transverse acoustic level leads to overestimation of the extent of the tumor.

Some studies have shown that small T1 esophageal carcinomas cannot be definitely assigned to the mucosa or submucosa using conventional EUS, which is in contrast to our own experience. However, the distinction is essential for assessing whether endoscopic mucosal resection of these small tumors is possible. Whether a T1 carcinoma has only infiltrated the mucosa or has already penetrated into the submucosa has substantial prognostic relevance. In patients with submucosal tumor invasion, and depending on the depth of submucosal infiltration, the rate of lymph-node metastases is much higher in comparison with those who only have mucosal invasion. T1 tumors with submucosal invasion are therefore not suitable for primary endoscopic therapy. Clear differentiation between T2 and T3 esophageal carcinomas is also challenging in relation to the prognosis and surgical strategy. Peritumoral edema or inflammatory infiltration, or both, can give tumors a hypoechoic margin that is difficult to distinguish

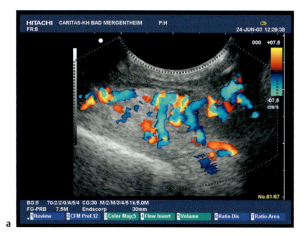
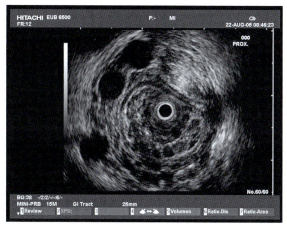
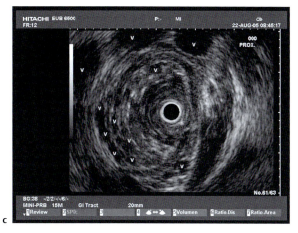
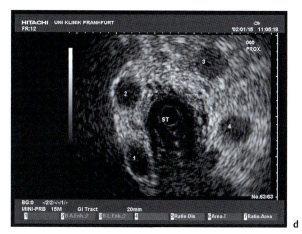

Fig. 13.6a–d Esophageal varices. Conventional EUS with color Doppler is helpful for identifying submucosal or extramural esophageal varices (**a**). Esophageal varices can also be detected with miniprobe EUS, demonstrating extramural vessels (**a, b**), intramucosal varices (**c**), and thrombosed vessels after therapy (**d**). ST, stomach.

from the tumor itself. Elastography may be helpful for differentiating between soft inflammatory tissue and harder neoplastic infiltration. The malignant status of circumscribed esophageal lesions can only be assessed with histological examination of representative biopsies (as the gold standard). Attempts have been made to develop EUS criteria for malignancy, but the initial cancer diagnosis in the gastrointestinal tract is always established using a histological examination of endoscopic biopsies.

Operability is the deciding criterion in the assessment of malignant esophageal tumors. The reported accuracy of EUS for assessing the extent of tumors (T staging) is 80–90%, slightly higher than that in the stomach. EUS examination of the esophagus is an established diagnostic method that still provides the only way of distinguishing between the different layers of the esophageal wall.

Several publications have shown that EUS is superior not only to computed tomography (CT) but also to more recent imaging techniques such as positron-emission tomography (PET) (**Tables 13.2, 13.3** and **13.4**). CT of the chest and magnetic resonance imaging have a sensitivity of only around 40–60% for mediastinal lymph-node involvement; however, studies do vary. For mediastinal lymph-node involvement, thoracoscopic procedures for tissue biopsy carry a risk of complications in up to 35% of cases. PET has been shown to be beneficial for detecting metastatic disease; however, the detection rate for locoregional metastases is limited. A meta-analysis was recently conducted to examine the role of EUS in the staging of esophageal cancer for locoregional spread.[1]

■ T Stage

The sensitivity of EUS for T staging in esophageal carcinoma is 85–95%. However, there is some variation in the accuracy depending on the specific T stage.

In the meta-analysis mentioned above, the pooled sensitivity and specificity of EUS for diagnosing T1 cancer were 81.6% (95% CI, 77.8 to 84.9) and 99.4% (95% CI, 99.0 to 99.7), respectively. For T2 staging, EUS had a pooled

Table 13.2 Accuracy of T staging with endoscopic ultrasound (EUS) in comparison with computed tomography (CT) in patients with esophageal carcinomas or carcinomas of the gastroesophageal junction

First author	Patients	Method	T total (%)	T1 (%)	T2 (%)	T3 (%)	T4 (%)	Ref.
Botet	50	EUS	92	n.a.	n.a.	n.a.	n.a.	[2]
	42	CT	42	n.a.	n.a.	n.a.	n.a.	[2]
Ziegler	37	EUS	89	n.a.	n.a.	n.a.	n.a.	[3]
		CT	51	n.a.	n.a.	n.a.	n.a.	[3]
Kienle	117	EUS	69	63	52	77	50	[4]
	36	CT	33	100	26	36	–	[4]
Weaver	52	EUS	83	88[a]		85	40	[5]
		CT	77	70[a]		80	50	[5]

[a] = T1 and T2 together. n.a., not available

Table 13.3 Accuracy of N staging with endoscopic ultrasound (EUS) in comparison with computed tomography (CT) in patients with esophageal carcinomas or carcinomas of the gastroesophageal junction

First author	Patients	Method	N total (%)	N0 (%)	N1 (%)	N2 (%)	Ref.
Botet	50	EUS	88	n.a.	n.a.	n.a.	[2]
	42	CT	74	n.a.	n.a.	n.a.	[2]
Ziegler	37	EUS	69	n.a.	n.a.	n.a.	[3]
		CT	51	n.a.	n.a.	n.a.	[3]
Kienle	117	EUS	79	71	85[a]		[4]
	36	CT	67	47	84[a]		[4]
Weaver	52	EUS	81	68	83[a]		[5]
		CT	81	84	74[a]		[5]

[a] = N1 and N2 together. n.a., not available

Table 13.4 Comparison of endoscopic ultrasound (EUS) with other imaging procedures—computed tomography (CT) and positron-emission tomography (PET)—for local staging of esophageal cancer

Author	Patients	Method	T stage			N stage			Ref.
			Sensitivity	Specificity	Accuracy	Sensitivity	Specificity	Accuracy	
Räsänen	42	EUS	n.a.	n.a.	63%	89%	54%	75%	[6]
		CT	n.a.	n.a.	n.a.	47%	92%	66%	[6]
		PET	n.a.	n.a.	n.a.	37%	100%	63%	[6]
Flamen	43	EUS	42%	94%	71%	63%	88%	85%	[7]
		CT	41%	83%	64%	22%	96%	78%	[7]
		PET	74%	90%	82%	39%	97%	83%	[7]
Berger	Review	EUS	58–91%	82–99%	n.a.	77–89%	75–85%	n.a.	[8]
		CT	25%	94%	n.a.	11–77%	71–95%	n.a.	[8]
		PET	n.a.	n.a.	n.a.	28–39%	95–100%	n.a.	[8]

n.a., not available

Table 13.5 Accuracy of endoscopic ultrasound, with 95% confidence intervals, in diagnosing T-stage esophageal cancer

	Pooled sensitivity (%)	Pooled specificity (%)	Pooled LR+	Pooled LR–	Pooled DOR
T1	81.6 (77.8 to 84.9)	99.4 (99.0 to 99.7)	44.4 (15.5 to 127.4)	0.2 (0.2 to 0.4)	221.5 (118.5 to 413.9)
T2	81.4 (77.5 to 84.8)	96.3 (95.4 to 97.1)	16.6 (9.3 to 29.7)	0.2 (0.2 to 0.3)	90.7 (48.3 to 170.5)
T3	91.4 (89.5 to 93.0)	94.4 (93.1 to 95.5)	12.5 (7.7 to 20.3)	0.1 (0.1 to 0.2)	145.2 (90.3 to 233.4)
T4	92.4 (89.2 to 95.0)	97.4 (96.6 to 98.0)	25.4 (13.7 to 47.0)	0.1 (0.1 to 0.2)	250.0 (145.2 to 430.5)

LR+, positive likelihood ratio; LR–, negative likelihood ratio; DOR, diagnostic odds ratio.

sensitivity and specificity of 81.4% (95% CI, 77.5 to 84.8) and 96.3% (95% CI, 95.4 to 97.1), respectively. For T3 staging, EUS had a pooled sensitivity and specificity of 91.4% (95% CI, 89.5 to 93.0) and 94.4% (95% CI, 93.1 to 95.5), respectively. For diagnosing T4 cancer, EUS had a pooled sensitivity of 92.4% (95% CI, 89.2 to 95.0) and specificity of 97.4% (95% CI, 96.6 to 98.0). **Table 13.5** shows the pooled accuracy estimates of EUS for T staging in esophageal cancer.[1]

In addition, as EUS is not capable of differentiating between tumor infiltration and concomitant inflammatory reactions, overstaging on EUS continues to be a problem (**Figs. 13.7, 13.8, 13.9, 13.10, 13.11** and **13.12**).

■ N Stage

Studies have shown that EUS has a sensitivity of 70–80% for N staging in esophageal carcinoma.

EUS-guided fine-needle aspiration (FNA) can improve the results in the staging of esophageal carcinomas, as has been shown by several reports comparing the method with CT and with conventional EUS without FNA (**Tables 13.6** and **13.7**).

With FNA, the sensitivity of EUS for diagnosing N-stage cancer improved from 84.7% (95% CI, 82.9 to 86.4) to 96.7% (95% CI, 92.4 to 98.9). The specificity of EUS improved from

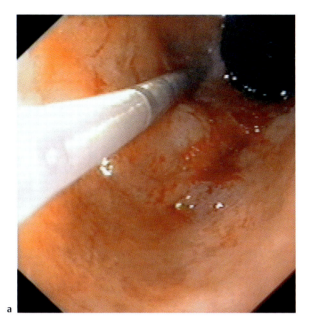

a

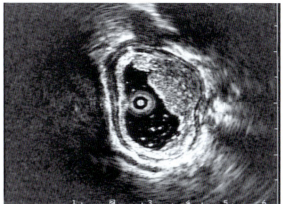

b

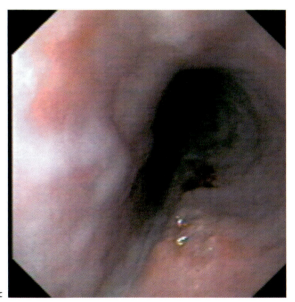

c

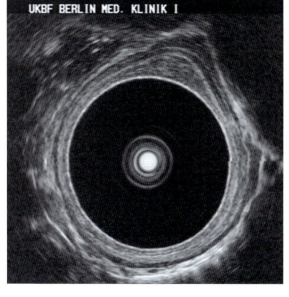

d

e

Fig. 13.7a–i T1 esophageal cancer, with mucosal and submucosal invasion.

a–d Ideally, the EUS miniprobe should be used under endoscopic vision without pressure. The EUS miniprobe provides unrivaled optical resolution.

e–g Other forms of T1 m (**e**) and T1sm tumors (**f, g**) are also shown. The morphology depends on the inflammatory reaction.

Fig. 13.7f–i ▷

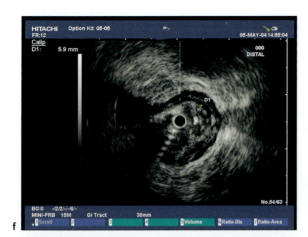

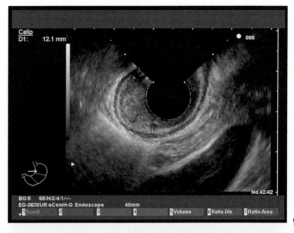

f

g

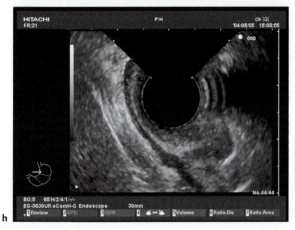

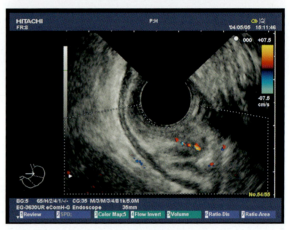

h

i

Fig. 13.7a–i (continued) **h, i** Hyperplastic polyps may not be distinguishable macroscopically (**h**); color Doppler imaging, demonstrating a normal vessel architecture, is helpful here (**i**).

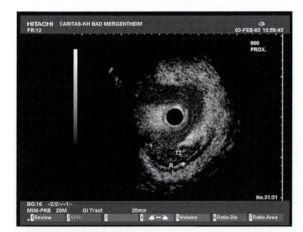

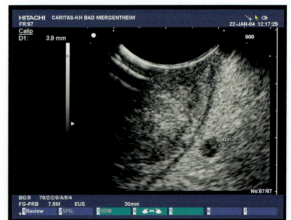

Fig. 13.8 EUS miniprobe findings in T2 esophageal cancer, with invasion of the submucosal (SM) and muscular layers (T2). In this case, the different depth of invasion is very well demonstrated. R, internal (ring) muscular layer; L, external (longitudinal) muscular layer. Due to the limited penetration with EUS miniprobes, adequate staging of periesophageal lymph nodes is not possible.

Fig. 13.9 T2N1 esophageal carcinoma. Due to the limited acoustic penetration of EUS miniprobes, adequate staging of periesophageal lymph nodes is not possible. Conventional EUS is therefore recommended for periesophageal lymph-node staging (as in the 4-mm periesophageal lymph node shown here). Conventional EUS also allows EUS-guided fine-needle aspiration of lymph nodes, particularly for assessment of celiac lymph-node metastases.

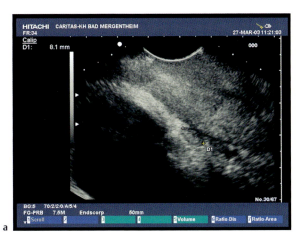
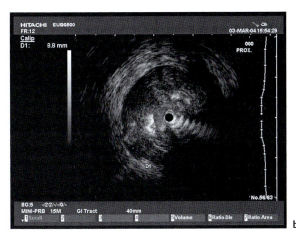

Fig. 13.10a, b T3 esophageal carcinoma. Tumor invasion into the periesophageal connective tissue can be detected reliably with conventional EUS (**a**, between the marks), as well as with the EUS miniprobe (**b**, between the marks). Inflammatory reactions and atypical vessels affecting the T3 stage need to be taken into consideration.

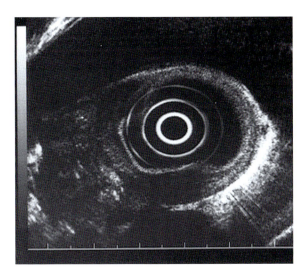

Fig. 13.11 T4 esophageal carcinoma. The T4 stage of esophageal carcinoma is defined as infiltration of the mediastinal vessels (such as the aorta, in this case) or infiltration of the heart.

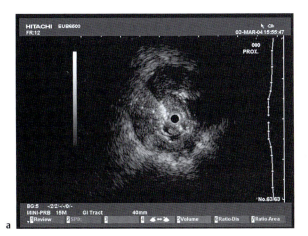
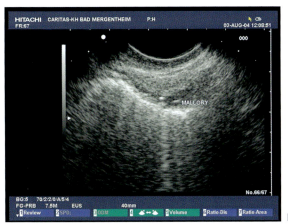

Fig. 13.12a, b EUS staging after dilation.
a Due to intramural bleeding and edema, EUS staging after dilation of malignant esophageal stenoses is not reliable, leading to an overstaging, as seen in this case in a patient with a T2 carcinoma.

b In a patient with a Mallory–Weiss lesion, air echoes are seen deep in the esophageal wall, showing that EUS staging is only of value in patients with histologically confirmed malignancies.

84.6% (95% CI, 83.2 to 85.9) to 95.5% (95% CI, 91.0 to 98.2) with FNA. The accuracy estimates for EUS alone and EUS with FNA are shown in **Table 13.8**.

■ Effect of Technology

EUS studies were grouped into three periods in order to standardize changes in EUS technology and changes in EUS criteria for tumor staging: 1986–1994, 1995–1999, and 2000–2006.[1] The pooled estimates of studies during these periods are shown in **Table 13.9**.

Table 13.6 Endoscopic ultrasound-guided fine-needle aspiration (EUS-FNA) of lymph nodes in the staging of esophageal carcinomas

Author	Patients	N stage			Ref.
		Sensitivity	Specificity	Accuracy	
Vasquez-Sequeiros	31	93%	100%	93%	9
Eloubeidi	51	98%	100%	98%	10
Parmar	20	100%	100%	100%	11
Murata	Review	81–97%	83–100%	83–97%	12
Vasquez-Sequeiros	124	83%	93%	87%	9

EUS as an imaging modality has high sensitivity and specificity for diagnosing N-stage esophageal cancer. This meta-analysis shows that FNA substantially improves the sensitivity (85–97%) and specificity (85–96%) of EUS for evaluating N-stage esophageal cancer. EUS with FNA should therefore be the diagnostic test of choice.

During the last 20 years, the specificity of EUS for diagnosing T-stage cancer has remained high. The method's sensitivity for T staging has also improved, particularly for early disease (T1), during the last 20 years, possibly due to improvements in imaging technology or training. For nodal staging, all the studies in which FNA was performed were from the most recent periods. The sensitivity and specificity of EUS alone for diagnosing N-stage cancer has not improved during the last 20 years. The meta-analysis shows that the sensitivity and specificity of EUS markedly improved with FNA.[1]

In summary, EUS has excellent sensitivity and specificity for accurately diagnosing T-stage esophageal cancer. EUS performs better with advanced (T4) than early (T1) disease. FNA substantially improves the sensitivity and specificity of EUS in evaluating N-stage esophageal cancers. EUS should be the test of choice for TN staging of esophageal cancer.

The accuracy of re-staging with EUS after chemoradiotherapy for esophageal and gastric tumors is currently a matter of controversy. After chemoradiotherapy, inflammatory and cicatricial processes cannot be distinguished

Table 13.7 Diagnostic value of endoscopic ultrasound-guided fine-needle aspiration (EUS-FNA) in N staging of esophageal carcinomas in comparison with other imaging procedures (EUS and CT)

Author	Patients	Method	Sensitivity	Specificity	Accuracy	Ref.
Parmar	20/40	EUS-FNA	100%	100%	100%	11
	40	EUS	100%	50%	90%	11
	40	CT	30%	67%	35%	11
Murata	Review	EUS-FNA	81–97%	83–100%	83–97%	12
		EUS	49–99%	33–99%	71–96%	12
Vasquez-Sequeiros	124	EUS-FNA	83%	93%	87%	9
		EUS	71%	79%	74%	9
		CT	29%	89%	51%	9
Chang	18	EUS-FNA	n.a.	n.a.	89%	13
		EUS	n.a.	n.a.	83%	13
		CT	n.a.	n.a.	56%	13

Table 13.8 Pooled estimate of accuracy of endoscopic ultrasound (EUS) alone and endoscopic ultrasound-guided fine-needle aspiration (EUS-FNA) in nodal staging of esophageal cancer, with 95% confidence intervals

	EUS	EUS-FNA
Studies	44	4
Pooled sensitivity (%)	84.7 (82.9 to 86.4)	96.7 (92.4 to 98.9)
Pooled specificity (%)	84.6 (83.2 to 85.9)	95.5 (91.0 to 98.2)
Positive likelihood ratio	3.3 (2.6 to 4.3)	7.3 (0.9 to 54.3)
Negative likelihood ratio	0.24 (0.9 to 0.3)	0.05 (0.01 to 0.64)
Diagnostic odds ratio	19.1 (12.7 to 28.5)	164.5 (4.5 to 6027.7)

Table 13.9 Accuracy of endoscopic ultrasound during the last 20 years in staging esophageal cancer, with 95% confidence intervals[1]

	Years	No. of studies	Pooled sensitivity (%)	Pooled specificity (%)	Pooled LR+	Pooled LR−	Pooled DOR
T1	1986–1944	17	80.4 (75.2 to 84.8)	99.2 (98.4 to 99.7)	41.5 (6.1 to 283.3)	0.25 (0.14 to 0.43)	181.9 (60.7 to 545.7)
	1995–1999	11	83.9 (76.0 to 90.0)	99.4 (98.4 to 99.8)	36.4 (18.5 to 71.6)	0.21 (0.09 to 0.47)	299.9 (107.8 to 834.1)
	2000–2006	8	82.4 (72.6 to 89.8)	100.0 (99.1 to 100.0)	59.5 (22.0 to 161.1)	0.27 (0.16 to 0.47)	261.2 (81.4 to 838.0)
T2	1986–1994	17	85.2 (80.2 to 89.4)	96.8 (95.5 to 97.8)	18.6 (5.9 to 58.6)	0.19 (0.12 to 0.30)	123.9 (47.7 to 322.0)
	1995–1999	13	86.8 (79.7 to 92.1)	97.4 (95.8 to 98.5)	16.9 (9.1 to 31.1)	0.20 (0.11 to 0.38)	139.5 (56.6 to 343.8)
	2000–2006	8	62.9 (52.0 to 72.9)	93.4 (90.4 to 95.6)	8.3 (4.3 to 15.9)	0.47 (0.34 to 0.64)	24.7 (9.1 to 67.4)
T3	1986–1994	18	90.8 (88.1 to 93.0)	94.6 (92.6 to 96.2)	13.9 (5.2 to 36.9)	0.12 (0.07 to 0.19)	157.7 (70.9 to 351.1)
	1995–1999	14	93.7 (90.0 to 96.3)	96.4 (94.5 to 97.7)	12.6 (7.6 to 20.9)	0.11 (0.08 to 0.17)	159.4 (77.9 to 326.2)
	2000–2006	8	89.9 (84.5 to 93.9)	90.0 (86.1 to 93.2)	7.0 (4.6 to 10.8)	0.11 (0.04 to 0.32)	100.9 (33.5 to 303.9)
T4	1986–1994	18	92.1 (87.9 to 95.2)	96.9 (95.6 to 97.9)	24.7 (8.4 to 72.7)	0.09 (0.04 to 0.23)	278.8 (97.2 to 799.9)
	1995–1999	14	89.2 (79.8 to 95.2)	98.0 (96.7 to 98.96)	22.2 (13.2 to 37.3)	0.23 (0.15 to 0.36)	227.1 (89.7 to 575.0)
	2000–2006	8	100.0 (91.8 to 100.0)	97.5 (95.4 to 98.8)	20.2 (8.8 to 46.3)	0.11 (0.04 to 0.29)	272.6 (73.4 to 1013.2)
N	1986–1994	17	88.0 (85.4 to 90.2)	85.2 (83.4 to 86.9)	3.6 (2.4 to 5.4)	0.2 (0.1 to 0.3)	27.6 (14.6 to 52.4)
	1995–1999	17	82.6 (78.0 to 85.9)	84.4 (81.6 to 86.9)	3.0 (2.1 to 4.5)	0.3 (0.2 to 0.4)	14.8 (7.5 to 29.3)
	2000–2005	10	81.6 (77.8 to 85.1)	82.4 (78.2 to 86.1)	3.4 (2.2 to 5.3)	0.3 (0.2 to 0.4)	14.9 (6.7 to 33.1)

LR+, positive likelihood ratio; LR−, negative likelihood ratio; DOR, diagnostic odds ratio.

from malignant infiltration, and routine EUS after radiotherapy is not at present accepted. However, local tumor recurrence in the anastomotic region after adequate previous surgery is an exception to this. As in primary tumor staging, local tumor recurrences also have to be confirmed histologically. Due to the underlying inflammatory and cicatricial changes, EUS of suspected local tumor recurrences has a relatively high level of sensitivity, but with low specificity.

Periesophageal structures can usually be assessed and even small lymph nodes can be detected. However, it has been shown that the morphology of lymph nodes that can be detected with EUS (their size, shape, acoustic pattern, and margins) is not sensitive enough to identify definite malignant infiltration. This is because there may be only microscopic malignant infiltration of the lymph nodes; on the other hand, peritumoral lymph nodes with inflammatory changes may meet the criteria for malignancy. These criteria are the number (more than three) and size (> 5 mm) of the lymph nodes; a round shape with a hypoechoic acoustic pattern; and precise delimitation from the surroundings.

EUS of the esophagus is useful for assessing the prognosis (for T staging, N staging, and providing the patient with information), for decision-making on whether curative or palliative surgery should be performed, and for assessing the effectiveness of preoperative (neoadjuvant) treatment (e.g., chemoradiotherapy).

The relationship between an esophageal cancer and the tracheal bifurcation can be clearly demonstrated. This relationship is important and has treatment implications. Depending on whether there are any distal metastases, preoperative neoadjuvant chemoradiotherapy is recommended for T3 lesions. In patients with distal metastases and tumor-related dysphagia, palliative stenting of the esophagus is beneficial. In severe stenoses of this type, which cannot be passed with conventional EUS devices, the thickness of the esophageal wall is usually more than 2 cm and in nearly all cases the tumors are in stages T3 or T4. It has been shown that traversing these stenoses with blind probes is of no practical value. Stenosis is strongly associated with advanced stages.[14]

Stomach

■ Orientation

In terms of its position, shape, and size, the stomach has a variable and rather longitudinal (rather than horizontal) alignment and lies on the left side and to the left of the spine. After it enters the stomach, the EUS device is rotated nearly 90° to the right. The lesser curvature of the stomach is in the 12-o'clock position and the anterior wall is in the 3-o'clock position.

As in passage from the cardia to the fundus, the position of the EUS device is changed completely when the angular notch is passed and the prepyloric antrum is entered (**Fig. 13.13**). An additional change is made in the position of the device after it has passed through the duodenal bulb, with the instrument being rotated to the left into its original position, as in the esophagus. Orientation in the deep duodenum, correlating with the body's axis, thus

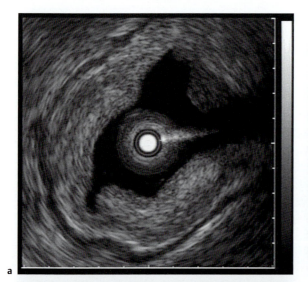

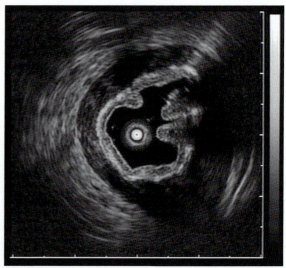

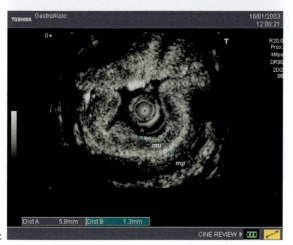

Fig. 13.13a–c The different layers of the gastric wall. The configuration of the gastric wall layers varies in different locations and with different EUS devices.
a Wall layers in the body of the stomach.
b, c Wall layers in the antrum, with an accentuated muscular layer (**b**) and using a different technique (**c**); ee, physical entrance echo; mu, mucosa; sm, submucosa; mp, muscularis propria.

resembles that in the esophagus, with the spine (the dorsal reference structure) in the 6-o'clock position, the kidney (the right lateral reference structure) in the 9-o'clock position, and the pancreatic head in the 3-o'clock position.

■ Optimizing the Examination

A 0.9% isotonic saline solution (300–500 mL) can be introduced into the stomach. However, some endoscopists prefer to work without filling the stomach with liquid. Simethicone (activated dimethicone) can be administered a few minutes before the examination to prevent intragastric foam. It is a matter of controversy whether the patient's position should be changed for assessment of the gastric fundus. For better assessment of the periduodenal structures (especially the pancreatic head), it is helpful to inflate the balloon at the echoendoscope's tip with water when it is in the duodenal bulb.

In most cases, additional external water-filling is not possible in the duodenum, but the internal duodenal fluid is sufficient. Because of their anatomical location and their air content, some areas of the duodenum and stomach (such as the cardia, fundus, parts of the anterior wall and antrum, the distal part of the duodenal bulb) are more difficult to evaluate. Repeated water-filling and suction of air bubbles, as well as changing the patient's position, is necessary for adequate examinations. For evaluation of the cardia, fundus, and lesser curvature of the stomach, it is sometimes necessary to position the patient with the head downward or on the right side, while avoiding aspiration.

Because of the variability of the stomach and duodenum, orthograde angling of the acoustic level is necessary in order to avoid misinterpreting artificial mural swelling in the duodenal or gastric wall. The effects of compression by the EUS device can lead to limited visualization of discrete mucosal lesions and should therefore also be avoided. For adequate evaluation of structures in the intestinal wall, it is essential to keep a fair distance from the target. A high-

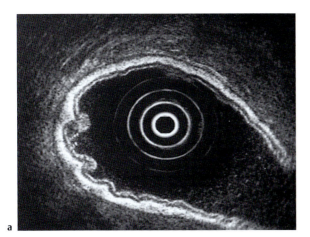

a

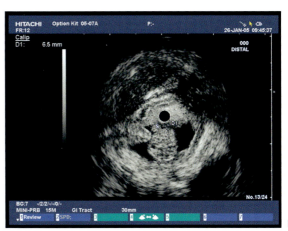

b

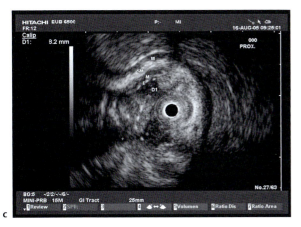

c

Fig. 13.14a–c Gastric polyp. EUS is of marginal value for evaluating small gastric polyps.
a With EUS, gastric polyps can be reliably assigned to the superficial mucosa layer, as shown in this case with an older Olympus UM-3 device.
b, c In contrast, a typical adenoma may be seen (**b**) or food (chyme) in **c**. E, superficial echo of the mucosa; M, mucosa; SM, submucosa; S, connection between the polyp and the mucosa.

frequency EUS miniprobe inserted through the endoscope's working channel and used without relevant compression is helpful for assessing smaller lesions.

■ Indications

The indications and examination criteria for evaluating the cardia and stomach are in principle similar to those for esophageal examinations. Due to the variable position of the stomach and consequently of the EUS device, the sensitivity and specificity of the method for diagnosing and staging gastric lesions are lower than in the esophagus.

■ Benign Gastric Lesions

Gastric polyps can be assigned to the superficial mucosa layer reliably with EUS (**Figs. 13.14** and **13.15**).

Definitive diagnosis and classification of a gastric polyp is only possible after complete removal and histological work-up of the polyp. Before endoscopic removal, transmural growth of larger polyps can be excluded with EUS.

Conventional EUS is only of marginal relevance for diagnosing gastric ulcers, as the diagnosis has to be confirmed histologically. In penetrating ulcers, malignant tumor growth may be simulated on EUS. Although a correlation has been demonstrated between the depth of penetration and the time to ulcer healing, the value of EUS for evaluating ulcer healing is a matter of controversy and the method ultimately has no practical relevance. By contrast, EUS is helpful for assessing transmural inflammation, fistulas, and abscess formation in Crohn disease.

In the evaluation of large folds in the stomach, suggestive findings can be detected by conventional EUS, but histological confirmation of the diagnosis remains obligatory. Foveolar hyperplasia of the stomach and Ménétrier disease, with swelling of only the two inner layers, have to be distinguished from other entities (such as diffuse gastric cancer, linitis plastica, and gastric lymphoma). Intramural vessels in patients with portal hypertension can be excluded with EUS. The value of EUS in relation to large gastric folds is that it allows intramural vessels to be excluded before endoscopic resection of a gastric fold (**Fig. 13.16**).

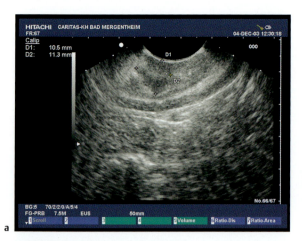

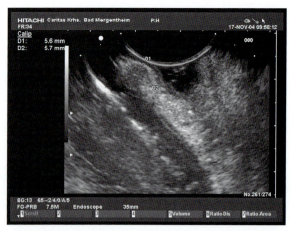

a

b

Fig. 13.15a, b Hyperplastic gastric polyps
a It is easy to assign a polyp to a specific layer with EUS (in this case, the mucosa).

b In this example, the hyperplastic polyp is only displayed at the tip of the fold.

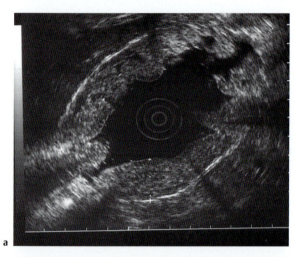

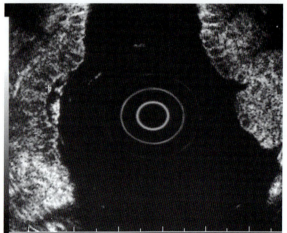

a

b

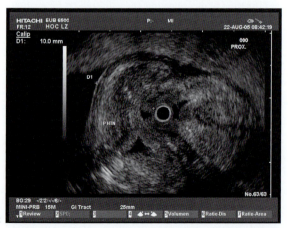

c

Fig. 13.16a–c Large-fold gastritis
a, b Ménétrier disease, with thickening of the mucosa and submucosa.
c Portal hypertension (PHTN).

■ Gastric Cancer

Gastric cancer is one of the most common cancers worldwide (and is the world's second leading cause of cancer-related deaths), although the numbers of patients in Germany are now declining. Treatment options for patients with gastric cancer depend mainly on an accurate evaluation of the stage of the cancer, which mainly depends on EUS. The advantage of EUS over other imaging modalities is its ability to differentiate the layers of gastric mucosa in almost all patients. The development of new, nonsurgical techniques at both ends of the range of conditions encountered (e.g., endoscopic mucosal resection and new palliative strategies) has also reinforced the need for accurate cancer staging. This raises the questions of which patients qualify for curative therapy and which patients qualify for palliative therapy. These issues are becoming increasingly important with improvements in nonsurgical treatment regimens. The prognosis for patients with gastric cancer is also determined by the extent of the tumor, and includes both nodal involvement and locoregional tumor extension beyond the gastric wall. The 5-year survival rate for patients with gastric cancer ranges from 5% to 95%, depending on the tumor stage. Surgery is the mainstay of curative therapy for gastric cancers. While patients with early localized disease clearly benefit from complete surgical resection, there is increasing evidence that multimodal treatment including chemoradiotherapy is superior to surgery alone for patients with resectable gastric cancer.[15–17] Early gastric cancer or superficially spreading carcinoma is defined as adenocarcinoma limited to the gastric mucosa or submucosa. Patients with early gastric cancer have a favorable prognosis, and the survival is > 90% after surgical resection.

A new TNM classification is now used for the staging of gastric cancer (**Tables 13.10** and **13.11**); the Laurén histological classification is also used (**Table 13.12**).

T1 lesions show infiltration into the mucosa and submucosa, but without invasion into the muscularis propria. In superficial T1 tumors with mucosal tumor growth, EUS can show inconspicuous gastric layers. A histologically confirmed gastric cancer without changes on EUS is therefore classified as stage T1. Stage T2 is defined as infiltration into the muscular layer (T2a) or into the subserosa (T2b), but differentiation between the muscular layer and the subserosa is not possible with ultrasound in patients who do not have ascites. Definitive differentiation between T2 and T3 tumors is therefore difficult. Stage T3 involves tumor infiltration through the serosa into the visceral peritoneum, without infiltration of neighboring organs. Stage T4 is defined by tumor invasion into neighboring organs (e.g., the colon, liver, and pancreas).

The new classification applies to carcinomas in which the disease has been histologically confirmed. A tumor with an epicenter within 5 cm of the esophagogastric junction and extension into the esophagus is classified and staged according to the esophageal scheme. All other

Table 13.10 TNM clinical classification

T	Primary tumor
TX	Primary tumor cannot be assessed
T0	No evidence of primary tumor
Tis	Carcinoma in situ: intraepithelial tumor without invasion of the lamina propria, high-grade dysplasia.
T1	Tumor invades lamina propria, muscularis, mucosae, or submucosa
	T1a Tumor invades lamina propria or muscularis mucosae
	T1b Tumor invades submucosa
T2	Tumor invades muscularis propria
T3	Tumor invades subserosa
T4	Tumor perforates serosa or invades adjacent structures[a, b]
	T4a Tumor perforates serosa
	T4b Tumor invades adjacent structures[a, b, c]
N	**Regional lymph nodes**
NX	Regional lymph nodes cannot be assessed
N0	No regional lymph node metastasis
N1	Metastasis in 1 or 2 regional lymph nodes
N2	Metastasis in 3–6 regional lymph nodes
N3	Metastasis in 7 or more regional lymph nodes
	N3a Metastasis in 7–15 regional lymph nodes
	N3b Metastasis in 16 or more regional lymph nodes
M	**Distant metastasis[d]**
M0	No distant metastasis
M1	Distant metastases

[a] The structures adjacent to the stomach are the spleen, transverse colon, liver, diaphragm, pancreas, abdominal wall, adrenal gland, kidney, small intestine, and retroperitoneum.
[b] Intramural extension to the duodenum or esophagus is classified by the depth of greatest invasion in any of these sites, including the stomach.
[c] Tumor that extends into the gastrocolic or gastrohepatic ligaments or into the greater or lesser omentum, without perforation of the visceral peritoneum, is T3.
[d] Distant metastasis includes peritoneal seeding, positive peritoneal cytology, and omental tumor that is not part of a continuous extension.

tumors, with an epicenter in the stomach more than 5 cm from the junction and with no extension into the esophagus, are staged using the gastric carcinoma scheme.

The following procedures are necessary for assessing T, N, and M categories:
- *T categories.* Physical examination, imaging, endoscopy, and/or surgical exploration
- *N categories.* Physical examination, imaging, and/or surgical exploration
- *M categories.* Physical examination, imaging, and/or surgical exploration

The regional lymph nodes in the stomach are: the perigastric nodes, along the lesser and greater curvatures; the nodes along the left gastric, common hepatic, splenic,

Table 13.11 Stage grouping

Stage 0	Tis	N0	M0
Stage IA	T1	N0	M0
Stage IB	T2	N0	M0
	T1	N1	M0
Stage IIA	T3	N0	M0
	T2	N1	M0
	T1	N2	M0
Stage IIB	T4a	N0	M0
	T3	N1	M0
	T1	N3	M0
Stage IIIB	T4b	N0, N1	M0
	T4a	N2	M0
	T3	N3	M0
Stage IIIC	T4a	N3	M0
	T4b	N2, N3	M0
Stage IV	Any T	Any N	M1

Table 13.12 The Laurén histological classification of gastric cancer

1	Not applicable (no adenocarcinoma, no signet ring cancer or dedifferentiated carcinoma)
2	Intestinal type (polypoid growth, well delimited, good prognosis) • Well differentiated • Moderately differentiated • Poorly differentiated
3	Diffuse type (infiltrative growth, poorly delimited)
4	Mixed type

and celiac arteries; and the hepatoduodenal nodes. Involvement of other intra-abdominal lymph nodes such as retropancreatic, mesenteric, and para-aortic is classified as distant metastasis.

Gastric cancers are normally hypoechoic, but hyperechoic tumors also occur.

Due to limited penetration depth, more distant lymph-node metastases cannot be diagnosed with EUS. EUS is superior to CT and transabdominal ultrasound in the staging of gastric cancer. The possibility of gastric wall metastases (e.g., from melanoma or ovarian carcinoma) should be considered. The accuracy of EUS in the staging of gastric cancers has been a matter of controversy. It should be borne in mind that EUS may underestimate the depth of invasion and may overestimate nodal invasion because of inflammation around the tumor or in the lymph nodes; underestimation of lymph-node infiltration may be due to the small size of infiltrated lymph nodes (< 5 mm). The EUS criteria for depth of tumor invasion and nodal metastasis have changed during the last 20 years, and advances in EUS technology have also been made. It is not clear whether these changes in EUS criteria and technology have had any impact on gastric cancer staging.

The sensitivity of EUS for T staging has also improved during the last 20 years, especially for early disease (T1). EUS is essential for identifying which patients qualify for curative therapy. However, EUS has not improved as an imaging modality for N staging, since up to 30% of lymph-node metastases are in lymph nodes < 5 mm. The specificity of both T and N staging have remained high over the last 20 years.

EUS is an accurate and minimally invasive diagnostic tool for evaluating the T stage in patients with gastric cancer. EUS results are more accurate with advanced disease than early disease.

After gastrectomy, EUS is helpful for detecting malignant infiltration of regional lymph nodes. In the diagnosis of local tumor recurrence, it needs to be borne in mind that inflammatory processes and connective tissue can lead to false-positive results. The problems with EUS in the stomach are the same here as in the esophagus.

In patients in whom surgical resection is contraindicated and in whom local endoscopic tumor removal is possible, EUS staging is of considerable value. EUS miniprobes are helpful in these cases in particular. Differentiation between the mucosal and submucosal T1 stages is possible, which is of considerable importance for curative endoscopic tumor therapy. The importance of perigastric lymph-node metastases in patients with T1 carcinomas was mentioned above. This is of great importance for planning endoscopic treatment and assessing the patients' prognosis.

Review of the Literature

Due to its high resolution, EUS is superior to other imaging modalities (especially CT) in the staging of malignant gastric tumors. This is especially true for T1 and T2 stage gastric cancer. With the increasing use of endoscopic mucosal resection in the treatment of early gastric cancer, endosonographic examination of the stomach is becoming increasingly important. In these cases, high-frequency miniprobes provide excellent resolution of the gastric wall, which helps in differentiating T1 carcinomas into several subtypes. This is helpful for identifying patients with early gastric cancer who are eligible for therapeutic endoscopic mucosal resection. Typical findings are shown in **Figs. 13.17, 13.18, 13.19, 13.20, 13.21, 13.22, 13.23, 13.24, 13.25** and **13.26.**

In a recently published meta-analysis, the pooled sensitivity and specificity for T1 were 88.1% (95% CI, 84.5 to 91.1) and 100.0% (95% CI, 99.7 to 100.0), respectively. For T2, the sensitivity was 82.3% (95% CI, 78.2 to 86.0) and the specificity was 95.6% (95% CI, 94.4 to 96.6). The pooled sensitivity for T3 was 89.7% (95% CI, 87.1 to 92.0) and the specificity was 94.7% (95% CI, 93.3 to 95.9). T4 had a pooled sensitivity of 99.2% (95% CI, 97.1 to 99.9) and a specificity of 96.7% (95% CI, 95.7 to 97.6). Pooled likelihood ratios and diagnostic odds ratios for various T stages are shown in **Table 13.13.** (The "diagnostic odds ratio" is defined as the odds of having a positive test in patients with the true anatomic stage of the disease in comparison with patients who do not have the disease). The pooled estimates for sensitivity, specificity, likelihood ratios, and diagnostic odds ratios computed using the random-effect model were similar to those with the fixed-effect model.[18]

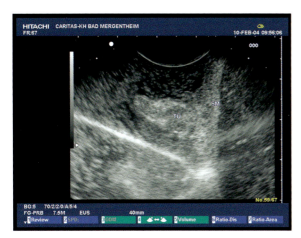

Fig. 13.17 Exophytic T1 gastric cancer. The tumor (TU) is well distinguished from the deeper muscular layer. Local endoscopic tumor therapy is technically possible. SM, submucosa.

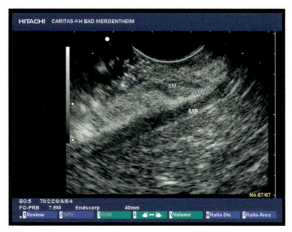

Fig. 13.18 Excavated T1 gastric cancer. The excavated form of gastric cancer seen here is associated with a poor prognosis and is difficult to classify in comparison with exophytic tumors, in which the underlying layers can be assessed precisely. Submucosal infiltration (SM) is seen in this case. MP, muscularis propria.

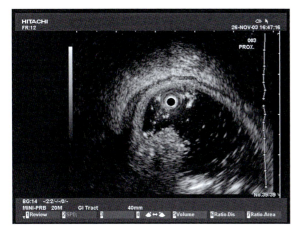

Fig. 13.19 T1 gastric cancer, imaged with an EUS miniprobe. The detailed resolution of superficial lesions is better with high-resolution miniprobes than with conventional EUS.

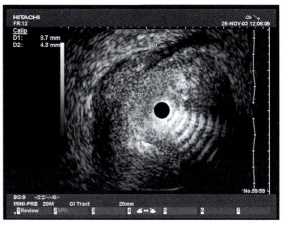

Fig. 13.20 T2 gastric cancer. The hypoechoic infiltration of the muscular layer is well visualized. There is no penetration through the gastric wall.

N stage

The pooled sensitivity and specificity for N1 were 58.2% (95% CI, 53.5 to 62.8) and 87.2% (95% CI, 84.4 to 89.7), respectively. N2 had a pooled sensitivity of 64.9% (95% CI, 60.8 to 68.8) and a specificity of 92.4% (95% CI, 89.9 to 94.4). Pooled likelihood ratios and diagnostic odds ratios for various N stages are shown in **Table 13.13**.[18]

M stage

The pooled sensitivity for diagnosing distal metastasis was 73.2% (95% CI, 63.2 to 81.7) in an analysis of four studies.[18] The specificity of EUS was 88.6% (95% CI, 84.8 to 91.7). The positive likelihood ratio for diagnosing distal metastasis was 17.2 (95% CI, 2.8 to 106.3) and the negative likelihood ratio was 0.4 (95% CI, 0.2 to 0.7).

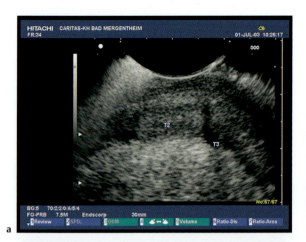

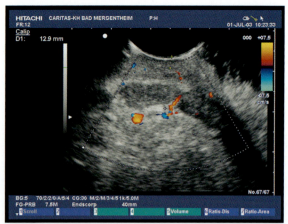

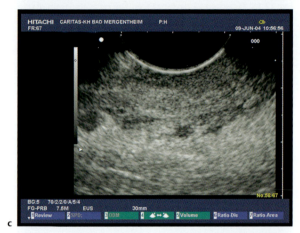

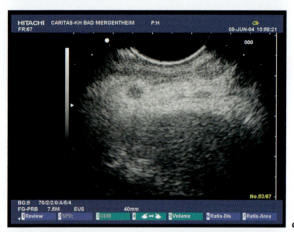

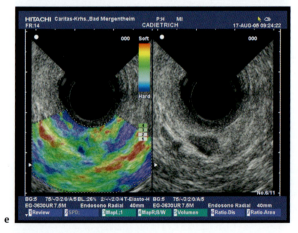

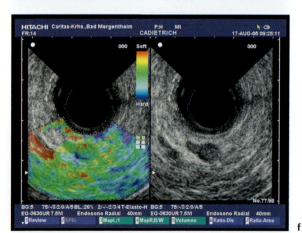

Fig. 13.21a–f T3 gastric cancer

a It can be difficult to distinguish between T2 and T3 gastric carcinomas with EUS alone, due to inflammatory reactions around the tumor.

b Color and power Doppler imaging can be helpful for detecting vessels and assessing tumor invasion.

c, d Another example, with lymph node infiltration in (**d**). Typically, there is no shift between the stomach and the surrounding tissue.

e, f Elastography is helpful and provides reproducible results for detecting circumscribed lymph-node infiltration.

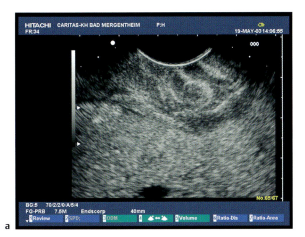

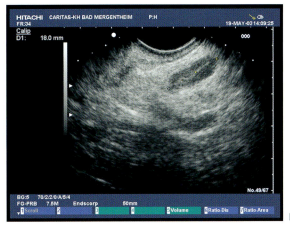

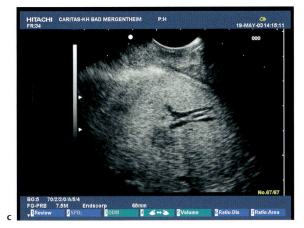

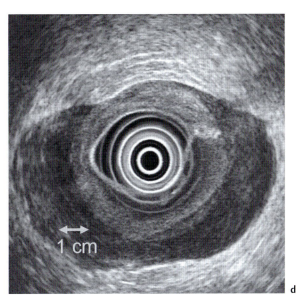

Fig. 13.22a–d T4N1 gastric cancer
a Tumor invasion into the pancreas (T4).
b Lymph-node metastases.
c A small liver metastasis with segmental biliary congestion.
d Linitis plastica.

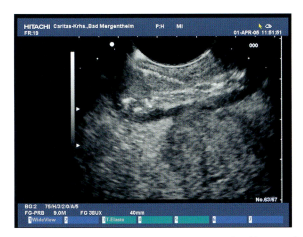

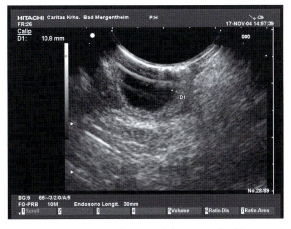

Fig. 13.23 EUS findings in peritoneal carcinosis, with infiltration of the serosa and muscularis propria by a tumor originating in the pancreas.

Fig. 13.24 An intramucosal metastasis from a small cell lung carcinoma is seen between the markers.

III Gastrointestinal Tract

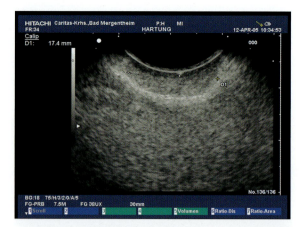

Fig. 13.25 A neuroendocrine tumor (between the markers), mimicking carcinoma of the stomach infiltrating the submucosa.

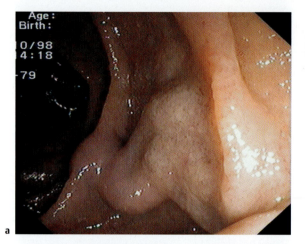

a

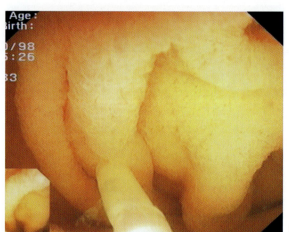

b

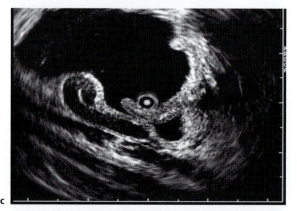

c

Fig. 13.26a–c Osler disease
a, b Vascular abnormalities in Osler disease can produce an impression resembling that of submucosal tumors.
c They can be very well detected with EUS.

Table 13.13 Accuracy of endoscopic ultrasound, with 95% confidence intervals, for diagnosing T and N stages in gastric cancer patients[18]

	Pooled sensitivity	Pooled specificity	Pooled LR+	Pooled LR–	Pooled DOR
T1	88.1% (84.5 to 91.1)	100.0% (99.7 to 100.0)	90.1 (48.9 to 165.7)	0.17 (0.10 to 0.28)	605.6 (296.8 to 1235.6)
T2	82.3% (78.2 to 86.0)	95.6% (94.4 to 96.6)	17.3 (10.9 to 27.5)	0.23 (0.17 to 0.29)	108.6 (56.6 to 208.1)
T3	89.7% (87.1 to 92.0)	94.7% (93.3 to 95.9)	14.3 (10.3 to 19.8)	0.13 (0.08 to 0.19)	144.4 (95.4 to 218.7)
T4	99.2% (97.1 to 99.9)	96.7% (95.7 to 97.6)	19.6 (14.1 to 27.2)	0.07 (0.04 to 0.12)	507.8 (247.5 to 1042.1)
N1	58.2% (53.5 to 62.8)	87.2% (84.4 to 89.7)	4.1 (2.4 to 7.1)	0.49 (0.41 to 0.58)	9.5 (5.3 to 16.9)
N2	64.9% (60.8 to 68.8)	92.4% (89.9 to 94.4)	6.7 (4.1 to 10.9)	0.39 (0.31 to 0.49)	26.6 (13.9 to 50.7)

LR+, positive likelihood ratio, LR–, negative likelihood ratio; DOR, diagnostic odds ratio.

Table 13.14 Accuracy of EUS, with 95% confidence intervals, for staging gastric cancers during the last 20 years

	Years	No. of studies	Pooled sensitivity	Pooled specificity	Pooled LR+	Pooled LR–	Pooled DOR
T1	1986–1994	12	56.3% (49.7 to 62.6)	89.1% (85.5 to 92.1)	4.6 (1.6 to 13.8)	0.51 (0.38 to 0.69)	9.3 (2.9 to 30.1)
	1995–1999	4	82.2% (67.9 to 92.0)	100.0% (97.9 to 100.0)	72.9 (18.2 to 288.8)	0.13 (0.03 to 0.68)	562.5 (92.0 to 3438.4)
	2000–2006	5	84.8% (71.1 to 93.7)	100.0% (98.9 to 100.0)	88.9 (25.3 to 312.4)	0.22 (0.13 to 0.38)	428.9 (96.6 to 1904.9)
T2	1986–1994	12	84.9% (79.8 to 89.2)	96.7% (95.4 to 97.8)	20.5 (14.8 to 28.4)	0.19 (0.13 to 0.30)	207.0 (109.5 to 391.6)
	1995–1999	4	74.4% (57.9 to 87.0)	90.9% (85.4 to 94.8)	6.7 (2.5 to 18.1)	0.33 (0.19 to 0.55)	23.7 (5.3 to 106.2)
	2000–2006	5	79.5% (70.8 to 86.5)	94.6% (91.3 to 96.9)	16.8 (5.3 to 53.8)	0.22 (0.12 to 0.38)	79.6 (22.9 to 277.2)
T3	1986–1994	12	89.6% (86.3 to 92.3)	95.3% (93.6 to 96.7)	15.5 (11.4 to 21.1)	0.12 (0.07 to 0.22)	160.2 (95.5 to 268.7)
	1995–1999	4	90.3% (80.1 to 96.4)	91.3% (85.8 to 95.2)	11.1 (3.5 to 35.4)	0.12 (0.06 to 0.25)	93.3 (30.6 to 284.6)
	2000–2006	5	89.8% (83.3 to 94.5)	94.8% (91.3 to 97.2)	13.9 (7.7 to 25.1)	0.12 (0.04 to 0.37)	154.7 (55.7 to 429.5)
T4	1986–1994	12	98.9% (95.9 to 99.9)	97.1% (95.9 to 98.0)	23.3 (14.6 to 37.4)	0.07 (0.04 to 0.14)	626.4 (256.1 to 1532.5)
	1995–1999	4	100% (92.5 to 100.0)	95.8% (91.5 to 98.3)	14.3 (7.6 to 26.9)	0.05 (0.01 to 0.18)	441.7 (85.6 to 2279.1)
	2000–2006	3	100.0% (87.2 to 100.0)	95.7% (91.9 to 98.0)	16.4 (7.9 to 33.9)	0.07 (0.02 to 0.33)	260.1 (43.7 to 1547.4)
N1	1986–1994	10	56.3% (49 to 62.6)	89.1% (85.5 to 92.1)	4.6 (1.6 to 13.6)	0.5 (0.4 to 0.7)	9.3 (2.9 to 30.1)
	1995–1999	4	64.6% (53.3 to 74.9)	83.5% (74.9 to 90.1)	3.6 (2.3 to 5.6)	0.5 (0.4 to 0.6)	8.8 (4.3 to 18.1)
	2000–2006	5	57.8% (49.0 to 66.20)	85.5% (79.3 to 90.4)	4.4 (2.9 to 6.6)	0.5 (0.3 to 0.7)	10.2 (4.8 to 21.8)
N2	1986–1994	10	70.6% (65.4 to 75.5)	94.7% (91.7 to 96.8)	11.0 (4.6 to 26.6)	0.3 (0.2 to 0.4)	63.9 (30.9 to 132.3)
	1995–1999	4	70.2% (59.9 to 79.2)	83.2% (74.1 to 90.1)	3.9 (2.5 to 6.1)	0.4 (0.3 to 0.5)	11.7 (5.6 to 24.1)
	2000–2006	4	49.0% (40.7 to 57.3)	93.0% (87.5 to 96.6)	6.4 (1.7 to 24.1)	0.6 (0.4 to 0.7)	12.7 (2.9 to 56.2)

■ Effect of Technology

EUS studies were grouped into three periods in order to standardize changes in EUS technology and also to standardize changes in the EUS criteria for tumor staging: 1986–1994, 1995–1999, and 2000–2006. The pooled estimates for studies during these periods of time are shown in **Table 13.14**.[18]

It should be noted that the majority of patients in the studies analyzed had adenocarcinomas, although patients with other types of gastric cancer could not be excluded from the study analysis.

The meta-analysis shows that the pooled sensitivity of EUS for tumor invasion (T stage) is high, and it is higher for advanced disease in comparison with early disease. The pooled specificity for depth of tumor invasion is very high for all the T stages. EUS has a high diagnostic odds ratio for

T staging. The negative likelihood ratio of a test is a measure of how good the test is at excluding a disease state. The lower the negative likelihood ratio, the better the test is at excluding a disease. The positive likelihood ratio is a measure of how well the same test identifies a disease state. For T staging, EUS has a low negative likelihood ratio for T4 disease in comparison with T1 disease and a high positive likelihood ratio for all T stages. This indicates that EUS is better at excluding T4 disease than T1 disease. Another way of looking at it is: if EUS diagnoses T2 disease, then the patient might still have anatomic T1 disease; but if EUS diagnoses T1 disease, then the patient probably truly has anatomic T1 disease and can receive curative therapy. This helps physicians offer endoscopic treatments such as endoscopic mucosal resection or endoscopic submucosal dissection with confidence for T1 gastric cancer as alternatives to curative surgery. For nodal staging of gastric cancers, all the pooled accuracy estimates of EUS are

Table 13.15 Accuracy of endoscopic ultrasound (EUS) for T staging of gastric cancer in comparison with computed tomography (CT)

Author	Patients	Method	T total	T1	T2	T3	T4	Ref.
Kuntz	82	EUS	n.a.	100%	81%	61%	100%	19
	Review	EUS	60–90%	n.a.	n.a.	n.a.	n.a.	19
	94	CT	58%		57%[a]	34%	75%	19
Habermann	51	EUS	86%	–	90%	79%	100%	20
		CT	76%	–	83%	63%	100%	20
Polkowski	88	EUS	63%	36%	55%	80%	33%	21
		CT	44%	18%	22%	56%	38%	21

[a] = T1 and T2 together. n.a., not available

Table 13.16 Accuracy of EUS in the staging (N-stage) of gastric cancer compared with CT

Author	Patients	Method	N total	N0	N1	N2	Ref.
Kuntz	82	EUS	n.a.	82%	89%[a]		19
	94	HCT	n.a.	48%	83%[a]		19
Habermann	51	EUS	90%	100%	83%	84%	20
		HCT	70%	84%	42%	74%	20
Polkowski	88	EUS	47%	64%	36%	43%	21
		HCT	52%	50%	54%	51%	21

[a] = N1 and N2 together. n.a., not available

higher for N2 (advanced disease) than for N1. The accuracy of EUS for diagnosing N stages is not high. It is also not clear whether using all the three criteria together or in combination for nodal involvement improves the diagnostic accuracy. The role of FNA in the nodal staging of gastric cancers could not be evaluated owing to the lack of a sufficient number of studies reporting such data. It can be expected that obtaining tissue with EUS-FNA will improve the accuracy, but further research is needed to establish this. Although there have also only been a few studies reporting data for distant metastases, the pooled specificity was high, but the sensitivity was not as high. As a diagnostic tool, EUS is not designed for investigating distant metastases.[18]

The available data support the recommendation that EUS should be strongly considered for staging, particularly as new curative and palliative endoscopic therapies are emerging as alternatives to surgery in gastric cancer.

The accuracy of EUS for T staging and N staging of gastric cancer in comparison with CT is summarized in **Tables 13.15** and **13.16**.

EUS of the Small Bowel

Due to the difficulty of diagnosing diseases in the small intestine, the value of EUS in evaluating these diseases is unclear. Correct staging and differential diagnosis of small-bowel diseases require adequate histological work-up, which is often only possible after surgical resection. The same principles apply as in EUS of the esophagus and stomach. In experienced hands, analogous decisions can therefore be reached easily. Some specific characteristics of neoplastic diseases in the small intestine are discussed below.

Despite the large surface area of the intestine and faster proliferation of the epithelial cells in comparison with the colon, benign tumors (30–50%) and malignant tumors (50–70%) in the small bowel are rare (< 5% of all gastrointestinal tumors, 0.1% of all malignant tumors; incidence one in 100 000). The incidence of colon cancer is more than 50 times higher. The available data on the frequency of tumors in the different parts of the small intestine are inconsistent. Distal (benign) tumors (in the ileum) are more frequent than proximally located tumors (in the duodenum and jejunum). However, the frequency of malignant intestinal tumors decreases from proximal to distal (duodenum 50%, jejunum 30%, ileum 20%). Adenocarcinomas, carcinoids, lymphomas, and sarcomas are the most frequently diagnosed malignant tumors in the small bowel. The frequency increases in older patients. Many possible etiological reasons for the relatively low incidence of these tumors have been discussed; in addition to the fast transit time and the low viscosity of the diluted intestinal fluid (low rate of bacteria, alkaline milieu), immunological factors (macrophages, T and B cells, IgA secretion) in the mucosa play an important role. Many (rare) diseases predispose to malignancies in the small intestine (**Tables 13.17, 13.18, 13.19** and **13.20**).

Table 13.17 Predisposing factors for the development of malignancies in the small intestine

Familial adenomatous polyposis
Genetically determined tumor diseases—e.g., hereditary nonpolyposis colorectal cancer (HNPCC) and multiple primary malignant neoplasia (MPMN)
Cowden syndrome
Peutz–Jeghers syndrome
Chronic inflammatory bowel diseases (e.g., Crohn disease) (predisposing factors: high inflammatory activity, involvement of the small bowel or isolated parts of the small bowel)
Celiac disease (treatment-resistant)
Hereditary or acquired immunodeficiency

Table 13.18 Benign tumors of the small intestine

Entity	Characteristics
Adenoma	Frequent epithelial tumor in the small bowel, frequency increasing from proximal to distal, risk of malignancy 30–50%; specific feature: familial polyposis syndromes
Leiomyoma	Frequent mesenchymal and symptomatic tumor in the small bowel (especially jejunum); leading symptom: occult bleeding and obstruction; *caution:* GIST
Lipoma	Predilection in the ileum; mostly asymptomatic
Hamartoma	E.g., Peutz–Jeghers syndrome, defined genetic defect (*LKB1/STK11* gene on chromosome 19 p); mucocutaneous, melanous pigments. Increased risk of malignancies (small bowel, colorectal cancer, pancreas, breast, and testicle). In hamartomas, no increased epithelial components are found
Others	Inflammatory pseudotumors (e.g., Crohn disease, postradiation enteritis)

GIST, gastrointestinal stromal tumor.

Table 13.19 Malignant tumors of the small intestine

Entity	Characteristics
Carcinoma	Frequent malignant tumor of the small bowel (> 50%). Predilection: duodenum and jejunum > ileum; association with Crohn disease and celiac disease; influence of genetic disorders (K-*ras*, erbB2, p53, etc.)
Sarcoma	Sarcomas develop from mesenchymal tissue (e.g., leiomyosarcoma from smooth muscle in the intestinal wall) and metastasize relatively early (e.g., to the liver). Treatment of choice: curative or palliative surgery, as benefit from chemotherapy or radiotherapy has not yet been established
Kaposi sarcoma	Frequent tumor in AIDS; mostly asymptomatic and diagnosed at endoscopy incidentally. Due to recurrent tumor manifestations, surgical resection is not promising
Others	Depending on the different tissue types, a large number of rare malignant tumors may be found in the small intestine

AIDS, acquired immune deficiency syndrome.

Table 13.20 Classification of benign and malignant tumors of the small intestine relative to the primary tissue. For gastrointestinal stromal tumors, see Chapter 14.

Tumor genesis	Benign	Malignant
Epithelial	Adenoma	Adenocarcinoma
Mesenchymal	Fibroma	Fibrosarcoma
Smooth muscle	Leiomyoma	Leiomyosarcoma
Fatty tissue	Lipoma	Liposarcoma
Blood vessels (see **Fig. 13.26**)	Hemangioma	Hemangiosarcoma, Kaposi sarcoma
Lymphatic vessels	Lymphangioma	Lymphangiosarcoma
Lymphatic tissue	Pseudolymphoma	Lymphoma
Neural tissue	Neurofibroma	Neurofibrosarcoma
Glia	Neurilemmoma	Neurofibrosarcoma
Enterochromaffin cells		Carcinoid, gastrinoma, insulinoma
Pluripotent stem cell	Hamartoma	Malignant mixed tumors (teratoma, adenocarcinoids, adenosquamous carcinoma)

Over 50% of tumors in the small intestine are asymptomatic. The most frequently observed findings are chronic (occult) bleeding, abdominal pain, and obstruction (ileus or subileus). Although 90% of patients have uncharacteristic symptoms at the time of diagnosis, small-intestinal tumors are normally diagnosed at an advanced stage of the disease (with intestinal bleeding, ileus, stenoses, invagination, perforation). Signs of invasive tumor disease should be noted (e.g., jaundice when there is biliary involvement).

Tumors of the small bowel are difficult to detect when endoscopically inaccessible parts of the small intestine are affected. Enteroclysis (Sellink) is the method with the best results. Only 50–60 cm of the proximal jejunum can be reached with push enteroscopy, so that the benefits of this method depend on the tumor location. High-resolution transabdominal ultrasound and CT can be very useful in specific cases, but definitive diagnosis can usually only be obtained by laparotomy. As in all other tumors, the prognosis with these lesions depends on the tumor stage, histology, grading, and available treatment modalities. The 5-year survival rates are lower in patients with adenocarcinomas and sarcomas in comparison with those with carcinoids and lymphomas.

References

1. Puli SR, Reddy JB, Bechtold ML, Antillon D, Ibdah JA, Antillon MR. Staging accuracy of esophageal cancer by endoscopic ultrasound: a meta-analysis and systematic review. World J Gastroenterol 2008;14(10):1479–1490.
2. Botet JF, Lightdale CJ, Zauber AG, et al. Preoperative staging of gastric cancer: comparison of endoscopic US and dynamic CT. Radiology 1991;181(2):426–432.
3. Ziegler K, Sanft C, Zeitz M, et al. Evaluation of endosonography in TN staging of oesophageal cancer. Gut 1991;32(1):16–20.
4. Kienle P, Buhl K, Kuntz C, et al. Prospective comparison of endoscopy, endosonography and computed tomography for staging of tumours of the oesophagus and gastric cardia. Digestion 2002;66(4):230–236.
5. Weaver SR, Blackshaw GR, Lewis WG, et al. Comparison of special interest computed tomography, endosonography and histopathological stage of oesophageal cancer. Clin Radiol 2004;59(6):499–504.
6. Räsänen JV, Sihvo EI, Knuuti MJ, et al. Prospective analysis of accuracy of positron emission tomography, computed tomography, and endoscopic ultrasonography in staging of adenocarcinoma of the esophagus and the esophagogastric junction. Ann Surg Oncol 2003;10(8):954–960.
7. Flamen P, Lerut A, Van Cutsem E, et al. Utility of positron emission tomography for the staging of patients with potentially operable esophageal carcinoma. J Clin Oncol 2000;18(18):3202–3210.
8. Berger AC, Scott WJ. Noninvasive staging of esophageal carcinoma. J Surg Res 2004;117(1):127–133.
9. Vazquez-Sequeiros E, Norton ID, Clain JE, et al. Impact of EUS-guided fine-needle aspiration on lymph node staging in patients with esophageal carcinoma. Gastrointest Endosc 2001;53(7):751–757.
10. Eloubeidi MA, Wallace MB, Reed CE, et al. The utility of EUS and EUS-guided fine needle aspiration in detecting celiac lymph node metastasis in patients with esophageal cancer: a single-center experience. Gastrointest Endosc 2001;54(6):714–719.
11. Parmar KS, Zwischenberger JB, Reeves AL, Waxman I. Clinical impact of endoscopic ultrasound-guided fine needle aspiration of celiac axis lymph nodes (M1a disease) in esophageal cancer. Ann Thorac Surg 2002;73(3):916–920, discussion 920–921.
12. Murata Y, Ohta M, Hayashi K, Ide H, Takasaki K. Preoperative evaluation of lymph node metastasis in esophageal cancer. Ann Thorac Cardiovasc Surg 2003;9(2):88–92.
13. Chang KJ, Soetikno RM, Bastas D, Tu C, Nguyen PT. Impact of endoscopic ultrasound combined with fine-needle aspiration biopsy in the management of esophageal cancer. Endoscopy 2003;35(11):962–966.
14. Puli SR, Reddy JB, Bechtold ML, Antillon MR, Ibdah JA. Accuracy of endoscopic ultrasound in the diagnosis of distal and celiac axis lymph node metastasis in esophageal cancer: a meta-analysis and systematic review. Dig Dis Sci 2008;53(9):2405–2414.
15. Cunningham D, Okines AF, Ashley S. Capecitabine and oxaliplatin for advanced esophagogastric cancer. N Engl J Med 2010;362(9):858–859.
16. Cunningham D, Oliveira J; ESMO Guidelines Working Group. Gastric cancer: ESMO clinical recommendations for diagnosis, treatment and follow-up. Ann Oncol 2008;19(Suppl 2):ii23–ii24.
17. Cunningham D, Allum WH, Stenning SP, et al; MAGIC Trial Participants. Perioperative chemotherapy versus surgery alone for resectable gastroesophageal cancer. N Engl J Med 2006;355(1):11–20.
18. Puli SR, Batapati Krishna Reddy J, Bechtold ML, Antillon MR, Ibdah JA. How good is endoscopic ultrasound for TNM staging of gastric cancers? A meta-analysis and systematic review. World J Gastroenterol 2008;14(25):4011–4019.
19. Kuntz C, Herfarth C. Imaging diagnosis for staging of gastric cancer. Semin Surg Oncol 1999;17(2):96–102.
20. Habermann CR, Weiss F, Riecken R, et al. Preoperative staging of gastric adenocarcinoma: comparison of helical CT and endoscopic US. Radiology 2004;230(2):465–471.
21. Polkowski M, Palucki J, Wronska E, Szawlowski A, Nasierowska-Guttmejer A, Butruk E. Endosonography versus helical computed tomography for locoregional staging of gastric cancer. Endoscopy 2004;36(7):617–623.

14 Endoscopic Ultrasound in Subepithelial Tumors of the Gastrointestinal Tract

C. Jenssen C.F. Dietrich

One of the classical indications for endoscopic ultrasonography (EUS) is the investigation of possible subepithelial tumors and the differential diagnosis, classification, and follow-up of these lesions.[1–5] There are no reliable data on the incidence of subepithelial tumors and other submucosal lesions of the gastrointestinal tract, since in the majority of cases they remain asymptomatic and undiagnosed throughout life. Postmortem and surgical studies have found mesenchymal esophageal tumors (leiomyomas) in up to 8% of cases,[6] and mesenchymal gastric tumors in half of all patients who died over the age of 50-years.[5] In one study, "seedling" mesenchymal tumors (0.2–12.0 mm) were found in more than 50% of 150 esophagogastric resections for esophageal cancer or carcinoma of the esophagogastric junction (one or two small gastrointestinal stromal tumors in 10% of cases and 1–13 leiomyomas in 47% of cases).[7]

Certainly, small subepithelial tumors are diagnosed much less frequently in living patients. One older endoscopic study described subepithelial gastric tumors in only 54 of 15 104 (0.36%) routine esophagogastroduodenoscopies (EGDs).[8] It can be assumed that with the increasing use of endoscopy and because of improved endoscopic imaging, they are now being discovered more often. One recent study in Asia found subepithelial tumors in 795 of 104 159 upper gastrointestinal endoscopies (0.76%)[9] and another in 188 of 5307 EGDs (3.5%).[10] Subepithelial tumors were the third most common esophageal disease in 6683 EGDs performed for screening purposes in a Korean center (0.6%).[11]

Subepithelial tumors of the gastrointestinal tract are usually an incidental finding and may be entirely unrelated to the clinical question that prompted the endoscopic examination in the first place (**Fig. 14.1**).[12–14] Over a period of 7 years, we carried out 346 endosonographic examinations for subepithelial lesions. In 87% of the examinations, the presenting symptoms did not correspond to the subepithelial lesion.[15] Symptomatic subepithelial tumors present with overt or obscure gastrointestinal hemorrhage (**Fig. 14.2**), pain, abdominal discomfort, dysphagia, or symptoms of intestinal obstruction (**Fig. 14.3**).[16–18,20]

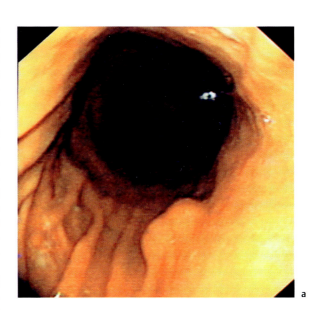

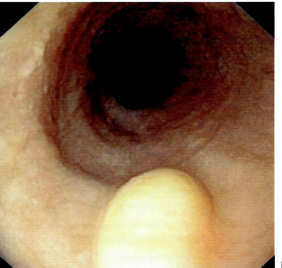

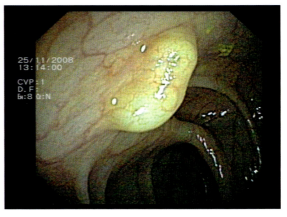

Fig. 14.1a–c Endoscopic view of small, asymptomatic gastrointestinal subepithelial tumors in the stomach (gastrointestinal stromal tumor, **a**), in the esophagus (granular cell tumor, **b**), and in the large intestine (leiomyoma, **c**).

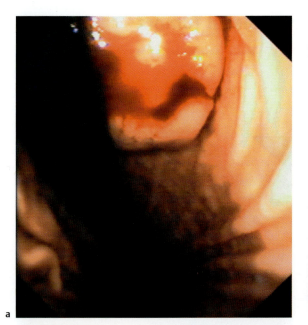

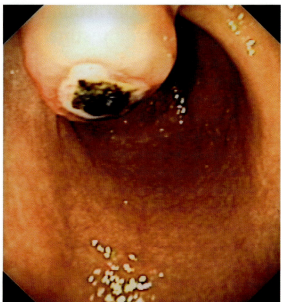

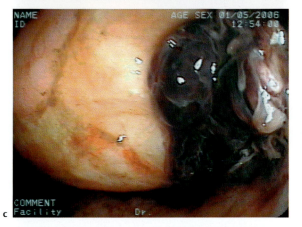

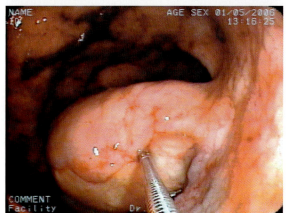

Fig. 14.2a–d Hemorrhage caused by subepithelial gastric tumors.
a Overt bleeding (retrograde view).
b Ulceration of a large gastrointestinal stromal tumor (GIST) with an adherent clot.

c, d A very large, ulcerated lipoma in the gastric body, causing severe gastrointestinal bleeding (**c** adherent clots; **d** extensive ulceration after removal of the clots). For the corresponding EUS image, see **Fig. 14.27e.**

The distribution of subepithelial tumors in the upper gastrointestinal tract is not uniform. In endoscopic series reporting on subepithelial tumors of the upper gastrointestinal tract, the stomach is the organ most frequently involved (in ≈ 60–70% of cases); ≈ 20–30% of subepithelial tumors are found in the esophagus, and fewer than 10% in the duodenum.[12,18,19] The endoscopic findings may vary from subtle protrusions to tiny polyps or large, protruding mass lesions (**Figs. 14.1, 14.2** and **14.3**).

As with radiographic methods, endoscopy is not capable of differentiating reliably between subepithelial tumors, intramural varices, and wall impressions caused by extraluminal lesions.[1,3,14,21–27] In addition, it is not possible to diagnose the lesion type, the depth and extent of an intra-

mural lesion, or whether neighboring organs are involved.[22,24,27] Endoscopic biopsy is usually unhelpful, as it only provides samples of the mucosa covering a subepithelial lesion, not tissue from the lesion itself. More invasive methods of tissue sampling, such as "buttonhole" or jumbo biopsies, have a low diagnostic yield and carry a high risk (**Fig. 14.4**).[28–30]

EUS is therefore an attractive noninvasive method in the investigation of subepithelial lesions of the gastrointestinal tract.[15,18,31]

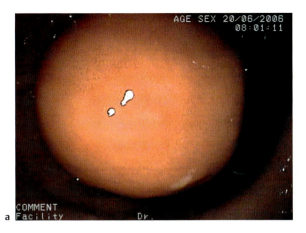

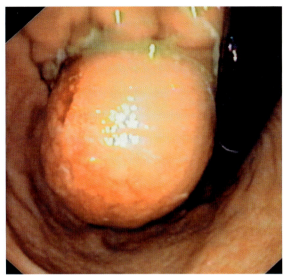

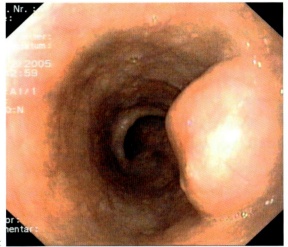

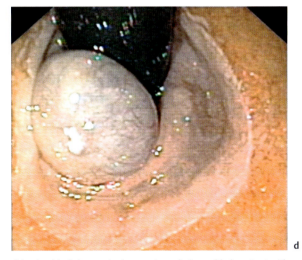

Fig. 14.3a–d Endoscopic view of large subepithelial gastrointestinal stromal tumors (GISTs) causing symptoms.
a, b Very large GISTs in the lesser curvature of the stomach (causing epigastric discomfort).
c A medium-sized subepithelial tumor in the esophagus (leiomyoma) in a patient with dysphagia.

d A subepithelial tumor in the gastric cardia in an elderly patient with dysphagia and recurrent regurgitation (cavernous hemangioma; retrograde view). For the corresponding EUS image, see **Fig. 14.20c, d**.

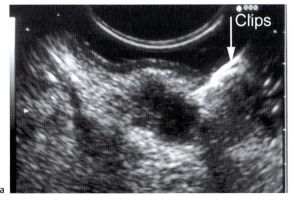

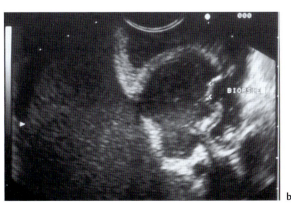

Fig. 14.4a, b Buttonhole biopsy of subepithelial gastric tumors.
a EUS view of a subepithelial neuroendocrine tumor, with hemoclips in place after hemorrhage.

b EUS view of a gastrointestinal stromal tumor (GIST) in the stomach, showing a superficial defect after biopsy. Clinically, there was recurrent bleeding from the biopsy site.

Table 14.1 Causes of wall protrusion/impression

	Chen et al. 2001[32] n = 238 (1993–2001)	Jenssen, Siebert (unpublished data, 2002–2007) n = 247
Patients with subepithelial tumors	183 (76.9%)	195 (79%)
Patients with wall impressions caused by extraluminal structures	55 (23.1%)	52 (21%)
Transient impression or not classified	6 (10.9%)	8/52 (15.4%)
Neighboring organs	32 (58.2%) (10 spleen, 6 splenic vessels, 9 gallbladder, 3 liver, 3 pancreas, 1 intestine)	30/52 (57.7%) (16 splenic vessels, 4 spleen, 4 aorta, 2 intestine, 1 pancreas, 2 liver, 1 uterus)
Benign lesions	12 (21.8%) (7 hepatic cysts, 2 hepatic hemangiomas, 1 splenic cyst, 2 pancreatic cysts)	9/52 (17.3%) (3 pancreatic cysts, 3 cases of gallbladder pathology: cholecystitis, hydrops, concealed gallbladder perforation, 1 hematoma; 1 liver cyst, 1 splenic tumor)
Malignant tumors	5 (9.1%) (3 hepatic tumors, 1 pancreatic tumor, 1 splenic tumor)	5/52 (9.6%) (2 pancreatic tumors, 1 splenic tumor, 1 liver tumor, 1 malignant lymphoma)

Subepithelial Tumors versus Extramural Impressions (Lesions Mimicking Subepithelial Tumors)

Endoscopic ultrasound is a highly reliable method for differentiating between subepithelial lesions and wall impressions caused by extramural lesions.[3,27,32–37] There is high interobserver agreement in the diagnosis of extramural lesions causing wall protrusion.[38] In comparison with other methods such as barium contrast, endoscopy with biopsy, and computed tomography (CT), EUS shows considerable superiority in the diagnosis of such lesions, and should therefore be regarded as the investigation of first choice.[21,23–25,39] There have been numerous studies reporting that among lesions endoscopically suspected to be subepithelial tumors, the proportion of extramural lesions causing wall impressions is in the range of 14–42%.[24,32,33,40,41] In our own patients, we found extramural impression effects in 17.6% (74 of 420) of endosonographic examinations conducted for suspected subepithelial tumors.[15] Extramural wall protrusions of this type are usually caused by neighboring structures such as the splenic artery, spleen, gallbladder, pancreas, liver, ovaries, uterus, or occasionally the intestine. More rarely, benign pathological changes in neighboring organs can cause wall impressions mimicking subepithelial tumors. In the upper gastrointestinal tract, such lesions may be cysts in the liver, pancreas, or spleen, mediastinal cysts, inflammatory lesions of the gallbladder or pancreas, benign tumors of the liver and spleen, adrenal gland adenomas, arteriovenous malformations, or arterial aneurysms. Only very rarely are external wall impressions caused by malignant tumors of the neighboring organs (e.g., carcinoma of the gallbladder, colon, pancreas, left adrenal gland, uterus or ovary, pleural, peritoneal and mediastinal malignancies, or lymphoma)[5,23,26,32,33,42,43] (**Table 14.1**, **Figs. 14.5**, **14.6**, **14.7** and **14.8**).

Pitfalls

- High-frequency ultrasound miniprobes have a limited depth of penetration. They make it possible to exclude subepithelial tumors, but they are often insufficient to allow detailed imaging and diagnosis of extramural structures which cause external wall impressions (**Fig. 14.9**).
- When using a curvilinear echoendoscope, it is possible to mistake a hypertrophied pyloric sphincter for a subepithelial tumor in the fourth hypoechoic layer, especially if the hypertrophy is asymmetrical (**Figs. 14.10** and **14.11**).
- Gastrointestinal stromal tumors (GISTs), especially in the stomach, may be connected to the fourth hypoechoic layer (tunica muscularis propria) only by a thin stalk, with the remainder of the tumor being located extraluminally (**Fig. 14.12**). Such tumors, especially epithelioid GISTs, are easily mistaken for a malignant lymph node, because their morphology and echogenicity may be very similar.[44,45] If a fine-needle biopsy of such a tumor is carried out in the expectation of obtaining material from a suspicious lymph node, there is a danger that a GIST may be wrongly diagnosed as a metastasis from an epithelial malignancy.[44]

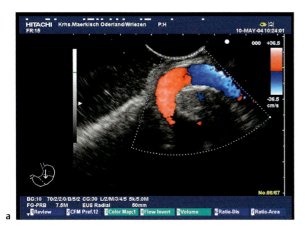

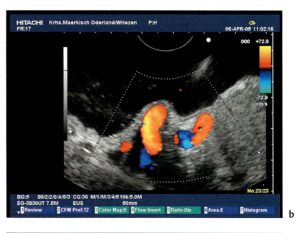

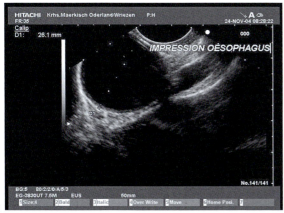

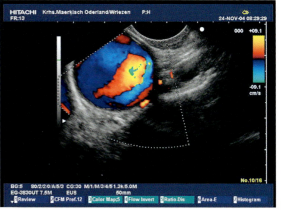

Fig. 14.5a–d Impressions on the gastric wall caused by adjacent vessels.
a, b Impressions on the gastric fundus made by elongated splenic arteries.

c, d An impression on the upper esophagus made by the aortic arch (**c**, gray-scale image; **d,** color-coded view).

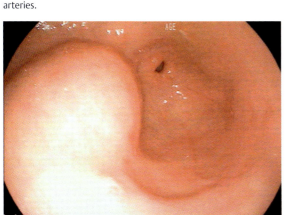

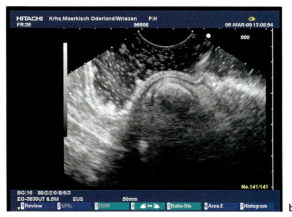

Fig. 14.6a–c Impressions on the gastric wall caused by gallbladder pathology.
a, b Concealed gallbladder perforation (**a** endoscopic view, **b** EUS image).
c A sludge-filled gallbladder, with wall thickening and small calcifications (chronic cholecystitis).

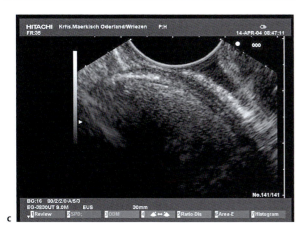

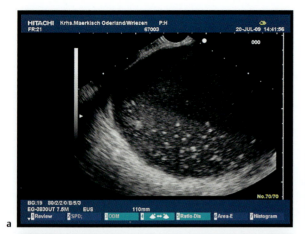

a

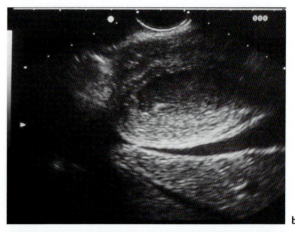

b

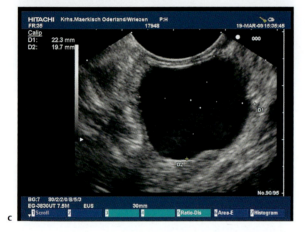

c

Fig. 14.7a–c Impressions on the gastric wall caused by cystic mass lesions.
a An infected pancreatic pseudocyst.
b Liver abscess in a patient with an acute attack of chronic pancreatitis.
c A cyst in the left liver lobe.

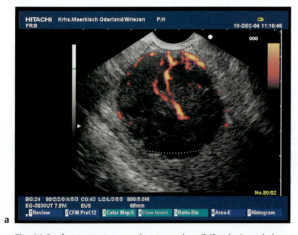

a

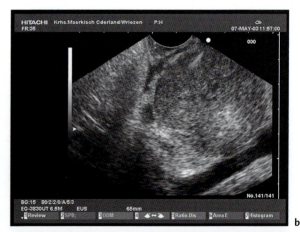

b

Fig. 14.8a, b Impressions on the stomach wall (fundus) made by a tumor of the spleen (**a**) and a large carcinoma in the pancreatic tail (**b**).

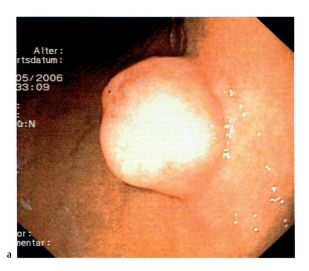

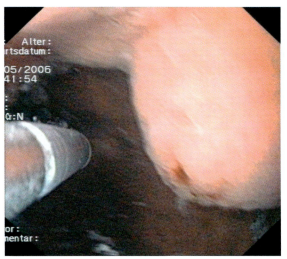

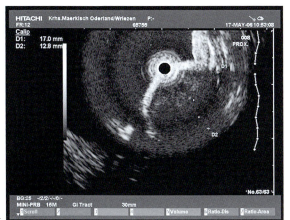

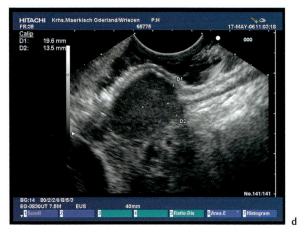

Fig. 14.9a–d A medium-sized gastrointestinal stromal tumor (GIST) in the stomach.
a Endoscopic view.
b, c Attempted examination with a high-frequency ultrasound mini-probe. Delineation of the layer of origin turned out to be impossible due to the limited penetration depth.

d The longitudinal echoendoscope (7.5 MHz) makes it possible to detect the origin of the hypoechoic subepithelial tumor, in the fourth echolayer (muscularis propria).

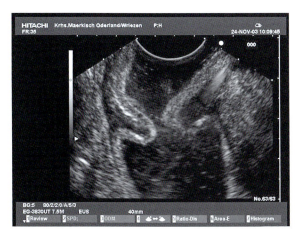

Fig. 14.10 Symmetric hypertrophy of the pyloric sphincter.

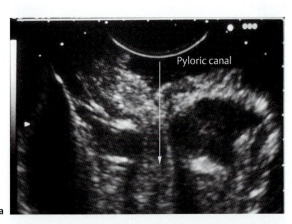
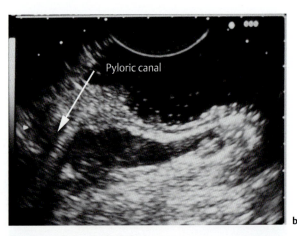

Fig. 14.11a, b Asymmetric hypertrophy of the pyloric sphincter (**a**, transverse view; **b**, longitudinal view).

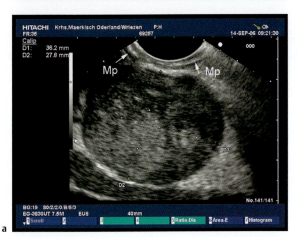
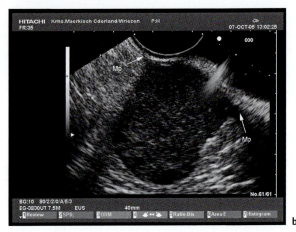

Fig. 14.12a, b Examples of gastrointestinal stromal tumors (GISTs) in the stomach, with predominantly extraluminal growth. Mp, muscularis propria.

Endosonographic Description and Classification of Subepithelial Lesions

All of the echoendoscopes currently available (mechanical and electronic radial echoendoscopes, electronic curvilinear-array echoendoscopes), as well as high-frequency miniprobes, provide detailed views of the wall structure of gastrointestinal organs and make it possible to determine from which layer of the wall subepithelial lesions originate[4,37,46,47] (**Fig. 14.13**). In addition, it is generally possible to measure the size of a lesion in two imaging planes. Two previous studies have demonstrated that EUS measures the subepithelial tumor size accurately in comparison with surgically resected specimens, with the exception of large lesions that extend beyond the sonographic penetration depth.[25,48]

Practical Hints

- Particularly important for follow-up studies: results obtained with radial scanning echoendoscopes (width and thickness) cannot be directly compared with measurements obtained with longitudinal scanning echoendoscopes (thickness and longitudinal diameter).
- High-frequency miniprobes are particularly useful in subepithelial lesions with a diameter of less than 20 mm, especially if an endoscopic therapeutic intervention is planned for the same session.[46,47,49–51]
- In the investigation of subepithelial tumors, EUS not only provides B-mode views of the lesion. In addition, it is also possible to study the perfusion of a lesion using color-coded duplex sonography[52] (**Fig. 14.14**) and to perform endoscopic ultrasound-guided fine-needle aspiration (EUS-FNA) (**Fig. 14.15**)[18,19,54–75,206] as well as EUS-guided Tru-Cut biopsies (EUS-TCB).[76–78] In addition, EUS-guided injection can be used to separate submucosal tumors from the muscular layer before endoscopic resection.[81] In selected cases, EUS has been used to assist in the obliteration of subepithelial vascular malformations[82] and for EUS-guided injection of ethanol or cyanoacrylate for treatment of bleeding GISTs.[83,84]

III Gastrointestinal Tract

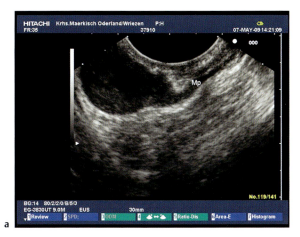

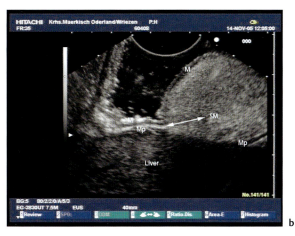

Fig. 14.13a, b Identifying the layer of origin of subepithelial tumors. **a** A gastric leiomyoma, originating from the fourth hypoechoic sonolayer. Mp, muscularis propria.

b A large gastric lipoma, originating from the third hyperechoic sonolayer (submucosa) and covered by the second hypoechoic sonolayer (mucosa). M, mucosa; Mp, muscularis propria; SM, submucosa.

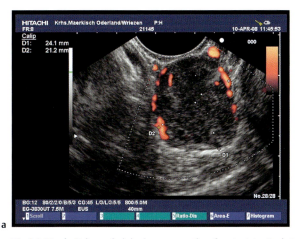

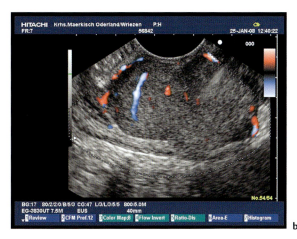

Fig. 14.14a, b Color-coded duplex sonography of gastrointestinal stromal tumors (GISTs) in the stomach.

- If the body of the stomach, the rectum, or the duodenum are being examined, we recommend filling the lumen of these organs in order to obtain adequate acoustic coupling. When the esophagus or gastric antrum are being examined, it may sometimes be helpful to use water-filled balloons.
- Good technique is essential to be able to measure the longitudinal extent of a tumor, to determine which mural layer it arises from, and to study its internal structure. Especially if a curvilinear-array echoendoscope is being used, one should remember to advance and retract slowly, to ensure optimal flexion of the tip of the endoscope, and to make certain that the endoscope attaches to the central longitudinal axis of the tumor.

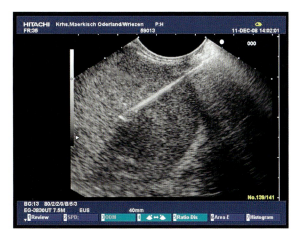

Fig. 14.15 EUS-guided fine-needle aspiration (EUS-FNA) of a hypoechoic subepithelial tumor (gastrointestinal stromal tumor) in the gastric body.

Table 14.2 Endoscopic ultrasound description of subepithelial lesions

Endoscopic findings
Localization
Changes in the mucosa in the area of the protrusion (e.g., erythema, lymphangiectasia, erosions, ulceration, blood clots, active bleeding, color) • Sessile versus pedunculated • Additional findings: central nidus, consistency, mobility, pillow sign, tenting
Endosonographic findings
Diameter measured in two orthogonal planes
Layer of origin (possible/not possible to determine; 2nd hypoechoic layer–3rd hyperechoic layer–4th hypoechoic layer; extramural)
Margin (smooth/irregular)
Can the lesion be distinguished from neighboring structures? (Yes/no; cannot be separated from ...; clearly infiltrates ...)
Are the covering layers intact? (No mucosal defect; localized mucosal defect, mucosal and submucosal defect = ulceration; ulceration extending into the tumor)
Solid; cystic; mixed solid and cystic
Echogenicity (anechoic, hypoechoic, hyperechoic/mixed echogenicity)
Texture (homogeneous, inhomogeneous—diffusely inhomogeneous versus inhomogeneous with defined internal structures)
Defined internal structures: echogenic strains; echogenic spots (without echo extinction); calcification (echogenic reflexes with echo extinction); tubular structures; cystic structures: solitary/some/multiple
Other findings
If possible: show presence of blood vessels on color-coded duplex sonography (CCDS); estimate perfusion with color power angio (CPA) mode: no/some/multiple perfusion signals
Suspicious-looking local or regional lymph nodes (morphology, location, number)
Any hepatic lesions (in the parts of the liver that are visible): morphology, location, number
Free fluid in the peritoneal cavity; pleural effusion

Table 14.3 Classification of subepithelial lesions

Vascular
Varices
Vascular malformations and hemangiomas
Cystic
Simple cysts (solitary or multiple)
Polycystic/septated cyst
Mixed solid cystic lesions
Solid
Hyperechoic (homogeneous, heterogeneous, inhomogeneous)
Hypoechoic (homogeneous, heterogeneous, inhomogeneous)
Mixed echogenicity (heterogeneous)

The endosonographic classification of subepithelial tumors is based on their outline, echogenicity, echohomogeneity, and internal echo pattern, as well as their demarcation from or infiltration of adjacent layers.[15] Their echogenicity is compared with the muscularis propria (low echogenicity), the submucosal layer (high echogenicity), and to the lumen of the organ being examined, which should be filled with water or with water-filled balloons and therefore be anechoic.[40,85] Some authors differentiate echogenicity in greater detail by also using the parenchyma of the spleen for comparison.[86] Further criteria that can be used to classify subepithelial tumors are the extent of compressibility using the tip of the echoendoscope, the presence of ulceration, the presence of sonomorphologically abnormal or enlarged lymph-nodes, and the presence of a connection between the intramural lesion and extramural structures[12,15,27,40,41] (**Table 14.2**).

Using electronic echoendoscopes with color-coded Doppler and color power angio functions makes it possible to assess the perfusion of subepithelial structures, which may sometimes simplify and accelerate the diagnostic process.[52,53] As a modification of the classification used by Hizawa et al.,[40] we suggest classifying subepithelial lesions according to the categories shown in **Table 14.3**.[15]

The criteria specified in **Tables 14.2** and **14.3** should enable the examiner to determine the type of lesion and to judge whether or not the lesion may have malignant potential. In addition, the criteria should be helpful in deciding which further investigations and therapeutic options may be indicated. Numerous examiners have attempted to correlate the histopathological characteristics of subepithelial lesions with specific sonomorphological findings (**Table 14.4**).

Pitfalls
• The degree of "echogenicity" is a very subjective criterion in relation to stromal tumors of the gastrointestinal tract. A study comparing the findings of five experienced endosonographers found very poor interobserver reproducibility, with a kappa value of 0.12.[87] • In small lesions close to the transducer (e.g., in the esophagus), it is very difficult to differentiate between anechogenicity and low echogenicity. This can lead to diagnostic errors (e.g., cyst versus leiomyoma)[88] (**Fig. 14.16**). • The echogenicity of subepithelial tumors depends on their cellular density—the higher this is, the lower the echogenicity—and also on the number and size of internal structures such as cysts or blood vessels. Numerous small cystic changes or small blood vessels evoke numerous interface reflections and can cause a paradoxically high echogenicity.[86,89,90] • Although no comparative studies have been published, the echogenicity of a lesion and its homogeneity appear to depend on the scanning frequency used, as well as on the various physical parameters and settings of the ultrasound system.

Table 14.4 Endoscopic ultrasound criteria in subepithelial lesions

Echogenicity	Type of lesion	Wall layers	Tumor characteristics
Anechoic	Cysts (various types)	3 (submucosa) extramural	Dorsal enhancement
	Varices	3 (submucosa) extramural	Vascular structure can be followed, perfusion imaging, perforating veins
	Lymphangioma	3 (submucosa)	Frequently polypoid and polycystic, no perfusion, compressible
	Cavernous hemangioma	3 (submucosa)	Polycystic appearance, perfusion visible
Hypoechoic	Gastrointestinal mesenchymal tumor (GIST, leiomyoma, schwannoma)	4 (muscularis propria) or 2 (muscularis mucosae)	Leiomyomas: usually in the esophagus and in the second hypoechoic layer of the lower gastrointestinal tract; GISTs: usually in the stomach
	Granular cell tumor (Abrikosov tumor)	3 (submucosa) and 4 (muscularis propria)	Usually homogeneous with smooth margin, usually < 20 mm, frequently in the esophagus
	Neuroendocrine tumors (carcinoids)	3 (submucosa), possibly no margin to layers 2 and 4	"Pepper-and-salt" appearance of inner texture, round, smooth margins, visible perfusion, usually in the rectum and duodenum
	Inflammatory fibroid polyps	2 (muscularis mucosae) and 3 (submucosa)	Usually with poorly defined margins, homogeneously low echogenicity, usually in the stomach
	Metastases	Do not respect layers	
	Submucosal cancer	Layers poorly defined or lost	Mixed homogeneity, possibly lymphadenopathy
	Lymphoma	Layers 2–4, separation lost	Multinodular, homogeneously low echogenicity, lymphadenopathy possible
	Rarely: amyloid, focal inflammation, endometriosis		
Hyperechoic	Lipoma, fibrolipoma	3 (submucosa)	Homogeneous echogenicity (possibly some slight irregularities)
Mixed echogenicity	Heterotopic pancreas	3 (submucosa)	Internal structure showing ducts or microcysts; central "umbilicuslike" indentation, usually in the gastric antrum
	Malignant mesenchymal tumors (GIST, leiomyosarcoma)	Usually 4 (muscularis propria) as origin, but often does not respect layers	Characteristic findings: containing cysts or hyperechoic structures, irregular margin, size > 40 mm, exophytic growth
	Fibrovascular polyp	3 (submucosa)	Polypoid
	Spontaneous esophageal hematoma	3 (submucosa)	Overall low echogenicity with discrete hyperechoic foci
	Wall abscess	3 (submucosa)	Possibly gaseous inclusions

GIST, gastrointestinal stromal tumor.

The diagnosis of vascular subepithelial lesions can usually also be made if color-coded Doppler sonography (CCDS) is not available.[91] If the diagnosis has not already been made by conventional endoscopy, varices can easily be recognized by following their course, by their compressibility, and by demonstration of extramural collateral vessels. However, the diagnosis can be made more quickly using CCDS, and additional information can be obtained—for example, a portosplenic thrombosis may be recognized (**Figs. 14.17, 14.18** and **14.19**).

Intramural cavernous hemangiomas are very rare,[92,93] but they can be diagnosed much more easily using CCDS (**Fig. 14.20**).

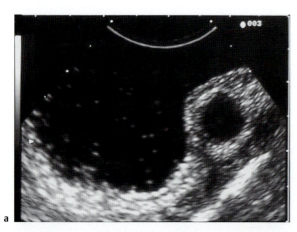

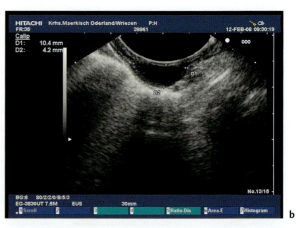

Fig. 14.16a, b It is difficult to distinguish between small, anechoic lesions and subepithelial tumors with low echogenicity. Are these cysts or solid, hypoechoic tumors in the gastric wall (**a**) or esophageal wall (**b**)?

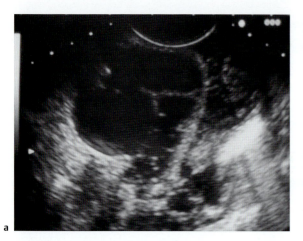

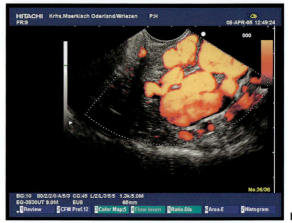

Fig. 14.17a, b Vascular subepithelial lesions: giant varices in the cardia.

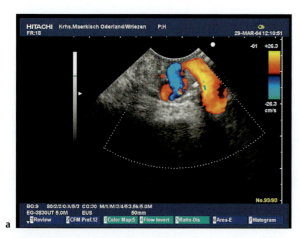

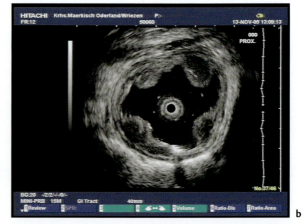

Fig. 14.18a, b Vascular subepithelial lesions
a Varices in the gastric body.

b Esophageal varices (15-MHz miniprobe).

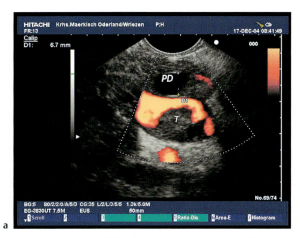

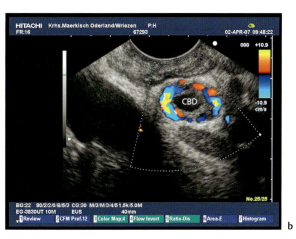

a

b

Fig. 14.19a, b a Portal thrombosis (T) as a consequence of an acute attack of chronic pancreatitis. PD, dilated pancreatic duct.

b Bile duct varices as a consequence of portal thrombosis in a patient with acute pancreatitis. CBD, common bile duct.

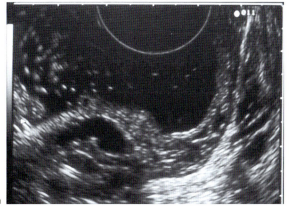

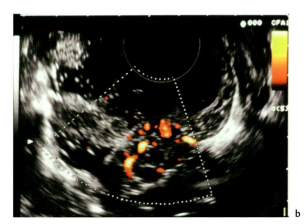

a

b

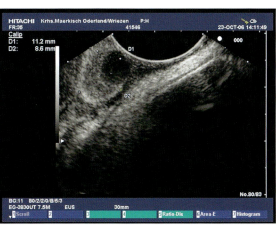

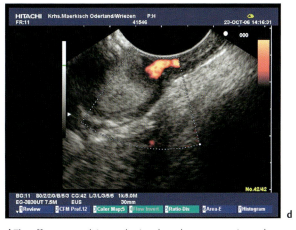

c

d

Fig. 14.20a–f Cavernous hemangioma
a–c A cavernous hemangioma in the rectum (**a, b**) and gastric cardia (**c**, B-mode image).

d The afferent vessel, imaged using the color-power angio mode.
Fig. 14.20e, f ▷

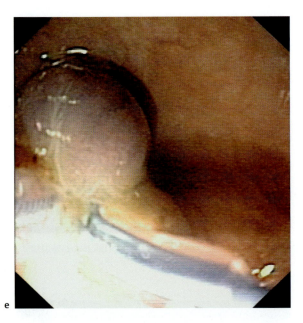

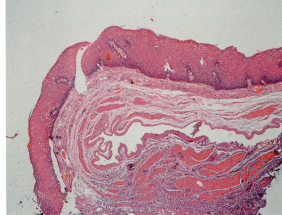

Fig. 14.20e, f (continued) **e** Endolooping and endoscopic resection of the lesion.
f Histological image of the resected specimen (hematoxylin–eosin, original magnification ×40). (Courtesy of S. Wagner, Königswusterhausen, Germany.)

Table 14.5 Endoscopic ultrasound of cystic subepithelial lesions

Simple cystic	Duplication cysts
	Bronchogenic cysts
	Heterotopic gastric mucosa
	Rare: • Brunner gland hamartoma • Mucocele • Intramural pancreatic pseudocyst • Abscess of the stomach wall (low echogenicity) • Pancreatic heterotopia
Multicystic	Lymphangioma
	Heterotopic gastric mucosa and gastritis cystica profunda
	Brunner gland hamartoma
Solid cystic	Pancreatic heterotopia
	Lymphangioma
	Rare: • Tuberculoma • GIST with cystic degeneration

■ Cystic and Mixed Solid Cystic Subepithelial Lesions

Anechoic nonvascular subepithelial lesions account for a large variety of underlying diagnoses. They may represent different types of cysts (bronchogenic cysts, duplication cysts),[55,94,95,103,104,106] mucosal heterotopia located in the submucosal layer,[40,101,116] Brunner gland hamartomas,[113–115] cystic lymphangiomas (lymphatic cysts),[89,101,108,110] or more rarely pancreatic heteroto-

pias,[111] mesenchymal tumors with cystic degeneration,[105,112] gastritis (colitis) cystica profunda,[117–119] tuberculomas, mural abscesses or empyema,[97–99,120–122] or mucoceles.[100,109]

This multitude of differential diagnoses makes it difficult to reach a confident diagnosis. To simplify the diagnostic process, the examiner should differentiate between simple cystic lesions, polycystic/septated lesions, and mixed solid cystic subepithelial lesions[15,40,101] (**Table 14.5**).

Simple submucosal cysts have been found endosonographically in the esophagus, in the stomach, in the duodenum, and near the cecal pole.[100,109] Simple submucosal cysts are round anechoic lesions with a smooth margin that can only be slightly compressed with the tip of the echoendoscope and which show dorsal enhancement. Occasionally, sedimented debris can be seen in the lumen of the cyst. Duplication cysts can usually be recognized through a duplicated wall, although this is not always visible. In appropriate cases, EUS-FNA can be helpful for further diagnostic and therapeutic management.[5,37,55,94–96,103–106]

Cystic and cavernous lymphangiomas are the most frequently encountered polycystic subepithelial lesions. They are usually found in the small and large intestine, more rarely in the stomach, and very rarely in the esophagus. They are benign lesions that consist of cavities or dilated lymphatic vessels situated in the submucosal or mucosal layers. Their inner wall is covered by an epithelial layer, and they are subdivided by irregular septal structures that consist of smooth muscle or connective tissue. Depending on their size and location, they may occasionally cause symptoms. Endoscopically, they usually appear as soft, broad-based polypoid structures, which are covered with normal or erythematous mucosa. They are easily compressible with forceps. In the duodenum and small intestine, it is often possible to find mucosal lymphangiectasia, evident from multiple dot-shaped whitish mucosal elevations. Somewhat more rarely, cystic lymphangiomas may have a pedicle.[107] Endosonographically, lymphangiomas are usually found in the third hyperechoic layer, although sessile lesions in particular may extend to the second hypoechoic layer. The endosonographic picture may vary depending on the size and number of the dilated lymphatic vessels and depending on the extent to which bundles of smooth muscle and connective tissue subdivide the lesion. If the lymphangioma consists of moderately dilated tortuous lymphatic vessels, or if it contains small cysts, EUS will usually show multiple hypoechoic or anechoic structures, possibly with hyperechoic subdivisions. Such lymphangiomas may also appear as simple or septated round or oval anechoic lesions in the third hyperechoic layer (**Fig. 14.21**). However, if the lymphatic vessels are very small (diameter < 1 mm), the lymphangioma will appear as a slightly inhomogeneous submucosal tumor with medium echogenicity.[89,101,107-110]

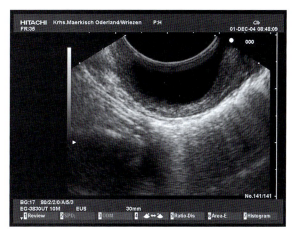

Fig. 14.21 A submucosal lymphangioma in the esophagus.

Heterotopia of the gastric mucosa, submucosal hyperplasia of Brunner glands, submucosal hamartomas, enteral cysts. A very similar appearance with the same endosonographic localization in layers 2 and 3 can be found for the different types of subepithelial heterotopia of the gastric, duodenal, and enteral mucosa (**Figs. 14.22** and **14.23**).[40,113-116] The range of endosonographic findings extends from simple submucosal cysts, which may also be multiple, through polycystic lesions with hyperechoic septa, to inhomogeneous hyperechoic submucosal tumors with small cystic areas. A special scenario is gastritis cystica profunda, which appears as a polycystic lesion and can often be found near the anastomosis after gastric surgery[117,118] (**Fig. 14.24**).

Endoscopically, these lesions appear as broad-based or stalked polyps. Subepithelial heterotopia of the gastric mucosa in Japanese patients is frequently (19–100%) associated with gastric cancer, particularly if multiple lesions are present. Occasionally, the carcinoma may arise from the subepithelial heterotopia (**Fig. 14.25**).[101,116-119,123,124]

Heterotopic pancreatic tissue (aberrant or ectopic pancreas). A further differential diagnosis of mixed solid cystic, heterogeneous solid, and rarely of cystic subepithelial lesions is heterotopic pancreas, which is usually located in the stomach, or more rarely in the esophagus, the small intestine, the duodenum, the papilla, or in other organs. Its incidence in autopsy series varies between 0.6% and 13.7%.[125] It is typically diagnosed incidentally during endoscopy, surgery, or postmortem examination. Rarely, it causes symptoms such as gastric outlet obstruction or intestinal obstruction, ulceration and bleeding, obstructive jaundice, ectopic pancreatitis, cystic

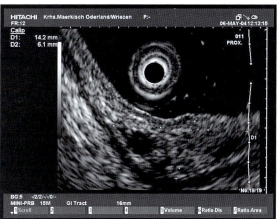

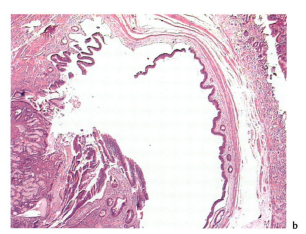

Fig. 14.22a, b Submucosal cystic heterotopia in the gastric mucosa, situated in the gastric antrum.
a Radial 15-MHz ultrasound miniprobe.
b Histological confirmation after endoscopic resection. (Histological image courtesy of S. Wagner and S. Bartho, Königswusterhausen, Germany).

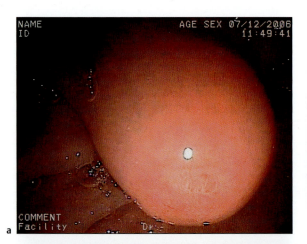

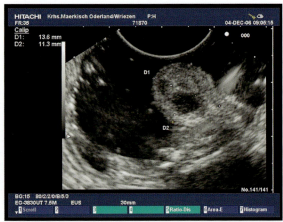

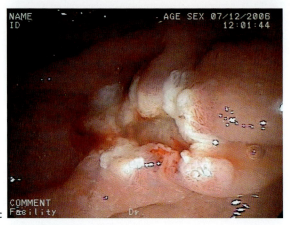

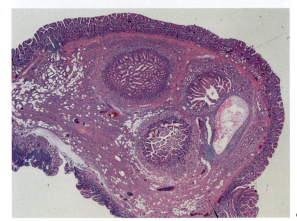

Fig. 14.23a–d A subepithelial solid cystic lesion in the descending duodenum, near the papilla.
a Endoscopic image.
b EUS image.

c Endoscopic snare resection.
d Histological diagnosis of an enterogenic cyst (hematoxylin–eosin, original magnification ×40). (Courtesy of S. Wagner, Königswusterhausen, Germany.)

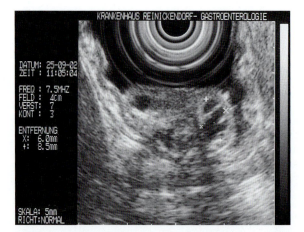

Fig. 14.24 Gastritis cystica profunda close to the anastomosis after a Billroth II gastrectomy (with a mechanical radial echoendoscope). (Courtesy of M. Mayr, Berlin).

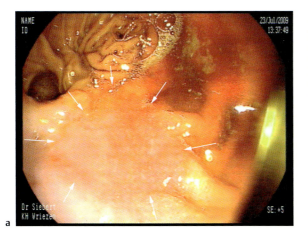
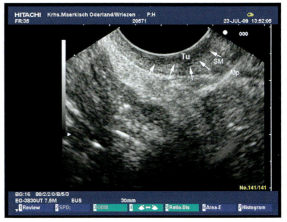
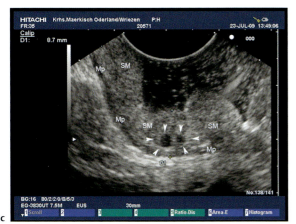
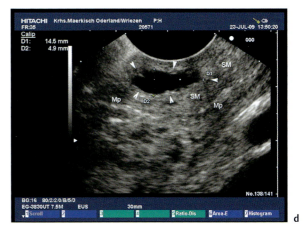

Fig. 14.25a–d Submucosal cysts in a patient presenting with cancer of the gastric remnant 20 years after partial gastric resection because of complicated ulcer disease.
a A flat-depressed lesion near the anastomosis (arrows): histologically confirmed adenocarcinoma.

b EUS image of the hypoechoic thickening of the mucosa, focally infiltrating the submucosal layer (arrows): stage T1a cancer. Mp, muscularis propria; SM, submucosa; Tu, tumor.
c, d EUS image of cysts (arrowheads) in the thickened submucosal layer of the gastric remnant. Mp, muscularis propria; SM, submucosa.

dystrophy, and pseudocyst development.[125–134] Adenocarcinoma, mucinous neoplasia, or neuroendocrine tumor arising within ectopic pancreas are very rare occurrences.[135–140,281] The endosonographic appearance is determined by the histological type of the lesion.[141,142] Type I heterotopia consists of complete pancreatic tissue (acini, ducts, Langerhans islets), type II of pancreatic tissue without any ducts, and type III of pancreatic ducts only. Heinrich type III ectopic pancreas is traditionally also known as adenomyoma.[143] Type III pancreatic heterotopia as well as pancreatic heterotopia with pseudocyst may appear as a simple or septated anechoic lesion with smooth margins, which is located in the third echogenic layer.[105,144] Heinrich types I and II pancreatic heterotopia appear as heterogeneous and hypoechoic subepithelial lesions with poorly defined margins, finely scattered hyperechoic spots, and occasionally calcifications, and in about one-third of cases with small cystic spaces and ductlike structures.[40,101,141,142,145] The irregular margins are caused by lobulated acinar tissue, and the mixed echogenicity is due

to ducts, small cysts, lobulated tissue, areas of fat, and bundles of muscle fibers.[141] A characteristic feature of submucosal pancreatic heterotopia is a thickening of the fourth layer adjacent to the mass. In a series of 10 pancreatic heterotopias located in the stomach that were studied both endosonographically and histologically, five were only located in the third echogenic layer (submucosa) and were easily differentiated from the fourth layer (separate type, **Fig. 14.26c, d, Fig. 14.50a**). In the remaining five cases, the lesion extended into the third echogenic and fourth hypoechoic layer (fusion type, **Fig. 14.26a, b**).[141] When the endoscopic findings (usually situated in the gastral antrum, central umbilication) are also taken into account, pancreatic heterotopia may be diagnosed endosonographically with a reasonable degree of certainty (**Fig. 14.26b, Fig. 14.50b**).[142,146] In a study of six patients, an endosonographically suspected diagnosis of pancreatic heterotopia was confirmed histologically in all cases after endoscopic resection.[88]

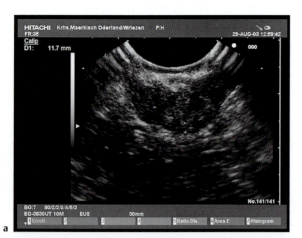

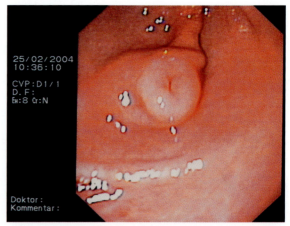

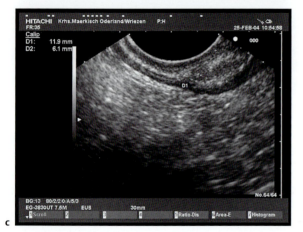

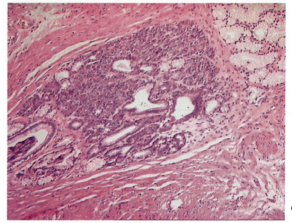

Fig. 14.26a–d Heterotopic pancreatic tissue in the stomach.
a The typical EUS features of the fusion type—i. e., with the muscular layer also affected, as confirmed histologically after surgical resection.
b–d The separate type—i. e., with only the submucosa affected.

b The endoscopic image, with central umbilication.
c The EUS appearance.
d Histological confirmation after endoscopic resection (histological image courtesy of S. Bartho and S. Wagner, Königswusterhausen, Germany).

Solid Subepithelial Lesions

Echogenic subepithelial tumors—lipomas, fibromas, and fibrovascular polyps. Lipomas are the most common echogenic subepithelial lesions. They usually appear as flat or sessile polypoid lesions, although they may have a stalk. They are classically located in the right colon, but can also appear in the stomach and duodenum. Frequently, an endosonographic examination is not required if the endoscopic findings are unequivocal (slightly yellow shimmering through the mucosa, pillow sign).[12,27] Endosonographically, lipomas appear as intensely hyperechoic, entirely homogeneous well-demarcated lesions located in the third echogenic layer (submucosa). Some inhomogeneities can sometimes be seen, particularly if the tumor is large[12,23,25,27,36,37,40,109,147] (**Fig. 14.27**).

Interobserver agreement for diagnosing a lipoma is good.[38] The differential diagnosis includes fibromas and, in the esophagus, fibrovascular polyps (fibrolipomas). The latter consist of a mixture of mesenchymal tissues and also contain fatty tissue. Only the lipomatous areas appear homogeneously echogenic, whereas the fibrous and muscular parts of these polyps show less echogenicity.[148]

In exceptional cases, inflammatory fibroid polyps (IFPs) may appear hyperechoic if numerous small blood vessels cause multiple interface reflections.[86,149]

Hypoechoic subepithelial tumors are a very heterogeneous group. In our own patients, 247 of 346 (71.4%) nonvascular subepithelial lesions showed low echogenicity.[15] They present the examiner with several problems. The range of diagnoses includes benign tumors such as leiomyomas, glomus tumors, granular cell tumors, schwannomas, pancreatic heterotopias, and inflammatory fibroid polyps (IFPs), but also includes (potentially) malignant lesions such as gastrointestinal stromal tumors (GISTs), neuroendocrine tumors, leiomyosarcomas, malignant lymphoma (**Fig. 14.28**), and submucosal metastases.[13] Very rarely, amyloidosis,[150] endometriosis,[63,109,151,152] cav-

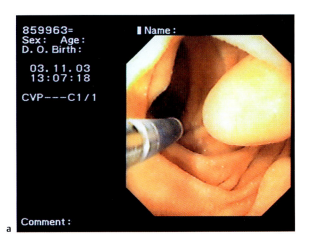

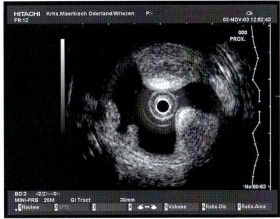

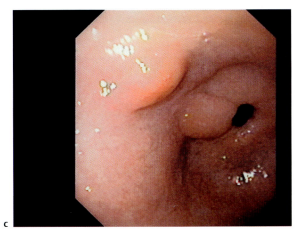

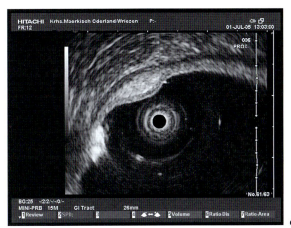

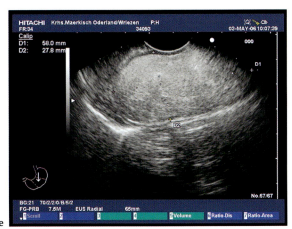

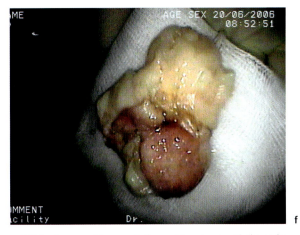

Fig. 14.27a–f Submucosal lipomas in the upper gastrointestinal tract.

a In the water-filled duodenal lumen, a radial 15-MHz ultrasound miniprobe has been introduced through the endoscope's working channel.

b The corresponding EUS image (15-MHz miniprobe).

c, d Flat submucosal lipomas in the gastric antrum, with the endoscopic view (**c**) and corresponding EUS image (15-MHz miniprobe) (**d**).

e, f A huge lipoma in the gastric body, with the EUS image (**e**) and endoscopically resected tumor (**f**). For the corresponding endoscopic images, see **Fig. 14.2c, d.**

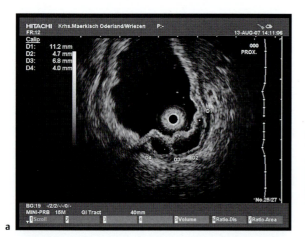

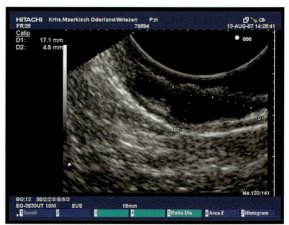

a

b

Fig. 14.28a, b Endosonographic images of a submucosal mantle cell lymphoma in the gastric body (images reproduced with permission from Jenssen and Dietrich[15]).

a Examination with the 15-MHz ultrasound miniprobe.
b With the longitudinal echoendoscope.

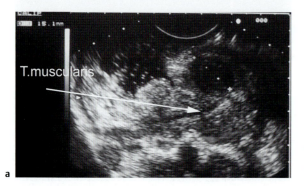

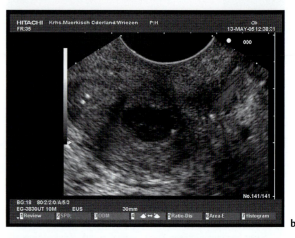

a

b

Fig. 14.29a, b Submucosal abscesses following acute episodes of chronic pancreatitis.

ernous hemangiomas,[92,93] tuberculosis, inflammatory tumors, and abscesses[98,99,122] (**Fig. 14.29**) may present as hypoechoic subepithelial lesions.

Gastrointestinal stromal tumors (GISTs) represent the largest group of mesenchymal tumors of the gastrointestinal tract and include tumors with a very variable clinicopathological spectrum and biological behavior. The most common locations are the stomach (60%), small bowel (30%), and duodenum (5%). Only small numbers of cases have been detected in the large bowel (< 5%), lower esophagus and appendix (< 1%), and in the omentum, mesenteries, or retroperitoneum.[153–155] In the early large endosonographic series,[21,23,25,36,37,39] hypoechoic mesenchymal tumors arising from one of the two muscular layers and histologically showing either a spindle cell or an epithelioid structure were either classified as myogenic tumors (leiomyomas, leiomyoblastomas, and leiomyosarcomas) or neurogenic tumors (schwannoma, neurofibroma). GISTs were only recognized as a separate entity fairly recently. They now can be differentiated from leiomyomas

and schwannomas by their immunohistochemical and genetic characteristics[20,75,102,153,155–157] (**Table 14.6**). GISTs are now defined as mesenchymal spindle cell, epithelioid, or rarely pleomorphic tumors of the gastrointestinal tract, which—in contrast to myogenic or neurogenic tumors—are driven by oncogenic, mutational gain-of-function activation of KIT or platelet-derived growth factor receptor-α (PDGFR-α). Most GISTs express KIT protein (stem cell factor receptor protein, CD117) (≈ 95%), the chloride channel protein DOG1 (> 95%), and CD34 (70%)[20,154,155,157,159–162] (**Table 14.6**). Histogenetically, these tumors probably originate from gastrointestinal pacemaker cells (interstitial cells of Cajal) or a pluripotent precursor cell. The relative risk of malignant behavior of a GIST primarily depends on the number of mitoses per 50 high-power fields (HPF), on its size, on certain types of mutation, and on its location in the gastrointestinal tract. If their anatomic site is not taken into consideration, only GISTs smaller than 5 cm and with a low mitotic index (< 5/50 HPFs) have a low risk of malignant behavior.[20,153,163] Taking the anatomic location into account, clinically malignant behavior is less frequent in

III Gastrointestinal Tract

Table 14.6 Gastrointestinal mesenchymal tumors: histological and immunohistochemical characterization (data from[16,154–157,160–162,173,175,176,244,291])

Myogenic tumors (leiomyoma, glomus tumor, leiomyosarcoma)

Leiomyoma: 75% spindle cell pattern, 25% epithelioid pattern; always benign; in the esophagus in almost all cases arising from the muscularis propria, in the large intestine preferentially from the muscularis mucosae

Immune phenotype:
- Positive: smooth muscle actin (SMA) (100%), desmin (100%)
- Negative: NSE, PGP9.5, S100, CD117, CD 34, DOG1, vimentin

Leiomyosarcoma: very rare, arising always from the muscularis propria

Immune phenotype:
- Positive: SMA (100%), desmin (63%)
- Occasionally positive: CD34
- Negative: CD117

Neurogenic tumors (peripheral nerve sheath tumors = schwannoma)

Rare, usually located in the stomach, very rarely in the esophagus or intestine

Nearly always benign

Typically spindle cell pattern, rarely epithelioid or plexiform pattern

Immune phenotype:
- Positive: S100 (100%), glial fibrillary acidic protein (64–100%), collagen type IV
- Occasionally positive: CD34
- Negative: SMA, desmin, CD117, DOG1

Gastrointestinal stromal tumor (GIST)

70–80% spindle cell type, 20–30% epithelioid type, 10% mixed type

c-kit mutations in 75–80%, PDGFRα mutations in 8%

<5% associated with tumor syndromes (neurofibromatosis type I/ von Recklinghausen disease, Carney triad, familial GIST syndrome)

Association with other malignancies (4.5–33%, mean 13%)

Inherent potential for malignant behavior (stomach 20–25%; small intestine, rectum: 40–50%)

Subgroup: gastrointestinal autonomic nerve tumor (GANT)

Occurrence: 60% stomach, 20–30% small intestine, 5% duodenum, 5% large intestine and rectum, <5% esophagus, 1% extraintestinal

Immune phenotype:
- Positive: CD117 (>90%), DOG1 (>90%), CD34 (overall 60–70%; rectum and esophagus: 95–100%; stomach: 80–85%; small intestine: 50%), vimentin
- Occasionally positive: SMA (20–40%)
- Negative: glial fibrillary acidic protein, desmin (<2%), S100 (<5%)

CD34, transmembrane sialomucin glycoprotein of unknown function; CD117, transmembrane tyrosine kinase receptor protein KIT; c-kit, c-kit proto-oncogene, coding for the transmembrane tyrosine kinase receptor protein KIT; DOG1 (discovered on GIST-1), antibody against a chloride channel protein (protein kinase C theta) of unknown function; NSE, neuron-specific enolase; PDGFRα, platelet-derived growth factor receptor α; PGP9.5, protein gene product 9.5; SMA, smooth muscle actin; S100, dimeric acidic calcium-binding protein, regulating calcium flux of nerve cells.

Table 14.7 Risk assessment of primary gastrointestinal stromal tumors (GISTs) in relation to tumor size and mitotic activity, according to Fletcher et al. 2002[163]

Risk of malignant behavior[a]	Tumor size (cm)	Number of mitoses per HPF[b]
Very low risk	<2	<5/50
Low risk	2–5	<5/50
Intermediate risk	<5	6–10/50
	5–10	<5/50
High risk	>5	>5/50
	>10	Any mitotic rate
	Any size	>10/50

[a] Defined as metastasis or tumor-related death.
[b] High-power field (HPF), defined as the area visible using 400x magnification level.

the case of gastral GISTs (20–25%) in comparison with GISTs located in the small intestine or rectum (40–50%)[154,155,164–166] (**Tables 14.7** and **14.8**).

Older reports need to be viewed in the light of the recent change in the classification of mesenchymal tumors of the gastrointestinal tract. A recent pathological study that examined archived tissue of subepithelial mesenchymal tumors of the gastrointestinal tract, previously classified as smooth-muscle tumors (leiomyomas and leiomyosarcomas), showed that with the exception of esophageal tumors, most of the lesions were actually GISTs.[154,196]

Epidemiological data on the frequency and the natural course of GIST are scarce. The incidence of clinically relevant GISTs is ≈ 10–20 per 1 million people. Most of the tumors are detected in individuals in the fifth or sixth decades of life.[16,155] A recent systematic review has shown that gastrointestinal bleeding is the most common presentation of GIST, with a pooled prevalence of 33%. Other common symptoms are abdominal pain (pooled prevalence 19%), iron-deficiency anemia (8.9%), palpable abdominal mass (6.9%), weight loss (4%), dysphagia (3%), and intestinal obstruction (3%).[17] In large population-based studies, only 15–30% of GISTs were discovered incidentally. On the other hand, very small GISTs (minute GISTs, microscopic GISTs, seedling GISTs, GIST tumorlets: 0.2–12.0 mm) are a very common finding in postmortem examinations and surgical resections of the proximal stomach and esophagogastric junction (9–35%), but not in intestinal resection specimens (≤0.1%) (**Fig. 14.30**).[7,158,167–170]

The clinical presentation of GISTs varies widely and includes incidentally found small benign tumors, tumors of uncertain prognosis, and clinically overt malignant tumors with predominantly hepatic and peritoneal metastases. Conversely, lymph-node metastases are exceedingly rare and occur preferentially in patients under the age of 40.[12,171]

Table 14.8 Risk assessment of primary gastrointestinal stromal tumors (GISTs) in relation to anatomic location, in addition to size and mitotic activity ([241,154 a])

Tumor parameters		Risk of progressive disease by location (%)[b]			
Size (cm)	Number of mitoses (per HPF)[c]	Stomach	Duodenum	Small intestine	Rectum
≤2	≤5/50	None (0)	None (0)	None (0)	None (0)
>2 to ≤5		Very low (1.9)	Low (8.3)	Low (4.3)	Low (8.5)
>5 to ≤10		Low (3.6)	n.a.[e]	Intermediate (24)	n.a.[e]
>10		Intermediate (10)	High (34)	High (52)	High (57)
≤2	>5/50	None (0)[d]	n.a.[e]	High (50)[d]	High (54)
>2 to ≤5		Intermediate (16)	High (50)	High (73)	High 52)
>5 to ≤10		High (55)	n.a.[e]	High (85)	n.a.[e]
>10		High (86)	High (86)	High (90)	High (71)

[a] Data are based on the follow-up observation of 1939 patients with GISTs (1055 gastric, 629 small intestinal, 144 duodenal, 111 rectal).
[b] Defined as metastasis or tumor-related death.
[c] High-power field (HPF), defined as the area visible using 400 × magnification level.
[d] Tumor categories with very few patients.
[e] Not available (n.a.) due to insufficient data.

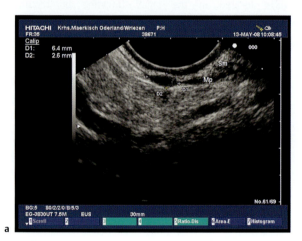 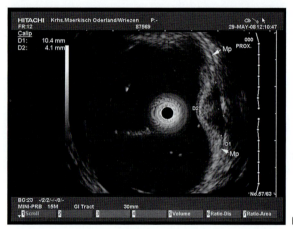

Fig. 14.30a, b "Seedling" mesenchymal subepithelial tumors of the stomach, ≤ 10 mm in size. Mp, muscularis propria; Sm, submucosa.

Leiomyomas (i.e., benign gastrointestinal mesenchymal tumors with muscular differentiation) are most often found in the esophagus, sometimes also in the gastric cardia and colon, and in rare cases in the stomach, small intestine, and rectum. They are related to the second hypoechoic layer (lamina muscularis mucosae) as well as to the fourth hypoechoic layer (tunica muscularis propria). Endosonographically, they appear as homogeneously hypoechoic, sometimes almost anechoic tumors with smooth margins. Occasionally, leiomyomas may contain calcifications (**Fig. 14.31**).[102,156,172,173,183–185,212,216,217]

Leiomyosarcomas are very rare in the gastrointestinal tract and occur in the intestine with a frequency of 2–10% of that of GISTs.[102,155,156,173,185,212,216,217]

Schwannomas (peripheral nerve sheath tumors) are the most infrequent subepithelial mesenchymal tumors of the gastrointestinal tract. Of 191 gastrointestinal mesenchy-

mal tumors evaluated by Kwon et al., only 12 (6.3%) were schwannomas.[174] They originate from the tunica muscularis propria and usually occur in the stomach (60–70%) or colon (20–30%), or rarely in the small intestine, rectum, and esophagus. With regard to their gross morphology, these S100-positive spindle cell, rarely epithelioid and in some cases plexiform tumors resemble GISTs. A peripheral lymphoid cuff is observed in almost all cases; a fibrous capsule, on the other hand, is rare. Gastrointestinal schwannomas always behave in a benign fashion.[156,174–177] Endosonography typically shows very hypoechoic, homogeneous, well-demarcated masses arising from the deep muscle layer with a marginal hypoechoic halo, corresponding to the lymphoid cuff.[178–180]

Depending on their size and age, leiomyomas, low-risk GISTs, and schwannomas may develop regressive changes that appear as anechoic or hyperechoic regions, and they may develop an irregular shape, which may make it diffi-

III Gastrointestinal Tract

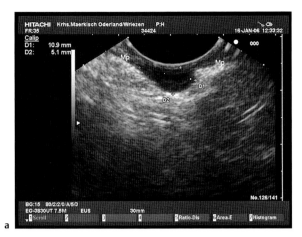
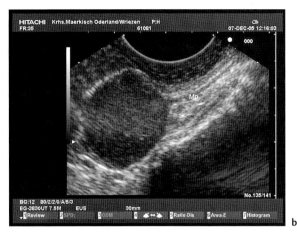

a

b

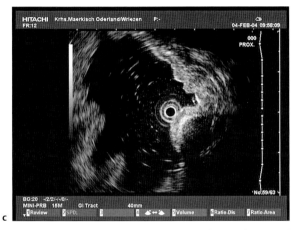
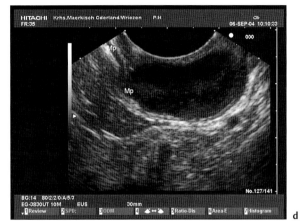

c

d

Fig. 14.31a–d Subepithelial leiomyomas in the esophagus and stomach.
a, b Hypoechoic, homogeneous tumors with smooth margins originating from the fourth echolayer in the esophagus. Mp, muscularis propria.

c A small subepithelial tumor in the gastric body, with extensive calcification and dorsal signal extinction, making it impossible to identify the layer of origin (15-MHz ultrasound miniprobe).
d A leiomyoma in the gastric cardia: very hypoechoic, middle-sized tumor, originating from the fourth sonographic layer. Mp, muscularis propria.

cult or impossible to differentiate them from malignant mesenchymal tumors.

Endosonographic differentiation of subepithelial mesenchymal tumors in the gastrointestinal tract. It is mandatory to distinguish between GISTs and other mesenchymal subepithelial tumors, as leiomyomas and schwannomas are truly benign and their clinical management therefore differs considerably from that of GISTs. However, only two studies, including 77 gastrointestinal mesenchymal tumors, have reported endosonographic differences between GISTs, myogenic, and neurogenic mesenchymal gastrointestinal tumors. A marginal halo is a common feature of both GISTs and schwannomas, but not of leiomyomas. GISTs are usually less hypoechoic than the normal tunica muscularis propria. By contrast, the echogenicity of leiomyomas and schwannomas is quite similar to that of the deep muscle layer. Inhomogeneity of the tumor, hyperechogenic spots and (only in one of the two studies)

lobulation of the tumor surface were observed more frequently in GISTs than in leiomyomas.[181,182] However, endosonographic criteria alone are not sufficient to distinguish reliably between GISTs and other mesenchymal tumors in the gastrointestinal tract.[12,18,27,34,182] In various studies, 74–83% of mesenchymal tumors in the esophagus were small muscle tumors (leiomyoma and very infrequently leiomyosarcoma).[75,157,173,185] Small mesenchymal tumors in the muscularis mucosae of the colon and rectum are always benign leiomyomas.[183] Conversely, a hypoechoic tumor of the stomach has a 69–94% likelihood of being diagnosed as a GIST on histopathological examination.[75,157,196] Similarly, subepithelial mesenchymal tumors in the duodenum (93%)[157,212] and small intestine (83–100%)[186] are most likely to be GISTs. The anatomic location is therefore a more important clue to the differential diagnosis of a hypoechoic tumor of the gastrointestinal tract than subtle differences in the endosonographic appearance.

Table 14.9 Endoscopic ultrasound diagnosis of hypoechoic subepithelial tumors relative to their anatomic location

Esophagus	Leiomyoma	Predominantly lower third, layer 4, rarely layer 2, homogeneous, very hypoechoic, smooth margins
	Abrikosov tumor	Usually layers 3 and 4, homogeneous with smooth margins, nearly always < 20 mm
	Very rare: GIST, leiomyosarcoma, IFP	
Stomach	GIST	Usually layers 2 and 4, more rarely "extramural," variable size and inhomogeneity
	Rare: leiomyoma, schwannoma, neuroendocrine tumor (carcinoid), IFP, metastases, submucosal cancer, lymphoma, pancreatic heterotopia	
	Very rare: leiomyosarcoma, focal inflammation	
Duodenum	Neuroendocrine tumor (carcinoid)	Small, slightly inhomogeneous, usually layers 2 and 3
	Rare: GIST, Abrikosov tumor	
	Very rare: IFP, metastases, lymphoma, amyloid	
Colon	Leiomyoma	Small, homogeneous with smooth margins, usually layer 2
	Rare: GIST, leiomyosarcoma, IFP, Abrikosov tumor, endometriosis	
	Very rare: metastases, lymphoma	
Rectum	Neuroendocrine tumor (carcinoid)	Small, slightly inhomogeneous, usually layers 2 and 3
	Leiomyoma	Small, homogeneous with smooth margins, usually layer 2
	Rare: GIST, leiomyosarcoma, local subepithelial cancer recurrences, Abrikosov tumor, endometriosis	

GIST, gastrointestinal stromal tumor, IFP: inflammatory fibroid polyp.

Pitfalls

- The endosonographic diagnosis of subepithelial tumors is influenced by subjective judgment and the examiner's experience. Observer agreement among 10 experienced sonographers was excellent for recognizing cystic lesions (κ 0.80) and external impression (κ 0.94) and was good for recognizing lipomas (κ 0.65). However, agreement was significantly lower for diagnosing leiomyomas (κ 0.53) and vascular structures (κ 0.54). Interobserver agreement was poor for diagnosing other subepithelial tumors (metastases, carcinoid, pancreatic heterotopia; κ 0.34).[38]
- Due to mucinous contents, some bronchogenic duplication cysts of the esophageal wall may appear hypoechoic, potentially giving rise to misdiagnosis of leiomyoma or leiomyosarcoma.[96]
- Flow velocities in cavernous hemangiomas may be so low that the correct diagnosis may be missed.[93]
- An atypical ultrastructure may lead to misclassification. Occasionally, lipomas may show a slightly inhomogeneous texture and GISTs may show medium echogenicity or cystic regions.[40,101] Pancreatic heterotopia may appear as a septated cyst[105] or may contain calcifications[145] and inflammatory fibroid polyps, and gastrointestinal lymphangiomas may appear hyperechoic.[86,89,90,149]

Practical Hints

- There is such a wide variety of hypoechoic subepithelial tumors that the examiner should refrain from trying to make a definite diagnosis of the tumor type. Instead, he or she should give a detailed description of the findings and offer a list of differential diagnoses. In one study in Asia including 205 histologically confirmed subepithelial tumors in the upper gastrointestinal tract, the EUS diagnosis was in agreement with the histologic diagnosis in only 53.7% of cases.[187]
- To date, the value of contrast-enhanced CCDS in diagnosing subepithelial lesions has not been sufficiently studied.[52] However, in our experience it does help differentiate between very hypoechoic solid lesions and anechoic cystic lesions. It also increases diagnostic certainty for cavernous hemangiomas.
- It is possible to increase the diagnostic yield by taking into account pathological and anatomical data such as the predilection sites for specific tumors, and endosonographic findings such as the layer of origin or the tumor outline (**Table 14.9**).

■ Hypoechoic Subepithelial Tumors of the Esophagus

Leiomyomas. In the esophagus, benign leiomyomas are both the most common subepithelial tumor and the most common mesenchymal tumor. Leiomyomas are typically located in the middle or lower third of the esophagus. Esophageal leiomyomas originate from the fourth hypoechoic layer (muscularis propria), and only rarely from the second hypoechoic layer (muscularis mucosae).[88,173,184] If a hypoechoic tumor is found in this location, the endosonographic diagnosis of a leiomyoma is most likely, particularly because leiomyomas outnumber GISTs by a factor of 3–9.[18,156,157,173,184,185] However, very small leiomyomas may be mistaken for intramural cysts, as they may appear almost anechoic (**Figs. 14.16** and **14.31a, d**). A Japanese study compared the endosonographic diagnosis of 26 endoscopically resected esophageal tumors (among which there were 19 leiomyomas) with the histological diagnosis. Two leiomyomas (with diameters of 8 mm and 20 mm) had been classified as cysts endosonographically, whereas a cyst with a diameter of 9 mm had been classified as a leiomyoma. For three leiomyomas, the endosonographic classification was uncertain, and one was thought to be a granular cell tumor.[88] Esophageal leiomyomas only rarely exceed a size of 30 mm, and they only very rarely have a stalk. Diffuse growth of multiple leiomyomas (esophageal leiomyomatosis) is sometimes observed.[173,184,188–190]

Granular cell tumors (also known as myoblastic myoma or Abrikosov tumor) are the second most common hypoechoic subepithelial tumor in the esophagus. The histogenetic origins of this rare tumor are possibly Schwann cells. Only 5–9% of granular cell tumors arise in the gastrointestinal tract, and they are then usually located in the esophagus. Immunohistochemically, the tumor is positive for S100 protein and normally also for neuron-specific enolase. These tumors are usually benign, and like leiomyomas they are usually found in the lower and middle third of the esophagus. Multiple tumors may occur. Endoscopically, granular cell tumors have a yellowish hue, but in contrast to lipomas their consistency is rather firm. Endosonographically, they appear as homogeneously hypoechoic lesions with a smooth margin, which rarely exceed a size of 20 mm. They can usually be found in the second hypoechoic layer (lamina muscularis mucosae) or the third echogenic layer (tunica submucosa)[191] (**Figs. 14.1b, 14.32** and **14.49c–e**).

However, high-frequency miniprobes may visualize a more heterogeneous echo texture and unclear margins, reflecting the mixture of laterally scattering tumor cells, fibrosis, and muscularis mucosae in granular cell tumors, and may therefore be useful for differentiating esophageal granular cell tumors from leiomyomas.[192] Malignant granular cell tumors are rare. They show infiltrative growth, are

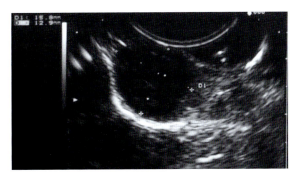

Fig. 14.32 A granular cell tumor in the esophagus. The tumor is displacing the surrounding tissues, but there is no infiltrative growth.

frequently larger than 40 mm, and tend to cause lymphatic metastases. These characteristics are easily recognized with endosonography.[191]

Inflammatory fibroid polyps (IFPs). Very rarely, the differential diagnosis for hypoechoic subepithelial tumors of the esophagus may include IFPs, which—as in the stomach—are located in the second and third layers and have poorly defined margins (**Fig. 14.33**).[193,194]

GISTs and leiomyosarcomas. Other rare differential diagnoses include GISTs and leiomyosarcomas.[195,239] Fewer than 5% of GISTs occur in the esophagus, which is thus one of the least common locations in which these are found. Only 9–25% of esophageal mesenchymal tumors are GISTs.[157,173,185] Like leiomyomas, GISTs may also originate from both muscular layers of the esophageal wall. The EUS features are not sufficient to differentiate esophageal GISTs from leiomyomas.[173] Leiomyosarcomas in the esophagus occur even more rarely than GISTs[173,185] (**Fig. 14.34**).

■ Hypoechoic Subepithelial Tumors of the Stomach

Gastrointestinal stromal tumors (GISTs). In contrast to the esophagus, GISTs are the most common hypoechoic subepithelial tumors in the stomach. Approximately 60% of GISTs are found in the stomach.[154,155,196] It can be assumed that papers published in the 1980s and 1990s that described the endosonographic characteristics of "leiomyomas," "leiomyoblastomas," and "leiomyosarcomas" of the stomach were probably referring to GISTs in the majority of cases.[21,23,25,36,37,39,87,197,198] The size of the lesions varies from a few millimeters to a few centimeters. While smaller tumors are often incidental findings (**Figs. 14.1a** and **14.30**), larger tumors may be symptomatic—e.g., they may cause gastrointestinal hemorrhage, pain, or obstruction (**Fig. 14.2a, b**).

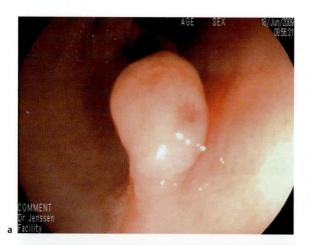

a

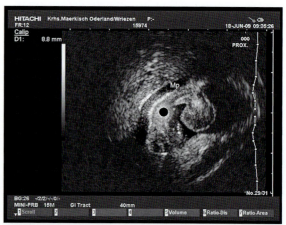

b

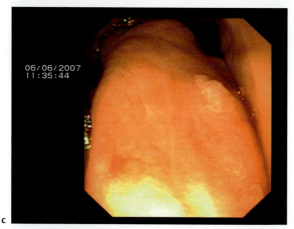

c

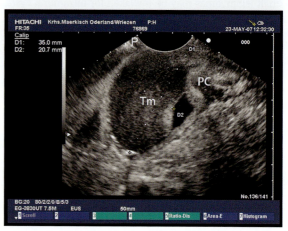

d

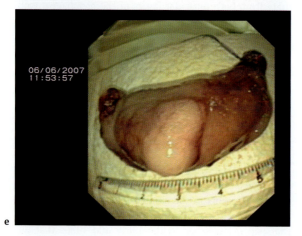

e

Fig. 14.33a–e Inflammatory fibroid polyps (IFPs) in the stomach.
a, b Small asymptomatic IFP in the stomach. Endoscopic image (**a**) and endosonographic image (**b**, 15-MHz ultrasound miniprobe). Mp, muscularis propria.
c, d A large IFP, causing vomiting due to recurrent obstruction of the pyloric channel. Endoscopic image (**c**) and EUS image (**d**) showing the large hypoechoic subepithelial tumor (Tm) protruding through the pyloric channel (PC) into the duodenal lumen.
e The endoscopically resected specimen.

GISTs can occur in all mural layers, although they usually originate from the fourth hypoechoic layer and less frequently from the second hypoechoic layer. GISTs that are mainly located extramurally have occasionally been observed. They are connected to the fourth hypoechoic layer only by a thin hypoechoic strand, which may easily be missed (**Figs. 14.12a, b** and **14.35**).[44]

Gastric leiomyomas are rare and are predominantly found in the region of the cardia (**Fig. 14.31c, d**).[156,196]

Gastric glomus tumors are benign tumors originating from modified smooth muscle cells of the glomus body. These very rare tumors arise from the fourth hypoechoic sonolayer, are hypoechoic and hypervascularized, and most often are localized in the gastric antrum. Immunohistochemically, they are positive for smooth muscle actin, collagen type IV, and calponin, but never for desmin, CD117, or S100.[57,199,201]

Schwannomas of the stomach are very rare.[156] They cannot be differentiated from GISTs endosonographically[180] (**Fig. 14.36**).

Inflammatory fibroid polyps (IFPs) are another rare differential diagnosis in hypoechoic subepithelial tumors of the stomach. They are situated in the submucosal layer and consist of acapsular loose perivascular connective tissue, which contains an eosinophilic inflammatory infiltrate.[86,90,149] To differentiate them from GISTs, it is important to bear in mind that IFPs are also positive for CD34, but do not express CD117 (**Fig. 14.33**).[102,153,156,196]

Kaposi sarcoma shares some macroscopic and histopathological features with GISTs. These tumors have a spindle cell pattern, express CD34 and sometimes CD117, but not DOG1. The clues to the diagnosis are the background of HIV infection, multiple occurrences, origin in the mucosal and submucosal layer, and positive immunohistochemistry for human herpesvirus 8 (HHV8).[202,204,205]

Neuroendocrine tumors ("carcinoids") of the stomach. The characteristics of these lesions are poorly defined margins, localization in the submucosal layer, and an inhomogeneous hypoechoic ("pepper-and-salt") appearance[40,147] (**Fig. 14.4a**).

Gastric metastases from malignant tumors, which in some 50% of cases may appear as subepithelial tumors endoscopically, and malignant lymphomas or gastric adenocarcinoma with purely submucosal polypoid growth, are also very rare[19,200,203,206–208] (**Figs. 14.28** and **14.37**).

■ Hypoechoic Subepithelial Tumors of the Duodenum and Small Intestine

No large reviews have been published on the prevalence and endosonographic characteristics of subepithelial tumors of the duodenum. One series described 114 subepithelial tumors of the gastrointestinal tract, all of which were examined with EUS, with the diagnosis subsequently being confirmed histologically. In this study, 27 tumors were seen in the duodenum, 15 of which originated from the Brunner glands and had a partially cystic appearance.[207] In a Chinese endosonographic study of 169 protruding duodenal lesions, 40 were identified as submucosal cysts and 67 as true subepithelial tumors. Twenty-five of the duodenal subepithelial tumors were Brunner adenomas, 19 were ectopic pancreas, 17 were GISTs, and six were lipomas.[209] In four endosonographic studies of hypoechoic subepithelial tumors of the duodenum, a

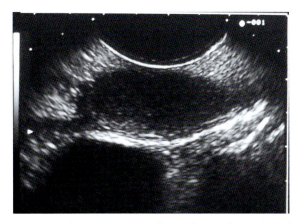

Fig. 14.34 A leiomyosarcoma in the esophagus. The esophageal lumen has been filled with simethicone (dimethicone) solution to improve visualization of the tumor.

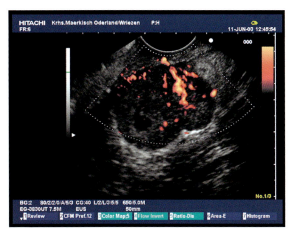

Fig. 14.35 A large extramural gastrointestinal stromal tumor (GIST) in the stomach, showing necrotic areas and obvious hyperperfusion.

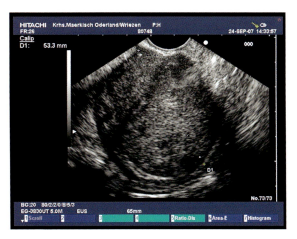

Fig. 14.36 Gastric schwannoma. The patient presented with severe gastrointestinal bleeding from ulceration of this very large tumor. The histological and immunohistochemical diagnosis was reached after surgical resection. (Further images are shown in **Fig. 14.54a–d**.)

III Gastrointestinal Tract

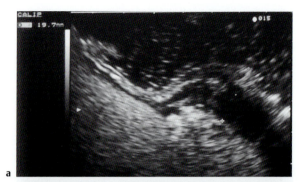

a

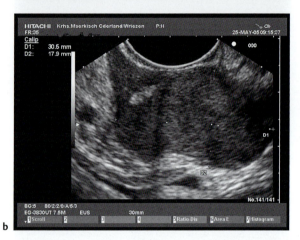

b

Fig. 14.37a–c Malignant subepithelial tumors in the stomach.
a A subepithelial hypoechoic T cell lymphoma in the stomach.
b, c Subepithelial metastases from an ovarian carcinoma (**b**, image from Jenssen et al.[200]) and pancreatic cancer (**c**).

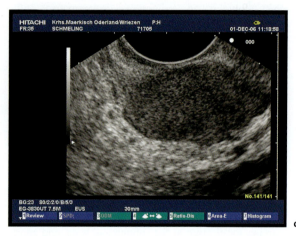

c

histological diagnosis was obtained for a total of 50 tumors. The authors found nine neuroendocrine tumors (carcinoid), one granular cell tumor, one leiomyoblastoma, one leiomyoma, one schwannoma, one inflammatory vascular polyp, and two lymphomas.[51,88,197,210] A case study described inflammatory fibroid polyps in the duodenum. Their endosonographic appearance was consistent with the known criteria for gastric IFPs.[211] The great majority of the rare mesenchymal tumors of the duodenum are gastrointestinal stromal tumors (GISTs) (**Fig. 14.38**); leiomyomas and leiomyosarcomas are very rare.[212] In the small intestine, hypoechoic tumors are GISTs in most cases. They outnumber smooth muscle tumors by a factor of 36.[172,186]

◼ Hypoechoic Subepithelial Tumors of the Colon and Rectum

Lipomas and lymphangiomas are the most common subepithelial tumors of the colon and rectum. However, in a study of 45 patients in whom a subepithelial tumor was suspected on endoscopy or radiography, there were 22 hypoechoic tumors that were diagnosed as six different tumor types—six leiomyomas and three leiomyosarcomas (possibly GISTs, in retrospect), seven cases of endometrio-

sis, two malignant lymphomas, three postoperative cancer recurrences, and one mucocele of the appendix.[109]

Gastrointestinal stromal tumors, schwannomas, or leiomyomas/leiomyosarcomas are endosonographically located in the fourth or second hypoechoic layer. Schwannomas of the colon and rectum are very rare and, independently of their size, they are always benign.[177,216] It is sometimes difficult or impossible to differentiate hypoechoic mesenchymal tumors from endometriosis of the colon, which may on occasion have a spindle-shaped appearance (**Fig. 14.39**).[109] Leiomyosarcomas of the colon and rectum occur much more rarely than GISTs and usually appear as large polypoid tumors. Leiomyosarcomas (or malignant GISTs) are larger than 40 mm, have a round or lobulated appearance, and in comparison with benign leiomyomas/GISTs have more inhomogeneities with echogenic foci.[109]

As elsewhere, differentiation of the different phenotypes of mesenchymal tumors in the lower gastrointestinal tract is only possible with immunohistochemical methods.[153,183,216,217]

There have been no endosonographic follow-up studies on hypoechoic mesenchymal tumors of the colon and rectum, and endosonographic markers of malignancy have not been described. The following details are therefore based on pathological and anatomical studies. Small hypoechoic mesenchymal tumors located in the muscularis mucosae are almost invariably benign leiomyomas (**Fig. 14.40**).[183] In contrast to the stomach, GISTs in the colon can only be regarded as low-risk if they measure less than 10 mm and have a low number of mitoses (< 5/50 HPFs).[216] In the rectum, GISTs measuring less than 20 mm with a low mitotic count have a low risk of malignany.[217]

Neuroendocrine tumors (carcinoids) are the predominant tumor type in the rectum. Endosonographically, they uniformly appear as well-demarcated, round hypoechoic tumors located in the submucosal layer, with the internal structure resembling a "pepper-and-salt" pattern. EUS is very helpful for treatment planning[51,213,214] (**Fig. 14.41**).

Granular cell tumors are very rare in the lower gastrointestinal tract. Their endosonographic appearance shows the same characteristics as in the esophagus.[215]

Endometriosis. In the rectum, endometriosis may appear as an extramural lesion, or—if it arises from a pelvic endometric nodulus—it may appear as a hypoechoic lesion that infiltrates the fourth hypoechoic layer or rarely the third echogenic layer[151,152,218,219] (**Fig. 14.39**).

Rectal cancer recurrences (**Fig. 14.42a**), submucosally growing rectal cancers (**Fig. 14.42b, c**), and lymphomas show irregular margins.

Amyloidosis is a rare diagnosis. Only one case of solitary amyloidosis localized in the transverse colon has been described, presenting as a homogeneously hypoechoic smooth oval lesion located in the third echogenic layer.[150]

Assessment of the Biological Behavior of Hypoechoic Subepithelial Tumors

The pathological and anatomical assessment of the behavior of mesenchymal tumors of the gastrointestinal tract is more difficult and less reliable than the pathological and anatomical assessment of the biological behavior of epithelial neoplasms. Differences between published studies are, among other things, largely due to relatively small numbers of patients, different follow-up periods, various definitions of the term "high-power field" (HPF). To a large extent, tumor behavior can be judged by the number of mitotic changes per 50 HPFs, the size of the tumor, and its location in the gastrointestinal tract (**Tables 14.7** and **14.8**). Further criteria are the presence of necrosis, markers of proliferation activity (Ki-67/MIB-1), specific mutations, expression of CD26, and telomerase activity.[60,154,155,159,165,166,220–223] In the upper gastrointestinal tract, only tumors measuring less than 50 mm and with a low number of mitoses (< 5/50 HPFs for GISTs and < 2/50 HPFs for leiomyomas) are deemed to have a benign

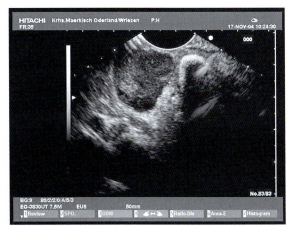

Fig. 14.38 A hypoechoic subepithelial duodenal tumor just below the papilla of Vater, coexisting with chronic calcifying pancreatitis. Histological examination after surgical resection showed that the lesion was a benign gastrointestinal stromal tumor (GIST), along with chronic pancreatitis.

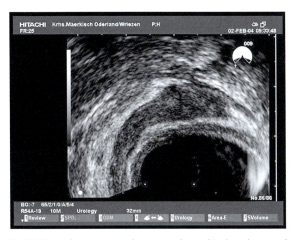

Fig. 14.39 Endometriosis in the rectum, located in the submucosal layer, is indistinguishable from the tunica muscularis.

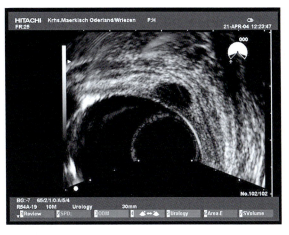

Fig. 14.40 A small, hypoechoic, homogeneous, and well-demarcated tumor in the second echolayer of the rectum (leiomyoma of the muscularis mucosae).

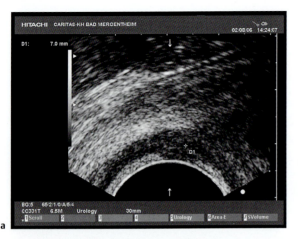

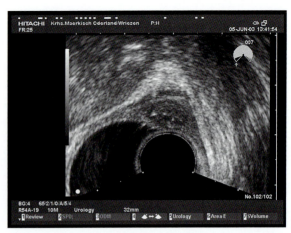

Fig. 14.41a, b Neuroendocrine tumors in the rectum.
a A hypoechoic tumor (7 mm, between the markers) is infiltrating the fourth echolayer, and endoscopic resection is therefore not possible.

b A well-demarcated, heterogeneous, hypoechoic tumor with a typical "pepper-and-salt" pattern, confined to the second hyperechoic (submucosal) echolayer. Endoscopic resection is feasible.

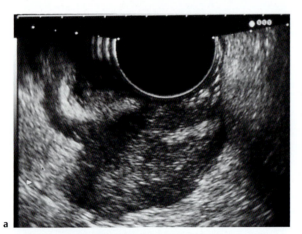

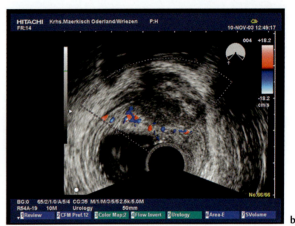

Fig. 14.42a–c Rectal cancer with subepithelial growth.
a Recurrent subepithelial rectal cancer, following a previous surgical resection.
b Rectal cancer of the signet-ring cell type, with subepithelial growth and infiltration beyond the deep muscle layer.
c Primary cancer in the anorectal transitional zone, with a subepithelial growth pattern and infiltration of the deep muscle layer.

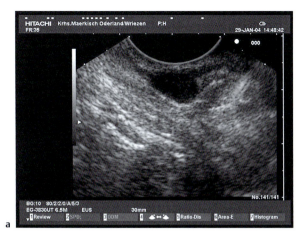
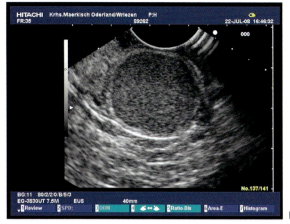
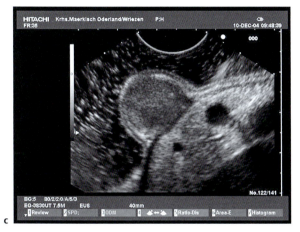
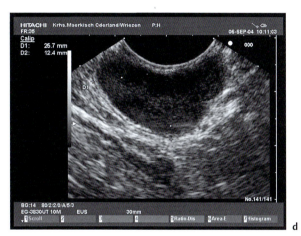

Fig. 14.43a–d Hypoechoic subepithelial tumors that are benign according to EUS criteria.

a An incidental finding in the gastric body. No external compression was visible on endoscopy.

b A minor external impression from a small, homogeneously hypoechoic tumor with smooth margins, arising from the tunica muscularis in the stomach.

c A small hypoechoic tumor in the gastric body, again arising from the tunica muscularis.

d A pseudopedunculated hypoechoic tumor in the upper stomach, with smooth margins, arising from the tunica muscularis of the cardia.

course (very low risk, low risk) (**Table 14.7**). Despite this, there have been a number of cases in which the histological features of gastrointestinal mesenchymal tumors supported a benign lesion, but in which the clinical course was malignant—specifically with the development of intraperitoneal dissemination and hepatic metastases. In addition, the number of mitoses and the degree of cell differentiation may vary within a mesenchymal tumor.[153,154,164–166] When these pathologic and anatomical difficulties are taken into account, it is easy to see that using EUS criteria alone to assess the biological behavior of hypoechoic tumors originating from the muscular layers of the gastrointestinal tract is problematic.[34] Despite these limitations, it has been possible in some series, in which the findings were verified histologically, to define criteria with some predictive value for assessing the biological behavior of mesenchymal subepithelial tumors[34,41,54,87,181,182,224–228] (**Table 14.10**).

In a study of 56 submucosal gastrointestinal mesenchymal tumors in which the endosonographic findings were controlled by histological assessments, hypoechoic subepithelial tumors with a diameter of less than 30 mm, a regular outline, and a homogeneous texture (**Fig. 14.43**) were always benign. However, 63% of the benign gastrointestinal mesenchymal tumors did not meet all three of these criteria for benign behavior.[226]

In the 10 larger endosonographic studies with histological controls, the following criteria were markers of malignancy: a diameter exceeding 30–40 mm, an irregular outline or local invasion, the presence of echogenic or cystic internal structures, an inhomogeneous echo pattern, and (only in two studies) the presence of enlarged local lymph nodes[34,40,41,87,182,207,224–228] (**Fig. 14.44**). In one study, endosonographic detection of significant tumor vessels turned out to be a predictive factor for malignant behavior (**Figs. 14.14, 14.35, 14.45b** and **14.46e, f**).[53]

III Gastrointestinal Tract

Table 14.10 Endoscopic ultrasound assessment of the biological behavior of gastrointestinal subepithelial tumors

First author, ref.	Benign	Criteria	Malignant	Evaluation
Chak 1997[87] n = 35 Gastrointestinal stromal cell tumors (GISTs)	≤40 mm Regular − −	Tumor size Extraluminal margin Cystic spaces >4 mm Echogenic foci >3 mm	>40 mm Irregular + +	Evaluation by 5 experts: • 2 of 3 main criteria for malignancy met: sensitivity 80–90% • No main criterion for malignancy met: specificity 89–100%
Palazzo 2000[226] n = 56 Histologically proven subepithelial mesenchymal tumors (22 malignant or borderline; 34 "benign leiomyoma")	≤30 mm Regular − − −	Tumor size Extraluminal margins[a, b] Cystic spaces >4 mm[a, b] Suspicious lymph nodes[b] Exophytic growth	>30 mm Irregular + + +	• All 3 main criteria for "benign" met: sensitivity 37%, specificity 100% • 1 of 3 main criteria for malignancy met: sensitivity 91%, specificity 88% • 2 of 3 main criteria for malignancy met: sensitivity 23%, specificity 100%
Will 2001[41] n = 41 (17 malignant)	≤40 mm Homogeneous −	Size Internal echo pattern Cystic/tubular internal structures	>40 mm Inhomogeneous +	• Both main criteria for malignancy met: sensitivity 71%, specificity 81%
Nickl 2002[225] n = 198 Hypoechoic subepithelial gastrointestinal tumors, 102 resected with surgical pathology in 64% of cases (74 GISTs; 9 "malignant," 31 of "indeterminate malignant potential," 34 "benign")	None <30 mm Regular, round or oval	Ulceration Size Contour	+ ≤30 mm Irregular	• Correlation of gastric location and malignancy • Resection of tumors with: ulceration, size >30 mm, irregular contour, no round or oval shape, suspicious regional lymph nodes → 100% of malignant tumors and >95% of borderline tumors diagnosed • No correlation between malignancy and hyperechogenic or hypoechoic foci
Rösch 2002[34] n = 84 Unselected subepithelial GI tumors (7 malignant)	≤30 mm Homogeneous Regular −	Tumor size Internal echo texture Extraluminal margin Lymph nodes >10 mm	>30 mm Inhomogeneous Irregular +	• ≤2 criteria for malignancy met: sensitivity 86%, specificity 80%
Brand 2002[224] n = 86 Unselected subepithelial GI tumors (20 malignant)	≤30 mm Homogeneous Regular	Tumor size Internal echo texture Extraluminal margin	>30 mm Inhomogeneous Irregular	• ≤2 criteria for malignancy met: sensitivity 80%, specificity 77%
Ando 2002[54] n = 23 GISTs (diagnosis by EUS-FNA)	≤50 mm − −	Tumor size Tumor margin Cystic spaces	>50 mm + +	• Tumor size >50 mm and one or both structural criteria for malignancy met: sensitivity 83%, specificity 76%

Table 14.10 (continued)

First author, ref.	Criteria	Benign	Malignant	Evaluation
Jeon 2007 n = 24[227] Histologically proven gastric GISTs (14 low risk, 7 intermediate risk, 3 high risk)	Tumor size	≤ 30 mm	> 30 mm	• Tumor size > 30 mm → prediction of intermediate or high-risk GIST: sensitivity 80%, specificity 79%
	Mucosal ulceration	–	+	
	Shape	Round, oval	Lobulated	
	Tumor margin	Regular	Irregular	
Kim 2009 [182] n = 43 Histologically proven gastric GISTs (33 very low and low risk = "benign"; 13 intermediate and high risk = "malignant")	Tumor size [a]	< 35 mm	≥ 35 mm	• Tumor size ≥ 35 mm → prediction of intermediate or high-risk GIST: sensitivity 92%, specificity 79% • Other criteria such as extraluminal growth, internal echo texture, cystic spaces, ulceration, lobulation were not predictive of malignant risk
	Tumor margin	Regular	Irregular	
Shah 2009[228] n = 26 Histologically proven GISTs (14 very low and low risk = "benign"; 12 intermediate and high risk = "malignant")	Tumor size	≤ 50 mm	> 50 mm	• All high-risk GISTs were > 50 mm, all low-risk GISTs ≤ 50 mm • If the 3 high-risk criteria other than size are used, the presence of all 3 features in tumors ≤ 50 mm is significantly associated with intermediate risk
	Extraluminal margin	Smooth	Irregular, lobular	
	Local invasion	–	+	
	Internal echo texture	Homogeneous	Inhomogeneous	

[a] Independently predictive of malignant potential in multivariate analysis.
[b] Most predictive (main) criteria for malignant or borderline subepithelial tumors.
GI, gastrointestinal; GIST, gastrointestinal stromal tumor.

An ex vivo analysis of five GISTs shortly after surgical resection found that hyperechoic foci or stranding around the periphery of the tumor on EUS were due to fibrotic changes; circumscribed echogenic areas represented areas of hyalinized necrosis, and cystic parts were found to be fluid-filled nonepithelialized cavities or older hemorrhages (**Fig. 14.45** and **14.46**).[50] More than 90% of malignant subepithelial mesenchymal tumors of the upper gastrointestinal tract show at least one of the criteria for malignancy mentioned above. However, these may also occur in a high percentage of benign tumors.[229] In the published series, the presence of two EUS criteria of malignancy (e.g., irregular outline and cystic internal structures, or an inhomogeneous echo pattern and size > 30–40 mm) was highly specific for malignant gastrointestinal mesenchymal tumors, but was not sufficiently sensitive to be able to diagnose malignant tumors reliably by endoscopic ultrasound (**Figs. 14.44, 14.45** and **14.46**).[34,40,41,182,207,224,226–229]

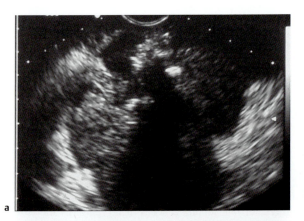

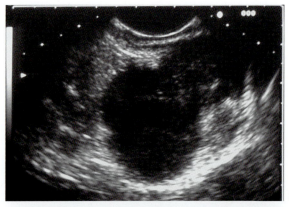

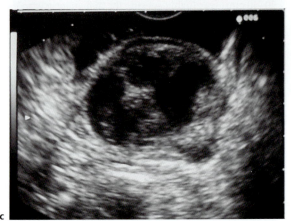

Fig. 14.44a–d Hypoechoic subepithelial tumors that are malignant according to EUS criteria.

a Duodenum: ulceration, size > 60 mm, with an inhomogeneous texture.

b Stomach: the endoscopic appearance and endoscopic biopsy suggested an anaplastic gastric carcinoma. The EUS findings led to a review and correction of the histological diagnosis to malignant gastrointestinal stromal tumor (GIST), and this was confirmed after surgical resection.

c Obvious inhomogeneities, with infiltrative growth. The histological diagnosis was borderline GIST.

d Some minor inhomogeneities, with definitely enlarged lymph nodes. Histological examination of the surgical specimen showed that it was a benign GIST.

Pitfalls

- The criteria for judging biological tumor behavior discussed above are very examiner-dependent. In the only published study to date, agreement between experienced observers in assessing biological behavior according to endosonographic criteria varied from unsatisfactory (cystic or echogenic internal structures) to moderate (heterogeneity, irregular outline).[38]

- Depending on size and age, benign leiomyomas and GISTs may develop an irregular outline and regressive changes, which appear as an inhomogeneous echo pattern or as anechoic or hypoechoic areas. These changes may make it difficult or impossible to distinguish these tumors from malignant mesenchymal tumors (**Figs. 14.45** and **14.46**).

- In our own series and in the series published by Ando et al.,[54] one malignant GIST tumor was found that according to the criteria presented by Palazzo et al.[226] would have been regarded as definitely benign: the tumor had a smooth margin, was homogeneously hypoechoic, and was smaller than 30 mm. However, the histological examination revealed definite malignant changes.

- The criteria for judging the biological behavior of mesenchymal tumors are almost exclusively based on tumors of the upper gastrointestinal tract. It is not known whether these can be generalized to the lower gastrointestinal tract. GISTs in the colon show biologically malignant behavior when they are larger than 10–20 mm.[216] In the series reported by Kameyama et al.,[109] it was not possible to distinguish "leiomyomas" (or benign GISTs) from "leiomyosarcomas" (or malignant GISTs) in the colon reliably using endoscopic ultrasound.

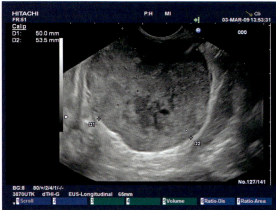

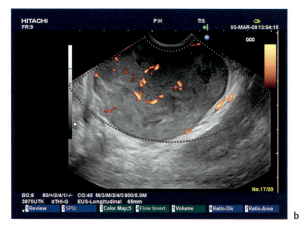

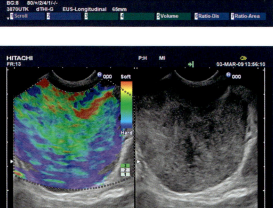

Fig. 14.45a–c a, b A large (53-mm) hypoechoic, inhomogeneous subepithelial tumor in the stomach (**a**), showing numerous vessels (**b**).

c Real-time elastography shows that the peripheral hyperechoic areas correlate with hard tumor tissue, whereas the central hypoechoic areas are relatively soft and may correspond to necrosis (image from Jenssen[246]). The tumor was resected surgically because of these EUS features, but histology and immunohistochemistry classified the tumor as a GIST with low malignant risk.

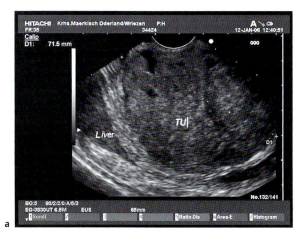

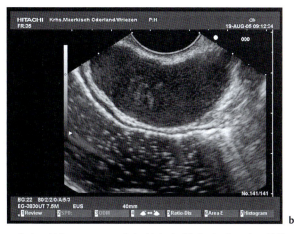

Fig. 14.46a–f Examples of hypoechoic subepithelial tumors in the stomach, in which assessment of the biological behavior based on EUS criteria led to equivocal results: size >40 mm (**a, c, e, f**), marginal or moderate inhomogeneities (**a–f**), lobulation (**c**), cystic areas (**d**), and marked vascularization (**e, f**). All of these tumors were found to be low-risk at surgical pathology. Mp, muscularis propria; Tu, tumor.

Fig. 14.46c–f ▷

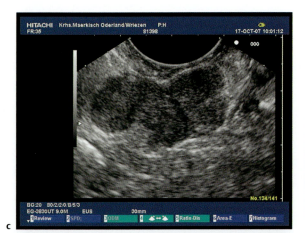

c

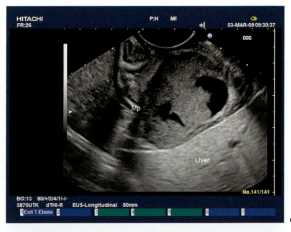

d

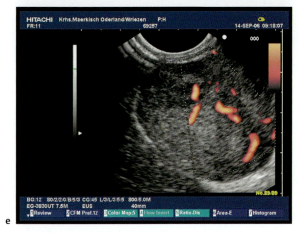

e

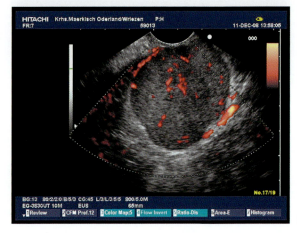

f

Fig. 14.46c–f (continued)

EUS-Guided Fine-Needle Aspiration (EUS-FNA) and Tru-Cut Biopsy (EUS-TCB)

As EUS imaging features alone are not sufficient for accurate differential diagnosis of hypoechoic and mixed echogenic subepithelial tumors in the gastrointestinal tract, or for assessing their biological behavior, histological analysis is necessary for definitive diagnosis. Percutaneous biopsy is not recommended in tumors suspected of being GISTs, due to the risk of tumor rupture and peritoneal dissemination of tumor cells. Endoscopic biopsy has a low yield and is associated with a notable risk of bleeding.[28–30]

Cytological diagnosis. Endoscopic ultrasound-guided fine-needle aspiration (EUS-FNA) is helpful for obtaining cytological material from lymph nodes and pancreatic tumors. Obtaining adequate specimens from subepithelial tumors with EUS-FNA is technically demanding, and in studies from the 1990s the sensitivity, specificity, and accuracy of cytological evaluation of intramural lesions was unacceptably low.[230,231] More recent studies have shown that EUS-FNA may provide a diagnosis of spindle cell or epithelioid neoplasms in the gastrointestinal wall on the basis of cytological smears, with satisfactory levels of sensitivity and specificity.[63,66,72] However, GISTs, schwannomas, and leiomyomas are difficult to distinguish from each other, as well as from contaminants from the gastrointestinal wall cytologically, as most of these tumors are composed of benign-appearing spindle cells. Smears from GISTs are more likely than leiomyomas to show occasional intact single cells with numerous stripped nuclei and to have cell groups with high cellularity.[74,232] There are only a few cytological characteristics that suggest malignancy, such as dominant single cells or very rarely pleomorphic or hyperchromatic nuclei. However, the cytological assessment of fine-needle aspirates is not sufficient for assessing the behavior of GISTs, in particular because the cytological appearance of an epithelioid GIST may mimic that of an adenocarcinoma or neuroendocrine tumor.[44,75,233]

Histological and immunohistochemical diagnosis. More recently, several studies have been published suggesting that the yield of EUS-guided biopsy in the diagnosis of solid subepithelial tumors can be improved by optimizing needles, aspiration techniques, and processing of the material (cell blocks and histological preparations). EUS-FNA with a modified sampling technique and EUS-TCB make it possible to obtain core tissue specimens from subepithelial tumors, which can then be examined histologically and immunohistochemically, providing a wider range of diagnostic options than cytological smears. Ando et al. used a 22-G aspiration needle to obtain core specimens from 23 gastrointestinal mesenchymal tumors with EUS guidance. They were able to assess the tumor phenotype and tumor behavior correctly by staining for CD117, CD34, smooth muscle actin (SMA), and S100 protein and by determining the number of mitoses and the Ki67 labeling index.[54] Similar results have been reported by other groups.[19,56–58,60,64,65,69,74,75,234,235] In hypoechoic subepithelial tumors, combinations of cytological and immunohistochemical criteria make it possible to differentiate between GISTs and neuroendocrine tumors,[237] gastric glomus tumors,[57,199,201] peripheral nerve sheath tumors,[62] leiomyosarcomas,[239] Abrikosov tumors,[238] and subepithelial metastases, for example.[19,200,203] It has also become possible to carry out mutational analysis of the KIT gene on material obtained by EUS-FNA.[67,235,236] Since myogenic, neurogenic, and undifferentiated gastrointestinal mesenchymal tumors behave differently, and because the numbers and types of mutation in the KIT or PDGFRα genes and the degree of malignancy of GISTs are closely corre-

lated,[155,221] it may in the future be easier to predict tumor behavior by using immunohistochemical and cytogenetic methods to study fine-needle aspirates.

Diagnostic yield with needle aspiration. Growing experience with EUS-FNA of subepithelial tumors has increased the rate at which adequate specimens are collected, and in some studies the method is now approaching the diagnostic yield of EUS-FNA of pancreatic mass lesions and lymph nodes. The weighted average for the pooled diagnostic yield of eight EUS-FNA studies (published since 2001 and each including more than 20 and a total of 523 patients with subepithelial tumors) was 73%.[19,54,64,68–70,72,73]

The usefulness and safety of EUS-guided Tru-Cut biopsy (EUS-TCB) and guillotine needles for obtaining tissue from subepithelial tumors under endosonographic guidance has also been tested successfully.[45,76–80,240] However, the diagnostic yield of EUS-TCB does not appear to be superior to that of EUS-FNA[78] (**Table 14.11**). In one recent prospective study, tumor tissue adequate for immunohistochemical diagnosis was obtained with EUS-TCB in 31 of 49 patients (63%) with hypoechoic gastric subepithelial tumors.[80]

Guidelines. In conclusion, EUS-guided biopsy is the preferred sampling technique for subepithelial tumors in the

Table 14.11 Diagnostic yield and accuracy of EUS-guided biopsy of subepithelial tumors of the gastrointestinal tract (studies including ≥ 10 cases)

First author, ref.	Lesions (n)	Needle type	Diagnostic yield / Diagnostic accuracy	Special features
Ando (2002)[54]	49 subepithelial tumors originating from the 4th echolayer (23 GISTs with surgical pathology)	22-G FNA	92%[a] (45/49) 91% (21/23 confirmed GISTs)[c], 100% (23/23 confirmed GISTs)[d]	Retrospective "malignant" (clinically malignant, ≥ 3 mitoses/10 HPFs) versus benign (< 3 mitoses/ 10 HPFs)
Fu (2002)[232]	10 GISTs with surgical pathology	22-G FNA	80% (8/10)[a] 80% (8/10)[e]	Retrospective; 2 of 10 cases misinterpreted as contaminants from the GI wall
Arantes (2004)[206]	10 subepithelial GI tumors (6 GISTs)	22-G FNA	80% (8/10)[b] 80% (8/10)[f]	Retrospective
Mallery (2004)[19]	93 solid subepithelial GI tumors, among them 59 mesenchymal neoplasms (37 GISTs)	19/22/25-G FNA	73% (68/93)[b] 79%[a] (if immunohistochemistry was needed based on initial smear results) No data on accuracy	Retrospective; lower diagnostic yield in isoechoic (43%) and hyperechoic (14%) than in hypoechoic lesions (81%)
Okubo (2004)[60]	14 gastric GISTs with surgical pathology	22-G FNA	100% (14/14)[e] 85.7% (12/14)[d]	Retrospective; "low-grade" GIST versus "high-grade" GIST
Van der Noot (2004)[63]	60 intramural and extramural mass lesions, among them 18 GISTs	22-G FNA	100% (60/60)[b] 89% (53/60)[f]	Retrospective; data given only for the whole study population (1 false-negative and 1 false-positive diagnosis of GIST)
Chen (2005)[66]	42 intramural and extramural mass lesions, among them 17 GISTs	22-G FNA	100% (42/42)[b] 98% (41/42)[f]	Prospective; data given only for the whole study population
Sasaki (2005)[61]	22 intramural and extramural mass lesions of the colon and rectum, among them 1 GIST	22-G FNA	95.5% (21/22)[a] No data on accuracy	Retrospective

Table 14.11 (continued)

First author, ref.	Lesions (n)	Needle type	Diagnostic yield Diagnostic accuracy	Special features
Mochizuki (2006)[71]	12 gastric GISTs with surgical pathology	22-G FNA	No data on yield 83.3% (10/12)[d]	Retrospective
Akahoshi (2007)[64]	53 gastrointestinal hypoechoic subepithelial tumors, 29 with surgical pathology (24 GISTs)	22-G FNA	82% (49/51 EUS-FNA, 2 were technically impossible)[a] 97% (28/29 with surgical pathology)[e]	Prospective; accuracy lower in small than in large tumors (≤ 2 cm: 71%, 2–4 cm: 86%; ≥ 4 cm: 100%)
Shah (2007)[73]	72 suspected gastric GISTs, 20 with surgical pathology (15 GISTs)	FNA	38.9% (28/72)[a], 50% (36/72)[b] 20%[e], 67%[f] (3/15 and 10/15 histologically confirmed GISTs, respectively)	Retrospective; relatively small tumors (mean size 27.6 mm)
Chatzipantelis (2008)[65]	17 gastric GISTs with surgical pathology	22-G FNA	No data on yield 100% (17/17)[e], 82.4% (14/17)[f]	Retrospective
Stelow (2008)[75]	95 subepithelial mesenchymal gastrointestinal tumors (29 with surgical pathology, among them 18 GISTs, 6 leiomyomas, 2 schwannomas, 1 glomus tumor, 1 granular cell tumor, and 1 carcinoid)	FNA	No data on yield 93.1% (27/29 with surgical pathology)[e]	Retrospective; data only from cases with sufficient cell block material
Hamerski (2008)[68]	66 solid subepithelial tumors of the upper GI tract (19 with surgical pathology, among them 13 GISTs)	FNA	68% (45/66)[b] 84%[e]	Retrospective; yield higher for gastric (75%) than for esophageal (43%) and for duodenal (25%) tumors; yield lower for lesions < 20 mm (45%) than for lesions ≥ 20 mm (80%)
Khan (2009)[70]	43 suspected GISTs (26 with surgical pathology)	22-G FNA	100% (43/43)[a] 86%[e]	Prospective; relatively large tumors (mean tumor size 72 × 52 mm)
Sepe (2009)[72]	37 histologically confirmed KIT-positive GISTs	19/22/25-G FNA	78.4%[b] 46.2% (6 of 13 patients with cell blocks)[e] No data on accuracy	Retrospective; sensitivity low only in very large tumors (≤ 2 cm 80%; 2–5 cm 87.5%; 5–10 cm 100%; ≥ 10 cm 0%) and nongastric GISTs (0% versus 84.4% for gastric GISTs)
Hoda (2009)[69]	112 suspected GISTs of the upper GI tract	22-G FNA 19-G TCB (only 15 patients)	83.9%[b] 61.6%[a] for EUS-FNA 46.7%[a] for EUS-TCB No data on accuracy	Retrospective; trend for diagnostic yield by size category
Polkowski (2009)[80]	49 hypoechoic gastric subepithelial tumors ≥ 20 mm (36 GISTs)	19-G TCB	63%[a] and 78%[b] No data on accuracy	Prospective 3.9% septic complications
Fernandez-Esparrach (2010)[78]	40 hypoechoic gastric subepithelial tumors ≥ 20 mm	22-G FNA and 19-G TCB	EUS-FNA: 52%[a] and 70%[b] EUS-TCB: 55%[a] and 60%[b] EUS-FNA + EUS-TCB: 77.5%[a] no data on accuracy	Prospective cross-over study; both EUS-FNA and EUS-TCB were performed in all patients

[a] Diagnostic yield for histopathological and immunohistochemical analysis (cell blocks, core specimens).
[b] Diagnostic yield for cytological and/or histological diagnosis without immunohistochemistry (smears, cell blocks, core specimens).
[c] Diagnostic accuracy for risk classification of GISTs based on histopathological evaluation of hematoxylin–eosin stains.
[d] Diagnostic accuracy for risk classification of GISTs based on additional Ki67 staining.
[e] Diagnostic accuracy for immunohistochemical diagnosis of GIST.
[f] Diagnostic accuracy for cytological diagnosis of GIST.
FNA, fine-needle aspiration; GI, gastrointestinal; GIST, gastrointestinal stromal tumor; HPF, high-power field; TCB, Tru-Cut biopsy.

III Gastrointestinal Tract

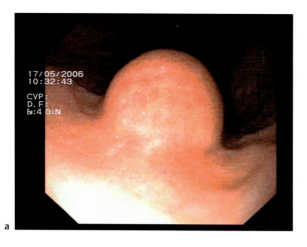
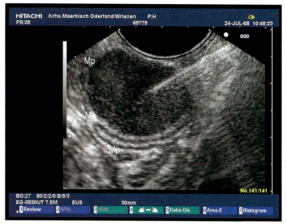

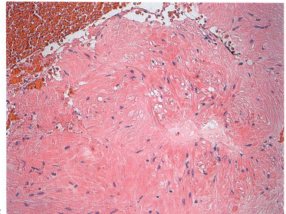
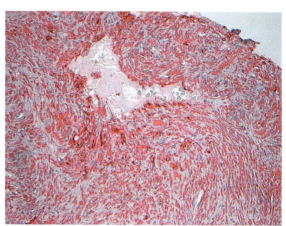

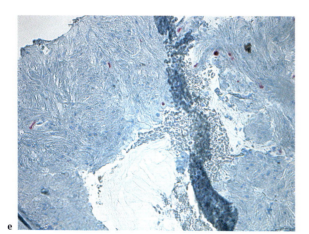

Fig. 14.47a–e a A medium-sized (20-mm) subepithelial tumor in the stomach (endoscopic image).
b EUS-FNA (19-G) of the hypoechoic and homogeneous tumor, which originates from the fourth hypoechoic sonolayer. Mp, muscularis propria.
c Hematoxylin–eosin staining (original magnification ×20) shows whorled fascicles of spindle cells.
d Strongly positive immunostaining for desmin is highly specific for leiomyoma.
e The MIB-1 staining index is below 1% (photomicrographs of the EUS-FNA specimen courtesy of M. Koch, Berlin, Germany). There is no indication for surgical resection of the benign gastric leiomyoma in this asymptomatic patient.

gastrointestinal tract suspected of being GISTs, according to the current guidelines.[241,242,243] To allow immunohistochemical phenotyping, the aim in EUS-guided biopsy of hypoechoic subepithelial gastrointestinal tumors should always be to sample core particles or to provide material for cell blocks. A limited panel of immunochemical stains (CD117, CD34, SMA, desmin, S100) together with hematoxylin–eosin (HE) staining has proved to be adequate for diagnosing most subepithelial gastrointestinal tumors (**Figs. 14.15, 14.47** and **14.48**).[75,244] A very acceptable level of interobserver agreement in interpreting CD117 immunostaining (κ values 0.72–0.93) and in determining Ki67 labeling indices (κ values 0.62–0.86) in GISTs and other spindle cell tumors of the gastrointestinal tract has been reported.[245]

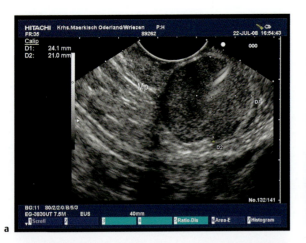

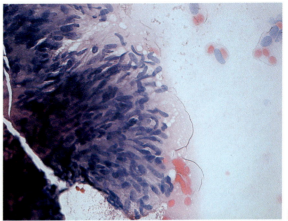

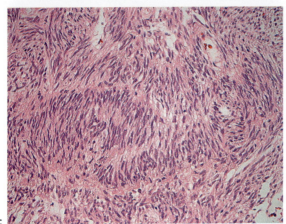

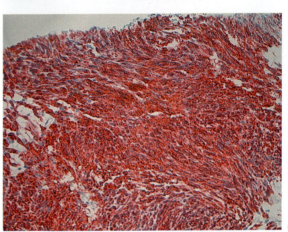

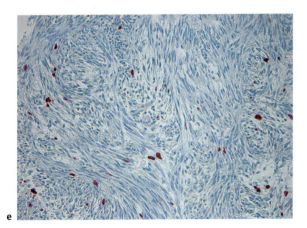

Fig. 14.48a–e a A medium-sized (24-mm) hypoechoic and homogeneous subepithelial tumor, originating from the fourth hypoechoic sonolayer in the gastric wall. There is no obvious difference in comparison with the tumor in **Fig. 14.47**. Mp, muscularis propria.
b Cytological smears obtained by EUS-FNA (19 G): a group of spindle cells with high cellularity and some single spindle cells with stripped nuclei (Papanicolaou, original magnification × 20).
c Fascicles of spindle-shaped tumor cells (hematoxylin–eosin, original magnification × 20).
d Positive immunostaining for CD117 (c-*kit*) confirms the diagnosis of gastrointestinal stromal tumor.
e The Ki67 (MIB-1) staining index is ≈ 2%, indicating low proliferative activity. Local surgical resection is indicated. (Photomicrographs of the EUS-FNA specimen courtesy of M. Koch, Berlin, Germany.)

Pitfalls and Practical Hints

- The diagnostic yields of EUS-FNA and EUS-TCB of subepithelial tumors reported in the literature vary widely, from 39% to 100% (**Table 14.11**). The ability to obtain adequate tissue samples with EUS-guided biopsy may be influenced by various factors—particularly the location of the tumor,[68,72,80] its size and shape,[64,68,69,72] the layer of origin,[72] and its echogenicity.[19]

- EUS-TCB does not increase the yield of EUS-FNA,[69,78] but a jumbo forceps biopsy may be diagnostic in the setting of an ulcerated subepithelial mass.[69]

- Almost all hypoechoic subepithelial tumors will be GISTs, leiomyomas, or peripheral nerve sheath tumors; approximately three-quarters of them are GISTs.[75,225] These tumors are easily diagnosed using a small battery of immunostains on material obtained with EUS-FNA or EUS-TCB. However, there are some rare and potentially difficult differential diagnoses. For example, 4–26% of GISTS are negative for KIT (CD117), but may show focal immunoreactivity against smooth muscle actin.[160–162,247–249] These KIT-negative GISTs are more likely to have epithelioid cell morphology. A large percentage harbor PDGFRα oncogenic mutations and appear to be associated with a poorer prognosis than KIT-positive GISTs.[248] Other diagnostic pitfalls may be rare cases of subepithelially growing malignant melanomas, cancer metastases, clear cell sarcomas, Kaposi sarcomas, desmoid-type fibromatoses, solitary fibrous tumors, inflammatory fibroid polyps, and neuroendocrine tumors, which may be composed of epithelioid or spindle cells and are immunoreactive with some of the antibodies used to characterize GISTs, leiomyomas, and schwannomas. These differential diagnoses can be solved by careful interpretation of hematoxylin–eosin sections and of the complete immunohistochemical panel, and by using antibodies to epithelial markers or specific antigens, to chromogranin, to β-catenin, to DOG1, and to PDGFRα in selected cases.[75,156,244]

- One of the two main criteria for the biological risk of GISTs is the number of mitoses per 50 HPFs (the mitotic index). Core particles obtained on EUS-FNA and EUS-TCB are too small to be used reliably to assess the mitotic index.[80] However, the presence of any mitosis in EUS-FNA specimens from GISTs is highly suggestive for a high-risk GIST, and in two studies a MIB-1 (Ki67) index >5% (or >3%) was found to be highly accurate for diagnosing a "malignant" GIST.[54,60]

- Severe complications of EUS-FNA and EUS-TCB of subepithelial tumors have been reported. Two case reports have been published describing gastrointestinal wall abscesses due to EUS-FNA of an esophageal leiomyoma and a duodenal GIST, respectively.[250,251] A recent study of the diagnostic yield and safety of EUS-TCB in patients with hypoechoic gastric subepithelial tumors reported two septic complications in 52 procedures (3.9%).[80] Two cases of immediate and delayed bleeding after EUS-TCB of gastric GISTs have also been reported.[252,253]

- Only 26% of 134 members of the EUS Special Interest Group of the American Society of Gastrointestinal Endoscopy (ASGE) who responded to an online survey of opinions and practices regarding the diagnosis and management of GISTs always carried out EUS-FNA on lesions suspicious for GISTs. Forty-seven percent only used EUS-FNA for selected lesions suspicious for GIST, and 27% rarely or never sample these tumors. More than 50% of the endosonographers surveyed believed that FNA is not helpful in distinguishing GISTs from other subepithelial lesions.[254] The results of this survey appear to reflect a lack of firm recommendations, poor awareness of the high level of accuracy of immunochemical phenotyping of subepithelial gastrointestinal tumors, and perhaps the inability of some centers to reproduce the satisfactory results reported in the literature.[73] An adequate sampling technique, a meticulous approach to the specimens obtained, and close collaboration and continuous, direct dialogue between the endosonographer and the cytopathologist are the cornerstones of diagnostic success.[255–257]

EUS-Guided Treatment of Subepithelial Lesions

With endoscopic ultrasound, it is possible to determine the layer of origin of subepithelial lesions reliably, both with radial high-frequency miniprobes[46,47,49,51,88,258,259] and with conventional echoendoscopes. This may also be useful for therapeutic interventions: some endoscopic resection techniques that were originally developed for removing epithelial lesions—particularly the techniques of endoscopic mucosal resection and endoscopic submucosal resection—can also be used with some technical variations to resect small subepithelial tumors arising from the second hypoechoic or third echogenic layer. With the exception of stalked tumors, most authors would regard a size of >20 mm (30 mm maximum) and a lack of separation from the fourth hypoechoic layer as a contraindication to endoscopic resection.[51,88,89,101,197,258,260,261] Various methods of resection have been described:[261,262] conventional snare resection of pedunculated subepithelial tumors, snare resection after prior submucosal injection with saline,[51,88,197,263–265] snare resection using a ligation device (**Fig. 14.49**),[265] endoscopic enucleation using a snare or an insulated-tip knife,[266–268] EUS-assisted endoscopic band ligation,[260,269,270] and partial snare resection ("unroofing") of cystic tumors.[101] In our department, we have successfully used the method of endoscopic submucosal tumor resection with a transparent cap[263] (first described by Inoue et al.[271] to resect flat mucosal neoplasms) or endoscopic band ligation followed by snare resection to treat several submucosal pancreatic heterotopias in the stomach and several other small tumors arising from the second hypoechoic or third echogenic layer of the esophagus and stomach (**Figs. 14.49** and **14.50**). It has been shown in principle that endoscopic submucosal resection (ESD) is feasible even for tumors arising from the deep muscle layer.[81,266–268] The decision on whether to resect a subepithelial tumor endoscopically depends on several considerations—in particular, the patient's symptoms, the endosonographic and endoscopic features of the tumor, its potential to cause complications, the patient's comorbidities, and local expertise and the availability of the various resection techniques. The endoscopic resection of subepi-

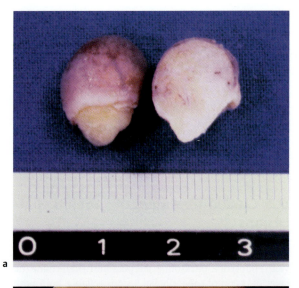

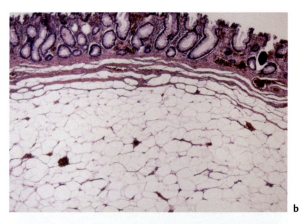

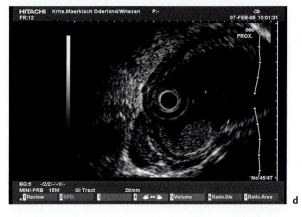

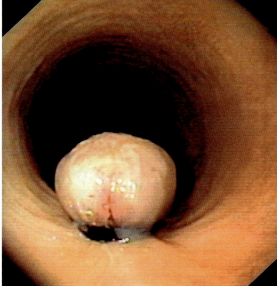

Fig. 14.49a–e Endoscopic resection of small submucosal tumors.
a A resected gastric lipoma.
b The corresponding histological specimen (courtesy of H. Martin, Berlin, Germany).
c An esophageal granular cell tumor after rubber-band ligation, before endoscopic snare resection.
d The EUS image (15-MHz ultrasound miniprobe).
e The corresponding histological specimen (courtesy of S. Bartho and S. Wagner, Königswusterhausen, Germany).

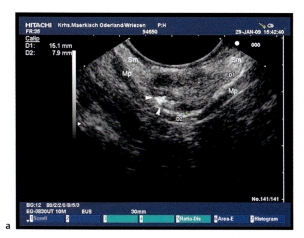

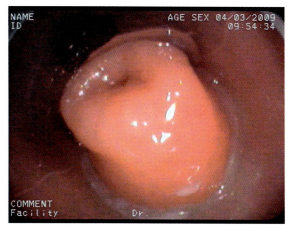

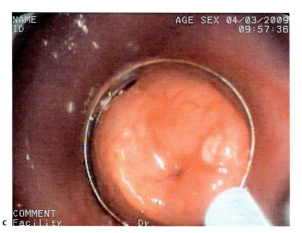

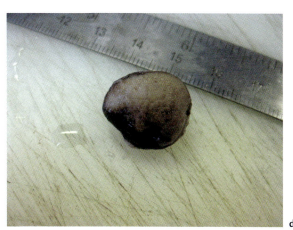

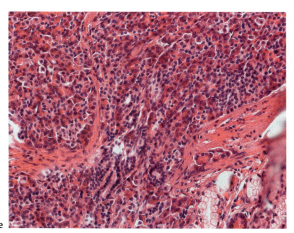

Fig. 14.50a–e Endoscopic resection of a small (15-mm), inhomogeneous, hypoechoic tumor with small peripheral calcifications (arrowheads), located in the third hyperechoic echolayer in the gastric antrum.

a The EUS image. EUS-FNA was not diagnostic. Mp, muscularis propria; Sm, submucosa.

b, c Endoscopic resection of the umbilicated tumor using a transparent hood.

d The resected specimen.

e Histological image (courtesy of S. Wagner, Königswusterhausen, Germany).

III Gastrointestinal Tract

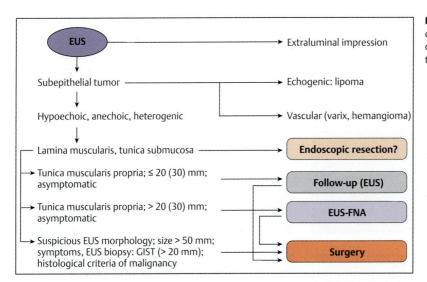

Fig. 14.51 Proposal for an EUS-based decision algorithm for the management of subepithelial tumors of the gastrointestinal tract (adapted from Jenssen[246]).

thelial tumors sometimes appears to be the most effective strategy for obtaining an unequivocal histopathological tissue diagnosis in comparison with EUS-FNA or jumbo biopsy.[28,29,265]

Pitfalls and Practical Hints

- Submucosal injection of normal saline may cause the mucosal surface to level off near the submucosal tumor if it is not done sufficiently close to the tunica muscularis and directly beneath the tumor. This may result in the resection being unsuccessful. If the subepithelial tumor extends to the fourth hypoechoic layer, the injection should therefore in selected cases either be performed with EUS guidance,[81] or, if done endoscopically, the length of the needle and the depth of the injection have to be adapted to the depth of the lesion. It may be useful to create a depot of physiological saline between the tunica muscularis and the tumor in order to minimize the trauma caused by coagulation and consequently the risk of perforation.
- The endoscopic resection of tumors arising from the tunica muscularis propria or infiltrating this layer is associated with a considerable risk of perforation.[267,272] These techniques are time-consuming, and radical resection of these tumors may in some cases also be technically impossible.[267,268] Complications following endoscopic resection of gastric GISTs may result in peritoneal dissemination of the disease.[272]

Diagnostic and Therapeutic Strategy for Subepithelial Lesions in the Gastrointestinal Tract

Endoscopic ultrasound plays a key role in management decisions regarding subepithelial tumors of the gastrointestinal tract. It should be used to exclude the presence of extramural impressions and varices, both of which may mimic subepithelial tumors. True subepithelial lesions should then be analyzed in accordance with a standardized protocol (**Table 14.2**) and, if possible, a diagnosis should be made. In special cases, EUS-guided biopsies may be of crucial importance in the decision-making process regarding treatment[246] (**Fig. 14.51**).

■ Symptomatic Subepithelial Tumors

If tumors are symptomatic (hemorrhage, pain, stenosis, endocrine activity), endoscopic or surgical treatment is always indicated. EUS-guided biopsy of symptomatic subepithelial tumors before resection is only recommended if there are criteria of primary unresectability or metastasis and neoadjuvant treatment is being considered.[70]

EUS may be useful for assessing whether a tumor can be resected endoscopically (**Fig. 14.52**), or which type of surgery should be performed. It is usually possible to resect a tumor endoscopically if its size does not exceed 20 mm (or 30 mm if in a suitable location) and if it is easily detachable from the fourth hypoechoic layer, perhaps after submucosal injection of physiological saline. Larger pedunculated subepithelial tumors may also be resected endoscopically. In such cases, our experience shows that it is useful to

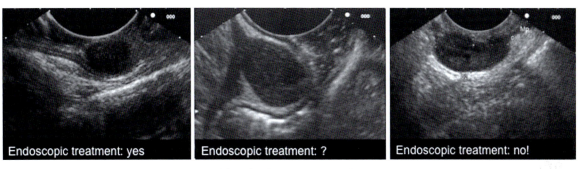

Fig. 14.52 Endosonographic assessment of the feasibility of endoscopic resection of subepithelial tumors.

assess the stalk with CCDS in order to estimate the risk of hemorrhage and initiate measures to reduce this risk (e.g., Endoloop). In some selected cases, special endoscopic techniques (en-bloc resection using insulated-tip knives) also make it possible to resect larger nonpedunculated subepithelial tumors.[267,268]

Surgical resection is the treatment of choice for tumors originating from the fourth echolayer of the gastrointestinal tract. The tumor should be removed en-bloc with a tumor-free margin, avoiding rupture and intraperitoneal dissemination.

EUS may provide the surgeon with preoperative information about the size and topography of the tumor, its depth of infiltration, and possibly the presence of enlarged lymph nodes. This information is helpful in deciding on the type of surgery required. In the case of gastric GISTs ≤50 mm, laparoscopic wedge resection with or without endoscopic assistance is the treatment of choice in most cases (**Fig. 14.53**). Open and sometimes extensive surgery, including partial or total gastrectomy, is necessary particularly in cases of very large tumors and in unfavorable locations (**Fig. 14.54**). Neoadjuvant imatinib treatment in some cases of nonresectable or metastatic GISTs may reduce the tumor size sufficiently to allow organ-preserving surgery.[16,71,241–243,262,273–278] Following resection of a GIST with a moderate or high risk of malignant behavior, adjuvant treatment with the tyrosine kinase inhibitor imatinib is recommended.[242,273,279]

■ Asymptomatic Subepithelial Tumors

The management of asymptomatic subepithelial tumors of the gastrointestinal tract is a matter of controversy, since 71% of subepithelial tumors are hypoechoic[15] and GISTs, with their uncertain malignant potential, constitute the largest group among these hypoechoic tumors.

The task of EUS is to differentiate between:
- Definitely benign lesions that do not require any treatment or follow-up
- Probably benign lesions, which should either be treated with endoscopic methods or followed up at regular intervals
- Potentially malignant lesions, which either require further investigation with EUS-FNA or EUS-TCB, or which require endoscopic or surgical resection
- Definitely or probably malignant lesions, which require complete surgical resection (**Fig. 14.51**)

In this scenario, EUS may reduce the use of cost-intensive, potentially dangerous, and often unhelpful further diagnostic procedures.[280]

Abstaining from treatment, biopsy, and surveillance. The only definitely benign subepithelial lesions that require neither treatment nor follow-up are typical lipomas. We can support the recommendation that submucosal cysts should be excluded from treatment or follow-up[41] only in the case of typical solitary monocystic lesions. The group of multiple cystic, polycystic, and solid cystic subepithelial tumors is large and heterogeneous. It includes various forms of cystic subepithelial heterotopia in the gastric mucosa, which may be associated with gastric cancer, some cases of pancreatic heterotopia, which very rarely may be associated with adenocarcinoma or neuroendocrine tumor, or may develop complications, and GISTs with cystic degeneration (see above). In subepithelial tumors of the stomach that arise from the second or third echolayer, measure up to 20 mm, and cannot be confidently diagnosed as simple lipomas or cysts, the threshold for proceeding to endoscopic resection should be low.[101] In such cases, EUS-FNA is unhelpful in deciding whether or not to operate. Endosonographic follow-up is an alternative option.

Endosonographic follow-up also appears to be a reasonable option in a subgroup of small hypoechoic subepithelial tumors[16,243,273] (**Table 14.12**). Data on the natural history of small, localized hypoechoic subepithelial tumors is limited. Four recent studies have reported on EUS surveillance of a pooled total of 157 subepithelial tumors with a maximum size of 30 mm originating from the fourth or second echolayer in the upper gastrointestinal tract over

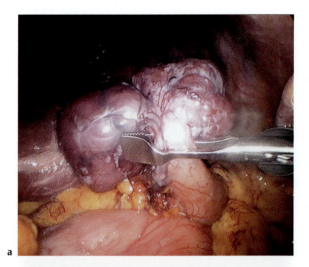

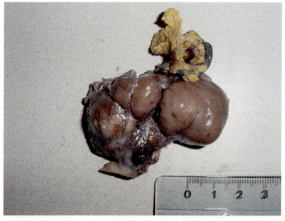

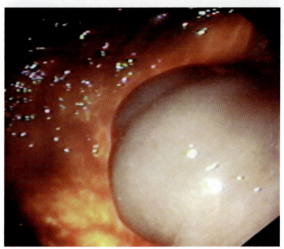

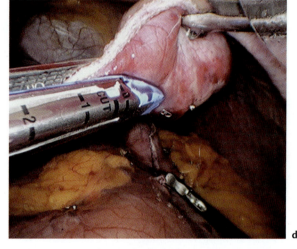

Fig. 14.53a–d Laparoscopic wedge resection of gastric gastrointestinal stromal tumors (GISTs) < 50 mm.
a A lobulated, extraluminally growing GIST, grasped with forceps.
b The resected specimen (intermediate-risk GIST).

c Endoscopic image of an intraluminally growing subepithelial tumor in the stomach, which was not visible with the surgical laparoscope (transillumination with the operating-room lamp).
d Assistance from a flexible endoscope facilitates laparoscopic wedge resection.

mean periods of 17–31 months. An increase in size and/or structural changes only occurred in 10.2–16.0% (pooled data: 19/157 = 12.1%) of these small subepithelial tumors with a "benign" EUS appearance. However, the definitions of "significant enlargement" used differed between the studies. Surgical pathology was available for 10 of the 19 tumors with significant enlargement. Only one tumor was a GIST with high malignant potential, five were GISTs with very low or low risk, two were schwannomas, and one was diagnosed as a gastric glomus tumor.[282–284,287] Data consistent with these findings were also provided by two studies with endoscopic surveillance of large groups of subepithelial tumors over periods of approximately 5 years, showing an increase in size in only two of 132 cases (1.5%) and 16 of 287 cases (5.5%), respectively.[9,10] A group in Israel reported follow-up data of 70 GISTs with

definite cytology or histology. Fourteen of 70 GISTs (20%) showed significant enlargement (> 1 mm/month). Increasing size was significantly more common with GISTs that were over 17 mm at the initial diagnosis.[285] Another group in the USA similarly found that a tumor size of > 20 mm at the index EUS and a suspicion of GIST or leiomyoma were predictive factors for significant size increases of subepithelial tumors in the gastrointestinal tract.[286]

In conclusion, the risk of following a surveillance strategy instead of endoscopic or surgical resection is very low in small (< 20 or 30 mm) hypoechoic subepithelial tumors with well-defined margins if they are homogeneous and if the layer of origin can be easily visualized without any signs of infiltration. In addition to this group of small hypoechoic subepithelial tumors, we would recommend endosonographic follow-up for cystic and mixed solid-

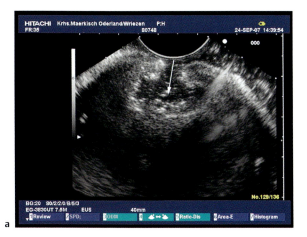
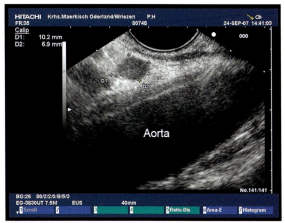

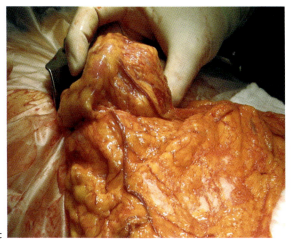
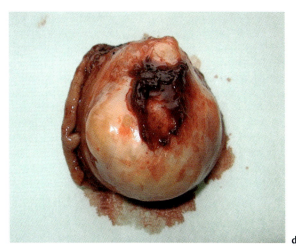

Fig. 14.54a–d Open resection of a bleeding hypoechoic subepithelial tumor in the stomach.
a A large ulceration (arrow) on the large tumor (>50 mm; cf. **Fig. 14.36**) in a patient who presented with severe upper gastrointestinal bleeding.

b Small hypoechoic perigastric lymph nodes close to the tumor site.
c Open surgical resection.
d The resected tumor, with a large ulceration.

Table 14.12 Criteria allowing EUS follow-up of hypoechoic and echocomplex subepithelial tumors

Asymptomatic patient (especially no hemorrhage, no intestinal obstruction)
Tumor size < 20 (30) mm[a]
Smooth margins, no signs of infiltrative growth, layer of origin clearly discernible
Homogeneous echo texture
No suspicious regional lymph nodes
During follow-up: no significant enlargement (e.g., >25% regardless of time interval or > 1 mm/month[b]), no change in structural EUS features, no symptoms
If (EUS-guided) biopsy was performed: no histological or cytological criteria of malignancy; histologically proven definitely benign tumors (e.g., schwannoma, leiomyoma, glomus tumor); histologically proven GIST (CD117 +) with a size of ≤ 20 (30) mm[a]

[a] Guidelines differ in their recommendations; the size threshold should be adjusted to the tumor location (20 mm for an extragastric location of a primary GIST), to age and to the individual surgical/interventional risk.
[b] There is no evidence-based definition of "significant enlargement."
GIST, gastrointestinal stromal tumor.

Table 14.13 Indications for surgical or endoscopic resection of hypoechoic and echocomplex subepithelial tumors

Tumor-related symptoms (especially hemorrhage or intestinal obstruction)
Tumor size ≥ 50 mm
≥ 2 EUS criteria of possible malignancy (tumor size ≥ 30 mm; irregular outer margins; inhomogeneous echo texture, particularly cystic spaces; infiltrative growth; suspicious regional lymph nodes)
During follow-up: significant enlargement (e.g., > 25% regardless of time interval or > 1 mm/month[b]), change in structural EUS features, tumor-related symptoms
If (EUS-guided) biopsy was performed: histological or cytological criteria of malignancy; histologically proven GIST (CD117 +) with a size of > 20 (30) mm[a]

[a] Guidelines differ in their recommendations; the size threshold should be adjusted to the tumor location (20 mm for an extragastric location of a primary GIST), to age and to the individual surgical/interventional risk.
[b] There is no evidence-based definition of "significant enlargement."
GIST, gastrointestinal stromal tumor.

cystic lesions (probable lymphangiomas, hemangiomas, pancreatic heterotopia, cystic hamartomas) that are not referred for histological investigation or endoscopic resection. A follow-up decision should be discussed with each patient on an individual basis,[41] as there are several problems with surveillance strategies. Firstly, there are no consistent and convincing definitions of "significant enlargement" or "rapid growth." Enlargement of > 25% along one diameter, regardless of the time interval,[282] or > 1 mm/month[285] both appear to be quite reasonable criteria. Secondly, both malignant and benign tumors may grow significantly. On the other hand, there is no definite proof that tumors that do not show rapid growth are not potentially malignant. Thirdly, optimal timing of EUS surveillance is still a matter of debate. An interval of 12 months appears to be adequate[243,283] and is used by 70% of the 134 endosonographers in the United States who responded to a recent survey of opinions and practices regarding diagnosis and management of GISTs.[254] The fourth and perhaps most serious problem with follow-up of subepithelial tumors is the clearly limited extent to which patients comply with surveillance examinations. In one prospective multicenter trial, a follow-up strategy for patients with hypoechoic subepithelial tumors without EUS features predictive of malignancy proved to be unsuccessful because of low patient compliance and lack of cost-effectiveness.[225] In one of the centers participating in the study, 54 of 97 patients scheduled for follow-up did not return for a second examination.[286] In the study by Lok et al., only 23 of 49 patients (46.9%) with small subepithelial tumors originating from the muscularis propria agreed to participate in surveillance.[284] An interesting alternative to endosonographic follow-up of subepithelial gastric tumors might be abdominal ultrasound surveillance. Three studies have shown that the great majority of subepithelial tumors of the stomach that have previously been diagnosed endoscopically or with EUS can be detected and measured using abdominal ultrasonography of the water-filled stomach (**Fig. 14.55**).[288–290]

When there is significant enlargement or distinct changes in the echo structure are seen during the follow-up, the tumor should be resected (**Table 14.13**).

Treatment decisions based on EUS-guided biopsy. If all subepithelial tumors that do not meet the above criteria for a benign tumor (**Table 14.10**) were surgically removed because of suspected malignancy, the prevalence of tumors that were found to be low-risk after resection would be unacceptably high (e.g., 65% in the report by Will et al.[41]). In our own patients, 31% (77/247) of hypoechoic subepithelial tumors met one of the EUS criteria for malignancy, and a further 31% (77/247) met at least two of these criteria[15] (**Figs. 14.45** and **14.46**). We would therefore suggest that in patients with asymptomatic subepithelial gastrointestinal tumors between 20 mm (30 mm) and 50 mm in size (not classified as lipomas or simple cysts) with no further endosonographic features of malignancy, therapeutic decisions should be based on the results of cytological and histological examinations (**Figs. 14.47, 14.48** and **14.51**). This is particularly worth considering if the risk of surgery is high or if the patient does not wish to undergo surgery. In such a scenario, it is important to try to obtain a core specimen (with EUS-FNA or EUS-TCB), as cytological smears in most cases are not sufficient for phenotyping and risk assessment of hypoechoic subepithelial tumors. Modern methods of investigation, such as immunohistochemistry and immunocytochemistry for determining the immunological phenotype and proliferative activity, and perhaps in the future also cytogenetic methods of analyzing mutations in the KIT gene, need to be included in the histopathologic and cytologic processing of the tissue samples obtained.

Resection. All asymptomatic subepithelial tumors that meet any of the following criteria definitely require resection: size > 50 mm; a significant increase in size or changes in structural EUS criteria during the follow-up period; development of symptoms during follow-up; two or more endosonographic features suggestive of malignancy (e.g., size ≥ 30 mm and an irregular outline); and cytolog-

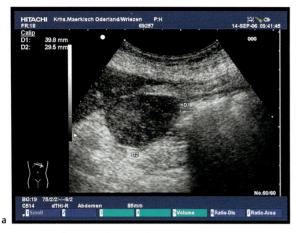
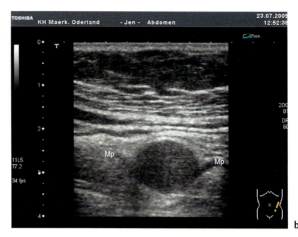

Fig. 14.55a,b Transabdominal ultrasound of gastrointestinal stromal tumors in the gastric wall (**a**; for the endosonographic image, see **Fig. 14.43**) and of the left colon (**b**). Mp, muscularis propria.

ical, histological, immunochemical, or cytogenetic criteria for a malignant neoplasm[15,41,243,273] (**Table 14.13**). With regard to histologically documented gastrointestinal stromal tumors, the latest guidelines recommend removal of all GISTs with diameters of ≥ 20 mm[241,273] or ≥ 30 mm.[243] The American Gastroenterological Association (AGA) also recommends resection of all tumors with endosonographic features suggestive of malignancy, regardless of their size.[243]

References

1. Gordon SJ, Rifkin MD, Goldberg BB. Endosonographic evaluation of mural abnormalities of the upper gastrointestinal tract. Gastrointest Endosc 1986;32(3):193–198.
2. Lambert R, Caletti G, Cho E, et al. International Workshop on the clinical impact of endoscopic ultrasound in gastroenterology. Endoscopy 2000;32(7):549–584.
3. Rifkin MD, Gordon SJ. Sonoendoscopic evaluation of extraesophageal and extragastric abnormalities: a review. Scand J Gastroenterol Suppl 1986;123:68–73.
4. Strohm WD, Classen M. Benign lesions of the upper GI tract by means of endoscopic ultrasonography. Scand J Gastroenterol Suppl 1986;123:41–46.
5. Van Stolk RU. Subepithelial lesions. In: Van Dam J, Sivak MV, eds. Gastrointestinal endosonography. Philadelphia: Saunders; 1999:153–165.
6. Takubo K, Nakagawa H, Tsuchiya S, Mitomo Y, Sasajima K, Shirota A. Seedling leiomyoma of the esophagus and esophagogastric junction zone. Hum Pathol 1981;12(11):1006–1010.
7. Abraham SC, Krasinskas AM, Hofstetter WL, Swisher SG, Wu TT. "Seedling" mesenchymal tumors (gastrointestinal stromal tumors and leiomyomas) are common incidental tumors of the esophagogastric junction. Am J Surg Pathol 2007;31(11):1629–1635.
8. Hedenbro JL, Ekelund M, Wetterberg P. Endoscopic diagnosis of submucosal gastric lesions. The results after routine endoscopy. Surg Endosc 1991;5(1):20–23.
9. Lee J-S, Son HJ, Kim YH, et al. Clinical course of subepithelial masses incidentally found by endoscopic examinations. Gastrointest Endosc 2007;65(5):AB167.
10. Imaoka H, Sawaki A, Mizuno N, et al. Incidence and clinical course of submucosal lesions of the stomach. Gastrointest Endosc 2005;61(5):AB167.
11. Yoo SS, Lee WH, Ha J, et al. The prevalence of esophageal disorders in the subjects examined for health screening. [Article in German] Korean J Gastroenterol 2007;50(5):306–312.
12. Hwang JH, Kimmey MB. The incidental upper gastrointestinal subepithelial mass. Gastroenterology 2004;126(1):301–307.
13. Ponsaing LG, Kiss K, Hansen MB. Classification of submucosal tumors in the gastrointestinal tract. World J Gastroenterol 2007;13(24):3311–3315.
14. Ponsaing LG, Kiss K, Loft A, Jensen LI, Hansen MB. Diagnostic procedures for submucosal tumors in the gastrointestinal tract. World J Gastroenterol 2007;13(24):3301–3310.
15. Jenssen C, Dietrich CF. Endoscopic ultrasound of gastrointestinal subepithelial lesions. Ultraschall Med 2008;29(3):236–256, quiz 257–264.
16. Sepe PS, Brugge WR. A guide for the diagnosis and management of gastrointestinal stromal cell tumors. Nat Rev Gastroenterol Hepatol 2009;6(6):363–371.
17. Scarpa M, Bertin M, Ruffolo C, Polese L, D'Amico DF, Angriman I. A systematic review on the clinical diagnosis of gastrointestinal stromal tumors. J Surg Oncol 2008;98(5):384–392.
18. Polkowski M. Endoscopic ultrasound and endoscopic ultrasound-guided fine-needle biopsy for the diagnosis of malignant submucosal tumors. Endoscopy 2005;37(7):635–645.
19. Mallery S, Lai R, Bardales R, Stelow E, Debol S, Stanley M. EUS-guided needle aspiration (EUS-FNA) in subepithelial GI-tract masses (SIGIM): results in 105 lesions. [abstract] Gastrointest Endosc 2004;59:AB234.
20. Davila RE, Faigel DO. GI stromal tumors. Gastrointest Endosc 2003;58(1):80–88.
21. Boyce GA, Sivak MV Jr, Rösch T, et al. Evaluation of submucosal upper gastrointestinal tract lesions by endoscopic ultrasound. Gastrointest Endosc 1991;37(4):449–454.

22. Faivre J, Bory R, Moulinier B. Benign tumors of oesophagus: value of endoscopy. Endoscopy 1978;10(4):264–268.

23. Rösch T, Classen M. Gastroenterologic Endosonography: Textbook and Atlas. Stuttgart: Thieme; 1992.

24. Rösch T, Kapfer B, Will U, et al. Endoscopy is not sufficient for a reliable diagnosis of upper GI submucosal tumors (SMT). [abstract] Gastrointest Endosc 1999;49:AB 212.

25. Rösch T, Lorenz R, Dancygier H, von Wickert A, Classen M. Endosonographic diagnosis of submucosal upper gastrointestinal tract tumors. Scand J Gastroenterol 1992; 27(1): 1–8.

26. Rösch T, Lorenz R, von Wichert A, Classen M. Gastric fundus impression caused by splenic vessels: detection by endoscopic ultrasound. Endoscopy 1991;23(2):85–87.

27. Hwang JH, Saunders MD, Rulyak SJ, Shaw S, Nietsch H, Kimmey MB. A prospective study comparing endoscopy and EUS in the evaluation of GI subepithelial masses. Gastrointest Endosc 2005;62(2):202–208.

28. Cantor MJ, Davila RE, Faigel DO. Yield of tissue sampling for subepithelial lesions evaluated by EUS: a comparison between forceps biopsies and endoscopic submucosal resection. Gastrointest Endosc 2006;64(1):29–34.

29. Hunt GC, Smith PP, Faigel DO. Yield of tissue sampling for submucosal lesions evaluated by EUS. Gastrointest Endosc 2003;57(1):68–72.

30. Rösch T, Kapfer B, Will U, et al. Endoscopic ultrasound (EUS) reduces the risk of large particle biopsy in upper GI submucosal lesions: a prospective study in 150 patients. [abstract] Gastrointest Endosc 1999;49:AB212.

31. Chung IK, Hawes RH. Advantages and limitations of endoscopic ultrasonography in the evaluation and management of patients with gastrointestinal submucosal tumors: a review. Rev Gastroenterol Disord 2007;7(4):179–192.

32. Chen TK, Wu CH, Lee CL, Lai YC, Yang SS, Tu TC. Endoscopic ultrasonography to study the causes of extragastric compression mimicking gastric submucosal tumor. J Formos Med Assoc 2001;100(11):758–761.

33. Motoo Y, Okai T, Ohta H, et al. Endoscopic ultrasonography in the diagnosis of extraluminal compressions mimicking gastric submucosal tumors. Endoscopy 1994;26(2): 239–242.

34. Rösch T, Kapfer B, Will U, et al; German EUS Club. Endoscopic ultrasonography. Accuracy of endoscopic ultrasonography in upper gastrointestinal submucosal lesions: a prospective multicenter study. Scand J Gastroenterol 2002;37(7):856–862.

35. Tio TL, Tytgat GN, den Hartog Jager FC. Endoscopic ultrasonography for the evaluation of smooth muscle tumors in the upper gastrointestinal tract: an experience with 42 cases. Gastrointest Endosc 1990;36(4):342–350.

36. Yasuda K, Nakajima M, Kawai K. Endoscopic ultrasonography in the diagnosis of submucosal tumor of the upper digestive tract. Scand J Gastroenterol Suppl 1986;123: 59–67.

37. Yasuda K, Nakajima M, Yoshida S, Kiyota K, Kawai K. The diagnosis of submucosal tumors of the stomach by endoscopic ultrasonography. Gastrointest Endosc 1989;35(1): 10–15.

38. Gress F, Schmitt C, Savides T, et al. Interobserver agreement for EUS in the evaluation and diagnosis of submucosal masses. Gastrointest Endosc 2001;53(1):71–76.

39. Rösch T. Endoscopic ultrasonography in upper gastrointestinal submucosal tumors: a literature review. Gastrointest Endosc Clin N Am 1995;5(3):609–614.

40. Hizawa K, Kawasaki M, Kouzuki T, et al. Endosonographic classifications of gastrointestinal submucosal tumors. Dig Endosc 2000;12:120–125.

41. Will U, Reinholz G, Bosseckert H. Wertigkeit der Endosonographie submuköser Tumore des oberen GIT. [abstract] Ultraschall Med 2001;22(Suppl):S118.

42. Shudo R, Yazaki Y, Sakurai S, et al. Adrenal adenoma mimicking a submucosal tumor of the stomach. Dig Endosc 2001;13:99–103.

43. Park JM, Kim J, Kim HI, Kim CS. Hepatic cyst misdiagnosed as a gastric submucosal tumor: a case report. World J Gastroenterol 2008;14(19):3092–3094.

44. Fritscher-Ravens A, Sriram PV, Schröder S, Topalidis T, Bohnacker S, Soehendra N. Stromal tumor as a pitfall in EUS-guided fine-needle aspiration cytology. Gastrointest Endosc 2000;51(6):746–749.

45. Fujisaki J, Chibai M. Endoscopic ultrasonography guided needle biopsy for submucosal tumors. Dig Endosc 2001; 13(Suppl 1):S57–S58.

46. Buscarini E, Stasi MD, Rossi S, et al. Endosonographic diagnosis of submucosal upper gastrointestinal tract lesions and large fold gastropathies by catheter ultrasound probe. Gastrointest Endosc 1999;49(2):184–191.

47. Xu GQ, Li YW, Han YM, et al. Miniature ultrasonic probes for diagnosis and treatment of digestive tract diseases. World J Gastroenterol 2004;10(13):1948–1953.

48. Murata Y, Yoshida M, Akimoto S, Ide H, Suzuki S, Hanyu F. Evaluation of endoscopic ultrasonography for the diagnosis of submucosal tumors of the esophagus. Surg Endosc 1988;2(2):51–58.

49. Koch J, Halvorsen RA Jr, Levenson SD, Cello JP. Prospective comparison of catheter-based endoscopic sonography versus standard endoscopic sonography: evaluation of gastrointestinal-wall abnormalities and staging of gastrointestinal malignancies. J Clin Ultrasound 2001;29(3):117–124.

50. Krinsky ML, Savides TJ, Behling CA. Ex-vivo correlation of endosonographic features with pathologic findings in gastric stromal tumors. [abstract] Gastrointest Endosc 2001; 53:AB170.

51. Waxman I, Saitoh Y, Raju GS, et al. High-frequency probe EUS-assisted endoscopic mucosal resection: a therapeutic strategy for submucosal tumors of the GI tract. Gastrointest Endosc 2002;55(1):44–49.

52. Niwa Y, Kobayashi S. Color Doppler-enhanced endoscopic ultrasonographic diagnosis of upper gastrointestinal submucosal lesions. Gastrointest Endosc 1998;47(1):95–96.

53. Săftoiu A, Vilmann P, Hassan H, Krag Jacobsen G. Utility of colour Doppler endoscopic ultrasound evaluation and guided therapy of submucosal tumours of the upper gastrointestinal tract. Ultraschall Med 2005;26(6):487–495.

54. Ando N, Goto H, Niwa Y, et al. The diagnosis of GI stromal tumors with EUS-guided fine needle aspiration with immunohistochemical analysis. Gastrointest Endosc 2002; 55(1):37–43.

55. Eloubeidi MA, Cohn M, Cerfolio RJ, et al. Endoscopic ultrasound-guided fine-needle aspiration in the diagnosis of foregut duplication cysts: the value of demonstrating detached ciliary tufts in cyst fluid. Cancer 2004; 102(4): 253–258.

56. Gu M, Ghafari S, Nguyen PT, Lin F. Cytologic diagnosis of gastrointestinal stromal tumors of the stomach by endoscopic ultrasound-guided fine-needle aspiration biopsy: cytomorphologic and immunohistochemical study of 12 cases. Diagn Cytopathol 2001;25(6):343–350.

57. Gu M, Nguyen PT, Cao S, Lin F. Diagnosis of gastric glomus tumor by endoscopic ultrasound-guided fine needle aspiration biopsy. A case report with cytologic, histologic and immunohistochemical studies. Acta Cytol 2002;46(3): 560–566.

58. Kinoshita K, Isozaki K, Tsutsui S, et al. Endoscopic ultrasonography-guided fine needle aspiration biopsy in follow-up patients with gastrointestinal stromal tumours. Eur J Gastroenterol Hepatol 2003;15(11):1189–1193.

59. Matsui M, Goto H, Niwa Y, Arisawa T, Hirooka Y, Hayakawa T. Preliminary results of fine needle aspiration biopsy histology in upper gastrointestinal submucosal tumors. Endoscopy 1998;30(9):750–755.

60. Okubo K, Yamao K, Nakamura T, et al. Endoscopic ultrasound-guided fine-needle aspiration biopsy for the diagnosis of gastrointestinal stromal tumors in the stomach. J Gastroenterol 2004;39(8):747–753.

61. Sasaki Y, Niwa Y, Hirooka Y, et al. The use of endoscopic ultrasound-guided fine-needle aspiration for investigation of submucosal and extrinsic masses of the colon and rectum. Endoscopy 2005;37(2):154–160.

62. Stelow EB, Lai R, Bardales RH, Linzie BM, Mallery S, Stanley MW. Endoscopic ultrasound-guided fine-needle aspiration cytology of peripheral nerve-sheath tumors. Diagn Cytopathol 2004;30(3):172–177.

63. Van der Noot MR III, Eloubeidi MA, Chen VK, et al. Diagnosis of gastrointestinal tract lesions by endoscopic ultrasound-guided fine-needle aspiration biopsy. Cancer 2004; 102(3):157–163.

64. Akahoshi K, Sumida Y, Matsui N, et al. Preoperative diagnosis of gastrointestinal stromal tumor by endoscopic ultrasound-guided fine needle aspiration. World J Gastroenterol 2007;13(14):2077–2082.

65. Chatzipantelis P, Salla C, Karoumpalis I, et al. Endoscopic ultrasound-guided fine needle aspiration biopsy in the diagnosis of gastrointestinal stromal tumors of the stomach. A study of 17 cases. J Gastrointestin Liver Dis 2008;17(1): 15–20.

66. Chen VK, Eloubeidi MA. Endoscopic ultrasound-guided fine-needle aspiration of intramural and extraintestinal mass lesions: diagnostic accuracy, complication assessment, and impact on management. Endoscopy 2005; 37(10):984–989.

67. Gomes AL, Bardales RH, Milanezi F, Reis RM, Schmitt F. Molecular analysis of c-Kit and PDGFRA in GISTs diagnosed by EUS. Am J Clin Pathol 2007;127(1):89–96.

68. Hamerski CM, Shergill AK, DeLusong MAA, et al. Yield of endoscopic ultrasound guided fine needle aspiration (EUS-FNA) in diagnosing submucosal lesions of the upper GI tract. Gastrointest Endosc 2008;67(5):AB222.

69. Hoda KM, Rodriguez SA, Faigel DO. EUS-guided sampling of suspected GI stromal tumors. Gastrointest Endosc 2009; 69(7):1218–1223.

70. Khan MA, Lu LP, Eloubeidi MA. Combined use of endoscopic ultrasonography (EUS) guided fine-needle aspiration (FNA) cytological analysis and immunohistochemistry for the diagnosis of gastrointestinal stromal tumors (GIST). Gastrointest Endosc 2009;69(5):AB338.

71. Mochizuki Y, Kodera Y, Fujiwara M, et al. Laparoscopic wedge resection for gastrointestinal stromal tumors of the stomach: initial experience. Surg Today 2006;36(4): 341–347.

72. Sepe PS, Moparty B, Pitman MB, Saltzman JR, Brugge WR. EUS-guided FNA for the diagnosis of GI stromal cell tumors:

73. sensitivity and cytologic yield. Gastrointest Endosc 2009;70(2):254–261.

73. Shah R, Early DS, Edmundowicz SA, Azar RR. The spectrum of subepithelial gastric lesions in a tertiary referral EUS practice. Gastrointest Endosc 2007;65(5):AB204.

74. Stelow EB, Stanley MW, Mallery S, Lai R, Linzie BM, Bardales RH. Endoscopic ultrasound-guided fine-needle aspiration findings of gastrointestinal leiomyomas and gastrointestinal stromal tumors. Am J Clin Pathol 2003;119(5):703–708.

75. Stelow EB, Murad FM, Debol SM, et al. A limited immunocytochemical panel for the distinction of subepithelial gastrointestinal mesenchymal neoplasms sampled by endoscopic ultrasound-guided fine-needle aspiration. Am J Clin Pathol 2008;129(2):219–225.

76. Yadav D, Levy MJ, Schwartz D, Jondal ML, Clain J, Wiersema MJ. EUS-guided trucut biopsy for diagnosis of an esophageal stromal tumor: case report. Gastrointest Endosc 2003;58(3):457–460.

77. Ribeiro A, Vernon S, Quintela P. EUS-guided trucut biopsy with immunohistochemical analysis of a gastric stromal tumor. Gastrointest Endosc 2004;60(4):645–648.

78. Fernandez-Esparrach G, Sendino O, Sole M, et al. Endoscopic ultrasound-guided fine-needle aspiration and trucut biopsy in the diagnosis of gastric stromal tumors: a randomized crossover study. Endoscopy 2010;42(4): 292–299.

79. Kipp BR, Pereira TC, Souza PC, Gleeson FC, Levy MJ, Clayton AC. Comparison of EUS-guided FNA and Trucut biopsy for diagnosing and staging abdominal and mediastinal neoplasms. Diagn Cytopathol 2009;37(8):549–556.

80. Polkowski M, Gerke W, Jarosz D, et al. Diagnostic yield and safety of endoscopic ultrasound-guided trucut [corrected] biopsy in patients with gastric submucosal tumors: a prospective study. Endoscopy 2009;41(4):329–334.

81. Sun S, Wang M, Sun S. Use of endoscopic ultrasound-guided injection in endoscopic resection of solid submucosal tumors. Endoscopy 2002;34(1):82–85.

82. Pedersen FM, Vilmann P, Bytzer P. Gastric arteriovenous malformation: Doppler EUS-guided diagnosis and therapy. Gastrointest Endosc 2002;55(4):597–599.

83. Günter E, Lingenfelser T, Eitelbach F, Müller H, Ell C. EUS-guided ethanol injection for treatment of a GI stromal tumor. Gastrointest Endosc 2003;57(1):113–115.

84. Levy MJ, Wong Kee Song LM, Farnell MB, Misra S, Sarr MG, Gostout CJ. Endoscopic ultrasound (EUS)-guided angiotherapy of refractory gastrointestinal bleeding. Am J Gastroenterol 2008;103(2):352–359.

85. Okanobu H, Hata J, Haruma K, et al. A classification system of echogenicity for gastrointestinal neoplasms. Digestion 2005;72(1):8–12.

86. Matsushita M, Hajiro K, Okazaki K, Takakuwa H. Gastric inflammatory fibroid polyps: endoscopic ultrasonographic analysis in comparison with the histology. Gastrointest Endosc 1997;46(1):53–57.

87. Chak A, Canto MI, Rösch T, et al. Endosonographic differentiation of benign and malignant stromal cell tumors. Gastrointest Endosc 1997;45(6):468–473.

88. Kojima T, Takahashi H, Parra-Blanco A, Kohsen K, Fujita R. Diagnosis of submucosal tumor of the upper GI tract by endoscopic resection. Gastrointest Endosc 1999;50(4): 516–522.

89. Hizawa K, Aoyagi K, Kurahara K, et al. Gastrointestinal lymphangioma: endosonographic demonstration and endoscopic removal. Gastrointest Endosc 1996;43(6): 620–624.

90. Matsushita M, Takakuwa H, Nishio A. Characteristic endosonographic features of gastric inflammatory fibroid polyps. Endoscopy 2001;33(8):729–730.

91. Kono K, Sekikawa T, Iino H, Ogawara T, Matsumoto Y. A case of arteriovenous malformation in the submucosal layer of the stomach. J Gastroenterol 1994;29(3):340–343.

92. Arafa UA, Fujiwara Y, Shiba M, Higuchi K, Wakasa K, Arakawa T. Endoscopic resection of a cavernous haemangioma of the stomach. Dig Liver Dis 2002;34(11):808–811.

93. Tominaga K, Arakawa T, Ando K, et al. Oesophageal cavernous haemangioma diagnosed histologically, not by endoscopic procedures. J Gastroenterol Hepatol 2000;15(2):215–219.

94. Fazel A, Moezardalan K, Varadarajulu S, Draganov P, Eloubeidi MA. The utility and the safety of EUS-guided FNA in the evaluation of duplication cysts. Gastrointest Endosc 2005;62(4):575–580.

95. Sato M, Irisawa A, Bhutani MS, et al. Gastric bronchogenic cyst diagnosed by endosonographically guided fine needle aspiration biopsy. J Clin Ultrasound 2008;36(4):237–239.

96. Westerterp M, van den Berg JG, van Lanschot JJ, Fockens P. Intramural bronchogenic cysts mimicking solid tumors. Endoscopy 2004;36(12):1119–1122.

97. Choong NW, Levy MJ, Rajan E, Kolars JC. Intramural gastric abscess: case history and review. Gastrointest Endosc 2003;58(4):627–629.

98. Soon MS, Yen HH, Soon A, Lin OS. Endoscopic ultrasonographic appearance of gastric emphysema. World J Gastroenterol 2005;11(11):1719–1721.

99. Will U, Masri R, Bosseckert H, Knopke A, Schönlebe J, Justus J. Gastric wall abscess, a rare endosonographic differential diagnosis of intramural tumors: successful endoscopic treatment. Endoscopy 1998;30(4):432–435.

100. Mizuma N, Kabemura T, Akahoshi K, et al. Endosonographic features of mucocele of the appendix: report of a case. Gastrointest Endosc 1997;46(6):549–552.

101. Hizawa K, Matsumoto T, Kouzuki T, Suekane H, Esaki M, Fujishima M. Cystic submucosal tumors in the gastrointestinal tract: endosonographic findings and endoscopic removal. Endoscopy 2000;32(9):712–714.

102. Miettinen M, Sobin LH, Sarlomo-Rikala M. Immunohistochemical spectrum of GISTs at different sites and their differential diagnosis with a reference to CD117 (KIT). Mod Pathol 2000;13(10):1134–1142.

103. Faigel DO, Burke A, Ginsberg GG, Stotland BR, Kadish SL, Kochman ML. The role of endoscopic ultrasound in the evaluation and management of foregut duplications. Gastrointest Endosc 1997;45(1):99–103.

104. Geller A, Wang KK, DiMagno EP. Diagnosis of foregut duplication cysts by endoscopic ultrasonography. Gastroenterology 1995;109(3):838–842.

105. Riyaz A, Cohen H. Ectopic pancreas presenting as a submucosal gastric antral tumor that was cystic on EUS. Gastrointest Endosc 2001;53(6):675–677.

106. Van Dam J, Rice TW, Sivak MV Jr. Endoscopic ultrasonography and endoscopically guided needle aspiration for the diagnosis of upper gastrointestinal tract foregut cysts. Am J Gastroenterol 1992;87(6):762–765.

107. Kim KM, Choi KY, Lee A, Kim BK. Lymphangioma of large intestine: report of ten cases with endoscopic and pathologic correlation. Gastrointest Endosc 2000;52(2):255–259.

108. Ishikawa N, Fuchigami T, Kikuchi Y, et al. EUS for gastric lymphangioma. Gastrointest Endosc 2000;52(6):798–800.

109. Kameyama H, Niwa Y, Arisawa T, Goto H, Hayakawa T. Endoscopic ultrasonography in the diagnosis of submucosal lesions of the large intestine. Gastrointest Endosc 1997;46(5):406–411.

110. Kochman ML, Wiersema MJ, Hawes RH, Canal D, Wiersema L. Preoperative diagnosis of cystic lymphangioma of the colon by endoscopic ultrasound. Gastrointest Endosc 1997;45(2):204–206.

111. Jovanovic I, Alempijevic T, Lukic S, et al. Cystic dystrophy in heterotopic pancreas of the duodenal wall. Dig Surg 2008;25(4):262–268.

112. Naitoh I, Okayama Y, Hirai M, et al. Exophytic pedunculated gastrointestinal stromal tumor with remarkable cystic change. J Gastroenterol 2003;38(12):1181–1184.

113. Changchien CS, Hsu CC, Hu TH. Endosonographic appearances of Brunner's gland hamartomas. J Clin Ultrasound 2001;29(4):243–246.

114. Kaufman DJ, Al Kharrat H, Weiss S, Robert M, Topazian M. EUS-guided endoscopic removal of a large Brunner's gland hamartoma. Gastrointest Endosc 2003;58(2):313–314.

115. Matsushita M, Hajiro K, Takakuwa H, Nishio A. Characteristic EUS appearance of Brunner's gland hamartoma. Gastrointest Endosc 1999;49(5):670–672.

116. Soon MS, Lin OS, Yeh KT. Gastric mucosal heterotopia in the gastric submucosa: an evaluation by EUS. Gastrointest Endosc 1999;49(4 Pt 1):534–537.

117. Okada M, Iizuka Y, Oh K, Murayama H, Maekawa T. Gastritis cystica profunda presenting as giant gastric mucosal folds: the role of endoscopic ultrasonography and mucosectomy in the diagnostic work-up. Gastrointest Endosc 1994; 40(5):640–644.

118. Shudo R, Horita K, Takahashi K, et al. A case of gastritis cystica polyposa showing a characteristic endoscopic ultrasonogram. Dig Endosc 2000;12:68–72.

119. Hizawa K, Suekane H, Kawasaki M, Yao T, Aoyagi K, Fujishima M. Diffuse cystic malformation and neoplasia-associated cystic formation in the stomach. Endosonographic features and diagnosis of tumor depth. J Clin Gastroenterol 1997;25(4):634–639.

120. Bodnár Z, Bubán T, Várvölgyi C. Submucosal tumor-like gastric wall abscess. Gastrointest Endosc 2004;59(4):599.

121. Chen CH, Yang CC, Yeh YH, Hwang MH. Gastric wall abscess presenting as a submucosal tumor: case report. Gastrointest Endosc 2003;57(7):959–962.

122. Kim SH, Park JH, Kang KH, et al. Gastric tuberculosis presenting as a submucosal tumor. Gastrointest Endosc 2005;61(2):319–322.

123. Niizawa M, Ishida H, Morikawa P, Watanabe H, Masamune O. Diffuse heterotopic submucosal cystic malformation of the stomach: ultrasonographic diagnosis. Gastrointest Radiol 1992;17(1):9–12.

124. Ohtsuka H, Ikeda M, Morozumi A, et al. Diagnosis of multiple submucosal cysts of the stomach by endoscopic ultrasonography. Dig Endosc 2001;13:207–211.

125. Armstrong CP, King PM, Dixon JM, Macleod IB. The clinical significance of heterotopic pancreas in the gastrointestinal tract. Br J Surg 1981;68(4):384–387.

126. Chen HL, Chang WH, Shih SC, Bair MJ, Lin SC. Changing pattern of ectopic pancreas: 22 years of experience in a medical center. J Formos Med Assoc 2008;107(12):932–936.

127. Chou SJ, Chou YW, Jan HC, Chen VT, Chen TH. Ectopic pancreas in the ampulla of vater with obstructive jaundice. A case report and review of literature. Dig Surg 2006;23(4):262–264.

128. Eisenberger CF, Gocht A, Knoefel WT, et al. Heterotopic pancreas—clinical presentation and pathology with review of the literature. Hepatogastroenterology 2004;51(57): 854–858.

129. Ormarsson OT, Gudmundsdottir I, Mårvik R. Diagnosis and treatment of gastric heterotopic pancreas. World J Surg 2006;30(9):1682–1689.

130. Rebours V, Lévy P, Vullierme MP, et al. Clinical and morphological features of duodenal cystic dystrophy in heterotopic pancreas. Am J Gastroenterol 2007;102(4):871–879.

131. Rimal D, Thapa SR, Munasinghe N, Chitre VV. Symptomatic gastric heterotopic pancreas: clinical presentation and review of the literature. Int J Surg 2008;6(6):e52–e54.

132. Shaib YH, Rabaa E, Feddersen RM, Jamal MM, Qaseem T. Gastric outlet obstruction secondary to heterotopic pancreas in the antrum: case report and review. Gastrointest Endosc 2001;54(4):527–530.

133. Wall I, Shah T, Tangorra M, Li JJ, Tenner S. Giant heterotopic pancreas presenting with massive upper gastrointestinal bleeding. Dig Dis Sci 2007;52(4):956–959.

134. Yuan Z, Chen J, Zheng Q, Huang XY, Yang Z, Tang J. Heterotopic pancreas in the gastrointestinal tract. World J Gastroenterol 2009;15(29):3701–3703.

135. Cárdenas CM, Domínguez I, Campuzano M, et al. Malignant insulinoma arising from intrasplenic heterotopic pancreas. JOP 2009;10(3):321–323.

136. Chetty R, Weinreb I. Gastric neuroendocrine carcinoma arising from heterotopic pancreatic tissue. J Clin Pathol 2004;57(3):314–317.

137. Emerson L, Layfield LJ, Rohr LR, Dayton MT. Adenocarcinoma arising in association with gastric heterotopic pancreas: A case report and review of the literature. J Surg Oncol 2004;87(1):53–57.

138. Jeong HY, Yang HW, Seo SW, et al. Adenocarcinoma arising from an ectopic pancreas in the stomach. Endoscopy 2002;34(12):1014–1017.

139. Phillips J, Katz A, Zopolsky P. Intraductal papillary mucinous neoplasm in an ectopic pancreas located in the gastric wall. Gastrointest Endosc 2006;64(5):814–815, discussion 815.

140. Tolentino LF, Lee H, Maung T, Stabile BE, Li K, French SW. Islet cell tumor arising from a heterotopic pancreas in the duodenal wall with ulceration. Exp Mol Pathol 2004;76(1):51–56.

141. Matsushita M, Hajiro K, Okazaki K, Takakuwa H. Gastric aberrant pancreas: EUS analysis in comparison with the histology. Gastrointest Endosc 1999;49(4 Pt 1):493–497.

142. Chen SH, Huang WH, Feng CL, et al. Clinical analysis of ectopic pancreas with endoscopic ultrasonography: an experience in a medical center. J Gastrointest Surg 2008; 12(5):877–881.

143. Heinrich H. Ein Beitrag zur Histologie des so genannten akzessorischen Pankreas. Virchows Arch Path Anat Physiol 1909;198:392–401.

144. Yen HH, Soon MS, Soon A. Heterotopic pancreas presenting as gastric submucosal cyst on endoscopic sonography. J Clin Ultrasound 2006;34(4):203–206.

145. Oka R, Okai T, Kitakata H, Ohta T. Heterotopic pancreas with calcification: a lesion mimicking leiomyosarcoma of the stomach. Gastrointest Endosc 2002;56(6):939–942.

146. Kim JH, Lim JS, Lee YC, et al. Endosonographic features of gastric ectopic pancreases distinguishable from mesenchymal tumors. J Gastroenterol Hepatol 2008;23(8 Pt 2): e301–e307.

147. Chak A. EUS in submucosal tumors. Gastrointest Endosc 2002; 56(4, Suppl):S43–S48.

148. Schuhmacher C, Becker K, Dittler HJ, Höfler H, Siewert JR, Stein HJ. Fibrovascular esophageal polyp as a diagnostic challenge. Dis Esophagus 2000;13(4):324–327.

149. Matsushita M, Okazaki K. Atypical EUS features of gastric inflammatory fibroid polyps. Gastrointest Endosc 2005; 61(4):637–638, author reply 638.

150. Watanabe T, Kato K, Sugitani M, et al. A case of solitary amyloidosis localized within the transverse colon presenting as a submucosal tumor. Gastrointest Endosc 1999; 49(5): 644–647.

151. Roseau G, Dumontier I, Palazzo L, et al. Rectosigmoid endometriosis: endoscopic ultrasound features and clinical implications. Endoscopy 2000;32(7):525–530.

152. Pishvaian AC, Ahlawat SK, Garvin D, Haddad NG. Role of EUS and EUS-guided FNA in the diagnosis of symptomatic rectosigmoid endometriosis. Gastrointest Endosc 2006; 63(2): 331–335.

153. Miettinen M, Lasota J. Gastrointestinal stromal tumors—definition, clinical, histological, immunohistochemical, and molecular genetic features and differential diagnosis. Virchows Arch 2001;438(1):1–12.

154. Miettinen M, Lasota J. Gastrointestinal stromal tumors: pathology and prognosis at different sites. Semin Diagn Pathol 2006;23(2):70–83.

155. Miettinen M, Lasota J. Gastrointestinal stromal tumors: review on morphology, molecular pathology, prognosis, and differential diagnosis. Arch Pathol Lab Med 2006;130(10): 1466–1478.

156. Abraham SC. Distinguishing gastrointestinal stromal tumors from their mimics: an update. Adv Anat Pathol 2007;14(3):178–188.

157. Ji F, Wang ZW, Wang LJ, Ning JW, Xu GQ. Clinicopathological characteristics of gastrointestinal mesenchymal tumors and diagnostic value of endoscopic ultrasonography. J Gastroenterol Hepatol 2008;23(8 Pt 2):e318–e324.

158. Agaimy A, Wünsch PH. Sporadic Cajal cell hyperplasia is common in resection specimens for distal oesophageal carcinoma. A retrospective review of 77 consecutive surgical resection specimens. Virchows Arch 2006;448(3): 288–294.

159. Debiec-Rychter M, Lasota J, Sarlomo-Rikala M, Kordek R, Miettinen M. Chromosomal aberrations in malignant gastrointestinal stromal tumors: correlation with c-KIT gene mutation. Cancer Genet Cytogenet 2001;128(1):24–30.

160. Espinosa I, Lee CH, Kim MK, et al. A novel monoclonal antibody against DOG1 is a sensitive and specific marker for gastrointestinal stromal tumors. Am J Surg Pathol 2008; 32(2):210–218.

161. Liegl B, Hornick JL, Corless CL, Fletcher CD. Monoclonal antibody DOG1.1 shows higher sensitivity than KIT in the diagnosis of gastrointestinal stromal tumors, including unusual subtypes. Am J Surg Pathol 2009;33(3):437–446.

162. Miettinen M, Wang ZF, Lasota J. DOG1 antibody in the differential diagnosis of gastrointestinal stromal tumors: a study of 1840 cases. Am J Surg Pathol 2009; 33(9): 1401–1408.

163. Fletcher CD, Berman JJ, Corless C, et al. Diagnosis of gastrointestinal stromal tumors: A consensus approach. Hum Pathol 2002;33(5):459–465.

164. DeMatteo RP, Lewis JJ, Leung D, Mudan SS, Woodruff JM, Brennan MF. Two hundred gastrointestinal stromal tumors: recurrence patterns and prognostic factors for survival. Ann Surg 2000;231(1):51–58.

165. DeMatteo RP, Gold JS, Saran L, et al. Tumor mitotic rate, size, and location independently predict recurrence after resec-

tion of primary gastrointestinal stromal tumor (GIST). Cancer 2008;112(3):608–615.

166. Emory TS, Sobin LH, Lukes L, Lee DH, O'Leary TJ. Prognosis of gastrointestinal smooth-muscle (stromal) tumors: dependence on anatomic site. Am J Surg Pathol 1999;23(1):82–87.

167. Agaimy A, Wünsch PH, Hofstaedter F, et al. Minute gastric sclerosing stromal tumors (GIST tumorlets) are common in adults and frequently show c-KIT mutations. Am J Surg Pathol 2007;31(1):113–120.

168. Agaimy A, Wünsch PH, Dirnhofer S, Bihl MP, Terracciano LM, Tornillo L. Microscopic gastrointestinal stromal tumors in esophageal and intestinal surgical resection specimens: a clinicopathologic, immunohistochemical, and molecular study of 19 lesions. Am J Surg Pathol 2008;32(6):867–873.

169. Chetty R. Small and microscopically detected gastrointestinal stromal tumours: an overview. Pathology 2008; 40(1):9–12.

170. Kawanowa K, Sakuma Y, Sakurai S, et al. High incidence of microscopic gastrointestinal stromal tumors in the stomach. Hum Pathol 2006;37(12):1527–1535.

171. Agaimy A, Wünsch PH. Lymph node metastasis in gastrointestinal stromal tumours (GIST) occurs preferentially in young patients < or =40 years: an overview based on our case material and the literature. Langenbecks Arch Surg 2009;394(2):375–381.

172. Miettinen M, Sobin LH, Lasota J. True smooth muscle tumors of the small intestine: a clinicopathologic, immunohistochemical, and molecular genetic study of 25 cases. Am J Surg Pathol 2009;33(3):430–436.

173. Zhu X, Zhang XQ, Li BM, Xu P, Zhang KH, Chen J. Esophageal mesenchymal tumors: endoscopy, pathology and immunohistochemistry. World J Gastroenterol 2007;13(5): 768–773.

174. Kwon MS, Lee SS, Ahn GH. Schwannomas of the gastrointestinal tract: clinicopathological features of 12 cases including a case of esophageal tumor compared with those of gastrointestinal stromal tumors and leiomyomas of the gastrointestinal tract. Pathol Res Pract 2002;198(9): 605–613.

175. Daimaru Y, Kido H, Hashimoto H, Enjoji M. Benign schwannoma of the gastrointestinal tract: a clinicopathologic and immunohistochemical study. Hum Pathol 1988;19(3): 257–264.

176. Hou YY, Tan YS, Xu JF, et al. Schwannoma of the gastrointestinal tract: a clinicopathological, immunohistochemical and ultrastructural study of 33 cases. Histopathology 2006;48(5):536–545.

177. Miettinen M, Shekitka KM, Sobin LH. Schwannomas in the colon and rectum: a clinicopathologic and immunohistochemical study of 20 cases. Am J Surg Pathol 2001; 25(7):846–855.

178. Hong HS, Ha HK, Won HJ, et al. Gastric schwannomas: radiological features with endoscopic and pathological correlation. Clin Radiol 2008;63(5):536–542.

179. Hou YY, Tan YS, Xu JF, et al. Schwannoma of the gastrointestinal tract: a clinicopathological, immunohistochemical and ultrastructural study of 33 cases. Histopathology 2006;48(5):536–545.

180. Jung MK, Jeon SW, Cho CM, et al. Gastric schwannomas: endosonographic characteristics. Abdom Imaging 2008; 33(4):388–390.

181. Okai T, Minamoto T, Ohtsubo K, et al. Endosonographic evaluation of c-kit-positive gastrointestinal stromal tumor. Abdom Imaging 2003;28(3):301–307.

182. Kim GH, Park Y, Kim S, et al. Is it possible to differentiate gastric GISTs from gastric leiomyomas by EUS? World J Gastroenterol 2009;15(27):3376–3381.

183. Miettinen M, Sarlomo-Rikala M, Sobin LH. Mesenchymal tumors of muscularis mucosae of colon and rectum are benign leiomyomas that should be separated from gastrointestinal stromal tumors—a clinicopathologic and immunohistochemical study of eighty-eight cases. Mod Pathol 2001;14(10):950–956.

184. Xu GQ, Zhang BL, Li YM, et al. Diagnostic value of endoscopic ultrasonography for gastrointestinal leiomyoma. World J Gastroenterol 2003;9(9):2088–2091.

185. Miettinen M, Sarlomo-Rikala M, Sobin LH, Lasota J. Esophageal stromal tumors: a clinicopathologic, immunohistochemical, and molecular genetic study of 17 cases and comparison with esophageal leiomyomas and leiomyosarcomas. Am J Surg Pathol 2000;24(2):211–222.

186. Miettinen M, Makhlouf H, Sobin LH, Lasota J. Gastrointestinal stromal tumors of the jejunum and ileum: a clinicopathologic, immunohistochemical, and molecular genetic study of 906 cases before imatinib with long-term follow-up. Am J Surg Pathol 2006;30(4):477–489.

187. Choi KD, Song HJ, Lee GH, et al. Role of endoscopic ultrasonography in pathologic diagnosis of upper gastrointestinal subepithelial lesions. Gastrointest Endosc 2007; 65(5): AB204.

188. Calabrese C, Fabbri A, Fusaroli P, Di Gaetano P, Miglioli M, Di Febo G. Diffuse esophageal leiomyomatosis: case report and review. Gastrointest Endosc 2002;55(4):590–593.

189. Kuo MJ, Yeh HZ, Chen GH, Jan YJ. Diffuse esophageal leiomyomatosis with a pedunculated polyp. J Gastroenterol 2004;39(12):1205–1209.

190. Sotoudehmanesh R, Ghafoori A, Mikaeli J, Tavangar SM, Moghaddam HM. Esophageal leiomyomatosis diagnosed by endoscopic ultrasound. Endoscopy 2005;37(3):281.

191. Palazzo L, Landi B, Cellier C, et al. Endosonographic features of esophageal granular cell tumors. Endoscopy 1997; 29(9):850–853.

192. Yazumi S, Takahashi R, Kajiyama T, et al. Comparison of histological analysis and endosonographic features in esophageal granular cell tumors. Dig Endosc 2003;15: 284–288.

193. Costa PM, Marques A, Távora, Oliveira E, Diaz M. Inflammatory fibroid polyp of the esophagus. Dis Esophagus 2000;13(1):75–79.

194. Devereaux BM, LeBlanc JK, Kesler K, et al. Giant fibrovascular polyp of the esophagus. Endoscopy 2003;35(11): 970–972.

195. Aimoto T, Sasajima K, Kyono S, et al. Leiomyosarcoma of the esophagus: report of a case and preoperative evaluation by CT scan, endoscopic ultrasonography and angiography. Gastroenterol Jpn 1992;27(6):773–779.

196. Miettinen M, Sobin LH, Lasota J. Gastrointestinal stromal tumors of the stomach: a clinicopathologic, immunohistochemical, and molecular genetic study of 1765 cases with long-term follow-up. Am J Surg Pathol 2005;29(1):52–68.

197. Kawamoto K, Yamada Y, Furukawa N, et al. Endoscopic submucosal tumorectomy for gastrointestinal submucosal tumors restricted to the submucosa: a new form of endoscopic minimal surgery. Gastrointest Endosc 1997;46(4): 311–317.

198. Nakazawa S, Yoshino J, Nakamura T, et al. Endoscopic ultrasonography of gastric myogenic tumor. A comparative study between histology and ultrasonography. J Ultrasound Med 1989;8(7):353–359.

199. Debol SM, Stanley MW, Mallery S, Sawinski E, Bardales RH. Glomus tumor of the stomach: cytologic diagnosis by endoscopic ultrasound-guided fine-needle aspiration. Diagn Cytopathol 2003;28(6):316–321.

200. Jenssen C, Schick B, Wagner S. Primary diagnosis of serous papillary ovarian carcinoma by EUS-guided fine-needle aspiration biopsy of a submucosal gastric tumor: A case report. [Article in German] Endosk Heute 2006;19:32–35.

201. Yan SL, Yeh YH, Chen CH, Yang CC, Kuo CL, Wu HS. Gastric glomus tumor: a hypervascular submucosal tumor on power Doppler endosonography. J Clin Ultrasound 2007; 35(3):164–168.

202. Parfitt JR, Rodriguez-Justo M, Feakins R, Novelli MR. Gastrointestinal Kaposi's sarcoma: CD117 expression and the potential for misdiagnosis as gastrointestinal stromal tumour. Histopathology 2008;52(7):816–823.

203. Sangha S, Gergeos F, Freter R, Paiva LL, Jacobson BC. Diagnosis of ovarian cancer metastatic to the stomach by EUS-guided FNA. Gastrointest Endosc 2003;58(6):933–935.

204. Zoller WG, Bogner JR, Powitz F, Liess H, Goebel FD. Endoscopic ultrasound in the diagnosis and staging of gastrointestinal Kaposi's sarcoma. Endoscopy 1995;27(2): 191–196.

205. Zoufaly A, Schmiedel S, Lohse AW, van Lunzen J. Intestinal Kaposi's sarcoma may mimic gastrointestinal stromal tumor in HIV infection. World J Gastroenterol 2007;13(33): 4514–4516.

206. Arantes V, Logroño R, Faruqi S, Ahmed I, Waxman I, Bhutani MS. Endoscopic sonographically guided fine-needle aspiration yield in submucosal tumors of the gastrointestinal tract. J Ultrasound Med 2004;23(9):1141–1150.

207. Kawamoto K, Yamada Y, Utsunomiya T, et al. Gastrointestinal submucosal tumors: evaluation with endoscopic US. Radiology 1997;205(3):733–740.

208. Oda I, Kondo H, Yamao T, et al. Metastatic tumors to the stomach: analysis of 54 patients diagnosed at endoscopy and 347 autopsy cases. Endoscopy 2001;33(6):507–510.

209. Xu GQ, Wu YQ, Wang LJ, Chen HT. Values of endoscopic ultrasonography for diagnosis and treatment of duodenal protruding lesions. J Zhejiang Univ Sci B 2008; 9(4): 329–334.

210. Inai M, Sakai M, Kajiyama T, et al. Endosonographic characterization of duodenal elevated lesions. Gastrointest Endosc 1996;44(6):714–719.

211. Soon MS, Lin OS. Inflammatory fibroid polyp of the duodenum. Surg Endosc 2000;14(1):86.

212. Miettinen M, Kopczynski J, Makhlouf HR, et al. Gastrointestinal stromal tumors, intramural leiomyomas, and leiomyosarcomas in the duodenum: a clinicopathologic, immunohistochemical, and molecular genetic study of 167 cases. Am J Surg Pathol 2003;27(5):625–641.

213. Fujishima H, Misawa T, Maruoka A, Yoshinaga M, Chijiiwa Y, Nawata H. Rectal carcinoid tumor: endoscopic ultrasonographic detection and endoscopic removal. Eur J Radiol 1993;16(3):198–200.

214. Matsumoto T, Iida M, Suekane H, Tominaga M, Yao T, Fujishima M. Endoscopic ultrasonography in rectal carcinoid tumors: contribution to selection of therapy. Gastrointest Endosc 1991;37(5):539–542.

215. Nakachi A, Miyazato H, Oshiro T, Shimoji H, Shiraishi M, Muto Y. Granular cell tumor of the rectum: a case report and review of the literature. J Gastroenterol 2000;35(8): 631–634.

216. Miettinen M, Sarlomo-Rikala M, Sobin LH, Lasota J. Gastrointestinal stromal tumors and leiomyosarcomas in the co-

lon: a clinicopathologic, immunohistochemical, and molecular genetic study of 44 cases. Am J Surg Pathol 2000; 24(10):1339–1352.

217. Miettinen M, Furlong M, Sarlomo-Rikala M, Burke A, Sobin LH, Lasota J. Gastrointestinal stromal tumors, intramural leiomyomas, and leiomyosarcomas in the rectum and anus: a clinicopathologic, immunohistochemical, and molecular genetic study of 144 cases. Am J Surg Pathol 2001; 25(9):1121–1133.

218. Delpy R, Barthet M, Gasmi M, et al. Value of endorectal ultrasonography for diagnosing rectovaginal septal endometriosis infiltrating the rectum. Endoscopy 2005;37(4): 357–361.

219. Ribeiro HS, Ribeiro PA, Rossini L, Rodrigues FC, Donadio N, Aoki T. Double-contrast barium enema and transrectal endoscopic ultrasonography in the diagnosis of intestinal deeply infiltrating endometriosis. J Minim Invasive Gynecol 2008;15(3):315–320.

220. Kawai J, Kodera Y, Fujiwara M, et al. Telomerase activity as prognostic factor in gastrointestinal stromal tumors of the stomach. Hepatogastroenterology 2005;52(63):959–964.

221. Lasota J, Stachura J, Miettinen M. GISTs with PDGFRA exon 14 mutations represent subset of clinically favorable gastric tumors with epithelioid morphology. Lab Invest 2006; 86(1):94–100.

222. Hata Y, Ishigami S, Natsugoe S, et al. P53 and MIB-1 expression in gastrointestinal stromal tumor (GIST) of the stomach. Hepatogastroenterology 2006;53(70):613–615.

223. Yamaguchi U, Nakayama R, Honda K, et al. Distinct gene expression-defined classes of gastrointestinal stromal tumor. J Clin Oncol 2008;26(25):4100–4108.

224. Brand B, Oesterhelweg L, Binmoeller KF, et al. Impact of endoscopic ultrasound for evaluation of submucosal lesions in gastrointestinal tract. Dig Liver Dis 2002;34(4): 290–297.

225. Nickl N, Gress F, McClave S, et al. Hypoechoic intramural tumor study: final report. [abstract] Gastrointest Endosc 2002;55:AB98.

226. Palazzo L, Landi B, Cellier C, Cuillerier E, Roseau G, Barbier JP. Endosonographic features predictive of benign and malignant gastrointestinal stromal cell tumours. Gut 2000;46(1): 88–92.

227. Jeon SW, Park YD, Chung YJ, et al. Gastrointestinal stromal tumors of the stomach: endosonographic differentiation in relation to histological risk. J Gastroenterol Hepatol 2007; 22(12):2069–2075.

228. Shah P, Gao F, Edmundowicz SA, Azar RR, Early DS. Predicting malignant potential of gastrointestinal stromal tumors using endoscopic ultrasound. Dig Dis Sci 2009;54(6): 1265–1269.

229. Hur BW, Chun HJ, Kang CD, et al. Reassessment of usefulness of EUS in differentiation of benign and malignant gastric stromal tumors which were diagnosed according to pathologic guidelines of Ackerman's surgical pathology. [abstract] Gastrointest Endosc 2000;51(4 Part 2):AB215.

230. Wiersema MJ, Vilmann P, Giovannini M, Chang KJ, Wiersema LM. Endosonography-guided fine-needle aspiration biopsy: diagnostic accuracy and complication assessment. Gastroenterology 1997;112(4):1087–1095.

231. Williams DB, Sahai AV, Aabakken L, et al. Endoscopic ultrasound guided fine needle aspiration biopsy: a large single centre experience. Gut 1999;44(5):720–726.

232. Fu K, Eloubeidi MA, Jhala NC, Jhala D, Chhieng DC, Eltoum IE. Diagnosis of gastrointestinal stromal tumor by endo-

scopic ultrasound-guided fine needle aspiration biopsy—a potential pitfall. Ann Diagn Pathol 2002;6(5):294–301.

233. Stelow EB, Bardales RH, Stanley MW. Pitfalls in endoscopic ultrasound-guided fine-needle aspiration and how to avoid them. Adv Anat Pathol 2005;12(2):62–73.

234. Hunt GC, Rader AE, Faigel DO. A comparison of EUS features between CD-117 positive GI stromal tumors and CD-117 negative GI spindle cell tumors. Gastrointest Endosc 2003; 57(4):469–474.

235. Rader AE, Avery A, Wait CL, McGreevey LS, Faigel D, Heinrich MC. Fine-needle aspiration biopsy diagnosis of gastrointestinal stromal tumors using morphology, immunocytochemistry, and mutational analysis of c-kit. Cancer 2001;93(4):269–275.

236. Pang NK, Chin SY, Nga ME, et al. Comparative validation of c-kit exon 11 mutation analysis on cytology samples and corresponding surgical resections of gastrointestinal stromal tumours. Cytopathology 2009;20(5):297–303.

237. Acs G, McGrath CM, Gupta PK. Duodenal carcinoid tumor: report of a case diagnosed by endoscopic ultrasound-guided fine-needle aspiration biopsy with immunocytochemical correlation. Diagn Cytopathol 2000;23(3):183–186.

238. Liu K, Madden JF, Olatidoye BA, Dodd LG. Features of benign granular cell tumor on fine needle aspiration. Acta Cytol 1999;43(4):552–557.

239. Stelow EB, Jones DR, Shami VM. Esophageal leiomyosarcoma diagnosed by endoscopic ultrasound-guided fine-needle aspiration. Diagn Cytopathol 2007;35(3):167–170.

240. Caletti GC, Brocchi E, Ferrari A, et al. Guillotine needle biopsy as a supplement to endosonography in the diagnosis of gastric submucosal tumors. Endoscopy 1991;23(5):251–254.

241. Demetri GD, Benjamin RS, Blanke CD, et al; NCCN Task Force. NCCN Task Force report: management of patients with gastrointestinal stromal tumor (GIST)—update of the NCCN clinical practice guidelines. J Natl Compr Canc Netw 2007;5(Suppl 2):S1–S29, quiz S30.

242. Demetri GD, Antonia S, Benjamin RS, et al. NCCN practice guidelines in oncology - v.2.2009. Soft tissue sarcoma. http://www.nccn.org/professionals/physicians_gls/PDF/sarcoma.pdf.

243. Hwang JH, Rulyak SD, Kimmey MB; American Gastroenterological Association Institute. American Gastroenterological Association Institute technical review on the management of gastric subepithelial masses. Gastroenterology 2006;130(7):2217–2228.

244. Yamaguchi U, Hasegawa T, Masuda T, et al. Differential diagnosis of gastrointestinal stromal tumor and other spindle cell tumors in the gastrointestinal tract based on immunohistochemical analysis. Virchows Arch 2004; 445(2):142–150.

245. Yamaguchi U, Hasegawa T, Sakurai S, et al. Interobserver variability in histologic recognition, interpretation of KIT immunostaining, and determining MIB-1 labeling indices in gastrointestinal stromal tumors and other spindle cell tumors of the gastrointestinal tract. Appl Immunohistochem Mol Morphol 2006;14(1):46–51.

246. Jenssen C. Diagnostic endosonography - state of the art 2009. Endosk Heute 2009;22:89–104.

247. Debiec-Rychter M, Wasag B, Stul M, et al. Gastrointestinal stromal tumours (GISTs) negative for KIT (CD117 antigen) immunoreactivity. J Pathol 2004;202(4):430–438.

248. Lee HE, Kim MA, Lee HS, Lee BL, Kim WH. Characteristics of KIT-negative gastrointestinal stromal tumours and diag-

nostic utility of protein kinase C theta immunostaining. J Clin Pathol 2008;61(6):722–729.

249. Medeiros F, Corless CL, Duensing A, et al. KIT-negative gastrointestinal stromal tumors: proof of concept and therapeutic implications. Am J Surg Pathol 2004;28(7):889–894.

250. DeWitt J, Al-Haddad M, Fogel E, et al. Endoscopic transduodenal drainage of an abscess arising after EUS-FNA of a duodenal GI stromal tumor. Gastrointest Endosc 2009;70(1):185–188.

251. Grandval P, Picon M, Coste P, Giovannini M, Thomas P, Lafon J. Infection of submucosal tumor after endosonography-guided needle biopsy. [Article in German] Gastroenterol Clin Biol 1999;23(5):566–568.

252. Inoue H, Mizuno N, Sawaki A, et al. Life-threatening delayed-onset bleeding after endoscopic ultrasound-guided 19-gauge Trucut needle biopsy of a gastric stromal tumor. Endoscopy 2006;38(Suppl 2):E38.

253. Varadarajulu S, Fraig M, Schmulewitz N, et al. Comparison of EUS-guided 19-gauge Trucut needle biopsy with EUS-guided fine-needle aspiration. Endoscopy 2004; 36(5):397–401.

254. Ha CY, Shah R, Chen J, Azar RR, Edmundowicz SA, Early DS. Diagnosis and management of GI stromal tumors by EUS-FNA: a survey of opinions and practices of endosonographers. Gastrointest Endosc 2009;69(6):1039–1044, e1.

255. Jenssen C, Möller K, Wagner S, Sarbia M. Endoscopic ultrasound-guided biopsy: diagnostic yield, pitfalls, quality management part 1: optimizing specimen collection and diagnostic efficiency. [Article in German] Z Gastroenterol 2008;46(6):590–600.

256. Jenssen C, Möller K, Wagner S, Sarbia M. Endoscopic ultrasound-guided biopsy: diagnostic yield, pitfalls, quality management. [Article in German] Z Gastroenterol 2008;46(9):897–908.

257. Jenssen C, Dietrich CF. Endoscopic ultrasound-guided fine-needle aspiration biopsy and trucut biopsy in gastroenterology - An overview. Best Pract Res Clin Gastroenterol 2009;23(5):743–759.

258. Nesje LB, Laerum OD, Svanes K, Ødegaard S. Subepithelial masses of the gastrointestinal tract evaluated by endoscopic ultrasonography. Eur J Ultrasound 2002;15(1-2):45–54.

259. Wallace MB, Hoffman BJ, Sahai AS, Inoue H, Van Velse A, Hawes RH. Imaging of esophageal tumors with a water-filled condom and a catheter US probe. Gastrointest Endosc 2000;51(5):597–600.

260. Chang KJ, Yoshinaka R, Nguyen P. Endoscopic ultrasound-assisted band ligation: a new technique for resection of submucosal tumors. Gastrointest Endosc 1996;44(6):720–722.

261. Shim CS, Jung IS. Endoscopic removal of submucosal tumors: preprocedure diagnosis, technical options, and results. Endoscopy 2005;37(7):646–654.

262. Ponsaing LG, Hansen MB. Therapeutic procedures for submucosal tumors in the gastrointestinal tract. World J Gastroenterol 2007;13(24):3316–3322.

263. Kajiyama T, Hajiro K, Sakai M, et al. Endoscopic resection of gastrointestinal submucosal lesions: a comparison between strip biopsy and aspiration lumpectomy. Gastrointest Endosc 1996;44(4):404–410.

264. Yasuda I, Tomita E, Nagura K, Nishigaki Y, Yamada O, Kachi H. Endoscopic removal of granular cell tumors. Gastrointest Endosc 1995;41(2):163–167.

265. Wehrmann T, Martchenko K, Nakamura M, Riphaus A, Stergiou N. Endoscopic resection of submucosal esophageal tumors: a prospective case series. Endoscopy 2004;36(9): 802–807.

266. Park YS, Park SW, Kim TI, et al. Endoscopic enucleation of upper-GI submucosal tumors by using an insulated-tip electrosurgical knife. Gastrointest Endosc 2004;59(3): 409–415.

267. Rösch T, Sarbia M, Schumacher B, et al. Attempted endoscopic en bloc resection of mucosal and submucosal tumors using insulated-tip knives: a pilot series. Endoscopy 2004; 36(9):788–801.

268. Lee IL, Lin PY, Tung SY, Shen CH, Wei KL, Wu CS. Endoscopic submucosal dissection for the treatment of intraluminal gastric subepithelial tumors originating from the muscularis propria layer. Endoscopy 2006;38(10):1024–1028.

269. Sun S, Ge N, Wang C, Wang M, Lü Q. Endoscopic band ligation of small gastric stromal tumors and follow-up by endoscopic ultrasonography. Surg Endosc 2007;21(4): 574–578.

270. Sun S, Ge N, Wang S, Liu X, Lü Q. EUS-assisted band ligation of small duodenal stromal tumors and follow-up by EUS. Gastrointest Endosc 2009;69(3 Pt 1):492–496.

271. Inoue H, Takeshita K, Hori H, Muraoka Y, Yoneshima H, Endo M. Endoscopic mucosal resection with a cap-fitted panendoscope for esophagus, stomach, and colon mucosal lesions. Gastrointest Endosc 1993;39(1):58–62.

272. Waterman AL, Grobmyer SR, Cance WG, Hochwald SN. Is endoscopic resection of gastric gastrointestinal stromal tumors safe? Am Surg 2008;74(12):1186–1189.

273. Casali PG, Jost L, Reichardt P, Schlemmer M, Blay JY; ESMO Guidelines Working Group. Gastrointestinal stromal tumors: ESMO clinical recommendations for diagnosis, treatment and follow-up. Ann Oncol 2008;19(Suppl 2): ii35–ii38.

274. Catena F, Di Battista M, Fusaroli P, et al. Laparoscopic treatment of gastric GIST: report of 21 cases and literature's review. J Gastrointest Surg 2008;12(3):561–568.

275. DeMatteo RP, Maki RG, Singer S, Gonen M, Brennan MF, Antonescu CR. Results of tyrosine kinase inhibitor therapy followed by surgical resection for metastatic gastrointestinal stromal tumor. Ann Surg 2007;245(3):347–352.

276. Ronellenfitsch U, Staiger W, Kähler G, Ströbel P, Schwarzbach M, Hohenberger P. Perioperative and oncological outcome of laparoscopic resection of gastrointestinal stromal tumour (GIST) of the stomach. Diagn Ther Endosc 2009; 2009:286138 .

277. Sexton JA, Pierce RA, Halpin VJ, et al. Laparoscopic gastric resection for gastrointestinal stromal tumors. Surg Endosc 2008;22(12):2583–2587.

278. Silberhumer GR, Hufschmid M, Wrba F, et al. Surgery for gastrointestinal stromal tumors of the stomach. J Gastrointest Surg 2009;13(7):1213–1219.

279. Dematteo RP, Ballman KV, Antonescu CR, et al; American College of Surgeons Oncology Group (ACOSOG) Intergroup Adjuvant GIST Study Team. Adjuvant imatinib mesylate after resection of localised, primary gastrointestinal stromal tumour: a randomised, double-blind, placebo-controlled trial. Lancet 2009;373(9669):1097–1104.

280. Sahai AV, Siess M, Kapfer B, et al. Endoscopic ultrasonography for upper gastrointestinal submucosal lesions: a cost minimization analysis with an international perspective. Am J Gastroenterol 2003;98(9):1989–1995.

281. Matsuki M, Gouda Y, Ando T, et al. Adenocarcinoma arising from aberrant pancreas in the stomach. J Gastroenterol 2005;40(6):652–656.

282. Bruno M, Carucci P, Repici A, et al. The natural history of gastrointestinal subepithelial tumors arising from muscularis propria: an endoscopic ultrasound survey. J Clin Gastroenterol 2009;43(9):821–825.

283. Gill KR, Camellini L, Conigliaro R, et al. The natural history of upper gastrointestinal subepithelial tumors: a multicenter endoscopic ultrasound survey. J Clin Gastroenterol 2009; 43(8):723–726.

284. Lok KH, Lai L, Yiu HL, Szeto ML, Leung SK. Endosonographic surveillance of small gastrointestinal tumors originating from muscularis propria. J Gastrointestin Liver Dis 2009; 18(2):177–180.

285. Lachter J, Bishara N, Rahimi E, Shiller M, Cohen H, Reshef R. EUS clarifies the natural history and ideal management of GISTs. Hepatogastroenterology 2008;55(86-87): 1653–1656.

286. Houssam E, Mardini HE, Murphy S, Grigorian A, Nickl NJ. Endoscopic ultrasound surveillance of submucosal tumors: Results of a single center experience. Gastrointest Endosc 2008;67(5):AB205.

287. Melzer E, Fidder H. The natural course of upper gastrointestinal submucosal tumors: an endoscopic ultrasound survey. Isr Med Assoc J 2000;2(6):430–432.

288. Futagami K, Hata J, Haruma K, et al. Extracorporeal ultrasound is an effective diagnostic alternative to endoscopic ultrasound for gastric submucosal tumours. Scand J Gastroenterol 2001;36(11):1222–1226.

289. Polkowski M, Palucki J, Butruk E. Transabdominal ultrasound for visualizing gastric submucosal tumors diagnosed by endosonography: can surveillance be simplified? Endoscopy 2002;34(12):979–983.

290. Tsai TL, Changchien CS, Hu TH, Hsiaw CM. Demonstration of gastric submucosal lesions by high-resolution transabdominal sonography. J Clin Ultrasound 2000;28(3):125–132.

291. Agaimy A, Wünsch PH, Sobin LH, Lasota J, Miettinen M. Occurrence of other malignancies in patients with gastrointestinal stromal tumors. Semin Diagn Pathol 2006; 23(2):120–129.

15 Endosonographic Diagnosis and Treatment Planning in Gastrointestinal Lymphoma

W. Fischbach, C.F. Dietrich

The gastrointestinal tract is by far the most frequent site of manifestation for extranodal non-Hodgkin lymphomas (NHLs). Primary gastrointestinal lymphomas are today regarded as an independent entity, and there are differences between gastric lymphomas and intestinal lymphomas with regard to etiology, histomorphology, and clinical course. The World Health Organization (WHO) classification, dating from 2002 (**Table 15.1**), deliberately avoids classification into low-grade and high-grade NHL.[1] However, a distinction of this type would still be useful from the clinical point of view. In its present form, the classification does take account of the fact that there is no conclusive evidence for the existence of a sequential development of high-grade lymphomas from low-grade ones.

More than 70% of primary gastrointestinal NHLs present as gastric lymphomas. In terms of numbers, marginal-zone B cell lymphomas (MZBCLs) of the mucosa-associated lymphoid tissue (MALT) type and diffuse large B cell lymphoma (DLBCLs) are predominant. The majority of intestinal lymphomas, which represent up to 20–30% of cases, are high-grade B cell and T cell lymphomas. Colonic lymphomas are a rarity, at 2%. Multiple-organ involvement in the gastrointestinal tract is seen in some 6% of cases.[2] The etiopathogenetic significance of *Helicobacter pylori* infection for the development of gastric MZBCL of MALT is well established, with convincing data from epidemiological, morphological, and molecular-biological studies, as well as animal experiments.[3] These insights have led to the use of eradication therapy as the treatment of first choice in patients with stage I MZBCL of MALT. Mucosal immune-regulatory changes resulting from untreated gluten-sensitive celiac disease or chronic infections, as well as congenital or acquired immune-deficiency syndromes, are recognized risk factors for intestinal lymphomas.

Clinical Presentation

The clinical picture of gastrointestinal lymphomas in nonspecific. It is characterized by abdominal discomfort, pain, vomiting, diarrhea, weight loss, and manifest or occult bleeding. However, gastric lymphomas are also quite often an incidental finding at endoscopy. In general, it can be stated that complications such as obstruction, perforation, or bleeding are extremely rare in gastric lymphomas but may occur in intestinal lymphomas—which may in part be due to the fact that diagnosing them is more difficult and consequently takes place later.

Diagnosis and Staging

The diagnostic procedure focuses on two aspects:
- Precise histological classification, typing, and grading of the lymphoma (MZBCL of MALT, DLBCL with or without MALT components, others (**Table 15.1**)
- Accurate clinical staging

These are the two decisive prognostic factors and determinants of treatment.[4,5] Careful endoscopic and biopsy diagnosis and accurate staging are the essential prerequisite for adequate treatment.

Gastric lymphomas are accessible to endoscopic viewing. Esophagogastroduodenoscopy is therefore of the utmost importance for diagnosis. In view of the nonspecific appearance of gastric lymphomas[6] and potential sources of error in diagnostic work-up with endoscopy and biopsy,[7] biopsy methods involving what is known as gastric mapping are required. This means:
- Taking 8–10 biopsies from suspicious areas
- Four-quadrant biopsies from normal-appearing mucosa in the antrum and gastric body
- Two biopsies from the fundus
- Rapid urease testing in the antrum and gastric body

Table 15.1 World Health Organization classification of gastrointestinal non-Hodgkin lymphomas[a]

B cell lymphomas
Marginal-zone B cell lymphoma of MALT
Follicular lymphoma (grades I–III)
Mantle cell lymphoma (lymphomatous polyposis)
Diffuse large B cell lymphoma with/without MALT-type components
Burkitt lymphoma
Immune deficiency-associated lymphoma
T cell lymphomas
Enteropathy-associated T cell lymphoma (EATCL)
Peripheral T cell-lymphoma (non-EATCL)

[a] Ulcerative jejunitis and celiac diseaselike T cell lymphoma are not mentioned in the WHO classification.
MALT, mucosa-associated lymphoid tissue.

This procedure ensures adequate histological, immunohistochemical, and molecular-biological diagnosis. As in the diagnosis of dysplasia, a second expert opinion from one of the reference centers in the lymphoma network should always be obtained. There are two consequences for everyday routine work. Firstly, the gastric mapping procedure usually requires a second endoscopy examination, since a biopsy technique of this type is not usually used during the initial investigation. Secondly, *H. pylori* eradication therapy should be postponed until the findings from the reference histology are available, since previous antibacterial treatment often makes a definitive diagnosis of lymphoma more difficult, or even impossible.

The particular difficulty with intestinal lymphomas lies in the limited endoscopic and biopsy access that was possible until very recently. This often made exploratory laparoscopy or laparotomy necessary for diagnostic or therapeutic reasons.

It can be expected that new methods such as double-balloon enteroscopy and capsule endoscopy (**Fig. 15.1**) will in the future allow improved noninvasive methods of diagnosing intestinal NHLs. In addition, capsule endoscopy makes it possible to identify the intestinal manifestation expected in some 6% of cases of gastric lymphoma when there is multiple-organ gastrointestinal involvement.[2] If a diagnosis of gastrointestinal lymphoma is established, various obligatory or optional (according to Fischbach et al.[8]) examinations follow to allow assessment of the spread of the lymphoma ("staging"):

- Endoscopic ultrasonography (EUS) (obligatory)
- Ileocolonoscopy (optional)
- Radiographic small-bowel double-contrast imaging or Sellink magnetic resonance imaging (optional)
- Cervical and abdominal ultrasonography (obligatory)
- Computed tomography of the abdomen (obligatory) and chest (optional in MZBCL of MALT and obligatory in diffuse large B cell lymphoma)
- Cytological and histological assessment of a bone-marrow puncture (optional in MZBCL of MALT and obligatory in DLBCL)

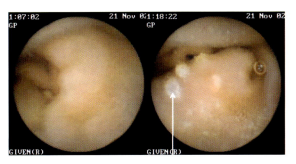

Fig. 15.1 Capsule endoscopy, demonstrating normal mucosa and a follicular lymphoma (arrow).

For staging, the Ann Arbor classification is still used, with Musshoff's modification and taking the Radaszkiewicz subclassification of stage I into account (**Table 15.2**). It would be desirable for the Paris staging system to become established, as it is more modern, is based on the TNM classification, and better reflects the specific characteristics of gastrointestinal lymphomas.[9]

Relevance of EUS

The prognostic relevance of the subclassification of stages I and II into stages I1, I2, and II1 (**Table 15.2**) has been confirmed.[5] EUS is the only imaging procedure that makes it possible to differentiate the gastric wall layers and that visualizes perigastric lymph nodes. EUS alone is now able to differentiate stages I and II into EI1 (T1 m/sm), EI2 (T2–4) and EII1 (T1–4 N1). EUS is therefore an obligatory part of the staging procedure for gastric lymphomas in both the current German S3 guideline "*H. pylori* and gastroduodenal ulcer disease"[8] and also in the forthcoming consensus report of the European Gastrointestinal Lymphoma Study Group (EGILS).

Table 15.2 Staging of primary gastrointestinal lymphomas

Ann Arbor system	Lugano system	TNM classification	Spread of lymphoma
E* I 1	I 1	T1 N0 M0	Mucosa, submucosa
E I 2	I 2	T2 N0 M0	Muscularis propria, subserosa
E I 2	I 2	T3 N0 M0	Serosal penetration
E I 2	II E**	T4 N0 M0	Infiltration of adjacent organs or tissues
E II 1	II 1 E	T1–4 N1 M0	Infiltration of regional lymph nodes (compartments I + II)
E II 2	II 1 E	T1–4 N2 M0	Infiltration of lymph nodes beyond the regional stations (compartment III), including retroperitoneal, mesenteric and para-aortic lymph nodes
III	–	T1–4 N3 M0	Infiltration of infradiaphragmatic and supradiaphragmatic lymph nodes
IV	IV	T1–4 N0–3 M1	Dissemination of the lymphoma

E*, primary extranodal location.
E**, infiltration of adjacent organs in continuity.

III Gastrointestinal Tract

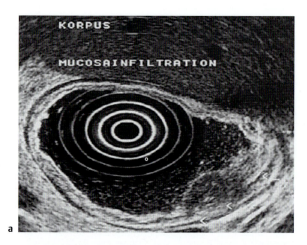

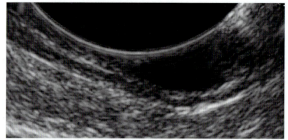

Fig. 15.2a, b Focal nodular (**a**) and more diffuse (**b**) infiltration of the gastric mucosa by a marginal-zone B cell lymphoma of the MALT type (stage I1 or T1).

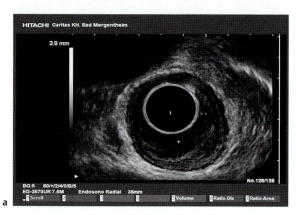

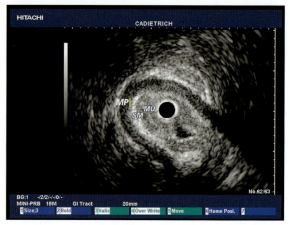

Fig. 15.3a, b **a** Circumscribed mucosal thickening of the gastric body by a marginal-zone B cell lymphoma of MALT type (stage I1 or T1). **b** Miniprobe. Normal gastric wall findings in the antrum. MU, mucosa; SM, submucosa; MP, muscularis propria.

The endosonographic appearance of gastric lymphomas varies depending on their shape. They may present as focal nodular infiltration of the mucosa (**Fig. 15.2**) or as diffuse, circumscribed mucosal thickening (**Fig. 15.3a**). In the latter case, the normal structure of the gastric wall in the antrum (**Fig. 15.3b**) can be clearly distinguished from the lymphoma in the gastric body. A mixed appearance, with thickened mucosa and focal loss of the normal gastric wall layers, can sometimes be seen (**Fig. 15.4**). Tumor growth through all of the wall layers (**Fig. 15.5**) is characteristic of stage I2 or T3 (**Table 15.2**); infiltration of adjacent organs or tissues (**Fig. 15.6**) represents stage I2 or T4; and involvement of perigastric lymph nodes (**Fig. 15.7**) represents stage II1 or T1–4N1. However, it should be mentioned that the endosonographic morphology is far from being specific for lymphoma. Scirrhous types of gastric cancer (linitis plastica), giant folds in patients with Ménétrier disease, inflammatory changes, or metastatic spread to the gastric wall may mimic endosonographically gastric lymphoma.

EUS has been regarded as the best method for local staging of gastric carcinoma for quite some time.[10] However, the endosonographic data on gastric lymphoma are in fact scarce and are mainly derived from a few prospective studies including only small numbers of patients.[11,12] In the era of surgical resection for gastric lymphoma, it was possible for EUS findings to be compared with the histopathological stage of the resected material as the gold standard.[7,13–18] These studies showed that EUS had high levels of diagnostic accuracy for both T and N staging (80–92% and 77–90%, respectively). However, the data were not confirmed in the German–Austrian multicenter study, which represented by far the largest series.[7,18] In this prospective study, EUS correctly classified the lymphoma in only 37 of 70 patients (53%). The sensitivity levels for defining the depth of lymphoma infiltration (59%) and the lymph-node status (71%) were unsatisfactory. What is the explanation for these discrepancies? In contrast to series from other single institutions or small numbers of centers with high levels of expertise in EUS, this study included 34 centers at a time (in the mid-1990s)

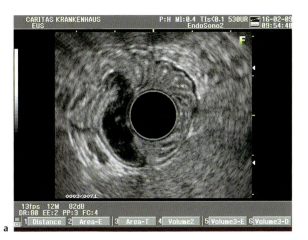
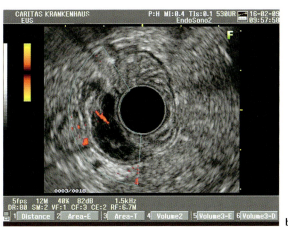

a

b

Fig. 15.4a, b Thickened mucosa (right) and focal loss of the normal gastric wall layers (left) due to a marginal-zone B cell lymphoma of MALT type (stage I2 or T2).

a B-mode.
b Color Doppler.

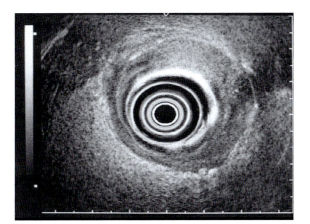
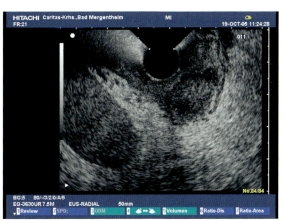

Fig. 15.5 Circular growth through all layers of the gastric wall by a marginal-zone B cell lymphoma of the MALT type (T3 here). Note the relationship of the tumor to the muscularis layer.

Fig. 15.6 Tumor growth through all layers of the gastric wall and continuous infiltration of adjacent tissues by a diffuse large B cell lymphoma (final diagnosis stage T4).

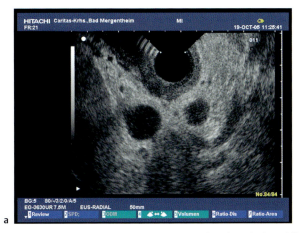
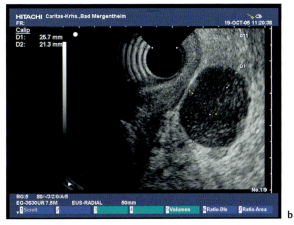

a

b

Fig. 15.7a, b Involvement of three perigastric lymph nodes by a diffuse large B cell lymphoma.

when experience with EUS was still generally low. Lesser expertise on the part of the investigators therefore appears to be the best explanation for the results of the multicenter trial. On the other hand, the results may also be a better reflection of clinical routine work at that time. However, quite high levels of interobserver variability in the staging of gastric lymphoma with EUS have been reported even among experts.[19]

Increasing experience, technical improvements such as the use of mini-echoendoscopes, elastography, and EUS-guided biopsies of perigastric lymph nodes will certainly further improve the accuracy of EUS. Miniprobes with higher ultrasound frequencies may provide results superior to those obtained with conventional EUS.[20,21] EUS elastography may provide additional information about the malignant status of lymph nodes in the same way as for metastatic carcinoma.[22,23] EUS-guided biopsies of perigastric lymph nodes may be able to clarify their malignant status, making it possible to differentiate stages EI and EII1 on a histological basis. However, for the same reasons as mentioned above, the value of EUS-guided biopsies of perigastric lymph nodes can only be indirectly estimated in relation to the treatment response and the course of the disease, against the background of treatment decisions based on EUS-guided biopsies. In summary, there is still no definitive proof of benefit from these new techniques in gastric lymphoma, and their value will probably remain unclear in view of the current strategy of nonsurgical treatment methods for gastric lymphomas. As conservative treatment strategies are now preferred, assessing the response to radiotherapy and chemotherapy will be a new challenge for EUS in the future. Sackmann and co-workers have shown that the regression of lymphoma after successful eradication of *H. pylori* can be reliably predicted with EUS,[24] and this finding has been confirmed by a Japanese group.[25] It remains to be seen whether the use of miniprobes will be capable of providing more precise information on the regression of lymphoma following therapy. EUS is of course not indicated in intestinal lymphomas.

Treatment Planning

In patients with stage I MZBCL of MALT, *H. pylori* eradication is the initial treatment of choice.[9] It leads to complete remission of the lymphoma in some 80% of cases. There was some doubt for a considerable period as to whether this does in fact represent long-term treatment success. However, long-term follow-up reports have now been published that impressively demonstrate that this is indeed the case and suggest that *H. pylori* eradication provides a genuine chance of a cure in the majority of these patients.[26,27]

Table 15.3 Summary of current treatment recommendations for gastric lymphoma

Stage	MZBCL of MALT	DLBCL
I 1 / 2	Hp eradication	R-CTx ± RTx (Hp eradication)
	If no response on Hp eradication or relapse: RTx	
	Minimal histological residuals: watch and wait	
II 1 / 2	RTx (Hp eradication)	R-CTx ± RTx
III / IV	R-CTx	R-CTx ± RTx

CTx, chemotherapy; DLBCL, diffuse large B cell lymphoma; Hp, *Helicobacter pylori*; MALT, mucosa-associated lymphoid tissue; MZBCL, marginal-zone B cell lymphoma; R, Rituximab; RTx, radiotherapy.

Most recently, it has also emerged that patients with minimal histological residues of MALT lymphoma after successful eradication therapy—i.e., normalization of the endoscopic findings but persistent residual lymphoma on histology—also have a favorable prognosis.[28,29] In these patients, a "watch-and-wait" strategy, with regular endoscopic and biopsy check-ups (every 3 months in the first year, every 4 months in the second year, then 6-monthly, and then annually after 5 years) is a well-justified approach, particularly since all of the other treatment options still remain open.[9]

For patients with *H. pylori*–negative recurrences of stage I/II gastric MZBCL of MALT, with an initially negative *H. pylori* status (including serological findings), and for patients in stage II, radiotherapy is the preferred option for treatment with curative intent. Radiation is as effective as surgical resection,[30] and offers a better quality of life.[31] Radiotherapy is now usually administered using the method of extended-field irradiation at a dosage of 30 Gy, with local saturation of the tumor region at 10 Gy. The rare patients (maximum 10%) with stage III/IV MZBCL of MALT should receive chemotherapy plus rituximab. Chemotherapy (cyclophosphamide, hydroxydaunomycin, Oncovin, and prednisone, CHOP) plus rituximab is also the treatment of choice for all stages of gastric DLBCL. The potential benefit of additional radiotherapy in these patients is an open question. There is considerable evidence that chemotherapy alone is as effective as combined chemoradiotherapy.[32] Radiotherapy can therefore probably be reserved for patients with initial bulky disease or with residual lymphoma after chemotherapy.

Complications such as endoscopically untreatable bleeding or perforation are the only indications that remain for surgical resection of gastric lymphomas.[9]

The current treatment recommendations for gastric lymphoma are summarized in **Table 15.3**. Clearly defined treatment recommendations such as those outlined for gastric lymphomas are not yet available for intestinal lymphomas.

References

1. Jaffe ES, Harris NL, Stein H, Vardiman JW, eds. Pathology and genetics of tumours of haematopoetic and lymphoid tissues. Lyons: IARC Press, 2002. (World Health Organization classification of tumours, 3).
2. Koch P, del Valle F, Berdel WE, et al; German Multicenter Study Group. Primary gastrointestinal non-Hodgkin's lymphoma: I. Anatomic and histologic distribution, clinical features, and survival data of 371 patients registered in the German Multicenter Study GIT NHL 01/92. J Clin Oncol 2001;19(18):3861–3873.
3. Fischbach W. Gastrointestinal lymphoma: etiology, pathogenesis and therapy. [Article in German] Internist (Berl) 2000;41(9):831–840.
4. Cogliatti SB, Schmid U, Schumacher U, et al. Primary B-cell gastric lymphoma: a clinicopathological study of 145 patients. Gastroenterology 1991;101(5):1159–1170.
5. Radaszkiewicz T, Dragosics B, Bauer P. Gastrointestinal malignant lymphomas of the mucosa-associated lymphoid tissue: factors relevant to prognosis. Gastroenterology 1992;102(5):1628–1638.
6. Kolve M, Fischbach W, Greiner A, Wilms K; German Gastrointestinal Lymphoma Study Group. Differences in endoscopic and clinicopathological features of primary and secondary gastric non-Hodgkin's lymphoma. Gastrointest Endosc 1999;49(3 Pt 1):307–315.
7. Fischbach W, Dragosics B, Kolve-Goebeler ME, et al; The German-Austrian Gastrointestinal Lymphoma Study Group. Primary gastric B-cell lymphoma: results of a prospective multicenter study. Gastroenterology 2000;119(5):1191–1202.
8. Fischbach W, Malfertheiner P, Hoffmann JC, et al. S3-guideline "Helicobacter pylori and gastroduodenal ulcer disease" [Article in German] Z Gastroenterol 2009;47:68–102.
9. Ruskoné-Fourmestraux A, Dragosics B, Morgner A, Wotherspoon A, De Jong D. Paris staging system for primary gastrointestinal lymphomas. Gut 2003;52(6):912–913.
10. Caletti G, Fusaroli P, Bocus P. Endoscopic ultrasonography. Digestion 1998;59(5):509–529.
11. Tio TL, den Hartog Jager FCA, Tijtgat GN. Endoscopic ultrasonography of non-Hodgkin lymphoma of the stomach. Gastroenterology 1986;91(2):401–408.
12. Bolondi L, Casanova P, Caletti GC, Grigioni W, Zani L, Barbara L. Primary gastric lymphoma versus gastric carcinoma: endoscopic US evaluation. Radiology 1987;165(3):821–826.
13. Fujishima H, Misawa T, Maruoka A, Chijiiwa Y, Sakai K, Nawata H. Staging and follow-up of primary gastric lymphoma by endoscopic ultrasonography. Am J Gastroenterol 1991;86(6):719–724.
14. Caletti GC, Ferrari A, Brocchi E, Barbara L. Accuracy of endoscopic ultrasonography in the diagnosis and staging of gastric cancer and lymphoma. Surgery 1993;113(1):14–27.
15. Palazzo L, Roseau G, Ruskone-Fourmestraux A, et al. Endoscopic ultrasonography in the local staging of primary gastric lymphoma. Endoscopy 1993;25(8):502–508.
16. Schüder G, Hildebrandt U, Kreissler-Haag D, Seitz G, Feifel G. Role of endosonography in the surgical management of non-Hodgkin's lymphoma of the stomach. Endoscopy 1993;25(8):509–512.
17. Suekane H, Iida M, Yao T, Matsumoto T, Masuda Y, Fujishima M. Endoscopic ultrasonography in primary gastric lymphoma: correlation with endoscopic and histologic findings. Gastrointest Endosc 1993;39(2):139–145.
18. Fischbach W, Goebeler-Kolve ME, Greiner A. Diagnostic accuracy of EUS in the local staging of primary gastric lymphoma: results of a prospective, multicenter study comparing EUS with histopathologic stage. Gastrointest Endosc 2002;56(5):696–700.
19. Fusaroli P, Buscarini E, Peyre S, et al. Interobserver agreement in staging gastric malt lymphoma by EUS. Gastrointest Endosc 2002;55(6):662–668.
20. Lügering N, Menzel J, Kucharzik T, et al. Impact of miniprobes compared to conventional endosonography in the staging of low-grade gastric malt lymphoma. Endoscopy 2001;33(10):832–837.
21. Yeh HZ, Chen GH, Chang WD, et al. Long-term follow up of gastric low-grade mucosa-associated lymphoid tissue lymphoma by endosonography emphasizing the application of a miniature ultrasound probe. J Gastroenterol Hepatol 2003;18(2):162–167.
22. Janssen J, Dietrich CF, Will U, Greiner L. Endosonographic elastography in the diagnosis of mediastinal lymph nodes. Endoscopy 2007;39(11):952–957.
23. Săftoiu A, Vilmann P, Ciurea T, et al. Dynamic analysis of EUS used for the differentiation of benign and malignant lymph nodes. Gastrointest Endosc 2007;66(2):291–300.
24. Sackmann M, Morgner A, Rudolph B, et al; MALT Lymphoma Study Group. Regression of gastric MALT lymphoma after eradication of Helicobacter pylori is predicted by endosonographic staging. Gastroenterology 1997;113(4):1087–1090.
25. Nakamura S, Matsumoto T, Suekane H, et al. Predictive value of endoscopic ultrasonography for regression of gastric low grade and high grade MALT lymphomas after eradication of Helicobacter pylori. Gut 2001;48(4):454–460.
26. Fischbach W, Goebeler-Kolve ME, Dragosics B, Greiner A, Stolte M. Long term outcome of patients with gastric marginal zone B cell lymphoma of mucosa associated lymphoid tissue (MALT) following exclusive Helicobacter pylori eradication therapy: experience from a large prospective series. Gut 2004;53(1):34–37.
27. Zullo A, Hassan C, Cristofari F, et al. Effects of Heicobacter pylori eradication on early stage gastric mucosa-associated lymphoid tissue lymphoma. Clin Gastroenterol Hepatol 2010 Feb; 8(2):105–110. Epub 2009 Jul 22.
28. Fischbach W, Goebeler-Kolve M, Starostik P, Greiner A, Müller-Hermelink HK. Minimal residual low-grade gastric MALT-type lymphoma after eradication of Helicobacter pylori. Lancet 2002;360(9332):547–548.
29. Fischbach W, Goebeler ME, Ruskone-Fourmestraux A, et al; EGILS (European Gastro-Intestinal Lymphoma Study) Group. Most patients with minimal histological residuals of gastric MALT lymphoma after successful eradication of Helicobacter pylori can be managed safely by a watch and wait strategy: experience from a large international series. Gut 2007;56(12):1685–1687.
30. Koch P, del Valle F, Berdel WE, et al; German Multicenter Study Group. Primary gastrointestinal non-Hodgkin's lymphoma: II. Combined surgical and conservative or conservative management only in localized gastric lymphoma—results of the prospective German Multicenter Study GIT NHL 01/92. J Clin Oncol 2001;19(18):3874–3883.
31. Fischbach W, Schramm S, Goebeler ME. Outcome and quality of life favor a conservative treatment of patients with primary gastric non-Hodgkin's lymphoma (NHL): Z Gastroenterol 2011;49:1–6.
32. Aviles A, Nambo MJ, Neri N, et al. Mucosa-associated lymphoid tissue (MALT) lymphoma of the stomach: results of a controlled clinical trial. Med. Oncol 2005;22:57–62.

16 Endoscopic Ultrasound in Chronic Pancreatitis

C. Jenssen, C.F. Dietrich

Difficulties in Diagnosing Chronic Pancreatitis

Establishing a definite diagnosis of chronic pancreatitis is a challenging task. The definition of the diagnosis itself is already problematic—for example, it is often not possible to differentiate clearly between recurrent attacks of acute pancreatitis and the early stages of chronic pancreatitis. The history and presenting symptoms may be nonspecific, which may result in up to four in every 10 patients being initially misdiagnosed as "nonspecific dyspepsia."[1] The correct diagnosis of chronic pancreatitis is, on average, only made 60 months after the original presentation.[2] Simple pancreatic function tests (e.g., fecal pancreatic elastase) and widely available noninvasive imaging methods such as abdominal ultrasonography and computed tomography (CT) are not sufficiently sensitive to diagnose the early stages of chronic pancreatitis. Percutaneous biopsy of the pancreas can be used to confirm a suspected diagnosis of chronic pancreatitis. However, it is a very invasive method, and since the extent of disease may vary widely within different areas of the pancreas, it may not necessarily be diagnostic. Its routine use is not recommended. Up to now, a combination of endoscopic retrograde cholangiopancreatography (ERCP) and the secretin–pancreozymin test has been regarded as the reference standard for diagnosing chronic pancreatitis.[3] However, ERCP does carry a considerable procedural risk, is unpleasant for the patient, and is very expensive.[4–6] Magnetic resonance cholangiopancreatography (MRCP) is so far not being used routinely, but it appears to be a promising method for the future.[7]

In chronic pancreatitis, functional deficits, morphological changes, and the degree of pain are not always closely correlated. The extent of changes in the pancreatic duct system and the extent of impairment of the exocrine function correlate closely in only about 75% to 80% of patients.[2,8] There are patients with severely damaged pancreatic ducts who have normal exocrine and endocrine pancreatic function, and some of these patients may be completely asymptomatic for years. In contrast, clinically significant impairment of pancreatic function does not have to be associated with severe ductal changes. Some 5–10% of patients with chronic pancreatitis are initially pain-free and only develop symptoms later on due to endocrine and exocrine dysfunction.[2,4,8]

It is difficult to judge the significance of mild or early changes in the pancreatic duct system and the pancreatic parenchyma, particularly because the normal appearance of the pancreas already varies widely with age. It may also be impossible to differentiate early chronic pancreatitis from scarring after acute pancreatitis, and from asymptomatic fibrosis of the pancreas.[3–5,9]

In up to 30% of cases of chronic pancreatitis or recurrent acute pancreatitis, it is not possible to determine the etiology of the disease, despite a detailed history and extensive investigations.[8,10] Even if a diagnosis of chronic pancreatitis is established, it may still be difficult to determine the exact nature of focal cystic or solid changes within the pancreas.[11]

The following imaging methods are available for diagnosing chronic pancreatitis and its complications:
- Radiographic methods: plain radiography, computed tomography (CT)
- Magnetic resonance imaging (MRI), magnetic resonance cholangiopancreatography (MRCP)
- Endoscopic methods: endoscopic retrograde cholangiopancreatography (ERCP), endoscopic ultrasonography (EUS)
- Abdominal ultrasonography (US), possibly with color-coded duplex sonography (CCDS). Chronic pancreatitis can be diagnosed with abdominal ultrasound in accordance with the criteria used in the Cambridge classification. This classification uses a combination of diagnostic criteria, each of which in itself is nonspecific (**Table 16.1**).[2,5,12,13]

In contrast to ERCP, which only allows investigation of the ductal system, ultrasound allows visualization of both the ductal system and of the pancreatic parenchyma. In addition, it is noninvasive, the patient is not exposed to X-rays, and, at least in theory, ultrasound should also be able to detect any complications of acute and chronic pancreatitis, particularly if it is used with CCDS .[13–22] However, in comparison with the reference standard of ERCP and the secretin–pancreozymin test, the sensitivity of abdominal ultrasound is relatively low (60–70%), to a large extent probably due to the retroperitoneal location of the pancreas.[5,16,17,23] The sensitivity of abdominal ultrasound is particularly low for diagnosing the early stages of chronic pancreatitis.

Table 16.1 The Cambridge classification of chronic pancreatitis for endoscopic retrograde cholangiopancreatography (ERCP) and abdominal ultrasonography/computed tomography (CT).[12,13] (Adapted from Glasbrenner et al.[5] and Lankisch[2])

Stage	ERCP	Abdominal ultrasonography, CT
Normal (0)	No pathological changes; good-quality study of the entire pancreatic duct system must be obtained	No pathological changes (main pancreatic duct < 2 mm, homogeneous parenchymal structure, normal size and shape)
Uncertain (1)	Normal main pancreatic duct, pathological changes in fewer than three side branches	One pathological change: • Main pancreatic duct 2–4 mm • Pancreas enlarged (up to twice normal size)
Mild (2)	Normal main pancreatic duct, pathological changes in more than three side branches	Two or more pathological changes: • Cysts < 10 mm • Irregular main pancreatic duct • Focal acute pancreatitis • Heterogeneous parenchymal structure • Hyperechoic pancreatic duct wall • Contour irregularities (pancreatic head or body)
Moderate (3)	As "mild," plus abnormal main pancreatic duct	All of the criteria mentioned above
Severe (4)	As "moderate," plus one or more of the following changes: • Cysts > 10 mm • Pancreas more than twice the normal size • Intraductal filling defects • Pancreatic duct calculi/calcifications • Duct obstruction (stricture) • Severe dilation or irregularities of the main pancreatic duct • Involvement of adjacent organs (ultrasound, CT)	

Endosonography of the Pancreas

In virtually all patients with normal upper gastrointestinal anatomy, EUS makes it possible to visualize the entire pancreas, the neighboring blood vessels, and the common bile duct from various scanning positions in the stomach and duodenum. This is not possible with abdominal ultrasound, and the local resolution provided by the endosonographic images is unsurpassed by any other imaging method. Despite there being some technical differences, this applies to both radial and curvilinear endosonography.[9,24–28] The large majority of published data were obtained with mechanical radial scanning echoendoscopes with a transducer frequency of 7.5 MHz. In addition, electronic curvilinear, and more recently electronic radial scanning echoendoscopes also allow visualization of the large vessels adjacent to the pancreas with CCDS, and, by using ultrasound contrast enhancement, they may show perfusion as well as pathological changes within the parenchyma of the pancreas.[29–38]

Because of the anatomical position of the stomach, the endosonographic appearance of the pancreas when viewed with a curvilinear-array transducer resembles its appearance when viewed with abdominal ultrasound. In addition, it is possible to view different planes of the pancreatic head by positioning the transducer in the duodenum[25,26,28,39] (**Fig. 16.1**).

In contrast to ERCP, with endosonography it is not only possible to view changes in the pancreatic duct, but changes in the parenchyma can also be taken into account

for diagnostic considerations. The procedural risk of EUS is, however, much lower than that of ERCP. Limitations may arise, as with ERCP, in patients with pyloric stenoses or after surgery, particularly after complete resection of the stomach.

The normal endosonographic appearance of the pancreas is characterized by specific criteria for size, contour, parenchyma, and ducts (**Table 16.2**).[9,25,26,28,40] However, since the imaging planes are less standardized than in CT, for example, the diameter of the pancreatic head has limited diagnostic significance.

To be able to diagnose pathological changes in the pancreas, it is also important to be aware of normal anatomic variants. For example, the width of the pancreatic duct and the echogenicity of the parenchyma increase with age.[9,43] Hyperechogenicity in the pancreatic parenchyma has been observed in ≈ 25% of EUS investigations and was found to be related to age, to a higher body mass index, liver steatosis, and to a regular intake of more than 14 g alcohol per week.[41,42] In addition, the ventral part (the embryological "ventral anlage") of the pancreas sonographically appears as a variably well-demarcated hypoechoic structure situated in the dorsal and inferior part of the pancreatic head, and may be detected in about 75% of patients undergoing EUS for nonpancreatic indications.[44] Detection of the ventral anlage on EUS is less likely in patients with diabetes mellitus, with the sonographic features of chronic pancreatitis, with a mass lesion in the pancreatic head, or with pancreas divisum[44–46] (**Fig. 16.2**).

With some experience, it is also possible to diagnose anatomic variants of the pancreatic duct. Pancreas divisum

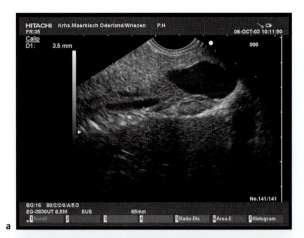

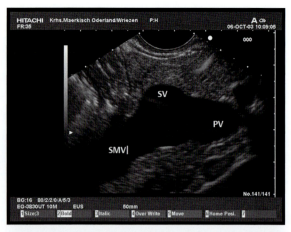

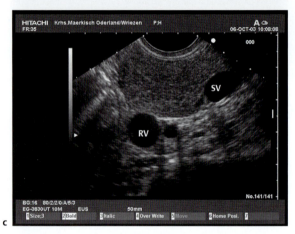

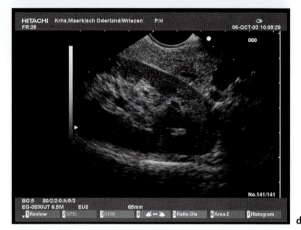

Fig. 16.1a–d The pancreas, viewed with a curvilinear-array echoendoscope.

a Seen from the gastric antrum, the confluence of the portal vein is a helpful anatomical landmark. The distal common bile duct and the main pancreatic duct are easily recognizable.

b The confluence of the portal vein and pancreatic neck. PV, portal vein; SMV, superior mesenteric vein; SV, splenic vein.

c View of the distal pancreatic body, seen from the gastric body. The splenic vein and splenic artery are anatomical landmarks. RV, left renal vein; SV, splenic vein.

d View of the pancreatic tail, adjacent to the left kidney, seen from the upper gastric body.

Table 16.2 Endoscopic ultrasonography of the pancreas: normal findings[9,25,26,28,40]

Characteristic	Normal appearance
Size	Measurements as for abdominal ultrasonography and CT: • Pancreatic head: 25–30 mm • Pancreatic body: up to 20 mm • Pancreatic tail: 20–30 mm
Contour	Smooth, fine, slightly hyperechoic outline of the pancreatic capsule. *Variant:* if the parenchyma is hyperechoic ("lipomatosis"), it is difficult to differentiate the pancreatic tissue from the peripancreatic fatty tissue
Parenchyma	Medium echogenicity, regular lobulation by fine, hyperechoic internal echo reflexes ("pepper-and-salt" appearance) *Variants:* With increasing echogenicity of the parenchyma, the physiological heterogeneity of the parenchyma is lost and replaced by a more homogeneous appearance.[41] The ventral part (embryological ventral anlage) of the pancreas can be differentiated as a variably well demarcated structure with lower echogenicity and variably regular lobulation
Pancreatic duct	Anechoic smooth linear structure, sometimes slightly hyperechoic contour, width <2 mm (in the pancreatic body)

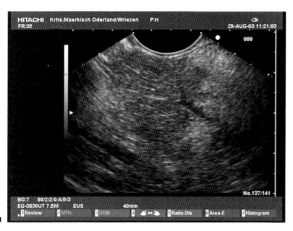
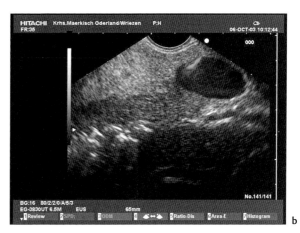

Fig. 16.2a, b The embryological ventral part of the pancreas, viewed with a curvilinear-array echoendoscope.
a Viewed from the descending part of the duodenum, the pancreatic duct is seen.

b Viewed from the gastric antrum, the confluence of the portal vein can be used for orientation.

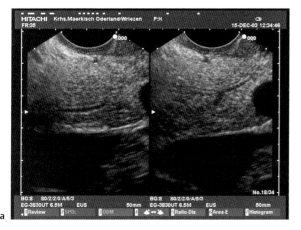
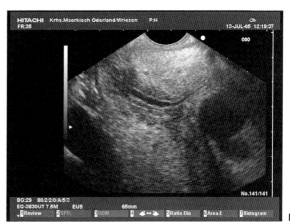

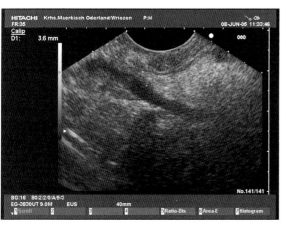

Fig. 16.3a–c Exclusion of pancreas divisum.
a, b Continuous visualization of the pancreatic duct from the ventral to the dorsal part of the pancreas.
c Pancreas divisum in a patient with recurrent acute pancreatitis: there is a separate orifice of the dorsal pancreatic duct at the minor papilla in pancreas divisum. Pancreas divisum can be confirmed and treated with endoscopic retrograde cholangiopancreatography.

is present if the course of the pancreatic duct cannot be followed from its origin at the ampulla of Vater through the ventral part to the dorsal part of the pancreas, or if the pancreatic duct cannot be visualized within the ventral part of the pancreas. Architectural distortion due to chronic pancreatitis may favor false-positive diagnoses of pancreas divisum.[47–49] It may also sometimes be possible to visualize the separate orifices of the common bile duct

at the major papilla and of the dorsal pancreatic duct at the minor papilla (**Fig. 16.3c**). Conversely, it is possible to exclude pancreas divisum reliably using endoscopic ultrasound if it is possible to follow the pancreatic duct continuously from the ventral to the dorsal pancreas, or between the papilla of Vater and the pancreatic neck[9,48,49] (**Figs. 16.2a** and **16.3a, b**).

Endosonographic Criteria for Chronic Pancreatitis

The endosonographic criteria for chronic pancreatitis follow the ultrasound criteria, which were developed by Jones et al.[13] and included in the Cambridge classification (see **Table 16.1**). The original 13 criteria developed in 1986 by Lees et al.[21,22] were revised and modified by Wiersema et al. in 1993.[50] In 30 patients in whom chronic pancreatitis had been confirmed by ERCP and/or an (intraductal) secretin test, calcifications and calculi in the pancreatic duct were found to have a positive predictive value of 100% for diagnosing chronic pancreatitis. From this study, the authors developed nine criteria, which now form the basis of most published studies on EUS in chronic pancreatitis. The five ductal criteria used by Wiersema et al. were dilation of the main pancreatic duct (MPD), calculi in the main pancreatic duct, dilated side branches, irregular ductal contour, and increased echogenicity of the main pancreatic duct wall; the four parenchymal criteria were hyperechoic foci, lobular pattern, focal hypoechoic areas, and parenchymal cysts[46,50] (**Figs. 16.4, 16.5, 16.6, 16.7, 16.8, 16.9 and 16.10**).

In their study of the different stages of chronic pancreatitis, Catalano et al.[51] modified the criteria developed by Wiersema et al.[50] slightly and added "inhomogeneous echo pattern" and "lobular outer gland margin," so that their classification included 11 criteria (the Milwaukee classification, with five ductal and six parenchymal criteria).[51]

There are a wide variety of views in the literature regarding the threshold number of criteria (within a range of one to five) required to diagnose chronic pancreatitis.[51-63] Some authors have suggested that a diagnosis of chronic pancreatitis can already be made if only one pathological feature is present, along with an appropriate clinical history.[51,53] Other groups have obtained high negative and positive predictive values for EUS if the threshold for

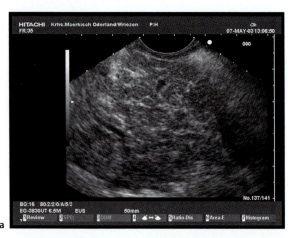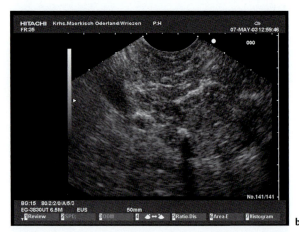

Fig. 16.4a, b Parenchymal criteria: inhomogeneities of pancreatic head (**a**) and body (**b**) caused by echogenic stranding, echogenic foci (with and without shadowing).

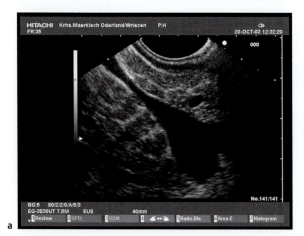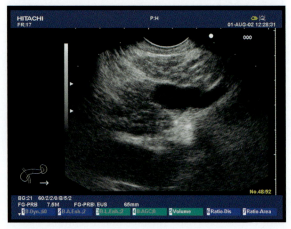

Fig. 16.5a, b Parenchymal criteria: lobularity with honeycombing; increased echogenicity and slight irregularity in the pancreatic capsule.

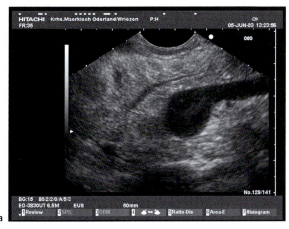
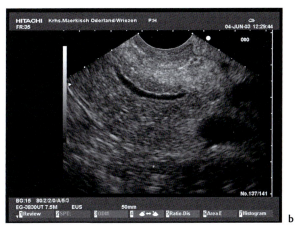

Fig. 16.6a, b Ductal criteria: hyperechoic and irregular main pancreatic duct (PD) contour in the pancreatic head and body (**a, b**); slight dilation of the PD in the pancreatic body.

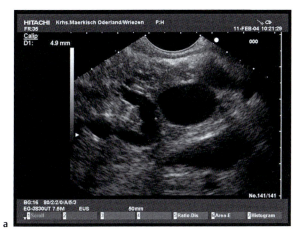
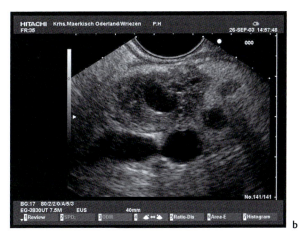

Fig. 16.7a, b Typical endosonographic appearance of chronic pancreatitis. Moderate dilation and irregular, hyperechoic contour of the main pancreatic duct (PD), inhomogeneous parenchyma with lobularity and stranding in the pancreatic head and neck (**a**); marked dilation, hyperechogenicity and irregular contour of the PD and of side branches in the pancreatic tail (**b**).

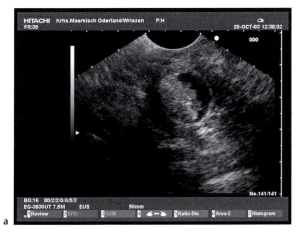
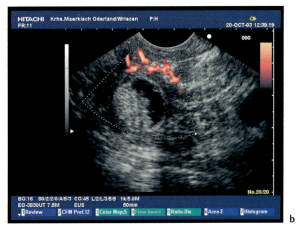

Fig. 16.8a, b Chronic pancreatitis with a small pseudocyst, which is partially filled with detritus.
a Very inhomogeneous parenchyma.
b Color power angio (CPA) mode. There is hyperperfusion around the margin of the pseudocyst.

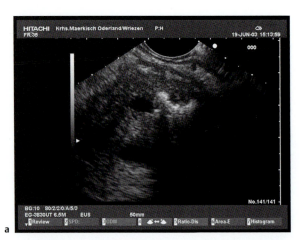
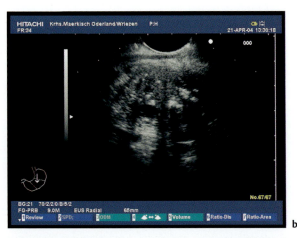

Fig. 16.9a, b Hyperechoic reflexes with shadowing can be differentiated into pancreatic stones (**a**) or parenchymal calcifications (**b**).

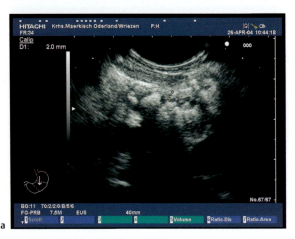
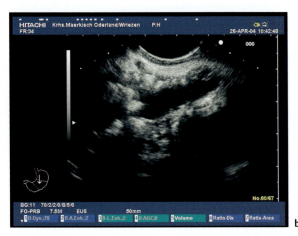

Fig. 16.10a, b Advanced chronic pancreatitis with calcifications, marked parenchymal atrophy, pancreatic stones (**a**), and marked dilation of the distal pancreatic duct (**b**).

"normal" was set at a maximum of two pathological criteria, and if at least five of nine pathological criteria have to be fulfilled to establish a diagnosis of "abnormal."[9,52, 58]

There are several further problems with using a threshold number of criteria for the EUS diagnosis of chronic pancreatitis.[9,40,52] Firstly, there are no consistent definitions of the various EUS features of chronic pancreatitis. Secondly, some features may be of much lesser diagnostic value if they are observed only in the relatively hypoechoic ventral pancreas and not in the body and the tail of the pancreas. Thirdly, some of the criteria used in various studies are related to each other—for example, ductal dilation and parenchymal atrophy (**Fig. 16.10**); echogenic stranding and honeycombing (see **Figs. 16.4** and **16.5**); hypoechoic parenchyma and increased echogenicity in the duct wall (see **Figs. 16.6b** and **16.7b**). However, in cases of extreme ductal ectasia and parenchymal atrophy, it is possible that some parenchymal criteria, such as echogenic foci and stranding, may not be visualized (**Fig. 16.10**). In such cases, the required threshold number of criteria may not be met, although the picture would clearly be that of advanced chronic pancreatitis. In other cases, a marked honeycomb pattern in the absence of ductal ectasia may make it difficult to recognize subtle ductal changes. All studies are in agreement that echogenic foci with shadowing (parenchymal calcifications) and ductal calculi provide the highest diagnostic power.[9,50–52] Further predictors of a diagnosis of chronic pancreatitis are the number of endosonographic parenchymal criteria and a clinical history of alcohol abuse.[52] So far, there have been no studies of the validity of the above criteria in larger groups of patients, and the criteria have only recently been correlated with clinical data such as age, sex, history of alcohol abuse, smoking, and clinical symptoms.[43,54–57]

Observer agreement between experienced examiners in making a diagnosis of chronic pancreatitis is moderate, both for radial systems[64,65] and for curvilinear EUS systems.[64] It is similar to the level of agreement in classifying hemorrhagic gastric ulcers using the Forrest classification. Only one study determined the agreement between radial and curvilinear systems and found it to be moderate.[64] To achieve sufficient competence in interpreting endosonographic findings in suspected chronic pancreatitis, in comparison with the consensus of a panel of experts, it has been suggested that it is necessary to undergo a supervised training program consisting of 15–40 examinations of patients with chronic pancreatitis.[66]

In an attempt to conclude controversies regarding the definition and threshold number of criteria, a group of experts in endosonography recently held a consensus meeting to define minor and major criteria (**Table 16.3**) and create a new EUS classification of chronic pancreatitis (**Table 16.4**).[67] After an extensive review of the literature, including thorough discussion of the definitions of each EUS feature, the 32 experts who took part in the Rosemont consensus meeting achieved a good level of interobserver reliability ($\kappa > 0.7$) for each feature.[67]

Table 16.3 Endoscopic ultrasound criteria for chronic pancreatitis (consensus criteria of the Rosemont classification)[67]

Parenchymal features
Hyperechoic foci with shadowing (≥ 2 mm)[a]
Lobularity (well-circumscribed, ≥ 5 mm structures with hyperechoic rim and relatively hypoechogenic center within the body and tail of pancreas) with honeycombing (≥ 3 contiguous lobules)[b]
Lobularity without honeycombing (≥ 3 noncontiguous lobules)[c]
Hyperechoic foci without shadowing (≥ 3; ≥ 2 mm)
Cysts (anechoic, round/elliptic, ≥ 2 mm in short axis)[c]
Stranding (≥ 3 hyperechoic lines, ≥ 3 mm in at least two different directions with respect to the imaged plane, not restricted to the ventral anlage)[c]
Ductal features
Main pancreatic duct (MPD) calculi (echogenic structures within the MPD with acoustic shadowing)[a]
Irregular MPD contour (body and tail)[c]
Dilated side branches (≥ 3; width ≥ 1 mm; body and tail)[c]
MPD dilation (≥ 3.5 mm body; > 1.5 mm tail)[c]
Hyperechoic MPD margin ($> 50\%$ of MPD in body and tail, both borderlines of MPD)[c]

[a] Major A criterion.
[b] Major B criterion.
[c] Minor criteria.

Comparison of Methods: Is EUS More Sensitive than ERCP for Diagnosing Chronic Pancreatitis?

On the basis of the criteria discussed in the previous section, the sensitivity of EUS for diagnosing chronic pancreatitis is at least as good as that of ERCP, which is commonly regarded as the morphological reference standard, and it appears to be superior to that of other imaging methods (US, CT, MRI/MRCP) (**Table 16.5**).[7,50,53,59,60,62,68,69] However, more detailed comparison is difficult, for several reasons. Firstly, many of the endosonographic studies investigated highly selected patients, who were frequently suffering from severe chronic pancreatitis. Secondly, the diagnostic reference standard used differs between studies, with diagnostic methods used including ERCP,[52,53,70–72] indirect pancreatic function test (PFT),[70] a combination of ERCP and the secretin test,[51] direct PFTs alone,[58,62,63,80] or a combination of different tests together

Table 16.4 Rosemont consensus criteria for the diagnosis of chronic pancreatitis (CP)[a] [67]

Consistent with CP	Suggestive of CP [a]	Indeterminate for CP [a]	Normal
A			
1 major A feature + ≥ 3 minor features	1 major A feature + 1 or 2 minor features	3 or 4 minor features + no major feature	1 or 2 minor features (excluded: cysts, MPD dilation, hyperechogenic foci, dilated side branches) + no major feature
B			
1 major A feature + major B feature (honeycombing)	Major B feature (honeycombing) + ≥ 3 minor features	Major B feature (honeycombing) +/– 1 or 2 minor features	
C			
2 major A features: (MPD calculi and echogenic foci with shadowing)	≥ 5 minor features		

[a] Diagnosis of CP requires confirmation by an additional imaging study (ERCP, CT, MRI) or a pancreatic function test.

Table 16.5 The accuracy of endoscopic ultrasound (EUS) in the diagnosis of CP, in comparison with endoscopic retrograde cholangiopancreatography (ERCP) in patients examined due to suspected pathology. The reference standards were either a combination of ERCP, pancreatic function test (PFT), and clinical criteria,[50,68,69] changes in the ERCP findings over time,[53] or direct secretin PFT[62]

First author, ref.	Sensitivity of EUS	Sensitivity of ERCP	Specificity of EUS	Specificity of ERCP	Patients (n)
Wiersema 1993[50]	80%	50%[a] 86%[b]	86%	–[c]	30
Giovannini 1994[69]	93%	76%	56%	–[c]	17
Buscail 1995[68] [d]	88%	74%	100%	100%	81
Kahl 2002[53]	100% [a]	80.7%[a]	–[e]	–[c]	130
Stevens 2008[62]	68%	72%	79%	76%	83

[a] Sensitivity for "early chronic pancreatitis".
[b] Sensitivity for all stages of chronic pancreatitis.
[c] No data given, ERCP was decisive part of the combined reference standard.
[d] Sensitivity of CT: 75%; of US: 58%; specificity of CT: 95%; of US: 75%.
[e] No data; the study did not include patients with no clinical suspicion of CP.

with clinical criteria.[50,60,61,68] However, it is well known that only a small proportion of patients with slightly abnormal findings on ERCP (Cambridge categories 1 and 2) meet any of the clinical criteria for chronic pancreatitis.[4] Four studies related endosonographic findings to the histology of resected pancreatic tissue, but did not compare EUS with other imaging techniques or PFT.[73–76] Other studies tried to relate the endosonographic diagnosis to cytological or histological findings obtained with endoscopic ultrasound-guided fine-needle aspiration (EUS-FNA)[70,77,78] or Tru-Cut biopsy (EUS-TCB).[78,79]

Several studies have shown that, in patients who meet the ERCP criteria for chronic pancreatitis (Cambridge classes 2–4), a mean of 4.4[52] or a median of six (range three to seven) out of nine[53] EUS criteria for chronic pancreatitis were present in the endosonographic examination.

Some studies have shown that, in patients with clinically suspected chronic pancreatitis, endosonography was able to identify changes consistent with this diagnosis, even though ERCP or CT did not show any signs of chronic pancreatitis.[50–53,59,71,72] For example, in a study of 43 patients with clinically suspected chronic pancreatitis, Nattermann et al.[71,72] found endosonographic criteria for chronic pancreatitis in 27 patients who had no changes in the pancreatic duct on ERCP. The combined results of the studies by Catalano et al.,[51] Sahai et al.,[52] and Wiersema et al.[50] show that 25% of patients with clinically suspected chronic pancreatitis and normal ERCP had abnormal findings on EUS. Similarly, 40% of patients with clinically suspected chronic pancreatitis and normal pancreatic function tests were found to have abnormalities on EUS.[4] In the study by Sahai et al., the 30 patients in whom ERCP did not support the clinically suspected diagnosis of chronic pancreatitis had a mean of 3.2 criteria of chronic pancreatitis on endosonography.[52] The most commonly observed endosonographic findings in patients with clinically suspected chronic pancreatitis but normal ductography (on ERCP) were parenchymal inhomogeneities (lobularity,

honeycomb pattern), increased echogenicity of the MPD wall, and changes in the contour of the pancreas. However, since the above studies used a cross-sectional design with no follow-up, the significance of abnormal endosonographic findings in patients with suspected chronic pancreatitis but normal ERCP findings and/or PFT remains controversial. There is still uncertainty regarding whether EUS can be used reliably to diagnose early chronic pancreatitis.[4,9,40,46,54,74,80] This is partly due to the fact that some of the ultrasound and endosonographic criteria for chronic pancreatitis may also be present in asymptomatic individuals with no clinical symptoms of pancreatic disease, either with or without a history of alcohol abuse.[43,54–57,82] However, the significance of abnormal findings on EUS in the presence of a normal ERCP may be different in symptomatic patients who have a history of alcohol abuse. In a region with a high prevalence of chronic pancreatitis, Kahl et al. studied a group of 38 patients with a history of chronic alcohol abuse and recurring upper abdominal pain who had at least one (median two) of the endosonographic (parenchymal) changes of chronic pancreatitis, but whose initial ERCP showed no ductal changes. After a median follow-up of 18 months, 22 of the patients (68.8%) developed changes typical of chronic pancreatitis on ERCP. The authors concluded that EUS may be more sensitive than ERCP for diagnosing early chronic pancreatitis, but that the endosonographic findings have to be interpreted against the background of the clinical history.[53] Very similar conclusions were drawn from the clinical and CT follow-up of a small group of 16 patients in whom there was a strong clinical suspicion of chronic pancreatitis and in whom CT, MRI, or ERCP had initially been nondiagnostic. EUS correctly diagnosed chronic pancreatitis in 13 patients and in a further two patients yielded alternative diagnoses (autoimmune pancreatitis and MPD stricture of uncertain origin).[59] Another study reported that in a cohort of 127 patients with dyspepsia but no clinical markers of pancreatic disease, approximately half met at least four of the pathological endosonographic criteria for chronic pancreatitis.[1] On the other hand, there are conflicting results with direct PFT and EUS in the investigation of patients with suspected minimal changes in chronic pancreatitis.[58,62,63,80] In view of the conflicting data and conclusions of the above studies, it is difficult to interpret the significance of such findings as long as no follow-up data for this population are available. It has been proposed that in diagnostically uncertain cases (endosonographic parenchymal criteria met, but normal ERCP; suspicion of autoimmune pancreatitis), cytological or histological examination using EUS-FNA[70,78,81] or EUS-TCB[78,83] may be helpful. However, since pancreatic EUS-guided biopsy carries a considerable risk, especially in patients with a history of pancreatitis,[84,85] EUS-FNA in particular has a limited diagnostic yield,[77,78,86] and a definite cytological or histological diagnosis of chronic pancreatitis may only have a limited influence on the clinical management, the diagnostic value of EUS-FNA and EUS-TCB remains to be determined.

In summary, then, the studies currently available suggest that EUS is at least as sensitive as ERCP in the diagnosis of chronic pancreatitis and that it should be the diagnostic imaging method of first choice. However, the normal appearance of the pancreas may be very variable, particularly in elderly patients. In addition, it may be difficult or impossible to differentiate between residual changes of acute pancreatitis, alcohol-induced toxic fibrosis of the pancreas, and chronic pancreatitis. As is also true for ERCP and pancreatic function tests, the specificity of EUS is highly dependent on the patient group studied, or, in individual cases, on the clinical setting. If the clinical findings and the patient's history are not taken into account, there may be a risk of overdiagnosing chronic pancreatitis when using EUS.[1,4,87,88]

A definite diagnosis of chronic pancreatitis can be made if the criteria of the Rosemont classification[67] are met. However, in patients younger than 60 without significant regular alcohol consumption, the detection of only three or more endosonographic criteria is highly predictive of chronic pancreatitis.[54,57] In such cases, further investigation is not required, and ERCP is only indicated for therapeutic interventions. Conversely, advanced chronic pancreatitis can be excluded if EUS only shows up to two minor pathological findings. ERCP, PFT, or other complex investigations for diagnosing chronic pancreatitis will probably be unhelpful and are not required. If the clinical presentation strongly suggests the presence of chronic pancreatitis (typical abdominal pain, chronic alcohol abuse), the presence of a limited number of endosonographic criteria is already suggestive for diagnosing early chronic pancreatitis. In such cases, in which EUS is suggestive of or only indeterminate for chronic pancreatitis, additional noninvasive imaging (especially MRI with MRCP),[60] direct PFT,[58,62,63,80] or measurement of interleukin-8 in pancreatic juice at the time of EUS,[61] or ERCP in selected cases, may be necessary in order to establish a definitive diagnosis.[67] EUS-guided biopsy may be helpful to prove an alternative diagnosis of autoimmune pancreatitis.[78,79] Long-term follow-up studies including symptomatic and asymptomatic patients with abnormal findings on EUS, but with normal ERCP and PFT, are needed.

If EUS is performed only shortly after an episode of acute pancreatitis—i.e., within 4 weeks of it—it is not possible to confirm or exclude a diagnosis of chronic pancreatitis reliably.[88]

Since the difference between acute recurrent pancreatitis and chronic pancreatitis is the progression of morphological and functional changes over time in chronic pancreatitis, the diagnosis may be more easily made by repeated endosonographic follow-up examinations than by more invasive tests.

Pitfalls

- *Anatomic variants.* A ventral anlage is recognized in up to three-quarters of endosonographic examinations. In comparison with the dorsal pancreas, the ventral pancreas tends to show lower echogenicity and a more inhomogeneous structure. It is possible to misinterpret this hypoechoic ventral pancreas as a tumor or as focal chronic pancreatitis.[9,44,46] In our experience, this is a common mistake in less experienced examiners.

- It may be difficult to differentiate the pancreas from visceral fatty tissue in patients with marked abdominal obesity (large amounts of visceral fat) who also have marked fatty changes in the pancreas.[9,41,42]

- Age-related changes in the pancreatic echo texture can be extremely variable. The pancreatic duct may become slightly ectatic, the echogenicity of the parenchyma and of the contours of the capsule and the ducts may increase, and the pancreas may develop an increasingly lobular structure. These changes cannot be differentiated from the changes in early chronic pancreatitis with certainty[9,43,46,57] (**Fig. 16.11**).

- Structural changes in the pancreatic parenchyma that would be consistent with an endosonographic diagnosis of chronic pancreatitis may be present in asymptomatic patients with a history of alcohol abuse, in heavy smokers, and in patients with nonspecific dyspepsia. In such cases, a diagnosis of chronic pancreatitis merely based on the EUS criteria may not necessarily be correct.[1,46,54–56,87]

- Hyperechogenic foci without shadowing, stranding, and a hyperechogenic or slightly irregular pancreatic duct wall are relatively nonspecific endosonographic findings, which may also be present in patients with no clinical markers of pancreatic disease. The duct wall is frequently hyperechoic in heavy smokers, and hyperechogenic foci are more common in men.[82,87] These changes, as well as an increased lobular parenchymal pattern, may also be found in patients with chronic alcohol abuse who have a diffusely fibrosed pancreas but no chronic pancreatitis[54–56,87] (**Fig. 16.11a**).

- Large calcifications and pancreatic calculi cause dorsal echo extinction and make it impossible to assess the pancreatic tissue situated dorsal to the calcification (**Figs. 16.9** and **16.10a**).

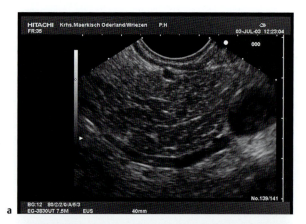

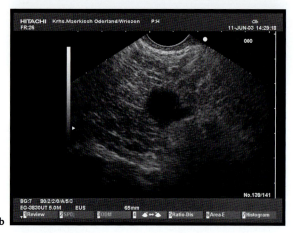

Fig. 16.11a, b Minimal changes in the echo texture of the pancreatic parenchyma.
a In a young patient with significant regular alcohol abuse.
b In an elderly woman with no clinical criteria for chronic pancreatitis.

Table 16.6 Suggested staging system for chronic pancreatitis (CP), based on the Cambridge classification (see Table 16.1; adapted from Jenssen and Dietrich 2005[40] and adjusted to the Rosemont classification (see Table 16.4)[67]

Cambridge class	Criteria
Class 0 (no CP)	0–2 features of the following: irregular MPD contour, hyperechoic MPD contour, lobularity without honeycombing, stranding
Class 1 (uncertain)[a]	≥ 1 feature of the following: cysts < 10 mm, dilation of MPD, hyperechogenic foci without shadowing, ≥ 3 side branches, lobularity with honeycombing, and ≥ 1 feature of the following: irregular MPD contour, hyperechoic MPD contour, lobularity without honeycombing, stranding *or:* 3–4 features of the following: irregular MPD contour, hyperechoic MPD contour, lobularity without honeycombing, stranding
Class 2 (mild CP)[a]	At least 5 features *including* dilation of ≥ 3 side branches *excluding* dilation of MPD, hyperechogenic foci with shadowing (parenchymal calcifications), MPD calculi, and/or cysts > 10 mm
Class 3 (moderate)	At least 5 features *including* obvious irregularities of the pancreatic duct (dilatation and/or variability of MPD, ≥ 3 dilated side branches) and lobularity with honeycombing *excluding* hyperechogenic foci with shadowing (parenchymal calcifications), MPD calculi and/or cysts > 10 mm, consistent with criteria of a typical pseudocyst
Class 4 (severe)	At least 7 features *including* hyperechogenic foci with shadowing (parenchymal calcifications), MPD calculi and/or cysts > 10 mm, consistent with criteria of a typical pseudocyst

[a] In the presence of a typical patient history and/or pathological pancreatic function test, a presumptive diagnosis of "early chronic pancreatitis" or "minimal-change chronic pancreatitis" is justified. Follow-up with EUS or another imaging method (especially magnetic resonance imaging or magnetic resonance cholangiopancreatography) is necessary.

Endosonographic Staging of Chronic Pancreatitis

EUS staging of chronic pancreatitis should follow the Cambridge classification.[12] There are no internationally consistent EUS staging systems. Nattermann and Dancygier qualitatively correlated the ERCP grades in the Cambridge classification with endosonographic findings, indirectly weighting the findings into minor and major criteria.[71,72] The endosonographic staging developed by Hollerbach et al. follows a similar principle.[70] In contrast, Catalano et al.[51] classified the presence of one or two of 11 endosono-

graphic criteria as mild chronic pancreatitis (Cambridge category 2), the presence of three to five of 11 criteria as moderate chronic pancreatitis (Cambridge category 3), and the presence of more than five of 11 criteria as severe chronic pancreatitis (Cambridge category 4). We have suggested a staging system that accounts not only for the number of EUS features, but also takes into account the different weighting of these features.[40] To make this compatible with the new Rosemont classification,[67] we have modified our proposal as outlined in **Table 16.6**.

Diagnosis of Complications of Chronic Pancreatitis

It is usually possible to diagnose the common sequelae of chronic pancreatitis or of acute recurrent pancreatitis, such as pancreatic pseudocysts, stenosis of the common bile duct, and portal or splenic vein thrombosis, using abdominal ultrasound or CT. Endosonography is therefore only rarely required.[14,16–19] CCDS is more sensitive than CT for diagnosing vascular complications.[15] However, if only abdominal ultrasound is used, it may still be difficult to demonstrate small pseudocysts or splenic vein thrombosis near the pancreatic tail, or, independently of the location,

partial or locally restricted portal vein thrombosis. In patients in whom abdominal ultrasound is not diagnostic, endosonography with CCDS is often useful for showing thromboses and occlusions of the portal and splenic veins, as well as portosystemic shunts and gastric varices.[89–92] Ultrasound contrast enhancement can be used to improve the reliability of EUS in diagnosing portal and splenic vein thromboses. In our experience, endoscopic ultrasound with systems capable of CCDS and color power angio (CPA)—electronic curvilinear and radial-array systems—can now be regarded as the most sensitive method of diagnosing vascular complications of chronic and acute pancreatitis (**Figs. 16.12, 16.13, 16.14, 16.15, 16.16** and **16.17**).

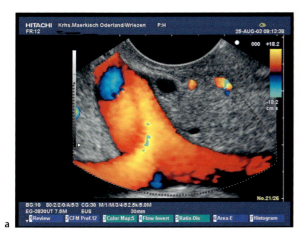

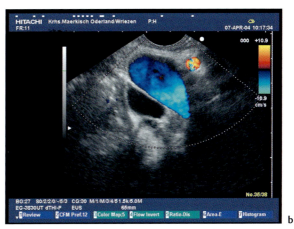

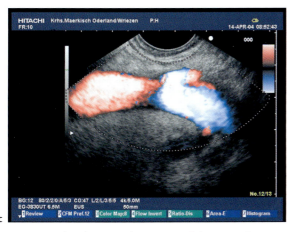

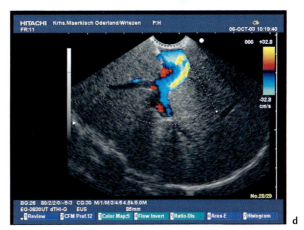

Fig. 16.12a–d Endosonographic imaging of the portosplenic vessels.
a The confluence of the portal vein.

b The portal vein in the portal region of the liver.
c The splenic vein within the pancreatic body.
d The splenic vessels in the hilar region of the spleen.

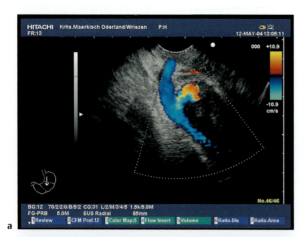

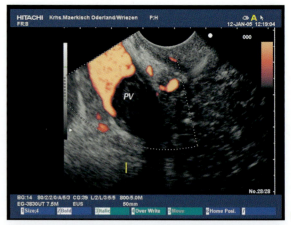

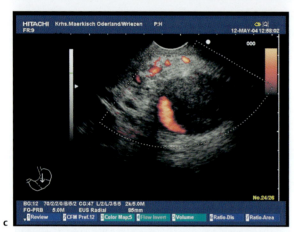

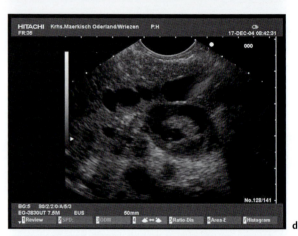

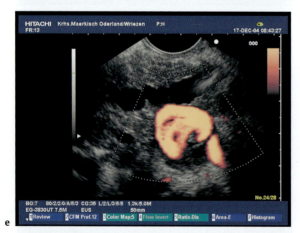

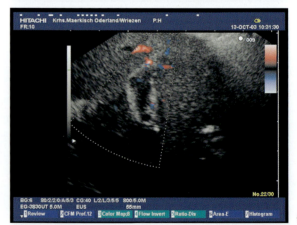

Fig. 16.13a–f Thrombosis of the portal vessels as a complication of chronic pancreatitis.

a, **b** Incomplete portal vein thrombosis with periduodenal collaterals. PV, portal vein.

c Dilated confluence of the portal vessels, with a large thrombus surrounded by some remaining blood flow.

d, **e** The confluence of the portal vessels with incomplete thrombosis; the dilation and irregular contour of the main pancreatic duct should be noted.

f Extension of a portal vein thrombus into an intrahepatic branch of the portal vein.

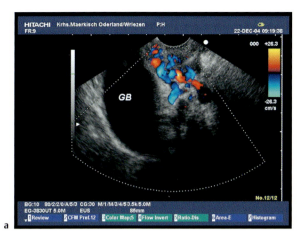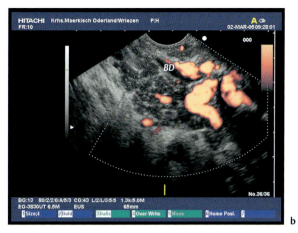

Fig. 16.14a, b Collaterals around the gallbladder (**a**) and around the common bile duct (**b**) in patients with chronic pancreatitis and thrombosis of the portal veins. BD, bile duct; GB, gallbladder.

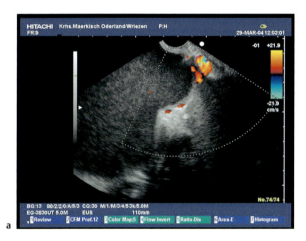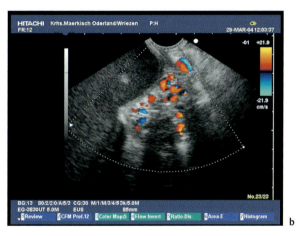

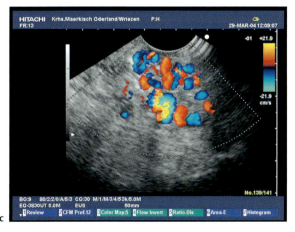

Fig. 16.15a–d a A space-occupying pseudocyst in the pancreatic tail.

b–d The lesion led to hilar splenic vein thrombosis, with hepatopetal and hepatofugal collaterals, cavernous transformation of the splenic vein (**b, c**), and gastric fundic varices (**d**).

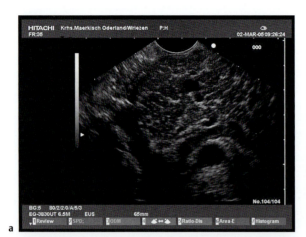

a

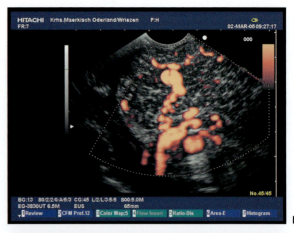

b

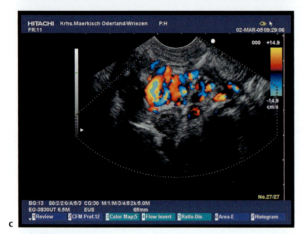

c

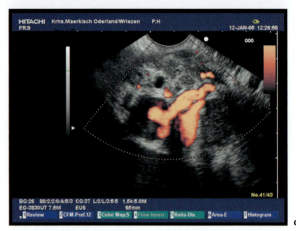

d

Fig. 16.16a–d Intrapancreatic hepatopetal collateralization in a patient with chronic pancreatitis and portosplenic thrombosis.
a Distinct parenchymal inhomogeneity in the pancreatic tail (echogenic foci without shadowing, stranding, lobularity with honeycombing, and also a suspicion of dilated side branches).

b Color power angio (CPA) mode reveals intrapancreatic collaterals, presumed to be dilated side branches.
c, d Color-coded duplex sonography (CCDS) also demonstrates peripancreatic collateral vessels (**c**) and the causative thrombosis of the splenic vein (**d**).

A detailed assessment of pancreatic pseudocysts and of post-pancreatitis abscesses is important, as it may have therapeutic implications (**Figs. 16.18** and **16.19**).

Tubular stenoses of the common bile duct and their underlying pathology can be reliably demonstrated with endoscopic ultrasound (**Fig. 16.20**).

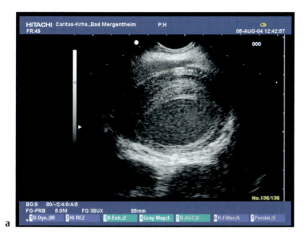

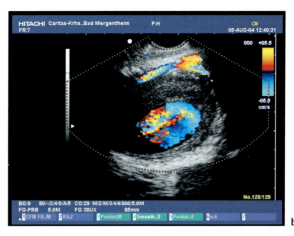

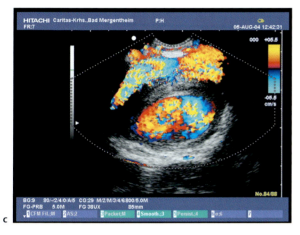

Fig. 16.17a–c A false aneurysm in chronic pancreatitis, with hemorrhage into a pseudocyst.
a Without color-coded duplex sonography (CCDS).
b With CCDS.
c After contrast enhancement by intravenous administration of the ultrasound contrast agent SonoVue.

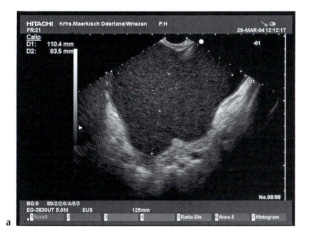

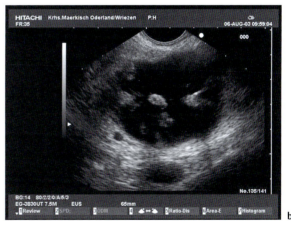

Fig. 16.18a, b Large pancreatic pseudocysts
a A pseudocyst containing finely dispersed hyperechoic reflexes.

b A pseudocyst filled with some hyperechoic debris.

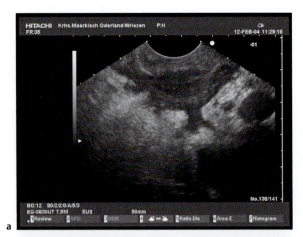

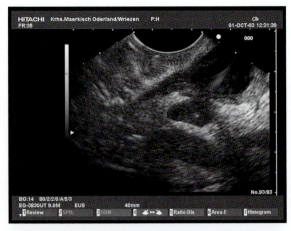

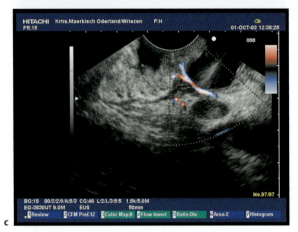

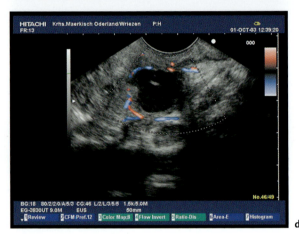

Fig. 16.19a–d A small mural pseudocyst in a patient with rim pancreatitis and recurrent pyloric stenosis.
a Hypoechoic material in the duodenopancreatic rim, with duodenal wall thickening.

b Periduodenal pseudocyst.
c, d A mural pseudocyst with perifocal vessels and an enlarged peripancreatic lymph node.

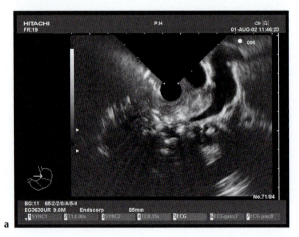

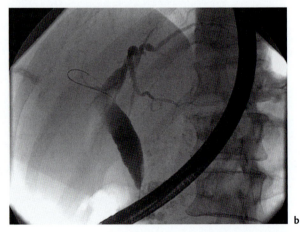

Fig. 16.20a, b a Endosonographic view of a tubular stenosis of the distal common bile duct in a patient with chronic calcifying pancreatitis.
b The corresponding endoscopic retrograde cholangiopancreatography (ERCP) view.

Etiological Information

EUS can provide etiological information only in patients with obstructive chronic pancreatitis (**Fig. 16.21**) or with idiopathic acute (recurrent) pancreatitis.[10,88,93–99] In a relatively large study, one-third of all patients with idiopathic acute (recurrent) pancreatitis who were examined with EUS and with ERCP and sphincter of Oddi manometry showed changes consistent with at least moderately severe chronic pancreatitis. An underlying tumor was found in 10% of the patients, and gallstones were present in a similar proportion.[10] Very similar results were found in an endosonographic study of 370 patients with primary and idiopathic acute recurrent pancreatitis.[88] More than four EUS criteria of chronic pancreatitis were found in 19.9% of patients with primary idiopathic acute pancreatitis and in 40.8% of patients with idiopathic acute recurrent pancreatitis. Other possible causes of idiopathic acute pancreatitis that were detected by EUS in this large group of patients included biliary sludge or stones (gallbladder or bile ducts, 13.5%), solid and cystic pancreatic neoplasms (3.5%), and pancreas divisum (7.3%).[88] Extraductal ultrasound (EDUS) using high-frequency miniprobes can be used to demonstrate pancreatic duct obstruction and its underlying causes, such as tumors of the papilla, ductal adenocarcinomas, intraductal papillary mucinous tumors (IPMTs), or obstructive calcifications and calculi[100] (**Fig. 16.22**).

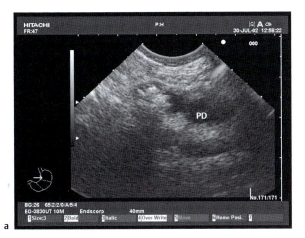
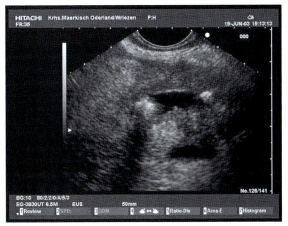

Fig. 16.21a, b Obstructive chronic pancreatitis caused by pancreatic duct stones. PD, pancreatic duct.

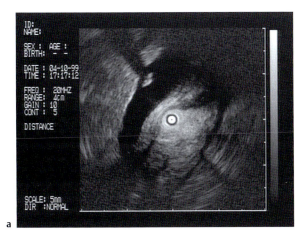
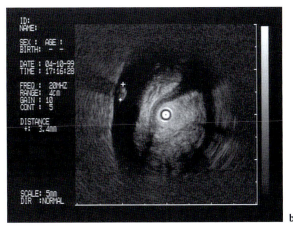

Fig. 16.22 a. b A small stone in the common bile duct, shown by extraductal endosonography (EDUS) with an endoscopic high-frequency miniprobe. Small stones of this type in undilated bile ducts may be missed on endoscopic retrograde cholangiopancreatography.

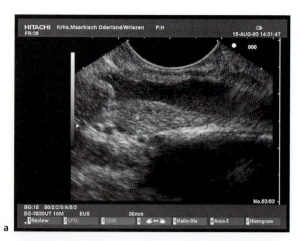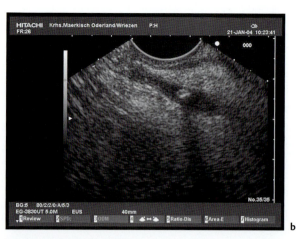

Fig. 16.23a, b Small common bile duct stones can be reliably visualized using endoscopic ultrasound.

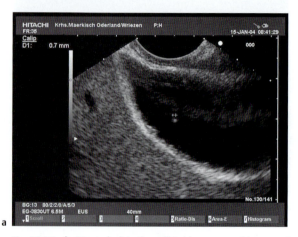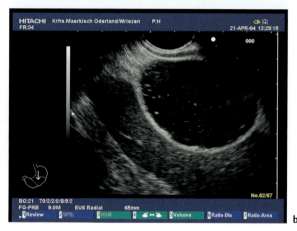

Fig. 16.24a, b Microcalculi in the gallbladder as a possible cause for pancreatitis—visualized by endoscopic ultrasound, but not visible on abdominal ultrasound.

EUS has been shown to have a high level of sensitivity for diagnosing calculi in the common bile duct, which are frequently responsible for causing acute recurrent pancreatitis, when mechanical radial scanners are used,[102–104] when EDUS with high-frequency miniprobes is used,[100,101] and recently also with electronic curvilinear scanners[105–108] (**Fig. 16.23**). In addition, endosonography can also demonstrate microcalculi in the gallbladder, which may sometimes not be visible on abdominal ultrasound[94,109] (**Fig. 16.24**).

EUS can be helpful in deciding whether or not invasive therapeutic interventions should be undertaken, and it may help avoid more risky and complex investigations such as ERCP and sphincter of Oddi manometry.[10,93,101,105,107,110] Secretin-stimulated EUS is superior to ERCP in diagnosing the causes of acute recurrent pancreatitis.[97] However, dynamic endosonography of the pancreas with secretin stimulation is not sufficiently sensitive to replace sphincter of Oddi manometry. Nevertheless, an obstructive cause of pancreatitis can be diagnosed reliably by observing that the diameter of the main pancreatic duct increases by at least 1 mm when stimulated with secretin. Similarly, occlusion of a pancreatic duct stent can be diagnosed using the same method.[111] An interesting observation was made in the only study published on this subject so far; Catalano et al. found that when using dynamic endosonography with secretin stimulation, they were able to identify patients with chronic pancreatitis and pancreas divisum who subsequently benefited from endoscopic stent placement.[111]

Practical Hints

- It is important to define the diagnostic aim of an EUS examination in chronic pancreatitis, bearing in mind the patient's individual clinical background.
- An endosonographic diagnosis of chronic pancreatitis should usually not be made only shortly (up to ≈ 4 weeks) after an acute attack of pancreatitis.[88] Diagnostic aims in such a situation might be exclusion of chronic pancreatitis; identification of the underlying etiology of the acute attack; diagnosis of complications.[75,99]

- Isolated changes in the ventral part of the pancreas[45] should not be used to make a diagnosis of chronic pancreatitis if the remainder of the pancreas appears normal.[9]
- A diagnosis of chronic pancreatitis must be made on the basis of the established EUS criteria, taking the patient's clinical background and history into account.[40,67]
- A complete endosonographic examination in acute recurrent pancreatitis or (suspected) chronic pancreatitis not only entails evaluation of the entire pancreas, but also assessment of the extrahepatic bile ducts and the portal vessels, if possible using CCDS and/or CPA.
- A full diagnostic evaluation should include a statement regarding whether the suspected diagnosis of chronic pancreatitis can be confirmed, the degree of diagnostic certainty according to the Rosemont classification,[67] and optionally the staging of severity in accordance with the Cambridge classification[40] (**Table 16.6**). In addition, the presence of possible complications of chronic pancreatitis should be determined, underlying etiological factors should be sought, and if appropriate, suggestions for therapeutic interventions should be offered.

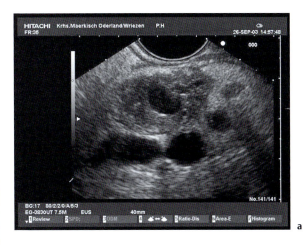

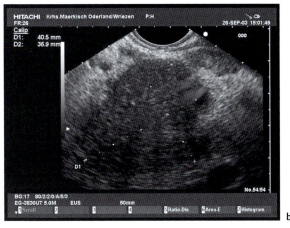

Fig. 16.25a, b a Changes consistent with chronic pancreatitis located in the pancreatic tail.
b The underlying cause is a large cancer in the pancreatic head.

Differential Diagnosis, Diagnostic Problems, and Pitfalls

Areas in which diagnostic difficulties may arise are in differentiating between neoplastic lesions and focal or segmental inflammatory masses, in the diagnostic interpretation of cystic lesions, and in the etiological diagnosis of ductal dilations.

■ Pancreatic Cancer versus Focal Inflammatory Masses

The life expectancy of patients with chronic pancreatitis is reduced.[112] They have an up to 19-fold increased risk of developing pancreatic cancer, which is most likely due to smoking being a common risk factor.[113–115] On the other hand, a proximal pancreatic tumor may well be the underlying reason for developing obstructive chronic pancreatitis. In a study of 103 patients with proven pancreatic cancer but no history of chronic pancreatitis, half of the patients had at least one of the endosonographic criteria for chronic pancreatitis—mostly dilation and a hyperechogenic wall in the main pancreatic duct. When at least four of the endosonographic criteria were found, 17% of the patients were diagnosed as having chronic pancreatitis in addition to their pancreatic cancer[116] (**Fig. 16.25**)

Approximately 50% of first-degree relatives of patients with familial pancreatic cancer have EUS findings of chronic pancreatitis.[117] Interestingly, Canto's group found a correlation in such high-risk individuals between endosonographic criteria of chronic pancreatitis and histolog-

ical criteria of parenchymal atrophy with multifocal duct-obstructive neoplastic precursor lesions such as pancreatic intraepithelial neoplasia (PanIn) and IPMN.[118] Because of the high risk of developing ductal pancreatic cancer in patients with hereditary chronic pancreatitis and in individuals from families with some hereditary cancer syndromes, EUS surveillance of these individuals is under evaluation. Some groups have reported a high detection rate with EUS of neoplastic precursor lesions (IPMN-like lesions), as well as of asymptomatic cancer in these high-risk individuals.[119-121] However, the interobserver reliability of EUS findings in familial pancreatic cancer kindreds is only fair to moderate,[122] and the clinical and economic effectiveness of EUS-based screening strategies are controversial.[117,123]

Focal inflammatory masses may mimic changes typical of pancreatic cancer on CT or ultrasound, and even on ERCP. Two large surgical studies found benign inflammatory lesions in 6–9% of patients who underwent surgery for lesions that even retrospectively appeared highly suspicious for pancreatic cancer.[124,125] A substantial proportion of these tumorlike forms of pancreatitis appear to belong to the only recently recognized clinical entity of autoimmune pancreatitis or lymphoplasmacytic sclerosing pancreatitis.[124–128] In a series of 442 patients who underwent pancreaticoduodenectomy,[124] 47 patients (10.6%) with histopathologically benign disease were identified, 40 of whom had undergone surgery due to a clinical suspicion of pancreatic malignancy. Fourteen patients turned out to have chronic pancreatitis (29.8%), and 11 patients (23.4%) were classified as having lymphoplasmacytic sclerosing pancreatitis.[124] The characteristic EUS findings for autoimmune pancreatitis include a diffusely or focal enlarged and hypoechoic pancreas that lacks the features of regular chronic pancreatitis (lobularity, heterogeneous foci). A hyperechoic, narrowed pancreatic duct and concentric wall thickening in the distal common bile duct, causing bile duct stenosis, are additional features frequently found in autoimmune pancreatitis. Pancreatic pseudocysts and peripancreatic fluid collections do not appear to be common findings in autoimmune pancreatitis. However, the endosonographic features of autoimmune pancreatitis are relatively heterogeneous, with no pathognomonic findings.[81,129,130] Whereas EUS-FNA has only very limited sensitivity for diagnosing autoimmune pancreatitis,[78,81,86] EUS-TCB in small series of patients did very well in obtaining a histological diagnosis (dense, mostly IgG4-positive lymphoplasmacellular infiltrations in the region of branch ducts and pancreatic venules) in patients with suspected autoimmune pancreatitis.[78,83]

Endosonography has been found to be a highly sensitive method of diagnosing solid pancreatic lesions in patients with or without chronic pancreatitis. However, differentiation between malignant and inflammatory lesions remains difficult[81,125,127,131–138] (**Figs. 16.26** and **16.27**). This is particularly true because markedly enlarged peripancreatic lymph nodes may also be present in chronic pancreatitis as well as in autoimmune pancreatitis,[81,129] and autoimmune pancreatitis may involve large vessels[81,128] (**Fig. 16.28**).

Nattermann et al. studied 12 different endosonographic criteria in 69 inflammatory lesions and 61 malignant tumors. They were unable to identify any characteristics that reliably allowed differentiation between the two types of lesion.[136] For example, the lesions showed irregular or indistinct margins with similar frequency (86% versus 84%). Rösch et al. found similar results.[138] Endosonographic changes that were more common in focal inflammatory lesions, though neither very sensitive nor specific, included coarsely speckled hyperechoic foci (23% versus 7%).[136] However, endosonographic criteria for infiltration of the duodenum or stomach, and for infiltration of neighboring vessels, were much less commonly found in focal inflammatory lesions: 7% versus 30% and 9% versus 39%, respectively.[136] In a small group of patients with both pancreatic cancer and chronic pancreatitis, the authors observed that, in contrast to inflammatory masses, the calcifications were limited to the periphery of the hypo-

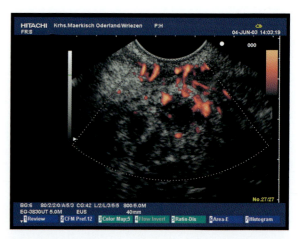

Fig. 16.26 Hypoechoic mass lesions in chronic pancreatitis may have numerous underlying diagnoses, and it is not possible to differentiate reliably between necrosis and carcinoma.

echoic tumors in all patients with cancerous masses[133] (**Figs. 16.25b** and **16.29a**).

It is possible to increase the diagnostic yield of endosonography markedly using contrast-enhanced CCDS or power Doppler.[30–38,139–141] As in recent findings in echo-enhanced ultrasonography,[140–146] adenocarcinomas of the pancreas appear almost exclusively hypoperfused endosonographically and may only occasionally show a hyperperfused rim[30–36,38,139,140] (**Fig. 16.27c, d**). Conversely, inflammatory lesions (but also neuroendocrine tumors, serous cystadenomas, mucinous tumors, and metastases from renal cell carcinomas) show obvious enhancement of the perfusion signal, certainly after application of echo-contrast enhancers[33,38,129,139–146] (**Figs. 16.27c, d** and **16.30**). Perfusion signals inside the mass lesion are only rarely observed in adenocarcinomas, regardless of whether abdominal ultrasound or endosonography is used.[30,33,38,139–142] Typically, the few vessels in the periphery of ductal cancer are only arteries with a high resistive index. In chronic pancreatitis, on the other hand, inflammatory tumors depict arterial vessels with normal resistive index and venous vessels as well[34–36] In autoimmune pancreatitis, echo enhancement also results in mild to marked enhancement of the pancreatic parenchyma and thickened wall of the distal common bile duct; the grade of vascularity in the lesion correlates with the pathological grade of inflammation and correlates inversely with the grade of fibrosis associated with autoimmune pancreatitis.[147] One differential diagnostic problem with contrast enhanced-EUS (CE-EUS) is that focal necrosis as a consequence of an acute attack of chronic pancreatitis is also characterized by an absence of perfusion signals inside the lesion, compared to pronounced vascular signals in the surrounding inflamed parenchyma (**Fig. 16.29**). Other auxiliary methods, such as real-time elastography and digital image analysis, also have limited value for differentiating

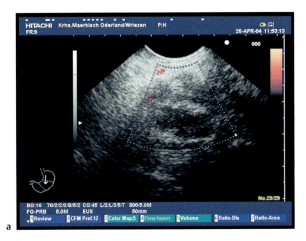

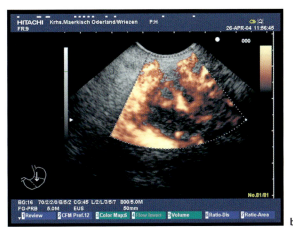

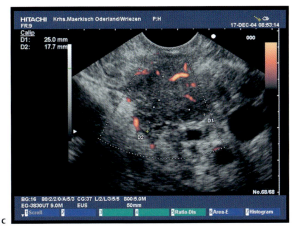

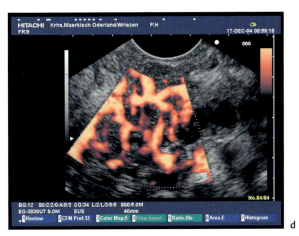

Fig. 16.27a–d Contrast-enhanced endosonography in patients with chronic pancreatitis and hypoechoic lesions in the pancreatic head. **a, b** After injection of only 0.6 mL of SonoVue, there is obvious enhancement of the pancreatic head, which is enlarged due to chronic inflammation. However, the hypoechoic lesion is spared, suggesting the presence of a small adenocarcinoma.

c, d In the second patient, there is enhancement of the entire hypoechoic lesion after injection of 2.5 mL SonoVue, suggesting an inflammatory pseudotumor.

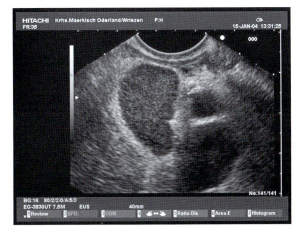

Fig. 16.28 An enlarged peripancreatic lymph node in a patient with chronic pancreatitis.

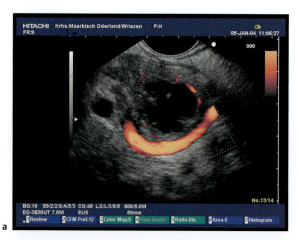

a

b

Fig. 16.29a, b Endoscopic ultrasound-guided fine-needle aspiration (EUS-FNA) in a patient with acute recurrent pancreatitis and a solid cystic mass lesion in the pancreatic tail. Turbid fluid was aspirated. The cytological and histological findings were typical of necrotic changes.

between inflammatory masses, organized necrosis, and neoplastic lesions.[148–153]

EUS-FNA generally has very high levels of sensitivity (80–95%) and specificity (> 90%) for diagnosing adenocarcinoma of the pancreas.[154–156] However, it is not capable of resolving the differential-diagnostic dilemma of hypoechoic mass lesions in patients with chronic pancreatitis. In such patients, the diagnostic sensitivity of EUS-FNA, even in highly specialized centers, has been reported to be between only 44% and 80%[131,135,157–162] (**Fig. 16.29**). Analysis of the K-*ras* point mutation and other molecular-genetic investigations,[161,164–166] as well as new immunohistochemical markers (14-3-3σ, mesothelin)[167] in specimens obtained with EUS-FNA may enhance the diagnostic accuracy in unclear cases.

We recommend that patients with chronic pancreatitis and a focal hypoechoic, hypoperfused lesion should be referred for surgery without delay if the clinical and imaging findings strongly suggest the presence of a resectable adenocarcinoma. Patients with chronic pancreatitis in whom CCDS shows a well-perfused lesion and in whom the CA19-9 level is low should undergo EUS-guided biopsy.[156] If this shows findings typical of chronic pancreatitis or autoimmune pancreatitis, we would suggest that as an alternative to surgery the patient might want to undergo further follow-up examinations, at least in the short term. One very recent study suggests that combining CE-EUS, EUS elastography and EUS-FNA is very promising for the differential diagnosis between chronic pseudotumoral pancreatitis and pancreatic cancer[168]. In our own experience, we have found that CE-EUS and EUS elastography help define the margins of the suspicious tumor, facilitating targeting of the lesion and thus increasing the diagnostic yield in patients with chronic pancreatitis and suspected adenocarcinoma (**Figs. 16.28** and **16.30**).

■ Pseudocyst versus Simple Cyst versus Cystic Neoplasia versus Pseudoaneurysm

If CCDS is used, it is relatively easy to differentiate between cystic lesions and pseudoaneurysms, both with US and with EUS (see **Fig. 16.17**). With mechanical radial echoendoscopes, this differentiation is not possible in some cases.

However, it is much more difficult—although extremely important, from the point of view of prognostic assessment and treatment—to differentiate between pseudocysts (80–90% of cystic pancreatic lesions), simple nonneoplastic cysts, and benign or malignant cystic neoplasms (serous or mucinous cystadenoma; mucinous cystadenocarcinoma; intraductal papillary mucinous tumors: ≈ 10–20% of cystic lesions in the pancreas) (**Fig. 16.31**; see also **Figs. 16.33** and **16.36**).

Lesions that occur only very rarely include cystic islet cell tumors, cystic lymphangiomas, solid pseudopapillary tumors, cystic teratomas, and paragangliomas or ganglioneuromas.[169–173] The incidence of pancreatic cystic lesions is much higher than previously reported. The widespread use of modern high-quality cross-sectional imaging and ultrasound has dramatically increased the number of patients in whom asymptomatic pancreatic cysts are discovered incidentally.[20,169,174]

A Japanese group have presented an endosonographic classification of cystic pancreatic lesions, consisting of six morphological subtypes: thick wall type; protruding tumor type; thick septal type; microcystic type; thin septal type; and simple type. Retrospectively, they were able to achieve reliable differentiation between neoplastic and nonneoplastic cystic pancreatic lesions using this classification.[175] A similarly reliable method of differentiation (with a sensitivity of 92%), which is only based on morphological criteria, has been presented by a group at the Mayo Clinic. They found that a wall thickness of 3 mm or

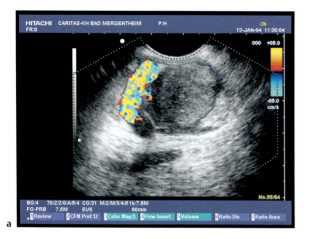

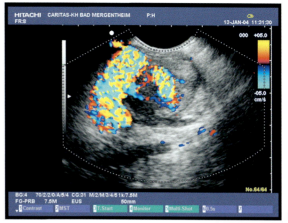

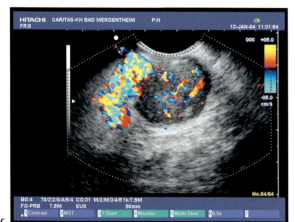

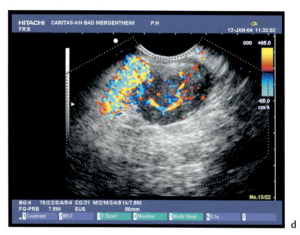

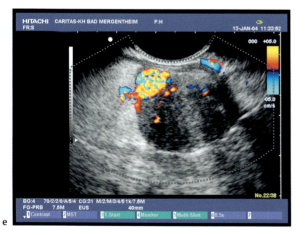

Fig. 16.30a–e A hypoechoic mass in the pancreatic tail, suspected to be adenocarcinoma.

a Color-coded duplex endoscopic ultrasound clearly delineates the splenic artery next to the mass lesion, but demonstrates no perfusion inside the lesion.

b–e Following intravenous injection of the contrast-enhancing agent SonoVue, several vascular signals are identified inside the lesion. After surgical resection, the histological examination excluded adenocarcinoma (the ultimate diagnosis was chronic pancreatitis).

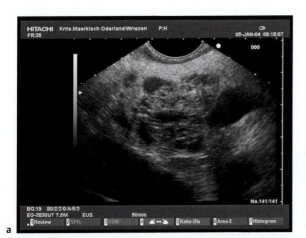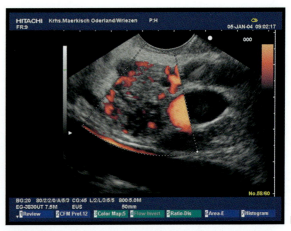

Fig. 16.31a, b Cystic mass lesions in the pancreas (serous microcystic adenoma).

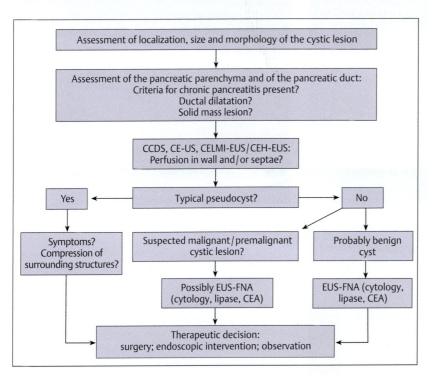

Fig. 16.32 Flow chart for the differential diagnosis of cystic lesions of the pancreas. CCDS, color-coded duplex sonography; CE-EUS, contrast-enhanced endoscopic ultrasound; CELMI-EUS, contrast-enhanced endoscopic ultrasound with low mechanical index; CEH-EUS, contrast-enhanced harmonic endoscopic ultrasound.

greater, macroseptation (all cyst compartments > 10 mm), the presence of mass or intratumoral growth, and cystic dilation of the main pancreatic duct were criteria for malignancy.[172] Similarly, Gress et al.[176] suggested that solid cystic or complex cystic mass lesions were typically malignant. Intraductal mucinous adenocarcinomas may sometimes also have hyperechogenic foci inside the solid part.[176] On the other hand, considerable interobserver disagreement has been reported among eight experienced endosonographers with regard to the diagnosis of neoplastic versus nonneoplastic cystic lesions, the specific type, and the specific EUS features of cystic pancreatic lesions.[177]

Small incidental simple pancreatic cysts that have initially been classified as benign do not undergo malignant change or cause morbidity or mortality, even if followed up for a long period.[178–180] There have been several prospective studies of cystic pancreatic lesions before surgical removal. In contrast to earlier studies, they found that several criteria—e.g., wall thickness, presence of septa, presence of solid parts, and lymphadenopathy—were not sufficiently reliable to differentiate between benign and malignant lesions if the patient's clinical history and the morphology of the pancreatic parenchyma were not known.[181–183] The sensitivity of diagnosing malignant and/or premalignant mucinous cysts can be increased by

Table 16.7 Morphological, cytological, and biochemical criteria for different cystic lesions of the pancreas. Data from [168–177,181–191,196–212,214–217]

Cystic lesion	EUS morphology	Cyst content and cytology	Biochemistry
Serous cystadenoma (SCA)	Microcystic, rarely macrocystic; thin septa, blood vessels within the septa	Thin, translucent fluid; small, cuboid epithelia containing glycogen	Lipase usually low; CEA low (<5 ng/mL)
Mucinous cystadenoma (MCA)	Macrocystic, thick septa, thick wall, potentially intramural tumor	Viscous fluid; fluid stains positive for mucin; mucinous columnar epithelial cells with variable atypia	CEA high: >192 ng/mL [183] >400 ng/mL [184] >480 ng/mL [190] >800 ng/mL [188] Predictive of malignancy: CEA >6000 ng/mL [190]
Intraductal papillary mucinous neoplasia (IPMN)	Dilation of the duct without stricture (main duct type), communication of cystic structures with MPD or side branches (branch duct type), probably non-anechoic contents and mural nodules, variable morphology Indicators of malignancy: • Cystic components >30 mm • Dilated MPD • Solid components • Mural nodules • Thick septa	Neoplastic mucinous cells: — Entrapped in a mucinous background (thick, colloidlike mucin in ≈50%) — Either single or arranged in loosely cohesive sheets, sometimes forming papillary formations IHC: MUC-1, MUC-2 Indicators of malignancy: • Necrosis • Epithelial cell clusters with hyperchromatic nuclei and a high nuclear-to-cytoplasmic ratio • Pale nuclei with parachromatin clearing	CEA variable high Lipase high Predictive of malignant IPMN: • CEA >120 ng/mL [217] • CEA >200 ng/mL [203] • CEA >2500 ng/mL [206] • CA 72.4 >40U/mL [203]
Pseudocyst	Simple cyst or cyst with thin septa, sometimes echogenic debris; changes in the pancreatic parenchyma	Thin, muddy-brown fluid; negative fluid staining for mucin; histiocytes, macrophages, neutrophils, but no epithelial cells	Lipase +++; CEA low (usually <5 ng/mL)
Simple cyst	Simple cyst or cyst with thin septa	Epithelial cells; no atypical cells	Lipase variable; CEA low
Cystic neuroendocrine tumor	Solid tumor with a large unilocular cyst	Thin, sometimes bloody fluid; monomorphic endocrine tumor cells, staining positive for chromogranin A and synaptophysin	No data
Solid pseudopapillary tumor (SPT)	Well-defined echo-poor (solid, mixed solid-cystic or cystic) tumor mainly of the pancreatic tail or body	Bloody fluid, sometimes with necrotic debris; monomorphic cells with round nuclei and eosinophilic, foamy cytoplasm with large, clear vacuoles; branching fragments with central capillaries and myxoid stroma; IHC: vimentin, α1-antitrypsin, α1-antichymotrypsin	No data

CA, cancer antigen; CEA, carcinoembryonic antigen; IHC, immunohistochemistry.

using a combination of endosonographic morphology, cytology of the fluid within the cyst, and the level of carcinoembryonic antigen (CEA)[170,171,173,174,183–191] (**Fig. 16.32**; **Table 16.7**). Measuring the CEA level in the fluid within the cyst has been found to be superior to measuring other tumor markers. However, there is considerable overlapping of CEA levels between the various types of pancreatic cystic lesion. The CEA cut-off levels reported in different studies vary substantially. CA19-9 may be nonspecifically raised in inflammatory processes.[173,188] The presence of high levels of pancreatic enzymes is typical of pseudocysts, but may also occur in cystic neoplasms that communicate with the pancreatic ducts.[173] In selected cases, injecting secretin during EUS may be useful for differentiating small

cystic lesions of the pancreas; this causes enlargement of pseudocysts that communicate with the pancreatic duct, but cystic neoplasms do not change in size.[192]

In the future, molecular analysis of DNA mutations in pancreatic cyst fluid may be helpful in the difficult differential diagnosis of cystic lesions of the pancreas.[193–195] In addition to biochemical, cytological, and molecular-genetic evaluations of the cystic fluid and other cost-intensive tests, we consider that morphological assessment of the entire pancreas and consideration of the clinical background (e.g., whether the patient has previously had episodes of acute pancreatitis or has a history of alcohol abuse) need to be taken into account and may well be more important[11,173,185–187] (**Fig. 16.32**).

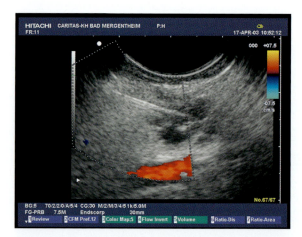

Fig. 16.33 Aspiration of a macrocystic adenoma of the pancreas.

However, it is important to remember that intraductal papillary mucinous neoplasms (IPMNs) may present with acute recurrent pancreatitis[196] and are accompanied by features of chronic pancreatitis in a high percentage of patients.[197] Doing without further investigation of a cystic pancreatic lesion is only acceptable if the clinical context, the (endo-)sonographic morphology of the pancreas and of the cystic lesion, and the findings of any other imaging examinations are taken into account, and if the lesion appears typical of a pseudocyst. If the diagnosis of a pseudocyst is uncertain, or if a cystic neoplasm is suspected, it depends on the degree of diagnostic uncertainty whether, before proceeding to surgery, the clinician may wish to undertake EUS-FNA of the contents of the cyst for cytological and biochemical studies[155–157,173,174,183–190,193–195, 198–212] (**Table 16.7**; **Fig. 16.33**).

In the case of EUS-FNA of cystic pancreatic lesions, antibiotic prophylaxis is mandatory.[171] The age of the patient is also an independent risk factor for malignancy and should be considered when making therapeutical decisions. However, the decision on whether to carry out surgical resec-

tion of a pancreatic cystic lesion has to weigh up the risk of surgery against the risk of malignancy.[173,174]

■ Dilation of the Main Pancreatic Duct

Dilation of the main pancreatic duct and its branches is one of the classical endosonographic characteristics of chronic pancreatitis and usually occurs together with an irregular, hyperechogenic duct contour.[9,40,50–52,67] In elderly people, mild dilation of the pancreatic ducts without any changes in the duct contour is frequent and can be regarded as normal[9,43] (see **Fig. 16.11b**). If the duct is clearly dilated, it is always necessary to look for an underlying tumor at the papilla or in the pancreatic head. Endoscopic ultrasound is the most suitable diagnostic method here[213] (**Fig. 16.34**).

In a large series of patients with pancreatic cancer who were studied prospectively for the presence of characteristics of chronic pancreatitis, a dilated pancreatic duct was present in just over half of the patients[116] (see **Fig. 16.25**). If the common bile duct and the pancreatic duct are both dilated from the level of the papilla, the differential diagnosis also includes benign stenosis of the papilla, adenomyomatosis, or obstruction by a stone[213] (**Fig. 16.35**, see also **Fig. 16.21**).

A further important differential diagnosis is an intraductal papillary mucinous neoplasm (IPMN). IPMNs are characterized by cystic lesions connected to the MPD (MD-IPMN) or branch ducts (BD-IPMN), with or without small polypoid structures in the wall of the pancreatic duct or cyst, duct dilation, and possibly solid lesions[171,173,196–208,214–217] (**Fig. 16.36**). Mural nodules, cystic components > 30 mm, marked dilation of the MPD, solid components, and thick septa are indicators of malignancy.[214–217] In such cases, endosonography-guided aspiration of the pancreatic duct with antibiotic protection (e.g., ciprofloxacin for 5 days, starting with the intervention), with biochemical and cytological investigation of the

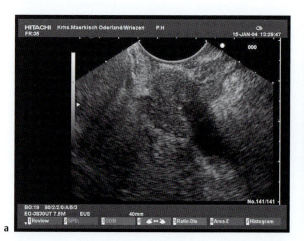 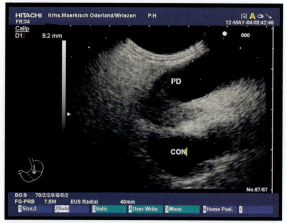

Fig. 16.34a, b Obvious dilation of the pancreatic duct in the presence of tumors of the papilla. CON, portal confluence; PD, pancreatic duct.

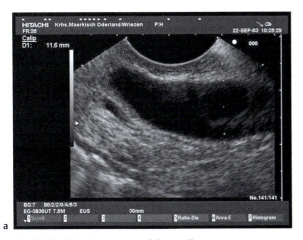

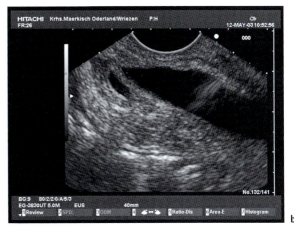

Fig. 16.35a, b Benign stenosis of the papilla.

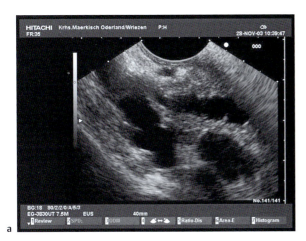

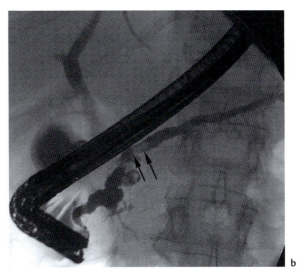

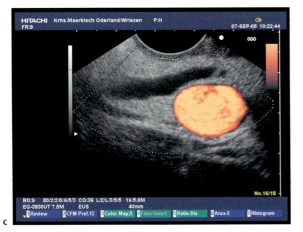

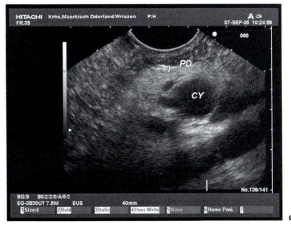

Fig. 16.36a–d Intraductal papillary mucinous tumors (IPMTs) of the pancreas.
a The corresponding EUS view of an IPMT of the main duct type.
b The corresponding ERCP view. There is obvious dilation of the pancreatic ducts, a bizarre pattern in the absence of any stenosis (endoscopic appearance of a fish-mouth papilla), and indistinct intraductal filling defects (arrows).

c, d An IPMT of the branch duct type. There is marked dilation of the smoothly outlined main pancreatic duct (**c**, color-coded: portal confluence). A small cystic (CY) lesion in the pancreatic body, communicating with a dilated side branch of the main pancreatic duct (**d**, PD).

Table 16.8 Endoscopic ultrasound (EUS)-guided therapeutic interventions in chronic pancreatitis[218–224,233–236]

EUS-guided intervention	Efficacy	Complications
EUS-assisted/guided pancreatic pseudocyst drainage	Several case series (≈ 400 patients) with high technical success (84–100%) and long-term clinical success (80–97%)	0–18% (bleeding, stent migration or occlusion, pseudocyst infection, pneumoperitoneum, perforation and peritonitis), safe also in cases of portal hypertension[233]
EUS-guided transmural necrosectomy and drainage of pancreatic necrosis/abscess	Several case series (more than 250 patients) with high technical success (77–100%) and long-term clinical success (80–93%)	0–31% (bleeding, stent migration or occlusion, pseudocyst infection, pneumoperitoneum, gallbladder puncture, perforation and peritonitis, air embolism) mortality up to 7.5% at 30 days[224]
EUS-guided celiac plexus block/ neurolysis	Several case series, retrospective and prospective (controlled) studies with moderate clinical success 59.45% (95% CI, 54.51 to 64.30) (data from meta-analysis of 9 studies with 376 patients: Puli et al. 2009[221]) Benefit diminishes with time EUS-guided celiac plexus block is more effective than CT-guided celiac plexus block in controlling pain in patients with chronic pancreatitis[234,235]	1.6% (major 0.5%)[a]–8.2% (major 0.6%)[b] (self-limited hypotension and diarrhea, retroperitoneal abscess, self-limited postprocedural pain, retroperitoneal bleeding)[236]
EUS-assisted or EUS-guided pancreatic duct drainage	5 case series (92 patients) with moderate-to-high technical (25–92%) and clinical success (69–78%)	14–25% (pancreatitis, bleeding, infection, pseudocyst, perforation)

[a] Complication rate of EUS-guided celiac plexus block in the prospective study by O'Toole and Schmulewitz (2009), n = 189 procedures.[236]
[b] Pooled complication rates of EUS-guided celiac plexus block in 6 studies (n = 170 procedures).[236]

Table 16.9 Diagnostic issues to be considered before endoscopic ultrasound (EUS)-guided or endoscopic drainage of a pancreatic pseudocyst

Is the lesion a typical pancreatic pseudocyst, or could the differential diagnosis include a cystic neoplasm, a pseudoaneurysm, or other benign cystic lesions?
Are the symptoms the patient is presenting with most likely due to the pseudocyst? (Size and location, anatomical relation to other structures, possible compression of neighboring structures)
Are there any diagnostic hints that the pseudocyst may be communicating with the pancreatic duct?
What is the location of the pseudocyst in relation to the wall of the stomach and the duodenum?
Is the pseudocyst (or post-pancreatic abscess) located in a parenchymal organ (spleen, liver)?
How thick is the wall of the pseudocyst? Are there blood vessels within the wall of the pseudocyst or within any septa (if present)?
Are there blood vessels or normal pancreatic parenchyma located between the pseudocyst and the gastrointestinal wall that might be injured during an aspiration?
Is left-sided portal hypertension present, for example with gastric varices?
Does the pseudocyst contain solid structures (sequestra) or sediment?
Are there clinical or endosonographic markers for a potential infection of the pseudocyst (abscess)?
Is additional exudate or free fluid present?

aspirate, has been found to be a safe method with a moderate diagnostic yield. If solid lesions of the pancreas are also present, these should be aspirated as well.[197–208]

The Contribution of EUS to the Treatment of Chronic Pancreatitis

Endoscopic ultrasonography has added several options and advantages to the armamentarium of therapeutic endoscopy for chronic pancreatitis. There is an expanding role for EUS in the planning and guidance of drainage procedures of pancreatic pseudocysts, abscesses, or infected necroses. Several other EUS-guided interventions in chronic pancreatitis have also recently been developed; **Table 16.8** provides an overview.[218–224]

The decision on whether to carry out EUS-guided or endoscopic drainage of a pancreatic pseudocyst depends on several different issues. Clinical and endosonographic findings, as well as potentially the findings of other investigations, influence which interventional method and specific methodology will be used (**Table 16.9**). For example, the interventional methods may differ depending on whether a pseudocyst, an infected pseudocyst, or necrotic tissue is present[222,223] (**Fig. 16.37**).

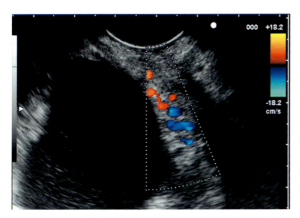

Fig. 16.37 Collateral vessels located between the wall of the pseudocyst and the stomach wall.

In a prospective study of 32 patients who were scheduled to undergo endoscopic drainage of a pancreatic pseudocyst, the endosonographic findings changed the therapeutic plan in more than one-third of the cases.[225] In our experience, one question that remains difficult to answer with endoscopic ultrasound is whether a pseudocyst is communicating with the pancreatic duct. We would therefore recommend that before endosonographic or endoscopic drainage of a pseudocyst, ERCP should be performed, providing the option of transpapillary drainage (**Fig. 16.38**).

Endoscopic ultrasound may also be helpful in planning other therapeutic interventions for chronic pancreatitis, particularly if ERCP is negative or shows an interruption of contrast within the duct during endoscopic retrograde pancreatography. In such cases, it is often possible to identify the reason for the interruption of the contrast medium by using endosonography.[226] It may be possible to differentiate between stones in the pancreatic duct and parenchymal calcifications, or to diagnose pancreas divisum. Endosonography can therefore make a useful contribution to the selection and planning of extracorporeal shock-wave lithotripsy (ESWL), surgical procedures, aggressive endoscopic interventions, or endosonography-guided drainage procedures in the common bile duct or main pancreatic duct.[218,227] In this context, the findings reported by Catalano et al.[111] are of interest; using dynamic secretin-stimulated endosonography in patients with pancreas divisum and a history of chronic pancreatitis, it was possible to identify patients capable of benefiting from endoscopic stent placement.

In selected patients with negative endoscopic retrograde pancreatography findings, it may be possible to use endosonography to puncture the pancreatic duct and inject contrast medium, thereby making pancreatography possible.[228,229] This technique allows subsequent EUS-guided transmural or EUS-assisted transpapillary drainage of the obstructed pancreatic duct in symptomatic patients in whom endoscopic retrograde access to the obstructed main pancreatic duct is not possible (see **Table 16.8**).[218–220]

Pitfalls

- Marked dilation of the pancreatic duct may be caused not only by chronic pancreatitis, but also by an intraductal mucinous tumor or by an obstructing proximal tumor of the pancreas or papilla (see **Figs. 16.34, 16.35** and **16.36**). Conversely, an obstructing proximal tumor of the pancreas or an IPMN may cause chronic pancreatitis.
- Enlarged lymph nodes may be present in chronic pancreatitis, autoimmune pancreatitis, or acute recurrent pancreatitis. However, they may also represent lymph-node metastases from a pancreatic carcinoma.[133] (see **Fig. 16.27**)
- Extension into neighboring structures is not always a sign of pancreatic cancer. It may also be present in chronic pancreatitis with focal inflammatory changes and in autoimmune pancreatitis.[81,134,136]
- In the presence of chronic pancreatitis, the diagnostic accuracy of EUS-guided biopsy for focal hypoechoic mass lesions or cystic lesions is too low to refrain from surgical intervention in patients with a suspicious lesion who are otherwise surgically fit.[135,157–163,173,174,184,197–212]

Practical Hints

- If the main pancreatic duct is dilated, its whole course, including the papilla, has to be inspected in detail. The examiner should particularly look for tumors at the papilla and near the ampulla, treatable benign obstructions of the pancreatic duct, associated cystic or solid mass lesions, and small protrusions indicating the presence of IPMN (see **Figs. 16.34, 16.35,** and **16.36**).
- If electronic curvilinear or radial echoendoscopes are used, CCDS—possibly with contrast enhancement (CE-EUS)—should always be used to look for thrombotic complications of chronic pancreatitis or acute recurrent pancreatitis (see **Figs. 16.12, 16.13, 16.14, 16.15, 16.16,** and **16.17**), to differentiate between cystic lesions and pseudoaneurysms and/or cavernomas of the portal vein (see **Fig. 16.17**), and possibly to improve the etiological diagnosis of solid or cystic mass lesions (see **Figs. 16.26** and **16.27**).
- In addition, CCDS should be used before endoscopic/endosonographic drainage of pseudocysts to identify interposed gastric or duodenal varices and extragastric collaterals (see **Figs. 16.15, 16.19,** and **16.37**). Exerting too much pressure with the transducer should be avoided.
- In the presence of chronic pancreatitis, the limitations of EUS-guided biopsy in the differential diagnosis of solid and cystic mass lesions should be borne in mind.
- Particular indications for EUS-guided biopsies (EUS-FNA, EUS-TCB) are as follows[156,173]:
  - To increase the probability of excluding malignant/premalignant changes in a lesion which, according to EUS and CE-EUS, is highly likely to be benign (for example, serous cystadenoma, focal inflammatory lesions, hemorrhagic pseudocyst)
  - Patients with a high clinical and endosonographic suspicion of an unresectable adenocarcinoma and/or pancreatic metastases in the presence of chronic pancreatitis (before palliative therapy)
  - Suspicion of borderline lesions (neuroendocrine tumors, mucinous cystadenoma, lymphoma) before surgical intervention or other specific treatment
  - Dilation of the pancreatic duct of unknown etiology (for example, to diagnose IPMN or ampullary neoplasia)

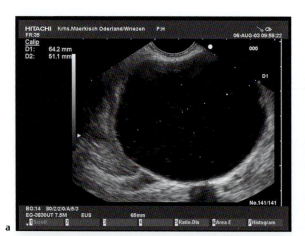

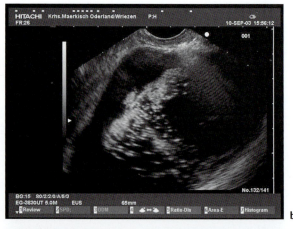

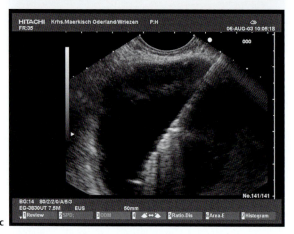

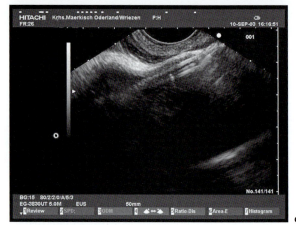

Fig. 16.38a–d Endoscopic ultrasound-guided drainage of a pseudo-cyst.
a There is close contact between the wall of the pseudocyst and the gastric wall.

b Incision with the electrosurgical needle.
c, d Insertion of a 10-Fr endoprosthesis via a guide wire.

• As patients with a long history of chronic pancreatitis have an increased risk of developing pancreatic cancer, new solid mass lesions should always be looked for in such cases. No validated recommendations are available at present for endosonographic follow-up in patients with moderate or severe chronic pancreatitis. Since the life expectancy in patients with chronic pancreatitis is reduced,[112] and since the surgical results in the treatment of pancreatic cancer are poor, it seems unlikely that regular endosonographic follow-up in patients with chronic pancreatitis would have a positive influence on the prognosis. However, in patients with additional risk factors (family history of pancreatic cancer, hereditary pancreatitis, smoking), one might want to consider regular follow-up from the age of 50 years.[119–121]

Conclusions

Particularly because of its lower complication rate in comparison with ERCP, EUS is playing an increasingly important role in the diagnosis and management of chronic pancreatitis—without, however, being able to solve all the diagnostic difficulties. Some authors have already declared that endosonography is the new reference standard for imaging in chronic pancreatitis.[5,230] This view is based on the method's high local imaging resolution, combined with its ability to allow assessment of both the pancreatic parenchyma and the structure of the pancreatic ducts. An international panel of experts has stated that EUS is a suitable method for the diagnosis of early chronic pancreatitis, for the etiological diagnosis of pancreatic duct stenosis, and for management planning in patients with pancreatic pseudocysts.[231] In addition, EUS also plays an important role in the diagnosis of idiopathic acute pancreatitis and autoimmune pancreatitis.

A study conducted in a Danish community hospital reported that over a 3-year period, suspected benign pancreaticobiliary disease was the most rapidly increasing indication for EUS. It was also the most common indication, ranking even higher than the staging of gastrointestinal and pancreatic tumors. Eighty-six percent of ERCPs scheduled for the investigation of suspected benign pancreaticobiliary disease were no longer considered to be required after EUS had been performed.[232]

With the exception of calcification, extreme caution should be exercised when interpreting isolated parenchymal abnormalities on EUS as an early sign of chronic pancreatitis. The clinical background and the results of further diagnostic tests—for example, MRCP, EUS-FNA or PFT—should always be taken into account.

Some weaknesses of EUS include differentiation between chronic pancreatitis and normal age-related changes; differentiation between chronic pancreatitis, residues of acute pancreatitis and diffuse alcohol-toxic fibrosis; and the diagnostic interpretation of hypoechoic pancreatic mass lesions, as well as cystic pancreatic lesions, in patients with chronic pancreatitis. In all of these diagnostic dilemmas, other imaging methods such as multidetector CT, MRI, MRCP, and positron-emission tomography (PET) are also unable to provide sufficient diagnostic accuracy. The decision on whether to investigate suspicious-looking solid or cystic lesions further using early surgical exploration, complex and invasive methods such as EUS-FNA, CE-EUS, or functional endosonography with secretin stimulation, has to be based on each patient's individual clinical background.

If EUS is to be widely used and if it is to be regarded as the reference standard for morphological imaging in the diagnosis of chronic pancreatitis, it will be necessary to adhere to internationally accepted definitions of the EUS features for chronic pancreatitis as well as to consensus criteria for diagnosis.[67] In addition, future examiners should be trained in centers with a considerable degree of expertise and experience in the diagnosis and management of chronic pancreatitis. In experienced hands, EUS has a considerable part to play in planning the management of pseudocysts, peripancreatic necrotic tissue, pancreatic duct obstruction, stenosis of the common bile duct, pancreatic lithiasis, and dysfunction of the sphincter of Oddi. In addition to providing a large amount of diagnostic information, EUS may also be used for carrying out therapeutic interventions.

References

1. Sahai AV, Mishra G, Penman ID, et al. EUS to detect evidence of pancreatic disease in patients with persistent or nonspecific dyspepsia. Gastrointest Endosc 2000;52(2):153–159.
2. Lankisch PG. Sicherheit bei der Diagnostik der chronischen Pankreatitis. Was ist wirklich erforderlich? [Article in German] Dtsch Med Wochenschr 2001;126:96–101.
3. Lankisch PG, Seidensticker F, Otto J, et al. Secretin-pancreozymin test (SPT) and endoscopic retrograde cholangiopancreatography (ERCP): both are necessary for diagnosing or excluding chronic pancreatitis. Pancreas 1996;12(2):149–152.
4. Forsmark CE. The diagnosis of chronic pancreatitis. Gastrointest Endosc 2000;52(2):293–298.
5. Glasbrenner B, Kahl S, Malfertheiner P. Modern diagnostics of chronic pancreatitis. Eur J Gastroenterol Hepatol 2002;14(9):935–941.
6. Hawes RH. Comparison of diagnostic modalities: EUS, ERCP, and fluid analysis. Gastrointest Endosc 1999;49(3 Pt 2):S74–S76.
7. Pungpapong S, Wallace MB, Woodward TA, Raimondo M. Accuracy of endoscopic ultrasonography and magnetic resonance cholangiopancreatography for the diagnosis of chronic pancreatitis. [abstract] Gastrointest Endosc 2005;61:AB298.
8. Lankisch PG, Assmus C, Maisonneuve P, Lowenfels AB. Epidemiology of pancreatic diseases in Lüneburg County. A study in a defined German population. Pancreatology 2002;2(5):469–477.
9. Sahai AV. EUS and chronic pancreatitis. Gastrointest Endosc 2002;56(4, Suppl):S76–S81.
10. Coyle WJ, Pineau BC, Tarnasky PR, et al. Evaluation of unexplained acute and acute recurrent pancreatitis using endoscopic retrograde cholangiopancreatography, sphincter of Oddi manometry and endoscopic ultrasound. Endoscopy 2002;34(8):617–623.
11. Hernandez LV, Bhutani MS. Endoscopic ultrasound and pancreatic cysts: a sticky situation! Am J Gastroenterol 2001;96(12):3229–3230.
12. Axon AT, Classen M, Cotton PB, Cremer M, Freeny PC, Lees WR. Pancreatography in chronic pancreatitis: international definitions. Gut 1984;25(10):1107–1112.
13. Jones SN, Lees WR, Frost RA. Diagnosis and grading of chronic pancreatitis by morphological criteria derived by ultrasound and pancreatography. Clin Radiol 1988;39(1):43–48.
14. Dietrich CF, Becker D. Signalverstärkte Farbdopplersonographie des Abdomens. Constance, Germany: Schnetztor; 2002.
15. Dörffel T, Wruck T, Rückert RI, Romaniuk P, Dörffel Q, Wermke W. Vascular complications in acute pancreatitis assessed by color duplex ultrasonography. Pancreas 2000;21(2):126–133.
16. Martínez-Noguera A, D'Onofrio M. Ultrasonography of the pancreas. 1. Conventional imaging. Abdom Imaging 2007;32(2):136–149.
17. Hohl C, Schmidt T, Honnef D, Günther RW, Haage P. Ultrasonography of the pancreas. 2. Harmonic imaging. Abdom Imaging 2007;32(2):150–160.
18. Bertolotto M, D'Onofrio M, Martone E, Malagò R, Pozzi Mucelli R. Ultrasonography of the pancreas. 3. Doppler imaging. Abdom Imaging 2007;32(2):161–170.

19. D'Onofrio M, Zamboni G, Faccioli N, Capelli P, Pozzi Mucelli R. Ultrasonography of the pancreas. 4. Contrast-enhanced imaging. Abdom Imaging 2007;32(2):171–181.

20. Ikeda M, Sato T, Morozumi A, et al. Morphologic changes in the pancreas detected by screening ultrasonography in a mass survey, with special reference to main duct dilatation, cyst formation, and calcification. Pancreas 1994;9(4):508–512.

21. Lees WR. Endoscopic ultrasonography of chronic pancreatitis and pancreatic pseudocysts. Scand J Gastroenterol Suppl 1986;123:123–129.

22. Lees WR, Vallon AG, Denyer ME, Vahl SP, Cotton PB. Prospective study of ultrasonography in chronic pancreatic disease. BMJ 1979;1(6157):162–164.

23. Hollerbach S, Ruser J, Ochs A, Frick E, Schölmerich J. Current status of abdominal pancreatic ultrasound. A retrospective analysis of 585 pancreatic ultrasound examinations. [Article in German] Med Klin (Munich) 1994;89(1):7–13.

24. Noh KW, Pungpapong S, Raimondo M. Role of endosonography in non-malignant pancreatic diseases. World J Gastroenterol 2007;13(2):165–169.

25. Conway JD, Hawes RH. The expanding role of endoscopic ultrasound in pancreatic disease. Rev Gastroenterol Disord 2006;6(4):201–208.

26. Chaya CT, Bhutani MS. Ultrasonography of the pancreas. 6. Endoscopic imaging. Abdom Imaging 2007;32(2):191–199.

27. Niwa K, Hirooka Y, Niwa Y, et al. Comparison of image quality between electronic and mechanical radial scanning echoendoscopes in pancreatic diseases. J Gastroenterol Hepatol 2004;19(4):454–459.

28. Vilmann P, Hancke S. Endoscopic ultrasound scanning of the upper gastrointestinal tract using a curved linear array transducer: "the linear anatomy". Gastrointest Endosc Clin N Am 1995;5(3):507–521.

29. Dietrich CF, Ignee A, Frey H. Contrast-enhanced endoscopic ultrasound with low mechanical index: a new technique. Z Gastroenterol 2005;43(11):1219–1223.

30. Dietrich CF, Ignee A, Braden B, Barreiros AP, Ott M, Hocke M. Improved differentiation of pancreatic tumors using contrast-enhanced endoscopic ultrasound. Clin Gastroenterol Hepatol 2008;6(5):590–597, e1.

31. Hirooka Y, Goto H, Ito A, et al. Contrast-enhanced endoscopic ultrasonography in pancreatic diseases: a preliminary study. Am J Gastroenterol 1998;93(4):632–635.

32. Hirooka Y, Itoh A, Goto H. Contrast-enhanced endoscopic ultrasonography in the diagnosis of pancreato-biliary diseases. Dig Endosc 2004;16(Suppl 2):S245–S248.

33. Săftoiu A, Popescu C, Cazacu S, et al. Power Doppler endoscopic ultrasonography for the differential diagnosis between pancreatic cancer and pseudotumoral chronic pancreatitis. J Ultrasound Med 2006;25(3):363–372.

34. Hocke M, Schulze E, Gottschalk P, Topalidis T, Dietrich CF. Contrast-enhanced endoscopic ultrasound in discrimination between focal pancreatitis and pancreatic cancer. World J Gastroenterol 2006;12(2):246–250.

35. Hocke M, Ignee A, Topalidis T, Stallmach A, Dietrich CF. Contrast-enhanced endosonographic Doppler spectrum analysis is helpful in discrimination between focal chronic pancreatitis and pancreatic cancer. Pancreas 2007;35(3):286–288.

36. Hocke M, Schmidt C, Zimmer B, Topalidis T, Dietrich CF, Stallmach A. Contrast enhanced endosonography for improving differential diagnosis between chronic pancreatitis and pancreatic cancer. [Article in German] Dtsch Med Wochenschr 2008;133(38):1888–1892.

37. Kitano M, Sakamoto H, Matsui U, et al. A novel perfusion imaging technique of the pancreas: contrast-enhanced harmonic EUS (with video). Gastrointest Endosc 2008;67(1):141–150.

38. Sakamoto H, Kitano M, Suetomi Y, Maekawa K, Takeyama Y, Kudo M. Utility of contrast-enhanced endoscopic ultrasonography for diagnosis of small pancreatic carcinomas. Ultrasound Med Biol 2008;34(4):525–532.

39. Chang KJ, Erickson RA. A primer on linear array endosonographic anatomy. Gastrointest Endosc 1996;43(2 Pt 2):S43–S47.

40. Jenssen C, Dietrich CF. Endoscopic ultrasound in chronic pancreatitis. [Article in German] Z Gastroenterol 2005;43(8):737–749.

41. Lucido ML, Lai R, Guda NM, Mallery P. Hyperechoic pancreas (HEP) on EUS and associated patient factors. [abstract] Gastrointest Endosc 2005;61:AB290.

42. Al-Haddad M, Khashab M, Zyromski N, et al. Risk factors for hyperechogenic pancreas on endoscopic ultrasound: a case-control study. Pancreas 2009;38(6):672–675.

43. Rajan E, Clain JE, Levy MJ, et al. Age-related changes in the pancreas identified by EUS: a prospective evaluation. Gastrointest Endosc 2005;61(3):401–406.

44. Savides TJ, Gress FG, Zaidi SA, Ikenberry SO, Hawes RH. Detection of embryologic ventral pancreatic parenchyma with endoscopic ultrasound. Gastrointest Endosc 1996;43(1):14–19.

45. Lucido ML, Lai R, Guda NM, Mallery P. Factors associated with detection of the ventral anlage (VA) on EUS. [abstract] Gastrointest Endosc 2005;61:AB290.

46. Wiersema MJ, Wiersema LM. Endosonography of the pancreas: normal variation versus changes of early chronic pancreatitis. Gastrointest Endosc Clin N Am 1995;5(3):487–496.

47. Bhutani MS, Hoffman BJ, Hawes RH. Diagnosis of pancreas divisum by endoscopic ultrasonography. Endoscopy 1999;31(2):167–169.

48. Lai R, Freeman ML, Cass OW, Mallery S. Accurate diagnosis of pancreas divisum by linear-array endoscopic ultrasonography. Endoscopy 2004;36(8):705–709.

49. Tessier G, Sahai A. A prospective validation of multiple EUS criteria to diagnose or to exclude pancreas divisum: EUS can accurately exclude pancreas divisum, but ERCP is still required for a definitive diagnosis. [abstract] Gastrointest Endosc 2005;61:AB302.

50. Wiersema MJ, Hawes RH, Lehman GA, Kochman ML, Sherman S, Kopecky KK. Prospective evaluation of endoscopic ultrasonography and endoscopic retrograde cholangiopancreatography in patients with chronic abdominal pain of suspected pancreatic origin. Endoscopy 1993;25(9):555–564.

51. Catalano MF, Lahoti S, Geenen JE, Hogan WJ. Prospective evaluation of endoscopic ultrasonography, endoscopic retrograde pancreatography, and secretin test in the diagnosis of chronic pancreatitis. Gastrointest Endosc 1998;48(1):11–17.

52. Sahai AV, Zimmerman M, Aabakken L, et al. Prospective assessment of the ability of endoscopic ultrasound to diagnose, exclude, or establish the severity of chronic pancreatitis found by endoscopic retrograde cholangiopancreatography. Gastrointest Endosc 1998;48(1):18–25.

53. Kahl S, Glasbrenner B, Leodolter A, Pross M, Schulz HU, Malfertheiner P. EUS in the diagnosis of early chronic pancreatitis: a prospective follow-up study. Gastrointest Endosc 2002;55(4):507–511.

54. Thuler FP, Costa PP, Paulo GA, Nakao FS, Ardengh JC, Ferrari AP. Endoscopic ultrasonography and alcoholic patients: can one predict early pancreatic tissue abnormalities? JOP 2005;6(6):568–574.

55. Bhutani MS. Endoscopic ultrasonography: changes of chronic pancreatitis in asymptomatic and symptomatic alcoholic patients. J Ultrasound Med 1999;18(7):455–462.

56. Hastier P, Buckley MJ, Francois E, et al. A prospective study of pancreatic disease in patients with alcoholic cirrhosis: comparative diagnostic value of ERCP and EUS and long-term significance of isolated parenchymal abnormalities. Gastrointest Endosc 1999;49(6):705–709.

57. Vazquez-Sequeiros E, Boixeda D, Moreira V, Plaza AG. New endoscopic ultrasound (EUS) criteria for diagnosis of chronic pancreatitis (CP). [abstract] Gastrointest Endosc 2004;59:AB223.

58. Conwell DL, Zuccaro G, Purich E, et al. Comparison of endoscopic ultrasound chronic pancreatitis criteria to the endoscopic secretin-stimulated pancreatic function test. Dig Dis Sci 2007;52(5):1206–1210.

59. Morris-Stiff G, Webster P, Frost B, Lewis WG, Puntis MC, Roberts SA. Endoscopic ultrasound reliably identifies chronic pancreatitis when other imaging modalities have been non-diagnostic. JOP 2009;10(3):280–283.

60. Pungpapong S, Wallace MB, Woodward TA, Noh KW, Raimondo M. Accuracy of endoscopic ultrasonography and magnetic resonance cholangiopancreatography for the diagnosis of chronic pancreatitis: a prospective comparison study. J Clin Gastroenterol 2007;41(1):88–93.

61. Pungpapong S, Noh KW, Woodward TA, Wallace MB, Al-Haddad M, Raimondo M. Endoscopic ultrasound and IL-8 in pancreatic juice to diagnose chronic pancreatitis. Pancreatology 2007;7(5-6):491–496.

62. Stevens T, Conwell DL, Zuccaro G Jr, Vargo JJ, Dumot JA, Lopez R. Comparison of endoscopic ultrasound and endoscopic retrograde pancreatography for the prediction of pancreatic exocrine insufficiency. Dig Dis Sci 2008;53(4):1146–1151.

63. Stevens T, Dumot JA, Zuccaro G Jr, et al. Evaluation of duct-cell and acinar-cell function and endosonographic abnormalities in patients with suspected chronic pancreatitis. Clin Gastroenterol Hepatol 2009;7(1):114–119.

64. Lai R, Wiersema MJ, Sahai AV, et al. Blinded comparison of linear and radial endoscopic ultrasound (EUS) for the evaluation of chronic pancreatitis. [abstract] Gastrointest Endosc 2001;53:AB170.

65. Wallace MB, Hawes RH, Durkalski V, et al. The reliability of EUS for the diagnosis of chronic pancreatitis: interobserver agreement among experienced endosonographers. Gastrointest Endosc 2001;53(3):294–299.

66. Wallace MB, Affi A, Eloubeidi MA, et al. How much experience is required to correctly interpret EUS features of chronic pancreatitis? A multicenter prospective trial of third tier EUS trainees compared to a consensus of experts. [abstract] Gastrointest Endosc 2000;51:AB176.

67. Catalano MF, Sahai A, Levy M, et al. EUS-based criteria for the diagnosis of chronic pancreatitis: the Rosemont classification. Gastrointest Endosc 2009;69(7):1251–1261.

68. Buscail L, Escourrou J, Moreau J, et al. Endoscopic ultrasonography in chronic pancreatitis: a comparative prospective study with conventional ultrasonography, computed tomography, and ERCP. Pancreas 1995;10(3):251–257.

69. Giovannini M, Seitz JF. Endoscopic ultrasonography with a linear-type echoendoscope in the evaluation of 94 patients with pancreatobiliary disease. Endoscopy 1994;26(7):579–585.

70. Hollerbach S, Klamann A, Topalidis T, Schmiegel WH. Endoscopic ultrasonography (EUS) and fine-needle aspiration (FNA) cytology for diagnosis of chronic pancreatitis. Endoscopy 2001;33(10):824–831.

71. Nattermann C, Goldschmidt AJ, Dancygier H. Endosonography in chronic pancreatitis. A comparative study of endoscopic retrograde pancreatography and endoscopic sonography. [Article in German] Ultraschall Med 1992;13(6):263–270.

72. Nattermann C, Goldschmidt AJ, Dancygier H. Endosonography in chronic pancreatitis—a comparison between endoscopic retrograde pancreatography and endoscopic ultrasonography. Endoscopy 1993;25(9):565–570.

73. Zimmerman MJ, Mishra G, Lewin D, et al. Comparison of EUS findings with histopathology in chronic pancreatitis. [abstract] Gastrointest Endosc 1997;45:AB185.

74. Bhutani MS, Ahmed I, Verma D, Xiao SY, Brining D. An animal model for studying endoscopic ultrasound changes of early chronic pancreatitis with histologic correlation: a pilot study. Endoscopy 2009;41(4):352–356.

75. Chong AK, Hawes RH, Hoffman BJ, Adams DB, Lewin DN, Romagnuolo J. Diagnostic performance of EUS for chronic pancreatitis: a comparison with histopathology. Gastrointest Endosc 2007;65(6):808–814.

76. Varadarajulu S, Eltoum I, Tamhane A, Eloubeidi MA. Histopathologic correlates of noncalcific chronic pancreatitis by EUS: a prospective tissue characterization study. Gastrointest Endosc 2007;66(3):501–509.

77. Iglesias-García J, Abdulkader I, Lariño-Noia J, Forteza J, Dominguez-Muñoz JE. Histological evaluation of chronic pancreatitis by endoscopic ultrasound-guided fine needle biopsy. Gut 2006;55(11):1661–1662.

78. Mizuno N, Bhatia V, Hosoda W, et al. Histological diagnosis of autoimmune pancreatitis using EUS-guided trucut biopsy: a comparison study with EUS-FNA. J Gastroenterol 2009;44(7):742–750.

79. DeWitt J, McGreevy K, LeBlanc J, McHenry L, Cummings O, Sherman S. EUS-guided Trucut biopsy of suspected nonfocal chronic pancreatitis. Gastrointest Endosc 2005;62(1):76–84.

80. Chowdhury R, Bhutani MS, Mishra G, Toskes PP, Forsmark CE. Comparative analysis of direct pancreatic function testing versus morphological assessment by endoscopic ultrasonography for the evaluation of chronic unexplained abdominal pain of presumed pancreatic origin. Pancreas 2005;31(1):63–68.

81. Farrell JJ, Garber J, Sahani D, Brugge WR. EUS findings in patients with autoimmune pancreatitis. Gastrointest Endosc 2004;60(6):927–936.

82. Jafri SF, Muthusamy R, Hernandez M, Chang KJ, Ngyen P. Prospective prevalence of endoscopic ultrasound (EUS) criteria for chronic pancreatitis (CP) in patients undergoing routine upper EUS. [abstract] Gastrointest Endosc 2001;53:AB168.

83. Levy MJ, Reddy RP, Wiersema MJ, et al. EUS-guided trucut biopsy in establishing autoimmune pancreatitis as the cause of obstructive jaundice. Gastrointest Endosc 2005;61(3):467–472.

84. Eloubeidi MA, Gress FG, Savides TJ, et al. Acute pancreatitis after EUS-guided FNA of solid pancreatic masses: a pooled analysis from EUS centers in the United States. Gastrointest Endosc 2004;60(3):385–389.

85. Jenssen C, Faiss S, Nürnberg D. Complications of endoscopic ultrasound and endoscopic ultrasound-guided interventions - results of a survey among German centers. [Article in German] Z Gastroenterol 2008;46(10):1177–1184.

86. Deshpande V, Mino-Kenudson M, Brugge WR, et al. Endoscopic ultrasound guided fine needle aspiration biopsy of autoimmune pancreatitis: diagnostic criteria and pitfalls. Am J Surg Pathol 2005;29(11):1464–1471.

87. Yusoff IF, Sahai AV. A prospective, quantitative assessment of the effect of ethanol and other variables on the endosonographic appearance of the pancreas. Clin Gastroenterol Hepatol 2004;2(5):405–409.

88. Yusoff IF, Raymond G, Sahai AV. A prospective comparison of the yield of EUS in primary vs. recurrent idiopathic acute pancreatitis. Gastrointest Endosc 2004;60(5):673–678.

89. Lai L, Brugge WR. Endoscopic ultrasound is a sensitive and specific test to diagnose portal venous system thrombosis (PVST). Am J Gastroenterol 2004;99(1):40–44.

90. Lewis JD, Faigel DO, Morris JB, Siegelman ES, Kochman ML. Splenic vein thrombosis secondary to focal pancreatitis diagnosed by endoscopic ultrasonography. J Clin Gastroenterol 1998;26(1):54–56.

91. Wiersema MJ, Chak A, Kopecky KK, Wiersema LM. Duplex Doppler endosonography in the diagnosis of splenic vein, portal vein, and portosystemic shunt thrombosis. Gastrointest Endosc 1995;42(1):19–26.

92. Sato T, Yamazaki K, Akaike J, Toyota J, Karino Y, Ohmura T. Clinical and endoscopic features of gastric varices secondary to splenic vein occlusion. Hepatol Res 2008;38(11): 1076–1082.

93. Frossard JL, Sosa-Valencia L, Amouyal G, Marty O, Hadengue A , Amouyal P. Usefulness of endoscopic ultrasonography in patients with "idiopathic" acute pancreatitis. Am J Med 2000;109(3):196–200.

94. Liu CL, Lo CM, Chan JK, Poon RT, Fan ST. EUS for detection of occult cholelithiasis in patients with idiopathic pancreatitis. Gastrointest Endosc 2000;51(1):28–32.

95. Norton SA, Alderson D. Endoscopic ultrasonography in the evaluation of idiopathic acute pancreatitis. Br J Surg 2000;87(12):1650–1655.

96. Tandon M, Topazian M. Endoscopic ultrasound in idiopathic acute pancreatitis. Am J Gastroenterol 2001;96(3): 705–709.

97. Mariani A, Arcidiacono PG, Curioni S, Giussani A, Testoni PA. Diagnostic yield of ERCP and secretin-enhanced MRCP and EUS in patients with acute recurrent pancreatitis of unknown aetiology. Dig Liver Dis 2009;41(10):753–758.

98. Morris-Stiff G, Al-Allak A, Frost B, Lewis WG, Puntis MC, Roberts A. Does endoscopic ultrasound have anything to offer in the diagnosis of idiopathic acute pancreatitis? JOP 2009;10(2):143–146.

99. Petrone MC, Arcidiacono PG, Testoni PA. Endoscopic ultrasonography for evaluating patients with recurrent pancreatitis. World J Gastroenterol 2008;14(7):1016–1022.

100. Seifert H, Wehrmann T, Hilgers R, Gouder S, Braden B, Dietrich CF. Catheter probe extraductal EUS reliably detects distal common bile duct abnormalities. Gastrointest Endosc 2004;60(1):61–67.

101. Wehrmann T, Martchenko K, Riphaus A. Catheter probe extraductal ultrasonography vs. conventional endoscopic ultrasonography for detection of bile duct stones. Endoscopy 2009;41(2):133–137.

102. Canto MI, Chak A, Stellato T, Sivak MV Jr. Endoscopic ultrasonography versus cholangiography for the diagnosis of choledocholithiasis. Gastrointest Endosc 1998;47(6): 439–448.

103. Palazzo L, O'toole D. EUS in common bile duct stones. Gastrointest Endosc 2002; 56(4, Suppl):S49–S57.

104. Prat F, Amouyal G, Amouyal P, et al. Prospective controlled study of endoscopic ultrasonography and endoscopic retrograde cholangiography in patients with suspected common-bileduct lithiasis. Lancet 1996;347(8994):75–79.

105. Kohut M, Nowak A, Nowakowska-Dulawa E, Marek T, Kaczor R. Endosonography with linear array instead of endoscopic retrograde cholangiography as the diagnostic tool in patients with moderate suspicion of common bile duct stones. World J Gastroenterol 2003;9(3):612–614.

106. Kohut M, Nowakowska-Duława E, Marek T, Kaczor R, Nowak A. Accuracy of linear endoscopic ultrasonography in the evaluation of patients with suspected common bile duct stones. Endoscopy 2002;34(4):299–303.

107. Janssen J, Halboos A, Greiner L. EUS accurately predicts the need for therapeutic ERCP in patients with a low probability of biliary obstruction. Gastrointest Endosc 2008;68(3): 470–476.

108. Lachter J, Rubin A, Shiller M, et al. Linear EUS for bile duct stones. Gastrointest Endosc 2000;51(1):51–54.

109. Thorbøll J, Vilmann P, Jacobsen B, Hassan H. Endoscopic ultrasonography in detection of cholelithiasis in patients with biliary pain and negative transabdominal ultrasonography. Scand J Gastroenterol 2004;39(3):267–269.

110. Lévy P, Boruchowicz A, Hastier P, et al. Diagnostic criteria in predicting a biliary origin of acute pancreatitis in the era of endoscopic ultrasound: multicentre prospective evaluation of 213 patients. Pancreatology 2005;5(4-5):450–456.

111. Catalano MF, Lahoti S, Alcocer E, Geenen JE, Hogan WJ. Dynamic imaging of the pancreas using real-time endoscopic ultrasonography with secretin stimulation. Gastrointest Endosc 1998;48(6):580–587.

112. Lowenfels AB, Maisonneuve P, Cavallini G, et al; International Pancreatitis Study Group. Prognosis of chronic pancreatitis: an international multicenter study. Am J Gastroenterol 1994;89(9):1467–1471.

113. Lowenfels AB, Maisonneuve P, Cavallini G, et al; International Pancreatitis Study Group. Pancreatitis and the risk of pancreatic cancer. N Engl J Med 1993;328(20):1433–1437.

114. Lowenfels AB, Maisonneuve P, Lankisch PG. Chronic pancreatitis and other risk factors for pancreatic cancer. Gastroenterol Clin North Am 1999;28(3):673–685.

115. Talamini G, Falconi M, Bassi C, et al. Incidence of cancer in the course of chronic pancreatitis. Am J Gastroenterol 1999;94(5):1253–1260.

116. Parasher G, Alasadi R, Chang KJ, Ngyen PT. Endoscopic ultrasound (EUS) changes of chronic pancreatitis (CP) are common among patients with pancreatic cancer. [abstract] Gastrointest Endosc 2002;55:AB250.

117. Rubenstein JH, Scheiman JM, Anderson MA. A clinical and economic evaluation of endoscopic ultrasound for patients at risk for familial pancreatic adenocarcinoma. Pancreatology 2007;7(5-6):514–525.

118. Brune K, Abe T, Canto M, et al. Multifocal neoplastic precursor lesions associated with lobular atrophy of the pancreas in patients having a strong family history of pancreatic cancer. Am J Surg Pathol 2006;30(9):1067–1076.

119. Canto MI, Goggins M, Yeo CJ, et al. Screening for pancreatic neoplasia in high-risk individuals: an EUS-based approach. Clin Gastroenterol Hepatol 2004;2(7):606–621.

120. Canto MI, Goggins M, Hruban RH, et al. Screening for early pancreatic neoplasia in high-risk individuals: a prospective

controlled study. Clin Gastroenterol Hepatol 2006; 4(6):766–781, quiz 665.

121. Poley JW, Kluijt I, Gouma DJ, et al. The yield of first-time endoscopic ultrasonography in screening individuals at a high risk of developing pancreatic cancer. Am J Gastroenterol 2009;104(9):2175–2181.

122. Topazian M, Enders F, Kimmey M, et al. Interobserver agreement for EUS findings in familial pancreatic-cancer kindreds. Gastrointest Endosc 2007;66(1):62–67.

123. Rulyak SJ, Kimmey MB, Veenstra DL, Brentnall TA. Cost-effectiveness of pancreatic cancer screening in familial pancreatic cancer kindreds. Gastrointest Endosc 2003;57(1): 23–29.

124. Abraham SC, Wilentz RE, Yeo CJ, et al. Pancreaticoduodenectomy (Whipple resections) in patients without malignancy: are they all 'chronic pancreatitis'? Am J Surg Pathol 2003;27(1):110–120.

125. van Gulik TM, Reeders JW, Bosma A, et al. Incidence and clinical findings of benign, inflammatory disease in patients resected for presumed pancreatic head cancer. Gastrointest Endosc 1997;46(5):417–423.

126. Notohara K, Burgart LJ, Yadav D, Chari S, Smyrk TC. Idiopathic chronic pancreatitis with periductal lymphoplasmacytic infiltration: clinicopathologic features of 35 cases. Am J Surg Pathol 2003;27(8):1119–1127.

127. Weber SM, Cubukcu-Dimopulo O, Palesty JA, et al. Lymphoplasmacytic sclerosing pancreatitis: inflammatory mimic of pancreatic carcinoma. J Gastrointest Surg 2003;7(1): 129–137, discussion 137–139.

128. Finkelberg DL, Sahani D, Deshpande V, Brugge WR. Autoimmune pancreatitis. N Engl J Med 2006;355(25): 2670–2676.

129. Hoki N, Mizuno N, Sawaki A, et al. Diagnosis of autoimmune pancreatitis using endoscopic ultrasonography. J Gastroenterol 2009;44(2):154–159.

130. Sahani DV, Kalva SP, Farrell J, et al. Autoimmune pancreatitis: imaging features. Radiology 2004;233(2):345–352.

131. Baron PL, Aabakken LE, Cole DJ, et al. Differentiation of benign from malignant pancreatic masses by endoscopic ultrasound. Ann Surg Oncol 1997;4(8):639–643.

132. Barthet M, Hastier P, Buckley MJ, et al. Eosinophilic pancreatitis mimicking pancreatic neoplasia: EUS and ERCP findings—is nonsurgical diagnosis possible? Pancreas 1998;17(4):419–422.

133. Barthet M, Portal I, Boujaoude J, Bernard JP, Sahel J. Endoscopic ultrasonographic diagnosis of pancreatic cancer complicating chronic pancreatitis. Endoscopy 1996; 28(6): 487–491.

134. Brand B, Pfaff T, Binmoeller KF, et al. Endoscopic ultrasound for differential diagnosis of focal pancreatic lesions, confirmed by surgery. Scand J Gastroenterol 2000;35(11): 1221–1228.

135. Canto MIF, Kantsevoy SV, Smith CL, McClelland L, Kalloo AN. Tumor versus pseudotumor? A prospective study of factors associated with missed cancers and nondiagnostic EUS-FNA in patients with pancreatobiliary lesions. [abstract] Gastrointest Endosc 2000;51:AB170.

136. Nattermann C, Goldschmidt AJ, Dancygier H. Endosonography in the assessment of pancreatic tumors. A comparison of the endosonographic findings of carcinomas and segmental inflammatory changes. [Article in German] Dtsch Med Wochenschr 1995;120(46):1571–1576.

137. Okai T, Fujii T, Ida M, Ueda H, Sawabu N. EUS and ERCP features of nonalcoholic duct-destructive, mass-forming pancreatitis before and after treatment with prednisolone. Abdom Imaging 2002;27(1):74–76.

138. Rösch T, Lorenz R, Braig C, et al. Endoscopic ultrasound in pancreatic tumor diagnosis. Gastrointest Endosc 1991; 37(3):347–352.

139. Becker D, Strobel D, Bernatik T, Hahn EG. Echo-enhanced color- and power-Doppler EUS for the discrimination between focal pancreatitis and pancreatic carcinoma. Gastrointest Endosc 2001;53(7):784–789.

140. Kato T, Tsukamoto Y, Naitoh Y, Hirooka Y, Furukawa T, Hayakawa T. Ultrasonographic and endoscopic ultrasonographic angiography in pancreatic mass lesions. Acta Radiol 1995;36(4):381–387.

141. Dietrich CF, Braden B, Hocke M, Ott M, Ignee A. Improved characterisation of solitary solid pancreatic tumours using contrast enhanced transabdominal ultrasound. J Cancer Res Clin Oncol 2008;134(6):635–643.

142. Ozawa Y, Numata K, Tanaka K, et al. Contrast-enhanced sonography of small pancreatic mass lesions. J Ultrasound Med 2002;21(9):983–991.

143. Rickes S, Malfertheiner P. Echo-enhanced sonography—an increasingly used procedure for the differentiation of pancreatic tumors. Dig Dis 2004;22(1):32–38.

144. Rickes S, Unkrodt K, Neye H, Ocran K, Lochs H, Wermke W. Differential diagnosis of frequent pancreatic tumours with echo-enhanced power-Doppler sonography - presentation of case reports. [Article in German] Z Gastroenterol 2002;40(4):235–240.

145. Rickes S, Unkrodt K, Neye H, Ocran KW, Wermke W. Differentiation of pancreatic tumours by conventional ultrasound, unenhanced and echo-enhanced power Doppler sonography. Scand J Gastroenterol 2002;37(11):1313–1320.

146. Rickes S, Unkrodt K, Ocran K, Neye H, Lochs H, Wermke W. Evaluation of Doppler ultrasonography criteria for the differential diagnosis of pancreatic tumors. [Article in German] Ultraschall Med 2000;21(6):253–258.

147. Numata K, Ozawa Y, Kobayashi N, et al. Contrast-enhanced sonography of autoimmune pancreatitis: comparison with pathologic findings. J Ultrasound Med 2004;23(2): 199–206.

148. Das A, Nguyen CC, Li F, Li B. Digital image analysis of EUS images accurately differentiates pancreatic cancer from chronic pancreatitis and normal tissue. Gastrointest Endosc 2008;67(6):861–867.

149. Giovannini M, Thomas B, Erwan B, et al. Endoscopic ultrasound elastography for evaluation of lymph nodes and pancreatic masses: a multicenter study. World J Gastroenterol 2009;15(13):1587–1593.

150. Janssen J, Schlörer E, Greiner L. EUS elastography of the pancreas: feasibility and pattern description of the normal pancreas, chronic pancreatitis, and focal pancreatic lesions. Gastrointest Endosc 2007;65(7):971–978.

151. Kumon RE, Olowe K, Faulx AL, et al. EUS spectrum analysis for in vivo characterization of pancreatic and lymph node tissue: a pilot study. Gastrointest Endosc 2007;66(6): 1096–1106.

152. Sãftoiu A, Vilmann P, Gorunescu F, et al. Neural network analysis of dynamic sequences of EUS elastography used for the differential diagnosis of chronic pancreatitis and pancreatic cancer. Gastrointest Endosc 2008;68(6):1086–1094.

153. Hirche TO, Ignee A, Barreiros AP, et al. Indications and limitations of endoscopic ultrasound elastography for evaluation of focal pancreatic lesions. Endoscopy 2008; 40(11):910–917.

154. Jenssen C, Möller K, Wagner S, Sarbia M. Endoscopic ultrasound-guided biopsy: diagnostic yield, pitfalls, quality management part 1: optimizing specimen collection and diagnostic efficiency. [Article in German] Z Gastroenterol 2008;46(6):590–600.

155. Jenssen C, Möller K, Wagner S, Sarbia M. Endoscopic ultrasound-guided biopsy: diagnostic yield, pitfalls, quality management. [Article in German] Z Gastroenterol 2008; 46(9):897–908.

156. Jenssen C, Dietrich CF. Endoscopic ultrasound-guided fine-needle aspiration biopsy and trucut biopsy in gastroenterology - An overview. Best Pract Res Clin Gastroenterol 2009;23(5):743–759.

157. Ardengh JC, Lopes CV, Campos AD, Pereira de Lima LF, Venco F, Módena JL. Endoscopic ultrasound and fine needle aspiration in chronic pancreatitis: differential diagnosis between pseudotumoral masses and pancreatic cancer. JOP 2007;8(4):413–421.

158. Fritscher-Ravens A, Brand L, Knöfel WT, et al. Comparison of endoscopic ultrasound-guided fine needle aspiration for focal pancreatic lesions in patients with normal parenchyma and chronic pancreatitis. Am J Gastroenterol 2002; 97(11):2768–2775.

159. Iordache S, Săftoiu A, Cazacu S, et al. Endoscopic ultrasound approach of pancreatic cancer in chronic pancreatitis patients in a tertiary referral centre. J Gastrointestin Liver Dis 2008;17(3):279–284.

160. Krishna NB, Mehra M, Reddy AV, Agarwal B. EUS/EUS-FNA for suspected pancreatic cancer: influence of chronic pancreatitis and clinical presentation with or without obstructive jaundice on performance characteristics. Gastrointest Endosc 2009;70(1):70–79.

161. Takahashi K, Yamao K, Okubo K, et al. Differential diagnosis of pancreatic cancer and focal pancreatitis by using EUS-guided FNA. Gastrointest Endosc 2005;61(1):76–79.

162. Varadarajulu S, Tamhane A, Eloubeidi MA. Yield of EUS-guided FNA of pancreatic masses in the presence or the absence of chronic pancreatitis. Gastrointest Endosc 2005; 62(5):728–736, quiz 751, 753.

163. Bournet B, Souque A, Senesse P, et al. Endoscopic ultrasound-guided fine-needle aspiration biopsy coupled with KRAS mutation assay to distinguish pancreatic cancer from pseudotumoral chronic pancreatitis. Endoscopy 2009; 41(6):552–557.

164. Khalid A, Nodit L, Zahid M, et al. Endoscopic ultrasound fine needle aspirate DNA analysis to differentiate malignant and benign pancreatic masses. Am J Gastroenterol 2006; 101(11):2493–2500.

165. Mishra G, Zhao Y, Sweeney J, et al. Determination of qualitative telomerase activity as an adjunct to the diagnosis of pancreatic adenocarcinoma by EUS-guided fine-needle aspiration. Gastrointest Endosc 2006;63(4):648–654.

166. Salek C, Benesova L, Zavoral M, et al. Evaluation of clinical relevance of examining K-ras, p16 and p53 mutations along with allelic losses at 9 p and 18q in EUS-guided fine needle aspiration samples of patients with chronic pancreatitis and pancreatic cancer. World J Gastroenterol 2007;13 (27):3714–3720.

167. Agarwal B, Ludwig OJ, Collins BT, Cortese C. Immunostaining as an adjunct to cytology for diagnosis of pancreatic adenocarcinoma. Clin Gastroenterol Hepatol 2008; 6(12):1425–1431.

168. Saftoiu A, Iordache SA, Gheonea DI, et al. Combined contrast-enhanced power Doppler and real-time sonoelastography performed during EUS, used in the differential diag-

nosis of focal pancreatic masses (with videos). Gastrointest Endosc 2010;72(4)739–747.

169. Brugge WR, Lauwers GY, Sahani D, Fernandez-del Castillo C, Warshaw AL. Cystic neoplasms of the pancreas. N Engl J Med 2004;351(12):1218–1226.

170. Hernandez LV, Mishra G, Forsmark C, et al. Role of endoscopic ultrasound (EUS) and EUS-guided fine needle aspiration in the diagnosis and treatment of cystic lesions of the pancreas. Pancreas 2002;25(3):222–228.

171. Jacobson BC, Baron TH, Adler DG, et al; American Society for Gastrointestinal Endoscopy. ASGE guideline: The role of endoscopy in the diagnosis and the management of cystic lesions and inflammatory fluid collections of the pancreas. Gastrointest Endosc 2005;61(3):363–370.

172. Sedlack R, Affi A, Vazquez-Sequeiros E, Norton ID, Clain JE, Wiersema MJ. Utility of EUS in the evaluation of cystic pancreatic lesions. Gastrointest Endosc 2002;56(4): 543–547.

173. Dietrich CF, Jenssen C, Allescher HD, Hocke M, Barreiros AP, Ignee A. Differential diagnosis of pancreatic lesions using endoscopic ultrasound. [Article in German] Z Gastroenterol 2008;46(6):601–617.

174. Brugge WR. Should all pancreatic cystic lesions be resected? Cyst-fluid analysis in the differential diagnosis of pancreatic cystic lesions: a meta-analysis. Gastrointest Endosc 2005;62(3):390–391.

175. Koito K, Namieno T, Nagakawa T, Shyonai T, Hirokawa N, Morita K. Solitary cystic tumor of the pancreas: EUS-pathologic correlation. Gastrointest Endosc 1997;45(3):268–276.

176. Gress F, Gottlieb K, Cummings O, Sherman S, Lehman G. Endoscopic ultrasound characteristics of mucinous cystic neoplasms of the pancreas. Am J Gastroenterol 2000; 95(4):961–965.

177. Ahmad NA, Kochman ML, Brensinger C, et al. Interobserver agreement among endosonographers for the diagnosis of neoplastic versus non-neoplastic pancreatic cystic lesions. Gastrointest Endosc 2003;58(1):59–64.

178. Handrich SJ, Hough DM, Fletcher JG, Sarr MG. The natural history of the incidentally discovered small simple pancreatic cyst: long-term follow-up and clinical implications. AJR Am J Roentgenol 2005;184(1):20–23.

179. Ikeda M, Sato T, Ochiai M, Morozumi A, Ainota T, Fujino MA. Ultrasonographic follow-up study of small pancreatic cysts of unknown etiology. Bildgebung 1993;60(4):209–214.

180. Brounts LR, Lehmann RK, Causey MW, Sebesta JA, Brown TA. Natural course and outcome of cystic lesions in the pancreas. Am J Surg 2009;197(5):619–622, discussion 622–623.

181. Ahmad NA, Kochman ML, Lewis JD, Ginsberg GG. Can EUS alone differentiate between malignant and benign cystic lesions of the pancreas? Am J Gastroenterol 2001;96(12): 3295–3300.

182. Brandwein SL, Farrell JJ, Centeno BA, Brugge WR. Detection and tumor staging of malignancy in cystic, intraductal, and solid tumors of the pancreas by EUS. Gastrointest Endosc 2001;53(7):722–727.

183. Brugge WR, Lewandrowski K, Lee-Lewandrowski E, et al. Diagnosis of pancreatic cystic neoplasms: a report of the cooperative pancreatic cyst study. Gastroenterology 2004; 126(5):1330–1336.

184. Frossard JL, Amouyal P, Amouyal G, et al. Performance of endosonography-guided fine needle aspiration and biopsy in the diagnosis of pancreatic cystic lesions. Am J Gastroenterol 2003;98(7):1516–1524.

185. Levy MJ, Clain JE. Evaluation and management of cystic pancreatic tumors: emphasis on the role of EUS FNA. Clin Gastroenterol Hepatol 2004;2(8):639–653.
186. O'Toole D, Palazzo L, Hammel P, et al. Macrocystic pancreatic cystadenoma: The role of EUS and cyst fluid analysis in distinguishing mucinous and serous lesions. Gastrointest Endosc 2004;59(7):823–829.
187. Sand JA, Hyoty MK, Mattila J, Dagorn JC, Nordback IH. Clinical assessment compared with cyst fluid analysis in the differential diagnosis of cystic lesions in the pancreas. Surgery 1996;119(3):275–280.
188. van der Waaij LA, van Dullemen HM, Porte RJ. Cyst fluid analysis in the differential diagnosis of pancreatic cystic lesions: a pooled analysis. Gastrointest Endosc 2005; 62(3):383–389.
189. Attasaranya S, Pais S, LeBlanc J, McHenry L, Sherman S, DeWitt JM. Endoscopic ultrasound-guided fine needle aspiration and cyst fluid analysis for pancreatic cysts. JOP 2007;8(5):553–563.
190. Linder JD, Geenen JE, Catalano MF. Cyst fluid analysis obtained by EUS-guided FNA in the evaluation of discrete cystic neoplasms of the pancreas: a prospective single-center experience. Gastrointest Endosc 2006;64(5): 697–702.
191. Song MH, Lee SK, Kim MH, et al. EUS in the evaluation of pancreatic cystic lesions. Gastrointest Endosc 2003;57(7): 891–896.
192. Ikeda M, Sato T, Ochiai M, Morozumi A, Nakamura T, Fujino MA. Morphological changes of small pancreatic cysts in response to secretin stimulation. Observation by endoscopic ultrasonography. Dig Dis Sci 1993;38(4):648–652.
193. Khalid A, Zahid M, Finkelstein SD, et al. Pancreatic cyst fluid DNA analysis in evaluating pancreatic cysts: a report of the PANDA study. Gastrointest Endosc 2009;69(6):1095–1102.
194. Shen J, Brugge WR, Dimaio CJ, Pitman MB. Molecular analysis of pancreatic cyst fluid: a comparative analysis with current practice of diagnosis. Cancer Cytopathol 2009; 117(3):217–227.
195. Sreenarasimhaiah J, Lara LF, Jazrawi SF, Barnett CC, Tang SJ. A comparative analysis of pancreas cyst fluid CEA and histology with DNA mutational analysis in the detection of mucin producing or malignant cysts. JOP 2009;10(2): 163–168.
196. Ringold DA, Shroff P, Sikka SK, et al. Pancreatitis is frequent among patients with side-branch intraductal papillary mucinous neoplasia diagnosed by EUS. Gastrointest Endosc 2009;70(3):488–494.
197. Aithal GP, Chen RY, Cunningham JT, et al. Accuracy of EUS for detection of intraductal papillary mucinous tumor of the pancreas. Gastrointest Endosc 2002;56(5):701–707.
198. Emerson RE, Randolph ML, Cramer HM. Endoscopic ultrasound-guided fine-needle aspiration cytology diagnosis of intraductal papillary mucinous neoplasm of the pancreas is highly predictive of pancreatic neoplasia. Diagn Cytopathol 2006;34(7):457–462.
199. Lai R, Stanley MW, Bardales R, Linzie B, Mallery S. Endoscopic ultrasound-guided pancreatic duct aspiration: diagnostic yield and safety. Endoscopy 2002;34(9):715–720.
200. Fernández-Esparrach G, Pellisé M, Solé M, et al. EUS FNA in intraductal papillary mucinous tumors of the pancreas. Hepatogastroenterology 2007;54(73):260–264.
201. Layfield LJ, Cramer H. Fine-needle aspiration cytology of intraductal papillary-mucinous tumors: a retrospective analysis. Diagn Cytopathol 2005;32(1):16–20.
202. Maire F, Couvelard A, Hammel P, et al. Intraductal papillary mucinous tumors of the pancreas: the preoperative value of cytologic and histopathologic diagnosis. Gastrointest Endosc 2003;58(5):701–706.
203. Maire F, Voitot H, Aubert A, et al. Intraductal papillary mucinous neoplasms of the pancreas: performance of pancreatic fluid analysis for positive diagnosis and the prediction of malignancy. Am J Gastroenterol 2008;103(11): 2871–2877.
204. Michaels PJ, Brachtel EF, Bounds BC, Brugge WR, Pitman MB. Intraductal papillary mucinous neoplasm of the pancreas: cytologic features predict histologic grade. Cancer 2006;108(3):163–173.
205. Pais SA, Attasaranya S, Leblanc JK, Sherman S, Schmidt CM, DeWitt J. Role of endoscopic ultrasound in the diagnosis of intraductal papillary mucinous neoplasms: correlation with surgical histopathology. Clin Gastroenterol Hepatol 2007;5(4):489–495.
206. Pitman MB, Michaels PJ, Deshpande V, Brugge WR, Bounds BC. Cytological and cyst fluid analysis of small (< or =3 cm) branch duct intraductal papillary mucinous neoplasms adds value to patient management decisions. Pancreatology 2008;8(3):277–284.
207. Salla C, Chatzipantelis P, Konstantinou P, et al. Endoscopic ultrasound-guided fine-needle aspiration cytology in the diagnosis of intraductal papillary mucinous neoplasms of the pancreas. A study of 8 cases. JOP 2007;8(6):715–724.
208. Solé M, Iglesias C, Fernández-Esparrach G, Colomo L, Pellisé M, Ginés A. Fine-needle aspiration cytology of intraductal papillary mucinous tumors of the pancreas. Cancer 2005;105(5):298–303.
209. Bardales RH, Centeno B, Mallery JS, et al. Endoscopic ultrasound-guided fine-needle aspiration cytology diagnosis of solid-pseudopapillary tumor of the pancreas: a rare neoplasm of elusive origin but characteristic cytomorphologic features. Am J Clin Pathol 2004;121(5):654–662.
210. Jani N, Dewitt J, Eloubeidi M, et al. Endoscopic ultrasound-guided fine-needle aspiration for diagnosis of solid pseudopapillary tumors of the pancreas: a multicenter experience. Endoscopy 2008;40(3):200–203.
211. Jhala N, Siegal GP, Jhala D. Large, clear cytoplasmic vacuolation: an under-recognized cytologic clue to distinguish solid pseudopapillary neoplasms of the pancreas from pancreatic endocrine neoplasms on fine-needle aspiration. Cancer 2008;114(4):249–254.
212. Salla C, Chatzipantelis P, Konstantinou P, Karoumpalis I, Pantazopoulou A, Dappola V. Endoscopic ultrasound-guided fine-needle aspiration cytology diagnosis of solid pseudopapillary tumor of the pancreas: a case report and literature review. World J Gastroenterol 2007;13(38): 5158–5163.
213. Will U, Bosseckert H, Meyer F. Correlation of endoscopic ultrasonography (EUS) for differential diagnostics between inflammatory and neoplastic lesions of the papilla of Vater and the peripapillary region with results of histologic investigation. Ultraschall Med 2008;29(3):275–280.
214. Ohno E, Hirooka Y, Itoh A, et al. Intraductal papillary mucinous neoplasms of the pancreas: differentiation of malignant and benign tumors by endoscopic ultrasound findings of mural nodules. Ann Surg 2009;249(4):628–634.
215. Kubo H, Chijiiwa Y, Akahoshi K, et al. Intraductal papillary-mucinous tumors of the pancreas: differential diagnosis between benign and malignant tumors by endoscopic ultrasonography. Am J Gastroenterol 2001;96(5):1429–1434.

216. Baba T, Yamaguchi T, Ishihara T, et al. Distinguishing benign from malignant intraductal papillary mucinous tumors of the pancreas by imaging techniques. Pancreas 2004; 29(3): 212–217.

217. Hirono S, Tani M, Kawai M, et al. Treatment strategy for intraductal papillary mucinous neoplasm of the pancreas based on malignant predictive factors. Arch Surg 2009; 144(4):345–349, discussion 349–350.

218. Will U. Therapeutic endosonography. [Article in German] Z Gastroenterol 2008;46(6):555–563.

219. Ginès A, Varadarajulu S, Napoleon B; EUS 2008 Working Group. EUS 2008 Working Group document: evaluation of EUS-guided pancreatic-duct drainage (with video). Gastrointest Endosc 2009; 69(2, Suppl):S43–S48.

220. Penman ID, Rösch T; EUS 2008 Working Group. EUS 2008 Working Group document: evaluation of EUS-guided celiac plexus neurolysis/block (with video). Gastrointest Endosc 2009; 69(2, Suppl):S28–S31.

221. Puli SR, Reddy JB, Bechtold ML, Antillon MR, Brugge WR. EUS-guided celiac plexus neurolysis for pain due to chronic pancreatitis or pancreatic cancer pain: a meta-analysis and systematic review. Dig Dis Sci 2009;54(11):2330–2337.

222. Seewald S, Ang TL, Teng KY, et al. Endoscopic ultrasound-guided drainage of abdominal abscesses and infected necrosis. Endoscopy 2009;41(2):166–174.

223. Seewald S, Ang TL, Kida M, Teng KY, Soehendra N; EUS 2008 Working Group. EUS 2008 Working Group document: evaluation of EUS-guided drainage of pancreatic-fluid collections (with video). Gastrointest Endosc 2009; 69(2, Suppl):S13–S21.

224. Seifert H, Biermer M, Schmitt W, et al. Transluminal endoscopic necrosectomy after acute pancreatitis: a multicentre study with long-term follow-up (the GEPARD Study). Gut 2009;58(9):1260–1266.

225. Fockens P, Johnson TG, van Dullemen HM, Huibregtse K, Tytgat GN. Endosonographic imaging of pancreatic pseudocysts before endoscopic transmural drainage. Gastrointest Endosc 1997;46(5):412–416.

226. Fazel A, Moezardalan K, Kalaghchi B, Forsmark C. The isolated pancreatic duct (PD) stricture with negative brush cytology: EUS for the detection of underlying malignancy. Gastrointest Endosc 2005;61:AB277.

227. Papanikolaou IS, Adler A, Neumann U, Neuhaus P, Rösch T. Endoscopic ultrasound in pancreatic disease—its influence on surgical decision-making. An update 2008. Pancreatology 2009;9(1-2):55–65.

228. Gress F, Ikenberry S, Sherman S, Lehman G. Endoscopic ultrasound-directed pancreatography. Gastrointest Endosc 1996;44(6):736–739.

229. Wiersema MJ, Sandusky D, Carr R, Wiersema LM, Erdel WC, Frederick PK. Endosonography-guided cholangiopancreatography. Gastrointest Endosc 1996;43(2 Pt 1):102–106.

230. Snady H. Endoscopic ultrasonography in benign pancreatic disease. Surg Clin North Am 2001;81(2):329–344.

231. Lambert R, Caletti G, Cho E, et al. International Workshop on the clinical impact of endoscopic ultrasound in gastroenterology. Endoscopy 2000;32(7):549–584.

232. Ainsworth AP, Mortensen MB, Durup J, Wamberg PA. Clinical impact of endoscopic ultrasonography at a county hospital. Endoscopy 2002;34(6):447–450.

233. Sriram PV, Kaffes AJ, Rao GV, Reddy DN. Endoscopic ultrasound-guided drainage of pancreatic pseudocysts complicated by portal hypertension or by intervening vessels. Endoscopy 2005;37(3):231–235.

234. Gress F, Schmitt C, Sherman S, Ikenberry S, Lehman G. A prospective randomized comparison of endoscopic ultrasound- and computed tomography-guided celiac plexus block for managing chronic pancreatitis pain. Am J Gastroenterol 1999;94(4):900–905.

235. Santosh D, Lakhtakia S, Gupta R, et al. Clinical trial: a randomized trial comparing fluoroscopy guided percutaneous technique vs. endoscopic ultrasound guided technique of coeliac plexus block for treatment of pain in chronic pancreatitis. Aliment Pharmacol Ther 2009;29(9): 979–984.

236. O'Toole TM, Schmulewitz N. Complication rates of EUS-guided celiac plexus blockade and neurolysis: results of a large case series. Endoscopy 2009;41(7):593–597.

17 Pancreatic Adenocarcinoma: the Role of Endoscopic Ultrasonography

P.G. Arcidiacono, S. Carrara

Pancreatic cancer is the fourth leading cause of cancer death in Western countries. It is unusual in persons under the age of 45, while after the age of 50 its frequency increases linearly. The increase in the incidence rate ranges from two per 100 000/year in patients aged 40–44, to 67 per 100 000/year in patients older than 75.[1] At the age of 70, the mortality due to pancreatic cancer is ≈ 60 deaths per 100 000 persons per year. Some 74 000 new cases of pancreatic cancers were diagnosed in 2000 in Europe.[2]

Screening in high-risk populations. Effective early detection and screening for average-risk populations are currently not available, but efforts are focusing on early screening of selected high-risk patients, who account for ≈ 10% of patients with pancreatic cancer. These high-risk groups include patients with chronic pancreatitis, kindreds with two or more first-degree relatives affected by pancreatic cancer, and patients with hereditary pancreatitis, Peutz–Jeghers syndrome, cystic fibrosis, familial breast cancer syndrome, and familial atypical multiple mole melanoma. At present, a multimodal screening approach involving endoscopic ultrasound, computed tomography, and/or magnetic resonance appears to be the most effective method of screening for pancreatic cancer in high-risk patients.[3,4]

Rulyak et al. investigated the cost-effectiveness of pancreatic cancer screening in familial pancreatic cancer patients. The authors compared one-time screening with endoscopic ultrasonography (EUS) for pancreatic dysplasia with no screening, in a hypothetical cohort of 100 members of families with pancreatic cancer. EUS was defined as abnormal if one or two of the following abnormalities were present: heterogeneous parenchyma with echogenic foci, hypoechoic nodules, hyperechoic main duct wall, or discrete masses. Patients with abnormal EUS underwent endoscopic retrograde cholangiopancreatography (ERCP), and if ERCP confirmed the abnormality, they underwent total pancreatectomy. This endoscopic screening approach was cost-effective, with an incremental cost-effectiveness ratio of $ 16 885 per life-year saved. Screening was more cost-effective as the probability of dysplasia and the sensitivity of EUS and ERCP increased. Screening was cost-effective if the prevalence of dysplasia was greater than 16% or the sensitivity of EUS was greater than 84%. In conclusion, endoscopic screening for carefully selected members of families with pancreatic cancer appears to increase patients' life expectancy in a cost-effective manner.[5]

Etiological and clinical information. Pancreatic cancers can arise from both the exocrine and endocrine cells. Among pancreatic tumors, ≈ 95% develop from the exocrine portion of the pancreas, including the ductal epithelium, acinar cells, connective tissue, and lymphatic tissue. Approximately 75% of pancreatic carcinomas occur in the head or neck of the pancreas, 15–20% occur in the body of the pancreas, and 5–10% occur in the tail. Typically, pancreatic cancer first metastasizes to regional lymph nodes, and then to the liver and less commonly to the lungs. It can also directly invade surrounding visceral organs such as the duodenum, stomach, and colon.

It spreads rapidly, is seldom detected in the early stages, and is extremely difficult to treat. Symptoms such as jaundice, abdominal pain, and weight loss may not appear until the disease is quite advanced. By that time, the cancer is likely to have spread to other tissues and surgical removal is no longer possible. This is why the conditions has been called the "silent killer."

The annual mortality rate approximates the annual incidence rate, reflecting the short survival time associated with pancreatic cancer.[6] Overall, fewer than 5% of patients are still alive 5 years after the diagnosis. The chances of achieving a 5-year survival are best with early diagnosis and treatment, although the odds are still slim. The EURO-CARE study analyzed the survival in 49 074 patients with pancreatic cancer at 1, 3, and 5 years from the diagnosis: the figures were 15.9%, 5.4%, and 4.1%, respectively.[7] The data were similar for men and women. The median survival time for patients with advanced cancer is ≈ 4–6 months.

For many years, little was known about the pancreas; it was one of the most difficult organs to study, due to its deep location in the abdomen, often inaccessible to traditional ultrasound, and too distant to biopsy. The complexity of pancreatic disease and the richness of the organ's anatomical relationships made the approach to this gland a challenge even for the best surgeons. Researchers are now beginning to understand the genetic basis and the pathogenesis of the disease, and imaging technologies are developing new and sophisticated methods of diagnosing and staging pancreatic cancer. Ultrasound, computed tomography (CT), and ERCP are the conventional radiologic modalities in the management of pancreatic cancer.

Endoscopic ultrasound was developed in the 1980s after high-frequency ultrasound transducers were combined with endoscopes to overcome the physical limitations of transabdominal ultrasonography (which is obstructed by fat, air, and bone). Initially, EUS was used to confirm and stage solid masses in which a suspicion of malignancy had been raised by other imaging techniques or in the clinical examination. As technology improved, dedicated accessories were developed, and endosonographers' experience grew, the application of EUS continued to expand. Its widespread use has revolutionized the management of pancreatic disease. It is now also used to diagnose and follow up benign or borderline diseases, and it is often required for evaluation of focal enlargement of the gland, in the absence of a definite mass with other imaging methods. It has been demonstrated that a CT finding of fullness or enlargement of the pancreas may be a sign of malignancy and that EUS may then be able to identify a mass.[8,9] In this case, fine-needle aspiration biopsy (FNA) is carried out with endosonographic guidance. A recent article has elucidated the potential benefits and drawbacks of EUS in the diagnosis, staging, and assessment of resectability of pancreatic cancer, from the origins of the technique up to the present day.[10]

The probe, which can be positioned in the esophagus, stomach, and duodenum, provides ultrasound images of the gastrointestinal wall, distinguishing the different parietal layers, and producing transmural images of the surrounding structures.

Two types of echoendoscope were initially developed: the radial-scanning instrument, with scans perpendicular to the scope's axis, providing radial 360° images similar to those of CT; and the convex linear-array instrument, with a scanning plane parallel to the longitudinal axis of the echoendoscope. The radial echoendoscope was first developed by the Olympus Corporation, while Pentax and Hitachi developed the convex linear-array probe, with an oblique forward optical view. No differences between the two types of instrument have been found with regard to the accuracy of pancreatic cancer staging.[11]

The linear-array echoendoscope is described in this chapter, as it is the instrument used for interventional procedures. It has a biopsy channel, the size of which varies from model to model. The probe is sheathed with a latex balloon that can be filled with water to allow acoustic coupling. The tip of the instrument is equipped with an elevator to angle the accessories exiting from the biopsy channel. The transducer operates at different frequencies, from 5 to 10 MHz. The frequency is inversely proportional to the penetration depth of ultrasound; at 5 MHz, the ultrasound penetrates ≈ 8 cm, while at 10 MHz the penetration field of ultrasound is ≈ 4 cm. The Hitachi console provides color and power Doppler images.

The patient is positioned in the left lateral decubitus position, as for any standard upper endoscopy procedure. Informed consent is obtained. Conscious sedation can be administered with midazolam and meperidine. The ideal condition is deep sedation with assistance from an anesthesiologist. The patient is monitored during and after the procedure.

Principles of the Technique

Examination of the pancreas starts from the proximal stomach. The most important landmark here is the descending aorta, with the emergence of the celiac trunk and, a few centimeters below, the superior mesenteric artery (**Fig. 17.1**).

The celiac trunk divides into three branches—the left gastric artery, the splenic artery, and the hepatic artery (**Fig. 17.2**). Just past the cardia, the tip of the echoendoscope is placed against the lesser curvature. From this point, a scan from the hepatic hilum (**Fig. 17.3**) with the

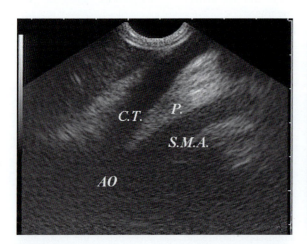

Fig. 17.1 The origin of the celiac trunk (CT) and superior mesenteric artery (SMA) from the aorta (AO); imaging from the proximal stomach. P, pancreas.

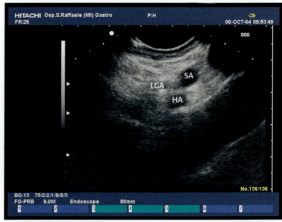

Fig. 17.2 The celiac trunk division with its branches, the left gastric artery (LGA), splenic artery (SA), and hepatic artery (HA).

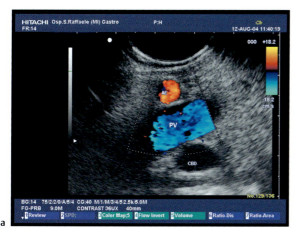
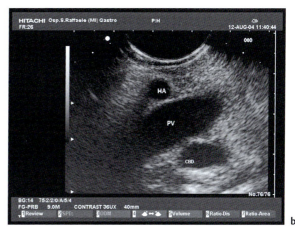

a   b

Fig. 17.3a, b a The hepatic hilum from the stomach. CBD, common bile duct; HA, hepatic artery; PV, portal vein. Color flow image.
b Without color flow.

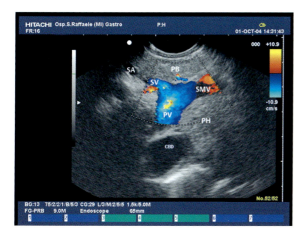
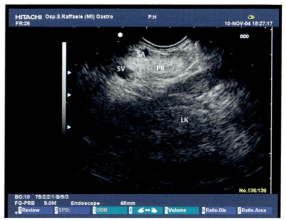

Fig. 17.4 The splenic vein (SV) and superior mesenteric vein (SMV) entering the confluence. CBD, common bile duct; PB, pancreatic body; PH, pancreatic head; PV, portal vein; SA, splenic artery.

Fig. 17.5 View of the pancreatic body (PB) from the stomach. The splenic vessels are important landmarks for visualizing the body and the tail of the pancreas. The splenic artery is proximal to the splenic vein. LK, left kidney; SA, splenic artery; SV, splenic vein.

portal vein as far as the splenomesenteric confluence (**Fig. 17.4**) is obtained by rotating the wrist clockwise on the instrument. The splenic vein and the splenic artery are important landmarks for imaging the body of the pancreas, where the main pancreatic duct is seen as two parallel hyperechoic lines; its lumen is usually virtual, but it may vary from 1 to 3 mm. (**Figs. 17.5** and **17.6**).

The splenic artery has a cephalic location, and its course is more serpiginous than that of the vein. The splenic vein is larger and oval in shape, while the artery is round. As the splenic vessels are followed along the posterior wall of the stomach to the splenic hilum, and as the tip is rotated more to the right, the tail of the pancreas is visualized as far as the spleen and, below, the left kidney. For the tail to be seen, the instrument has to be withdrawn slightly, as the tail courses upward and leftward. The pancreatic neck is imaged from the stomach as the tip is advanced further into the antrum. The main landmark, the superior mesen-

teric artery, imaged longitudinally, courses posterior to the pancreas, parallel to the splenomesenteric confluence. From this position, the probe displays the pancreatic neck and visualizes one of the most important crossroads for the staging of vascular involvement in patients with pancreatic cancer: the portal vein, the splenomesenteric confluence, with the splenic vein and the superior mesenteric vein, and the superior mesenteric artery (**Fig. 17.7**; see also **Fig. 17.4**).

If there is portal vein obstruction, collaterals may be seen along the gastric and duodenal wall; color Doppler is helpful for recognizing these vessels. The transducer is then advanced to the descending duodenum, past the ampulla of Vater, and the instrument is straightened into the short position. Air in the duodenal lumen is suctioned, and the latex balloon on the probe is inflated with water; the duodenal lumen may also be filled with water to improve acoustic coupling. From this position, a full scan

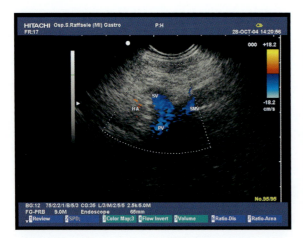

Fig. 17.6 The pancreatic body, with the splenic vein (SV) and the superior mesenteric vein (SMV) forming the portal vein (PV). HA, hepatic artery.

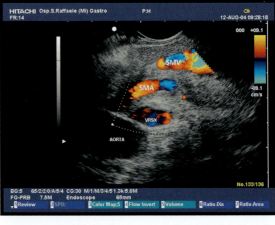

Fig. 17.7 A color flow image of the abdominal vessels from the posterior wall of the stomach. The pancreatic body is seen with the superior mesenteric artery (SMA) emerging from the aorta and the superior mesenteric vein (SMV), and the left renal vein (VRSX) crossing the aorta below the SMA.

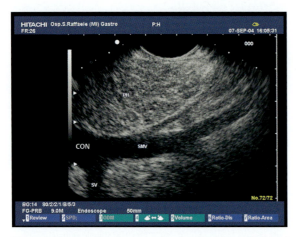

Fig. 17.8 The uncinate process seen from the duodenum. The portal confluence (CON) is seen with its vessels—the superior mesenteric vein (SMV) and splenic vein (SV). PH, pancreatic head.

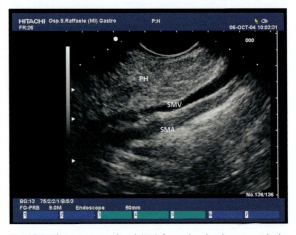

Fig. 17.9 The pancreatic head (PH) from the duodenum, with the mesenteric vessels, the superior mesenteric vein (SMV) and the superior mesenteric artery (SMA).

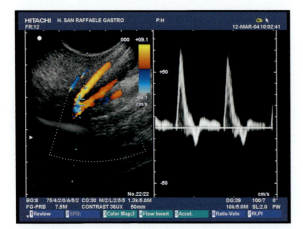

Fig. 17.10 A color and fast Fourier transform (FFT) Doppler image of the mesenteric vessels seen from the duodenum.

of the pancreatic head and uncinate process is obtained (**Fig. 17.8**)—from the mesenteric vessels (vein and artery), with the echoendoscope rotated to the right, to the aorta, with rotation to the left (**Figs. 17.9, 17.10,** and **17.11**).

The probe is maneuvered and withdrawn with fine movements. The superior mesenteric vein is followed as far as the confluence. Here, the neck of the pancreas is also visualized from the duodenum, and this image complements the previous scan obtained from the stomach. Two different areas of the pancreatic head can be identified, due to their different embryogenesis—the dorsal and the ventral pancreas. Their echogenicity differs; the ventral part may appear more hypoechoic, mimicking a pseudotumor, although its structure is homogeneous, while the dorsal part is more hyperechoic, as it is richer in interacinar fat tissue. The ampulla of Vater is seen as a hypoechoic,

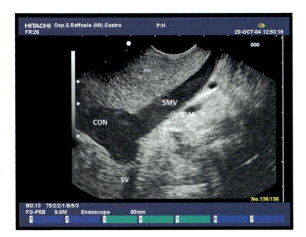

Fig. 17.11 The uncinate process with the veins and, more deeply, the superior mesenteric artery (SMA), which is located below the portal confluence (CON). PH, pancreatic head; SMV, superior mesenteric vein; SV, splenic vein.

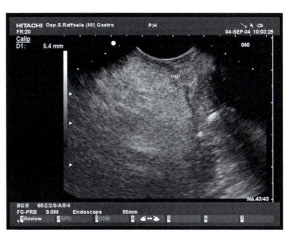

Fig. 17.12 Scanning of the normal papilla of Vater (PAP) from the duodenum.

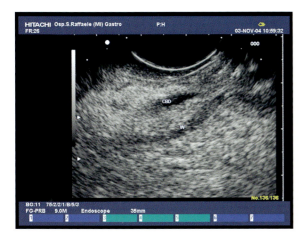

Fig. 17.13 View of the common bile duct (CBD) and distal pancreatic duct (Wirsung duct, W) in the pancreatic head from the descending duodenum. The two ducts are shown in a longitudinal section that passes into the papilla, the smooth, hypoechoic area on the right of the image.

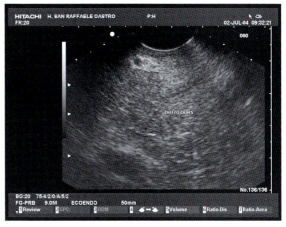

Fig. 17.14 A view of the Santorini duct (SD, the accessory pancreatic duct) from the descending duodenum. Once the papilla of Vater has been visualized, the transducer is withdrawn further, with fine movements; the minor papilla comes into view, and the Santorini duct can be followed into the pancreatic head.

well-delineated structure (**Fig. 17.12**), from which the two ducts—the common bile duct (upper) and the main pancreatic duct (lower)—can be traced and followed into the pancreatic head (**Fig. 17.13**). While the ampulla is being imaged, one must ensure that the probe is not pressed too hard against the duodenal wall, to avoid compression artifacts. The common bile duct can be followed as far as the hepatic hilum, with the tip being withdrawn and lifted. As the tip is withdrawn from the major ampulla, the minor ampulla and Santorini duct (the accessory pancreatic duct) are imaged (**Fig. 17.14**).

The normal pancreatic parenchyma has a characteristic homogeneous "salt-and-pepper" echo texture. Its echo structure is similar to that of the liver in young people. In older people and in the obese, it is more hyperechoic.

Staging

The prognosis in cancer depends on how advanced the tumor is at the time of diagnosis. Accurate staging is essential to allow the best treatment decisions to be made, particularly in selecting patients for surgery and patients for chemotherapy or palliative procedures.

Pancreatic adenocarcinoma is classified using the tumor, node, and metastases (TNM) staging system which was modified by the American Joint Committee on Cancer in 2002.[12] This classification assigns tumors that are invading the portal venous system (previously staged as T4) to T3. Although surgery is technically feasible, invasion of the portal vein, superior mesenteric vessels, and celiac trunk

Table 17.1 TNM staging

Tumor (T)	
TX	Primary tumor cannot be assessed
T0	No evidence of primary tumor
Tis	Carcinoma in situ
T1	Tumor limited to the pancreas, 2 cm or smaller in largest diameter
T2	Tumor limited to the pancreas, larger than 2 cm in largest diameter
T3	Tumor extension beyond the pancreas (i.e., duodenum, bile duct, portal or superior mesenteric vein) but not involving the celiac axis or superior mesenteric artery
T4	Tumor involves the celiac axis or superior mesenteric arteries
Regional lymph nodes (N)	
NX	Regional lymph nodes cannot be assessed
N0	No regional lymph-node metastasis
N1	Regional lymph-node metastasis
Distant metastasis (M)	
MX	Distant metastasis cannot be assessed
M0	No distant metastasis
M1	Distant metastasis

Table 17.2 The results of TNM staging system can be grouped into these stages

Stage 0	Tis, N0, M0	The tumor is confined to the top layers of pancreatic duct cells and has not invaded deeper tissues. It has not spread outside of the pancreas. These tumors are sometimes referred to as pancreatic carcinoma in situ or pancreatic intraepithelial neoplasia III (PanIn III)
Stage IA	T1, N0, M0	The tumor is confined to the pancreas and is less than 2 cm in size. It has not spread to nearby lymph nodes or distant sites
Stage IB	T2, N0, M0	The tumor is confined to the pancreas and is larger than 2 cm in size. It has not spread to nearby lymph nodes or distant sites
Stage IIA	T3, N0, M0	The tumor is growing outside the pancreas but not into large blood vessels. It has not spread to nearby lymph nodes or distant sites
Stage IIB	T1–3, N1, M0	The tumor is either confined to the pancreas or is growing outside the pancreas, but not into nearby large blood vessels or major nerves. It has spread to nearby lymph nodes, but not to distant sites
Stage III	T4, any N, M0	The tumor is growing outside the pancreas into nearby large blood vessels or major nerves. It may or may not have spread to nearby lymph nodes. It has not spread to distant sites
Stage IV	Any T, any N, M1	The tumor has spread to distant sites

usually precludes surgical resection[13] (**Tables 17.1** and **17.2**).

Older and more recent imaging modalities are available to help in the diagnosis of pancreatic carcinoma: transabdominal ultrasonography (TUS), CT, EUS, magnetic resonance imaging (MRI), ERCP, and positron-emission tomography (PET). EUS is one of the most sensitive techniques for detecting pancreatic masses, with a high accuracy rate that varies from 78% to 94% for T staging and from 64% to 82% for N staging.[14–16]

Many studies have examined the role of EUS in the detection of suspected pancreatic masses not defined by cross-sectional imaging techniques, and it has been found that EUS has better sensitivity for lesions less than 3 cm in size, with the best advantage for lesions less than 2 cm in size.[17] In a review article, Hunt and Faigel pooled data from four studies, comparing the accuracy of EUS and helical CT in the evaluation of pancreatic cancer.[18] They noted that EUS detected more tumors (97% versus 73%), that it was more accurate for determining tumor resectability (91% versus 73%) and that it was more sensitive for detecting vascular involvement (91% versus 64%). However, newer and more sophisticated multiphase helical CT scans have shown better accuracy for detecting small cancers (< 2 cm), with a sensitivity of 97% and a specificity of 100%.[19]

DeWitt et al. compared endoscopic ultrasonography with multidetector CT for detecting and staging pancreatic cancer and concluded that EUS was superior for tumor detection (98% versus 86%; $P = 0.01$), but equivalent to multidetector CT for nodal staging and determination of resectability (88% versus 92%).[20] Detection of lesions 25 mm or smaller in size did not significantly differ between EUS and multidetector CT (89% versus 53%; $P = 0.077$). In patients who underwent surgery, the overall accuracy of EUS staging was superior to that of CT (67% versus 41%; $P = 0.007$).

T stage. The T stage reflects the tumor characteristics and invasion of adjacent structures. The tumor is usually imaged as a focal, hypoechoic mass. Lesions of huge dimensions are inhomogeneous due to fibrosis and necrotic tissue, and they may have anechoic foci and poorly defined margins. Small cancers (< 2 cm) are more homogeneous, with smooth borders. There is a clear demarcation between the hypoechogenicity of the tumor and the surrounding, healthy pancreatic tissue or fat tissue. Tumors with a homogeneous echo texture, similar to that of the surrounding pancreas, with only a mild hypoechoic pattern, are often well-differentiated, less aggressive cancers (**Fig. 17.15**).

Usually, there are no calcifications in a tumor arising from a "healthy" pancreas, while cancers originating from chronic pancreatitis may be surrounded by calcifications. The endosonographer has to recognize an area with less calcification in the context of chronic pancreatitis, as this is suspicious for malignancy and a biopsy has to be directed toward the area. If there is diffuse enlargement of the gland, lymphoma has to be included in the differential diagnosis; lymphomas are often huge and multifocal, with an ultrasound pattern similar to that of acute pancreatitis. In describing the T stage, the endosonographer has to note the size of the tumor and its relationship with the surrounding organs, particularly with the duodenum, the stomach, and the common bile duct. The parietal layers of the duodenum have to be observed in order to exclude invasion if there is a tumor of the pancreatic head. In this case, the normal layered architecture of the duodenal wall is lost and replaced with hypoechoic tissue. Dilation of the main pancreatic duct is a sign that may suggest the presence of an obstructing mass downstream. The dilated duct is different from that observed in chronic pancreatitis and shows uniform, regular dilation. Tumors in the head of the pancreas are usually diagnosed earlier than those in the body or tail, because of the close relationship with the common bile duct and the subsequent obstructive jaundice (**Fig. 17.16**).

The differential diagnosis of a pancreatic solid mass has to include inflammatory masses such as chronic and autoimmune pancreatitis, and other kinds of tumor. Clinical, laboratory, and imaging tests have to be evaluated in order to reach the final diagnosis, and FNA has to be performed if there is a strong suspicion of cancer. Some centers have suggested that biopsies should not be carried out in lesions that will undergo surgery. The surgeons argue that a negative cytological result may be a sampling error that will not preclude surgery. On the other hand, passage of the needle into a tumor may contaminate the peritoneum with tumor cells. The risk of carcinomatous seeding secondary to EUS-guided FNA is very low; the needle path is short, and the tract passed by the needle is also resected at the time of surgery.[21] EUS-FNA through the duodenum does not breach the peritoneal cavity, and this should prevent peritoneal seeding. Another aspect in favor of EUS-FNA is the need to obtain cytological identification of a tumor mass before neoadjuvant therapy is started.

Despite the good resolution of EUS, pancreatic cancer may be missed with the method in certain conditions: chronic pancreatitis with a severely inhomogeneous echo texture; diffuse infiltration by the tumor; a prominent ventral/dorsal split; and in patients who have had a recent episode of acute pancreatitis (< 4 weeks), in whom edema may conceal a focal lesion. These factors have been reported in a recent study by Bhutani and colleagues.[22]

The accuracy of T staging is also affected by the peritumoral inflammation and by large tumors that cause ultrasound attenuation. Various studies have shown that EUS is more accurate in cancers less than 3 cm in size.[23]

Echo-enhancing intravenous contrast media have been used to help differentiate between benign inflammatory pseudotumoral masses and pancreatic cancer. The initial studies were carried out with transabdominal ultrasound, with good results being reported. Marked hyperperfusion was seen in cases of neuroendocrine tumors or inflammatory lesions, whereas pancreatic carcinoma typically

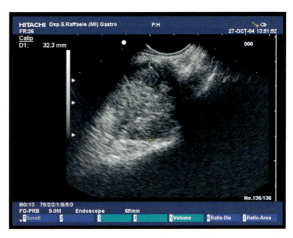

Fig. 17.15 A lesion 3 cm in size in the head of the pancreas. The larger the lesion, the more inhomogeneous the echo texture.

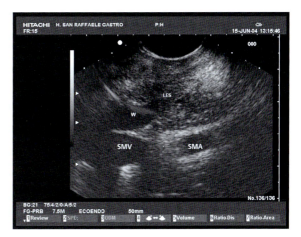

Fig. 17.16 A pancreatic head lesion (LES) occluding the main pancreatic duct (Wirsung duct, W), which is dilated. SMA, superior mesenteric artery; SMV, superior mesenteric vein.

showed a hypoperfused pattern.[24,25] Contrast agents are now also being used for EUS examinations.[26] They consist of stabilized microbubbles that range in size from 2 to 8 µm (the size of an erythrocyte) and have outer shells to prevent coagulation and aggregation. They can therefore be injected intravenously with no risk of thrombosis, and they cross the pulmonary capillaries in the same way that blood cells do. The presence of contrast in the bloodstream increases the ultrasonographic signal intensity and consequently the sensitivity of the equipment for detecting small vessels with slow flow. The contrast medium is injected as an intravenous bolus, and enhancement persists for ≈ 3–5 minutes. This new technique is safe, involving no risk of pancreatitis, no risk of thrombosis, and does not expose the patient to ionizing radiation. It is useful for differentiating between an inflammatory pancreatic mass and a ductal carcinoma, and it can be used to guide biopsies in an area of suspicion.

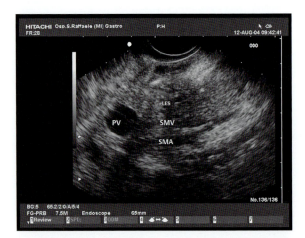

Fig. 17.17 A pancreatic lesion (LES) occluding the superior mesenteric vein (SMV). A cuff of hypoechoic tissue is visible around the superior mesenteric artery (SMA). PV, portal vein.

The second step, after the identification and description of the primary lesion, is the evaluation of vascular structures surrounding the pancreas. This is one of the most important criteria for resectability in pancreatic cancer (**Fig. 17.17**). Since its very beginnings, EUS has been regarded as the most accurate preoperative method for evaluating tumor resectability. The criteria for assessing vascular invasion have been examined by Brugge et al.[27] and Snady et al.,[28] with an accuracy of 55–94% being reported. When assessing vascular involvement, the endosonographer has to note:

- Any loss of interface between the tumor and the vessel wall
- The presence of tumor in the vessel lumen (seen as echoic material)
- Collateral vessels
- Irregularity in the vessel wall

If there is an intact hyperechoic interface between the tumor and the vessel, one can be sure that the tumor does not involve the vessel, while complete encasement of the vessel by the tumor is a sign of involvement. Initial studies demonstrated the high sensitivity and specificity of EUS for assessing vascular invasion; however, most of these studies suffered from a bias, in that EUS was compared with surgical palpation in unresectable cancers. This surgical method is extremely subjective and it is susceptible to interobserver variability.[13–15] More recent studies have found that EUS is not so accurate for predicting resectability. In a blinded re-evaluation of videotapes, Rösch et al. found that the ultrasound features of vascular invasion did not show sensitivity and specificity values greater than 80%.[29] Recent reports have focused on reassessing the accuracy of EUS for predicting vascular involvement. The only gold standard for comparison with EUS assessment of invasion is the surgical specimen, with histological analysis. Aslanian and colleagues compared

EUS with vascular resection and histological evidence of vascular invasion in 30 resected pancreatic cancers.[30] They found that EUS had poor predictive accuracy for diagnosing vascular invasion. The sensitivity, specificity, positive predictive value, and negative predictive value were 63%, 64%, 43%, and 80%, respectively, for vascular adherence, and 50%, 58%, 28%, and 82%, respectively, for vascular invasion. The loss of a hyperechoic interface between the tumor and the vessel, previously regarded as a major criterion for vascular invasion, was found to be a poor predictor of vascular involvement. Peritumoral inflammatory tissue may be one of the causes of endosonographic overdiagnosis of vascular invasion. What appears to be vascular adherence may be only fibrosis and edema, seen as a smooth hypoechoic area. On the other hand, CT sometimes underdiagnoses vascular involvement. The two methods are therefore complementary; EUS provides an opportunity for biopsies to be taken and CT provides broad imaging of the abdomen, making it possible to diagnose distant metastases. The authors conclude that if sonographic features of vascular invasion are absent, EUS usually excludes involvement of the portal confluence, but when sonographic signs of vascular involvement are present, they may not be reliable for diagnosis. Dilated and collateral veins may sometimes be seen in patients with invasion or thrombosis of the portal vein system.

The assessment of vascular invasion may be more difficult in the arteries, particularly with the superior mesenteric artery, which is deeper and more distant from the probe; in this case, the accuracy of EUS is lower than that for detecting portal or splenic veins.[27–29] This difficulty is thought to be due to the fact that arteries are smaller than veins and have a more tortuous course, which is difficult to follow along its entire path. Arteries often show signs of encasement, rather than clear invasion with tumoral growth in their lumen, perhaps because the vessel walls are thicker than those in venous structures (**Fig. 17.18**).

N stage. The accuracy of EUS for N staging lies in the range of 64–82%.[16] Although EUS is highly sensitive for detecting regional lymph nodes, it has difficulties in distinguishing between malignant and inflammatory adenopathy. Catalano et al.[31] suggested some predictive features of malignancy: lymph nodes are considered malignant when they have a round shape and are homogeneous and hypoechoic, with sharp margins, and if they have a diameter of 10 mm or more. Loss of the hyperechoic center is a sign of malignancy. A lymph node with an elongated shape that is heterogeneous and hyperechoic is usually reactive, but it may sometimes have micrometastases that are not detectable with ultrasound; in this case, the endosonographic features of malignancy are not sufficient to allow prediction of the real nature of the enlarged node, and EUS-FNA is needed in order to resolve the issue (**Fig. 17.19**).

The main node stations to image are the perigastric, periduodenal, and celiac nodes, and the hepatic hilum. Mediastinal adenopathy, detected in ≈5% of patients with pancreatobiliary cancer, has prognostic value and precludes surgical resection in patients with pancreatic cancer.[32] The endosonographer should therefore routinely explore the mediastinal stations.

M stage. As far as M staging is concerned, EUS is not capable of identifying distant metastases, but it is useful for detecting ascites and metastases in the left hepatic lobe.

EUS-Guided Fine-Needle Aspiration Biopsy

EUS allows high-resolution images of lesions and is an accurate tool for diagnosing pancreatic masses, but it has a major limitation—its low specificity ($\approx 75\%$)[33] and inability to differentiate between malignant and inflammatory pancreatic masses. The specificity of EUS can be significantly increased by using EUS-guided FNA. Since the first studies of the technique, EUS-FNA has been found to have a high specificity (100%) and accuracy rate (95%).[34] It has been shown to have a relatively low complication rate, with a major complication rate of 1%,[35] and a low risk of tumor seeding. EUS-FNA through the duodenum has the advantage of not passing through the peritoneal cavity, which should prevent peritoneal seeding; moreover, in cases of resectable tumors, the area through which the needle has passed is removed.

The necessity of obtaining a cytologic or histologic sample in order to diagnose pancreatic cancer before surgery remains controversial. In a review on the use of EUS in pancreatic cancer, Varadarajulu and Eloubeidi listed the indications for the EUS-FNA (**Table 17.3**).[36]

Tissue diagnosis is almost always required in unresectable cancers before chemotherapy, radiotherapy (whether

Table 17.3 Indications for endoscopic ultrasound-guided fine-needle aspiration (EUS-FNA)[32]

To document a diagnosis of malignancy in a patient with an unresectable mass as a prerequisite for adjuvant chemotherapy or radiotherapy
To exclude other tumor types such as lymphoma, small cell metastasis, or neuroendocrine cancer that may require a different management strategy
To determine a diagnosis in patients who are reluctant to undergo major surgery without a definitive diagnosis
To document the absence of malignancy when the pretest probability of malignancy is low

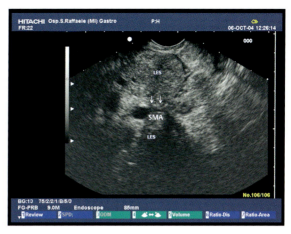

Fig. 17.18 A huge pancreatic lesion (LES), with infiltration (arrows) into the superior mesenteric artery (SMA).

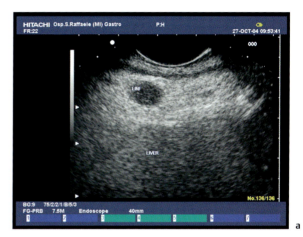

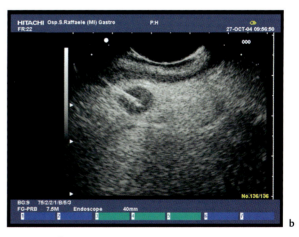

Fig. 17.19a, b
a A peripancreatic lymph node (LINF) with a malignant appearance.
b EUS-guided fine-needle aspiration of the node.

palliative or neoadjuvant), or nonsurgical palliative treatment for obstructive jaundice are started. The histological nature of a pancreatic tumor can also change the management approach; for example, a pancreatic lymphoma may require medical treatment rather than surgery.

Guidelines for Managing Pancreatic Cancer

In 2005, five British societies of gastroenterologists, radiologists, and surgeons presented guidelines for the management of patients with pancreatic cancer.[37] The recommendations have been assessed using evidence-based criteria (grade A, at least one randomized control trial: Ia, Ib; grade B, well-conducted clinical studies: IIa, IIb, III; and grade C, respected opinions, but without directly applicable good-quality clinical studies: IV).

The guidelines recommend that a clinical presentation suggesting cancer of the pancreas should lead first to transabdominal ultrasound of the pancreas, liver, and bile duct (grade B). When a diagnosis of pancreatic malignancy is suspected on the basis of clinical symptoms and/or abdominal ultrasound findings, selective use of CT and/or MRI and magnetic resonance cholangiopancreatography (MRCP), and occasionally magnetic resonance angiography (MRA), will accurately delineate the tumor size, infiltration, and presence of metastatic disease in the majority of cases (grade B). Where available, endosonography and/or laparoscopy with laparoscopic ultrasonography may be appropriate in selected cases (grade B). ERCP should only be used if a surgical procedure is necessary (e.g., biliary stenting). The guidelines also list all the services that the centers need to provide in order to be recognized as cancer units.

- Attempts should be made to obtain a tissue diagnosis during the course of investigative endoscopic procedures (grade C).
- Failure to obtain histological confirmation of a suspected diagnosis of malignancy does not exclude the presence of a tumor and should not delay appropriate surgical treatment (grade C).
- Efforts should be made to obtain a tissue diagnosis in patients selected for palliative forms of treatment (grade C).
- Transperitoneal techniques for obtaining a tissue diagnosis have limited sensitivity in patients with potentially resectable tumors and should be avoided in such patients (grade C).

Endoscopic Ultrasound Elastography

Elastography has recently been introduced as a technique that can be used during EUS to assess tissue elasticity and which may be useful for distinguishing between benign and malignant nodules.[38–40] Specialized software is provided for the ultrasound equipment, and the image can be switched from conventional B-mode to elastography by pushing a button. EUS elastography imaging is easy to use in routine practice and does not excessively prolong the time required for standard EUS.

An elastographic scoring system has been established on the basis of previous studies:[38]

- Score 1 is assigned when the image shows a homogeneous soft tissue area (green), corresponding to normal tissue.
- Score 2 is assigned when the image indicates heterogeneous soft tissue (green, yellow, and red), corresponding to fibrosis or inflammatory tissue (pancreatitis).
- Score 3 is assigned when the image shows mixed colors or a honeycomb elastographic pattern—indicating mixed hard and soft tissue and making interpretation difficult, but often related to malignant masses.
- Score 4 is assigned when the image displays a small, soft (green) central area surrounded by mainly hard (blue) tissue, corresponding to a malignant hypervascularized lesion (neuroendocrine tumors).
- Score 5 is assigned to lesions showing mainly hard (blue) tissue with areas of heterogeneous soft tissue (green, red), representing zones of necrosis in advanced malignant lesions (adenocarcinoma) (**Fig. 17.20**).

A recent multicenter study has focused on the role of EUS elastography in the evaluation of pancreatic masses and lymph nodes. The authors concluded that this new technique may be reserved as a second-line examination to help characterize pancreatic masses after negative EUS-FNA.[41] When scores 1 and 2 are interpreted as benign and scores 3, 4, and 5 as malignant, the sensitivity, specificity, and positive and negative predictive values of EUS elastography for differentiating between benign and malignant pancreatic masses were 92.3%, 80.0%, 93.3%, and 77.4%, respectively, with a global accuracy rate of 89.2% for this new technology.

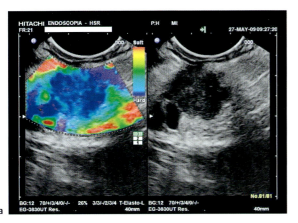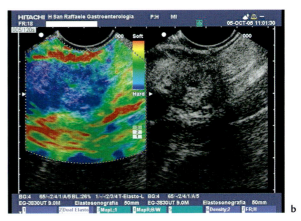

Fig. 17.20a, b Comparison between standard EUS (on the right) and EUS-elastography (on the left): the solid tumor of the pancreas is seen as a blue area; expression of an increased stiffness of the tissues.

EUS-FNA Technique

Lesions located in the pancreatic head and uncinate process are biopsied from the duodenum, while those located in the body and tail are biopsied from the stomach. Color Doppler is used to image the lesion and surrounding structures, in order to avoid vascular structures along the needle path.

Once the target lesion has been visualized, with the transducer in a steady position, the tip is pushed against the gastrointestinal wall and the up–down and left–right wheels are locked. Keeping a steady position is often easier from the duodenum, for pancreatic head cancer, than from the stomach, for cancers of the pancreatic body and tail. A biopsy from the stomach may require more energy and a firm hit, as the gastric folds present resistance to needle passage. The needle can be easily introduced if the procedure is carried out in a straight position. If the tip is flexed too much or the echoendoscope is looped, advancement of the needle is difficult and may be dangerous for the instrument. Excessive pushing of the needle may cause a hole in the endoscope's working channel. In this case, the instrument should be withdrawn and straightened until needle passage becomes easier, without resistance. Most pancreatic solid tumors are as hard as stone, due to the desmoplastic reaction typical of these cancers, and strong needle penetration is necessary.

The needle used for EUS-FNA is equipped with a stylet covered by a protective spiral sheath. The stylet prevents the needle from clogging due to tissue or blood as it is advanced into the target lesion. During the FNA procedure, the catheter is inserted into the biopsy channel. Before the puncture, the stylet is withdrawn a few millimeters to expose the sharp tip of the needle. The tip is then advanced with real-time endoscopic ultrasound guidance until the needle tip is seen within the lesion. The needle appears as a hyperechoic line; artifacts due to reflections produced by the metal are easily recognized. If the needle is not fully visualized, fine adjustments of the transducer position usually restore the correct image. Once the lesion has been penetrated, the stylet is advanced to the original position to clean the needle of cells or clots that have entered during the passage through the gastrointestinal wall. The stylet is then removed, suction is applied through a 10-mL syringe, and the needle is moved to and fro 5–10 times inside the lesion. The suction is then released, the needle is retracted into the catheter, and the entire catheter is removed from the echoendoscope. The aspirate is placed on glass slides for smears using Papanicolaou and Wright–Giemsa stains.

The presence of a cytology technician or cytopathologist in the endoscopy room during the procedure is important for assessing the adequacy of the specimen after each pass. This helps the endosonographer decide whether further passes are needed. The number of passes needed to provide an adequate sample is still a matter of controversy. An average of three or four passes appears to provide definitive cytologic diagnosis.[42,43] In a technological review on EUS-FNA, Erickson clearly explains the advantages, disadvantages, and complications of the procedure.[44] There appear to be no clinical or EUS features predictive of the number of passes needed. The major determinant of FNA pass numbers appears to be the degree of tumor differentiation; some cases in which 10 or more passes were needed in well-differentiated cancers have been reported[45] (**Figs. 17.21** and **17.22**).

Ductal and parenchymal changes have been observed in patients with pancreatic or biliary stents, due to edema and fibrosis, resulting in abnormalities in echogenicity and texture of the tissue surrounding the stent (**Fig. 17.23**). As a foreign body, the plastic or metal stent creates a fibrotic reaction around the duct, altering the diagnostic value of endosonography and making FNA more difficult. Air in the biliary ducts cause interference and reverberations, and the stent may cause shadowing that conceals the

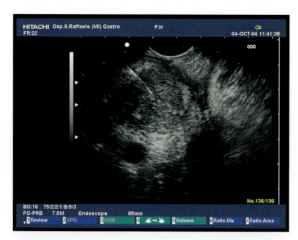

Fig. 17.21 EUS-guided fine-needle aspiration biopsy of a mass in the head of the pancreas. The lesion is hypoechoic, with defined margins. The needle is visible as a hyperechoic line.

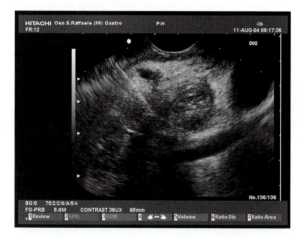

Fig. 17.22 EUS-guided fine-needle aspiration of a tumor in the head of the pancreas.

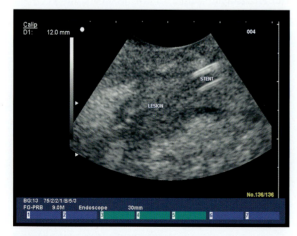

Fig. 17.23 A malignant lesion in the pancreatic head, with a stent placed in the bile duct. The stent appears as two parallel hyperechoic lines. The lesion does not have defined margins and may be difficult to distinguish from the edema caused by the stent.

surrounding tissues. This condition is known to create artifacts and fibrosis that make it more difficult to carry out FNA, as the needle has to touch hard tissue and it sometimes has to pass through the stent. Despite the method's high level of accuracy, its low negative predictive value (NPV) limits the usefulness of EUS-FNA in these cases. Even in the presence of a negative cytological result, malignancy cannot be ruled out, particularly if clinical and laboratory tests are strongly suspicious for cancer. Agarwal et al.[46] reported an NPV of 22% with EUS-FNA in patients with obstructive jaundice and biliary strictures. In seven of the eight patients with false-negative results, a plastic stent had previously been placed in the bile duct. In addition, indeterminate biliary strictures may also be benign, without a clearly defined mass. In these cases, the edema caused by stent placement may resemble a focal lesion. Despite these difficulties, we consider that EUS-FNA is an important tool for reaching a cytological diagnosis, even in patients with biliary or pancreatic stents; the availability of a cytology technician is very important in these cases.

EUS-FNA is not only a prognostic indicator, but also has a substantial impact on cost savings. It can avoid the need for major surgery in unresectable patients and it is helpful in the management of patients (establishing the need for palliative treatment, chemotherapy, or minimally invasive procedures). In a study on the clinical value of EUS-FNA, Chang et al. showed that it led to cost savings of approximately $3300 per patient, due to the avoidance of surgery.[34]

In conclusion, EUS and CT scanning are complementary methods in the diagnosis and staging of pancreatic cancer. Technological developments have provided EUS with new accessories to improve the diagnosis, such as contrast enhancement and most importantly the option of carrying out guided fine-needle aspiration biopsies. EUS is now emerging not only as a purely imaging technique, but also as method of guiding the delivery of new forms of treatment for pancreatic cancer, and it can be helpful in the palliative treatment of pancreatic cancer. New therapeutic applications of EUS, such as injection therapy with genetic or immunological agents and radiofrequency therapy, have yet to be fully assessed in large multicenter trials in order to define their real clinical value.

References

1. Ferlay J, Bray F, Sankila R, et al. Cancer incidence, mortality and prevalence in the European Union. Lyons: IARC Press; 1999.
2. Ferlay J, Bray F, Pisani P, Parkin DM. Cancer incidence, mortality and prevalence worldwide, version 1.0. Lyons: IARC Press. IARC Cancer Base No. 5, 2001.
3. Canto MI, Goggins M, Yeo CJ, et al. Screening for pancreatic neoplasia in high-risk individuals: an EUS-based approach. Clin Gastroenterol Hepatol 2004;2(7):606–621.

4. Klapman J, Malafa MP. Early detection of pancreatic cancer: why, who, and how to screen. Cancer Contr 2008;15(4): 280–287.

5. Rulyak SJ, Kimmey MB, Veenstra DL, Brentnall TA. Cost-effectiveness of pancreatic cancer screening in familial pancreatic cancer kindreds. Gastrointest Endosc 2003;57(1): 23–29.

6. Coleman MP, Babb P, Daniecki P, et al. Cancer survival trends in England and Wales, 1971–1995: deprivation and NHS region. Studies in medical and population subjects No. 61. London: The Stationery Office; 1999.

7. Roazzi P, Capocaccia R, Santaquilani M, Carrani E; EURO-CARE Working Group. Electronic availability of EURO-CARE-3 data: a tool for further analysis. Ann Oncol 2003; 14(Suppl 5):v150–v155.

8. Horwath JD, Gerke H, Acosta RD. Focal or diffuse "fullness" of the pankreas on CT. Usually benign, but EUS plus/minus FNA is warranted to identify malignancy. JOP 2009 Jan 8;10(1):37–42.

9. Ho S, Bonasera RJ, Pollack BJ. A single-center experience of endoscopic ultrasonography for enlarged pancreas on computed tomography. Clin Gastroenterol Hepatol 2006 Jan;4(1):98–103.

10. Chang DK, Nguyen NQ, Merrett ND, Dixson H, Leong RW, Biankin AV. Role of endoscopic ultrasound in pancreatic cancer. Expert Rev Gastroenterol Hepatol 2009;3(3): 293–303.

11. Gress F, Savides T, Cummings O, et al. Radial scanning and linear array endosonography for staging pancreatic cancer: a prospective randomized comparison. Gastrointest Endosc 1997;45(2):138–142.

12. Exocrine pancreas. American Joint Committee on Cancer: AJCC Cancer Staging Manual. 6th ed. New York: Springer; 2002:157–164.

13. Rosch T, Lorenz R, Braig C, Classen M. Endoscopic ultrasonography in diagnosis and staging of pancreatic and biliary tumors. Endoscopy 1992;24:304–308.

14. Gress FG, Hawes RH, Savides TJ, et al. Role of EUS in the preoperative staging of pancreatic cancer: a large single-center experience. Gastrointest Endosc 1999;50(6): 786–791.

15. Palazzo L, Roseau G, Gayet B, et al. Endoscopic ultrasonography in the diagnosis and staging of pancreatic adenocarcinoma. Results of a prospective study with comparison to ultrasonography and CT scan. Endoscopy 1993;25(2): 143–150.

16. Yasuda K, Mukai H, Nakajima M, Kawai K. Staging of pancreatic carcinoma by endoscopic ultrasonography. Endoscopy 1993;25(2):151–155.

17. Rösch T, Braig C, Gain T, et al. Staging of pancreatic and ampullary carcinoma by endoscopic ultrasonography. Comparison with conventional sonography, computed tomography, and angiography. Gastroenterology 1992; 102(1):188–199.

18. Hunt GC, Faigel DO. Assessment of EUS for diagnosing, staging, and determining resectability of pancreatic cancer: a review. Gastrointest Endosc 2002;55(2):232–237.

19. Bronstein YL, Loyer EM, Kaur H, et al. Detection of small pancreatic tumors with multiphasic helical CT. AJR Am J Roentgenol 2004;182(3):619–623.

20. DeWitt J, Devereaux B, Chriswell M, et al. Comparison of endoscopic ultrasonography and multidetector computed tomography for detecting and staging pancreatic cancer. Ann Intern Med 2004;141(10):753–763.

21. Micames C, Jowell PS, White R, et al. Lower frequency of peritoneal carcinomatosis in patients with pancreatic cancer diagnosed by EUS-guided FNA vs. percutaneous FNA. Gastrointest Endosc 2003;58(5):690–695.

22. Bhutani MS, Gress FG, Giovannini M, et al; No Endosonographic Detection of Tumor (NEST) Study. The No Endosonographic Detection of Tumor (NEST) Study: a case series of pancreatic cancers missed on endoscopic ultrasonography. Endoscopy 2004;36(5):385–389.

23. Nakaizumi A, Uehara H, Iishi H, et al. Endoscopic ultrasonography in diagnosis and staging of pancreatic cancer. Dig Dis Sci 1995;40(3):696–700.

24. Rickes S, Malfertheiner P. Echo-enhanced sonography—an increasingly used procedure for the differentiation of pancreatic tumors. Dig Dis 2004;22(1):32–38.

25. D'Onofrio M, Mansueto G, Falconi M, Procacci C. Neuroendocrine pancreatic tumor: value of contrast enhanced ultrasonography. Abdom Imaging 2004;29(2):246–258.

26. Becker D, Strobel D, Bernatik T, Hahn EG. Echo-enhanced color- and power-Doppler EUS for the discrimination between focal pancreatitis and pancreatic carcinoma. Gastrointest Endosc 2001;53(7):784–789.

27. Brugge WR, Lee MJ, Kelsey PB, Schapiro RH, Warshaw AL. The use of EUS to diagnose malignant portal venous system invasion by pancreatic cancer. Gastrointest Endosc 1996; 43(6):561–567.

28. Snady H, Bruckner H, Siegel J, Cooperman A, Neff R, Kiefer L. Endoscopic ultrasonographic criteria of vascular invasion by potentially resectable pancreatic tumors. Gastrointest Endosc 1994;40(3):326–333.

29. Rösch T, Dittler HJ, Strobel K, et al. Endoscopic ultrasound criteria for vascular invasion in the staging of cancer of the head of the pancreas: a blind reevaluation of videotapes. Gastrointest Endosc 2000;52(4):469–477.

30. Aslanian H, Salem R, Lee J, Andersen D, Robert M, Topazian M . EUS diagnosis of vascular invasion in pancreatic cancer: surgical and histologic correlates. Am J Gastroenterol 2005;100(6):1381–1385.

31. Catalano MF, Sivak MV Jr, Rice T, Gragg LA, Van Dam J. Endosonographic features predictive of lymph node metastasis. Gastrointest Endosc 1994;40(4):442–446.

32. Agarwal B, Gogia S, Eloubeidi MA, Correa AM, Ho L, Collins BT. Malignant mediastinal lymphadenopathy detected by staging EUS in patients with pancreaticobiliary cancer. Gastrointest Endosc 2005;61(7):849–853.

33. Rösch T, Lorenz R, Braig C, et al. Endoscopic ultrasound in pancreatic tumor diagnosis. Gastrointest Endosc 1991; 37(3):347–352.

34. Chang KJ, Nguyen P, Erickson RA, Durbin TE, Katz KD. The clinical utility of endoscopic ultrasound-guided fine-needle aspiration in the diagnosis and staging of pancreatic carcinoma. Gastrointest Endosc 1997;45(5):387–393.

35. Eloubeidi MA, Chen VK, Eltoum IA, et al. Endoscopic ultrasound-guided fine needle aspiration biopsy of patients with suspected pancreatic cancer: diagnostic accuracy and acute and 30-day complications. Am. J Gastroenterol 2003;98:2663–2668.

36. Varadarajulu S, Eloubeidi MA. Frequency and significance of acute intracystic hemorrhage during EUS-FNA of cystic lesions of the pancreas. Gastrointest Endosc 2004; 60(4):631–635.

37. Pancreatic Section, British Society of Gastroenterology; Pancreatic Society of Great Britain and Ireland; Association of Upper Gastrointestinal Surgeons of Great Britain and Ireland; Royal College of Pathologists; Special Interest

Group for Gastro-Intestinal Radiology. Guidelines for the management of patients with pancreatic cancer periampullary and ampullary carcinomas. Gut 2005;54(Suppl 5): v1–v16.

38. Giovannini M, Hookey LC, Bories E, Pesenti C, Monges G, Delpero JR. Endoscopic ultrasound elastography: the first step towards virtual biopsy? Preliminary results in 49 patients. Endoscopy 2006;38(4):344–348.

39. Janssen J, Schlörer E, Greiner L. EUS elastography of the pancreas: feasibility and pattern description of the normal pancreas, chronic pancreatitis, and focal pancreatic lesions. Gastrointest Endosc 2007;65(7):971–978.

40. Săftoiu A, Vilman P. Endoscopic ultrasound elastography— a new imaging technique for the visualization of tissue elasticity distribution. J Gastrointestin Liver Dis 2006;15(2): 161–165.

41. Giovannini M, Thomas B, Erwan B, et al. Endoscopic ultrasound elastography for evaluation of lymph nodes and pancreatic masses: a multicenter study. World J Gastroenterol 2009;15(13):1587–1593.

42. Erickson RA, Sayage-Rabie L, Beissner RS. Factors predicting the number of EUS-guided fine-needle passes for diagnosis of pancreatic malignancies. Gastrointest Endosc 2000; 51(2):184–190.

43. Wiersema MJ, Vilmann P, Giovannini M, Chang KJ, Wiersema LM. Endosonography-guided fine-needle aspiration biopsy: diagnostic accuracy and complication assessment. Gastroenterology 1997;112(4):1087–1095.

44. Erickson RA. EUS-guided FNA. Gastrointest Endosc 2004; 60(2):267–279.

45. Lin F, Staerkel G. Cytologic criteria for well differentiated adenocarcinoma of the pancreas in fine-needle aspiration biopsy specimens. Cancer 2003;99(1):44–50.

46. Agarwal B, Abu-Hamda E, Molke KL, Correa AM, Ho L. Endoscopic ultrasound-guided fine needle aspiration and multidetector spiral CT in the diagnosis of pancreatic cancer. Am J Gastroenterol 2004;99(5):844–850.

18 Benign and Malignant (Cystic) Tumors of the Pancreas

C.F. Dietrich, C. Jenssen

Various types of benign and malignant cystic tumor can occur in the pancreas. Cystic lesions in the pancreas can be divided pathologically into retention cysts, pseudocysts, and cystic neoplasms. Distinguishing between the various types of lesion has important prognostic and therapeutic implications. Cystic lesions of the pancreas are associated with systemic disease (e.g., cystic fibrosis and von Hippel–Lindau disease). In the latter, the reported incidence is ≈ 10–20%. In a recent study, 77% of 158 consecutive patients had lesions in the pancreas, including cysts, serous cystadenomas, and neuroendocrine tumors. Most patients had no symptoms related to peptide hormone secretion. As a result, many of these lesions are diagnosed incidentally in surveillance examinations—for example, for renal tumors. Anatomic or intensive biochemical studies reveal pancreatic tumors in up to 80% of patients with multiple endocrine neoplasia type 1. The World Health Organization (WHO) classification of pancreatic tumors is summarized in **Table 18.1**.

Simple cysts. Simple (true or retention) cysts of the pancreas are often small, fluid-containing spaces lined with normal duct and centroacinar cells. They are usually incidental findings with no clinical significance and can be left untreated. They are found in about 25% of patients with cystic fibrosis.[1] In sharp contrast to other parenchymal organs (kidney, liver), simple cysts in the pancreas are a very rare finding. Other uncommon benign cysts of the pancreas are benign mucinous cysts and lymphoepithelial cysts.

Pseudocysts. Pancreatic pseudocysts develop as a result of pancreatic inflammation and necrosis. Most pseudocysts communicate with the pancreatic ductal system and contain high concentrations of enzymes. The walls of pseudocysts are formed by adjacent structures and consist of fibrous and granulation tissue and are therefore not lined with normal duct and centroacinar cells. The lack of an epithelial lining thus distinguishes pseudocysts from true cystic lesions of the pancreas. A pseudocyst should be suspected in patients with a recent history of pancreatitis and an elevated serum amylase concentration, when the lesion contains enzyme-rich watery fluid and communicates with the pancreatic duct as assessed by endoscopic retrograde cholangiopancreatography (ERCP). The diagnostic implications of pancreatic pseudocysts are described in the respective sections below.

When a diagnosis of pseudocyst is made, the management is mostly determined by the symptoms. Asymptomatic pseudocysts that are not increasing in size can be monitored, even if they are large. Symptoms should be treated either with resection (for lesions in the body or tail of the pancreas) or drainage (for lesions anywhere in the pancreas). Drainage can be carried out with endoscopic ultrasound (EUS) guidance, either into the stomach or (less favorably) into the duodenum or via the percutaneous route.[2–10] Pseudocysts can also be drained surgically by anastomosing the stomach, duodenum, or jejunum to the cyst wall. The therapeutic implications mainly depend on the locally available expertise and clinicians' preferences, since none of the methods has been shown to be superior to the others. EUS management is discussed in Chapter 19.

EUS in acute pancreatitis (**Fig. 18.1**) is performed routinely to demonstrate the biliary etiology, but has rarely been used to assess the degree of necrosis.

Table 18.1 The World Health Organization (WHO) classification of pancreatic tumors

Benign
Serous cystadenoma
Mucinous cystadenoma
Intraductal papillary mucinous adenoma
Mature teratoma
Borderline
Mucinous cystic tumor with moderate dysplasia
Intraductal mucinous papillary tumor with moderate dysplasia
Solid pseudopapillary tumor
Malignant
Highly ductal dysplasia, carcinoma in situ
Ductal adenocarcinoma
Serous cystadenocarcinoma
Mucinous cystadenocarcinoma
Intraductal papillary mucinous carcinoma
Acinar cell carcinoma
Solid pseudopapillary carcinoma
Pancreatic blastoma
Osteoclasts similar to giant cell tumor
Mixed carcinoma

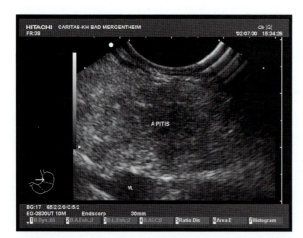
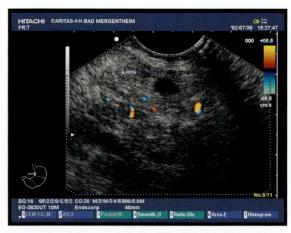

Fig. 18.1a, b Acute pancreatitis. Exudates and necrosis can be delineated with high-resolution EUS, using color Doppler imaging.

Cystic Neoplasms

More than 25 different types of cystic pancreatic neoplasm have now been described, most of which are very rare. Four of these types account for at least two-thirds of all cystic neoplasms in the pancreas:
- Intraductal papillary mucinous neoplasm (IPMN)
- Serous cystic neoplasm (SCN; microcystic serous cystadenoma; oligocystic/macrocystic cystadenoma)
- Mucinous cystic neoplasm (MCN; cystadenoma/cystadenocarcinoma)
- Solid pseudopapillary neoplasm (SPN; also known as papillary cystic neoplasm, solid pseudopapillary tumor, or Frantz–Gruber tumor)[11,12]

Epidemiology. Older statistics showed that mucinous cystadenoma is the most common type of cystic pancreatic neoplasm and that serous cystadenoma is the second most common. Papillary cystic neoplasm (or tumor, also known as solid pseudopapillary neoplasm or tumor) is the least common type of pancreatic cystic neoplasm.[13,14] However, recent data show that IPMN is by far the most common cystic neoplasm in the pancreas, accounting for around one-third of cystic neoplasms. Cystic lesions of the pancreas, even when found incidentally, may have a malignant potential and require diagnostic evaluation regardless of their size.[11,12]

Diagnosis. The EUS findings by themselves are not accurate enough to diagnose the type of cystic lesion of the pancreas definitively, or to determine its malignant potential in all cases. Endoscopic ultrasound-guided fine-needle aspiration (EUS-FNA) with assessment of lipase and tumor markers may increase the accuracy (see Chapters 16 and 17).[15–18]

Cytology. Cytological analysis of the cyst fluid obtained using EUS-FNA lacks sensitivity, but has a high level of specificity for malignancies and mucinous cystic neoplasms. Measurement of cyst fluid amylase, lipase, and various tumor markers such as carcinoembryonic antigen (CEA) and CA19-9 is clinically useful. One study examined 341 patients who underwent EUS-FNA of pancreatic cystic lesions. Cyst fluid was analyzed for CEA, CA72-4, CA125, CA19-9, and CA15-3. A histological diagnosis was obtained in 112 patients who underwent surgical resection (68 with mucinous lesions, seven with serous, 27 with inflammatory, five with endocrine, and five with other types of cystic lesion). Using a cut-off value of 192 ng/mL, CEA levels were the most accurate method of differentiating between mucinous and nonmucinous cystic lesions (sensitivity 73%, specificity 84%). There was no combination of tests that provided greater accuracy than CEA alone.[19] In addition, biopsies may not be diagnostic, since such samples frequently do not contain cells that are representative of the entire cyst lining. The relatively low sensitivity and specificity levels raise questions about the reliability of these methods for assessing the need for surgery in individual patients.

Histology. Cytological examination of the cystic fluid may allow diagnosis if either glycogen-rich cells (suggesting serous cystadenoma) or mucin-containing cells (suggesting mucinous lesions) are present. However, false-negative cytology is not unusual, and mucus-secreting cells can be found in the normal pancreatic duct lining. In patients with suspected serous cystadenoma, a core biopsy for histology is required if the lesion appears solid, to avoid surgery (see Chapter 17).

Immunohistochemistry and molecular genetics. The accuracy of ultrasound-guided and EUS-guided biopsy can be enhanced using immunohistochemical tests (mucin

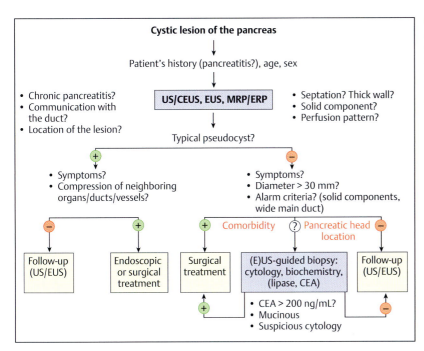

Fig. 18.2 Management of cystic pancreatic lesions. CEA, carcinoembryonic antigen; CEUS, contrast-enhanced ultrasound; ERP, endoscopic retrograde pancreatography; EUS, endoscopic ultrasonography; MRP, magnetic resonance pancreatography; US, ultrasound.

expression profile) and molecular genetic tests (K-*ras,* loss of heterozygosity; see Chapter 17).

The differential diagnosis of cystic pancreatic lesions is challenging. Diagnosis should be based on a combination of the patient's history, clinical data, endosonographic morphology, cytomorphological features, and biochemical analysis of cyst fluid. Taking a comprehensive view—including the patient's clinical data (sex, age, race, history of pancreatitis), morphological features on EUS and radiological studies (size, location, pancreatic duct dilation, wall thickness, ductal communication, mural protuberances, and solid components) and the results of EUS-guided biopsy (cytology, fluid markers)—is the key to achieving accurate differential diagnosis of cystic pancreatic lesions (**Table 18.2**) and for predicting their malignant potential (**Table 18.3**).[17,18]

Safety. FNA of cystic lesions is generally safe. Prophylactic antibiotics should be administered to patients undergoing EUS-FNA, ERCP, or endoscopic drainage procedures for (inflammatory) cystic lesions of the pancreas.

Differential diagnosis (**Table 18.2**). It is sometimes difficult to distinguish between pseudocysts and serous and mucinous tumors, as the latter may contain enzyme-rich fluid, communicate with the ductal system, and may be seen in patients with symptoms of recent pancreatitis.

Endoscopic ultrasound may make it possible to distinguish between serous and mucinous neoplasms by revealing a mass composed of either many tiny cysts (microcystic), showing a solid-appearing hypervascular tumor, or showing several large cysts (macrocystic). Serous cystadenomas typically have a central scar and central vessel,

similar to focal nodular hyperplasia in the liver. This finding can often also be seen with transabdominal ultrasonography. However, even with these findings, it is not possible to exclude the presence of a malignancy, especially a neuroendocrine tumor.[20]

Therapy. The EUS findings by themselves are not sufficiently accurate to diagnose the type of cystic lesion of the pancreas definitively or to determine its malignant potential in all cases, and surgery is therefore mandatory, depending on the patient's age and comorbidity. In patients with histologically confirmed serous cystadenomas, which are only accessible via the transabdominal route or using EUS-guided Tru-Cut biopsy,[21] careful follow-up may be possible. (**Fig. 18.2**)[22,23]

The management of patients with uncertain cystic lesions is difficult. In a study including 398 patients with cystadenomas from 73 institutions, 372 of whom underwent surgery, accurate preoperative diagnosis of the tumor type was achieved in only 20% of those who were ultimately diagnosed with serous cystadenomas, 30% of those with mucinous cystadenomas, and 29% of those with mucinous cystadenocarcinomas.[24] Many experts and pancreatic surgeons therefore recommend resection for even moderately suspicious lesions in the body and tail of the pancreas, and for highly suspicious lesions in the head of the gland.

There are currently no established endoscopic treatments for cystic neoplasms of the pancreas. EUS and ERCP should always be considered before surgical or percutaneous drainage of pancreatic pseudocysts, in order to optimize patient selection. In one prospective randomized study, EUS-guided ethanol lavage of unilocular cystic

III Gastrointestinal Tract

Table 18.2 Differential diagnosis of cystic pancreatic lesions

Type	Simple cyst	Pseudocyst	SCN	MD-IPMN	BD-IPMN	MCN	SPN
Age (y)	All ages	20–80	50–70	40–80	50–70	30–70	8–40
Sex	F:M 1:1	F:M 1:1	F:M 10:1	F:M 1:1	F:M 1:2	Almost exclusively F	F:M 10:1
Patient's history	Nonspecific	Pancreatitis	Nonspecific	Pancreatitis possible	Pancreatitis possible	Pain possible	Pain possible
Localization	Mostly head	No predilection	No predilection	Head: 80%	Head: >90%	Tail/body: 70%	Tail/body
Ductal communication	No	Variable	No	Yes	Yes	No	No
Typical morphological features	Small, smooth borders	Variable size, variable content (debris) Hyperechoic wall Coexistence of typical morphological features of chronic pancreatitis	No definable cyst wall/capsule, tiny septa Type 1 (75%): pseudosolid, microcystic, stellate scar Type 2 (>20%): Oligocystic/ macrocystic, no stellate scar Type 3 (von Hippel–Lindau): multilocular	Ductal dilation without stenosis, wall protrusions (pancreatobiliary type), mucinous content and papilla (intestinal type), hypoechoic wall/patulous papilla; in pancreatic body and tail features of chronic pancreatitis	Multilocular (clusters of small cysts) Communication with ductal structures	Unilocular (rarely multilocular) Focal thickening of the cyst wall, solid components, parietal nodules	Large solid tumor with clear borders, regressive changes and variable cystic components
Vascularity	None	None	High	High	High	High	High
Cyst fluid analysis	Clear fluid Viscosity low Lipase variable CEA low	Dirty fluid Viscosity low Lipase high CEA low	Clear fluid Viscosity low Lipase low CEA low	Clear fluid Viscosity high Lipase high CEA variable	Clear fluid Viscosity variable Lipase high CEA variable	Clear fluid Viscosity high Lipase low CEA high	Bloody fluid Viscosity low Lipase low CEA low
Typical cytological features	Epithelial cells without any atypia	Histiocytes, macrophages, no epithelial cells	Small, cuboid glycogen-positive cells	Mucinous epithelial cells with variable atypia	Mucinous epithelial cells with variable atypia	Mucinous epithelial cells with variable atypia	Monomorphic cells with round nuclei and foamy cytoplasm, branching papillae, myxoid and fibrovascular stroma
Immunohisto-chemistry	PAS	–	–	CDX2, MUC2, MUC5 (intestinal type) MUC1, MUC5 (pancreatobiliary type)	MUC5 (gastric type)		Vimentin, NSE, α_1-antitrypsin, progesterone receptor
Malignant potential	No	No	Very low (<5%)	High (10–50%) Pancreatobiliary type > intestinal type	Low (9–27%)	High	Low (5–15%)

BD-IPMN, branch duct intraductal papillary mucinous neoplasm; CEA, carcinoembryonic antigen; MCN, mucinous cystic neoplasm; MD-IPMN, main duct intraductal papillary mucinous neoplasm; PAS, periodic acid–Schiff; SCN, serous cystic neoplasm; SPN, solid pseudopapillary neoplasm.

Table 18.3 Criteria for the malignant potential of cystic pancreatic neoplasias (adapted from Dietrich et al.[17])

EUS criteria
Wall ≥ 3 mm or thick septa
Macroseptation (cystic components > 10 mm)
Solid parts or solid-cystic tumor
Focal thickening of the wall, mass extending beyond the duct wall
Wall protrusions
Cystic dilation of the main pancreatic duct > 10 mm
Lesion > 30 mm
Growth during follow-up
EUS-FNA criteria
High viscosity of the cyst fluid
High CEA level in the cyst fluid (variable cut-off values)
Presence of mucin in the cyst fluid (MUC1, MUC2 and MUC5AC)
Cytological or histological detection of mucinous epithelium
Cytological detection of nuclear atypia, necrosis, and significant background inflammation
Cytological or histological diagnosis of defined cystic neoplasia with malignant potential
K-ras mutation and loss of heterozygosity
High telomerase activity in cyst fluid

lesions of the pancreas was compared with saline solution lavage. EUS-guided ethanol lavage resulted in a greater reduction in the cyst size, but only led to complete disappearance of the cysts in one-third of the patients.[25]

◼ Mucinous Cystadenoma and Cystadenocarcinoma

Mucinous cystadenomas consist of one or more macrocystic spaces lined with mucus-secreting cells and are typically located in the body or tail of the pancreas. It is often difficult to make the diagnosis on the basis of biopsy or aspiration samples, as the cellular lining is frequently irregular. A mucinous lesion should be suspected when one or more macrocystic spaces containing mucin are found. Most of these mucinous tumors are malignant at time of diagnosis, and benign forms have a high potential for malignant transformation (**Figs. 18.3** and **18.4**). During ERCP, tissue sampling with brushing, and/or biopsy, and/or pancreatic fluid collection, should be performed whenever possible.

When the diagnosis of a mucinous cystadenoma is made, the lesion should be resected, due to the high potential for malignant change, but also depending on the patient's age and comorbidity. Distal pancreatectomy should be carried out for lesions in the tail or body of the pancreas, and patients with lesions in the pancreatic head should undergo pancreaticoduodenectomy.

Another type of mucinous tumor of the pancreas is intraductal papillary mucinous neoplasm (IPMN) or mucinous duct ectasia. The relationship between IPMNs (in

which an increasing incidence is being observed) and mucinous cystadenoma/cystadenocarcinomas is not yet clear.[20]

◼ Intraductal Papillary Mucinous Neoplasm

IPMNs were first described in 1982 in patients suspected of having pancreatic carcinoma who had a favorable outcome. A variety of confusing synonyms have been used—for example, mucinous ductal ectasia, mucin-producing carcinoma, intraductal mucin-producing tumor, intraductal papillary hyperplasia, intraductal papillary tumor, intraductal papillary neoplasm, etc. Intraductal papillary mucinous neoplasms show dilated ductal segments lined with mucus-secreting cells and may be located within the head of the pancreas or diffusely throughout the organ. IPMNs have been subclassified into a main duct type (MD-IPMN) and a branch duct type (BD-IPMN, often in the uncinate process) based on the anatomical involvement of the pancreatic duct. The malignant potential of MD-IPMNs is nearly as high as that of mucinous cystic neoplasms. The BD-IPMN subtype is associated with less aggressive histological features in comparison with the MD-IPMN subtype. Four subtypes of IPMN are currently distinguished: the intestinal type (common), a pancreatobiliary type (uncommon), and an oncocytic type (very rare) may be found in patients with MD-IPMN. The gastric type, which is the most common, corresponds to the BD-IPMN. These four types have special biological properties, which have prognostic implications. The majority of patients with IPMNs do not have invasive cancer at the time of

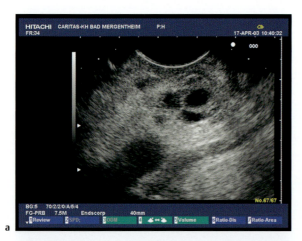
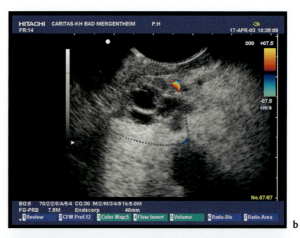
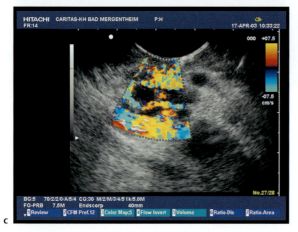
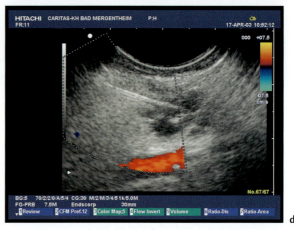

Fig. 18.3a–d Image of a partly solid and partly cystic mass, which was identified as a pseudocyst with an external transabdominal examination.
a B-mode.
b Color duplex ultrasonography.

c Vascularization of the tumor areas is identified after application of the echo contrast agent SonoVue.
d The tumor areas were aspirated in the same procedure. The cytological and histological diagnosis confirmed that the lesion was a mucinous cystadenoma, with no signs of malignancy.

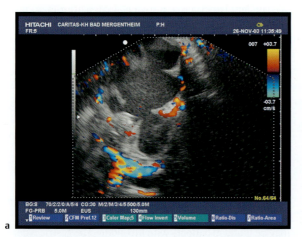
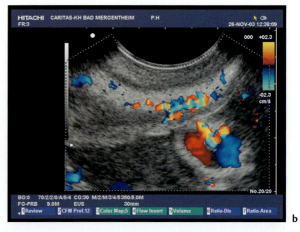

Fig. 18.4a–d Mucinous cystadenocarcinoma of the pancreas with mucus-containing cysts (**a**) and vascularized septa (**b**) and collaterals due to portal vein thrombosis (**c, d**).

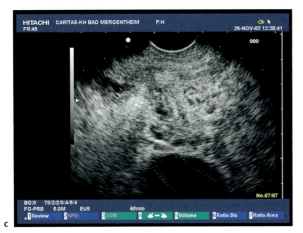

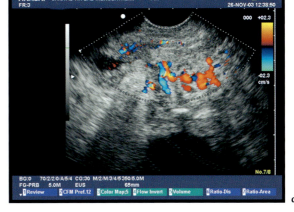

Fig. 18.4c, d (continued)

diagnosis, and the rate of progression appears to be slow (more than 5 years).[26–28]

Epidemiology. IPMNs have most commonly been described in men over the age of 60, some of whom have symptoms suggestive of chronic obstructive pancreatitis or acute recurrent pancreatitis due to intermittent obstruction of the pancreatic duct with mucus plugs. The etiology of IPMN is unclear. It has been described in association with familial adenomatous polyposis, Peutz–Jeghers syndrome, and other nonpancreatic tumors.

Diagnosis. There are three classic signs of MD-IPMN: a segmental or diffusely dilated main pancreatic duct without involvement of the common bile duct; a patulous ampullary orifice ("fishmouth"), frequently with mucus secretion (specific but not sensitive); and mural nodules. BD-IPMN is associated with multiple small cysts (5–20 mm) communicating with branch ducts. Dilation of the pancreatic duct to over 10 mm and cysts larger than 20 mm are suggestive of malignancy. Intraductal ultrasonography can be helpful for assessing the tumor extent in MD-IPMNs, but is rarely performed. EUS-FNA of the dilated pancreatic duct, including mural nodules and especially solid components of the tumor, may be helpful in the diagnosis (**Figs. 18.5** and **18.6**). Histopathological analysis tends to underestimate the tumor grade.[29]

Tumor markers are elevated in fewer than 25% of patients and are not helpful indicators of malignant transformation. Pancreatic secretions can be tested for molecular markers such as K-*ras,* P53, and telomerase activity, but the results have so far been inconsistent.

Differential diagnosis. The differential diagnosis of IPMN includes chronic obstructive pancreatitis, mucinous cystic tumors of the pancreas, and rarely pancreatic ductal adenocarcinoma.

Therapy. When an MD-IPMN is diagnosed, the lesion should be resected, due to the high potential for malignant change, but also depending on the patient's age and comorbidity and the type of lesion involved. BD-IPMNs less than 30 mm in diameter with a thin wall, without papillary wall protrusions, without thick septumlike structures, and without dilation of the main pancreatic duct progress very slowly. In view of the risks of pancreatic surgery, close monitoring—for example, with periodical EUS examinations—may be justified in patients with these lesions.[17,26,30]

Patients with recurrent pancreatitis caused by IPMN-induced intermittent obstruction should undergo resection of the mucous-secreting abnormal portion of the pancreas. Distal pancreatectomy, pancreaticoduodenectomy, or even total pancreatectomy, depending on the location and extent of the lesion, may be necessary. In our experience, patients with recurrent pancreatitis who are not suitable for surgery may benefit from endoscopic therapy.

■ Serous Cystadenoma

Microcystic pancreatic adenomas were formerly considered a rarity. Nowadays, with technological advances in the equipment, localized changes in the pancreas are much more frequently observed. In contrast to mucous cystadenomas and IPMNs, serous cystadenomas have a very low potential for malignant transformation. Tumors are distributed throughout the pancreas without predilection (**Fig. 18.7**). Histologically, the lesions typically consist of multiple small cysts lined with glycogen-rich cells, with a regular vascular architecture.

It has been found useful to remove larger cylinders of tissue, as the specimens obtained with EUS-FNA are only sufficient for determining malignancy, but not for classify-

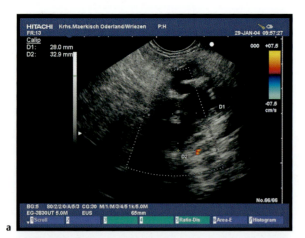
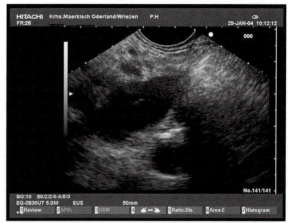
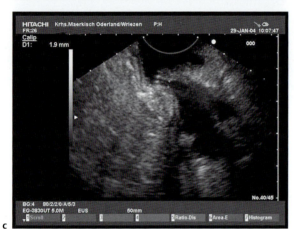
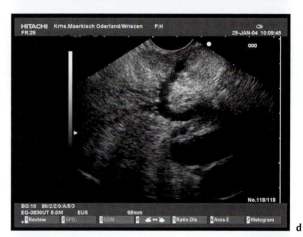
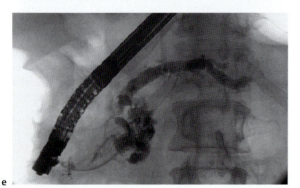
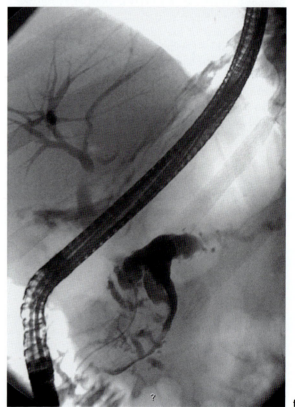

Fig. 18.5a–f Intraductal papillary mucinous neoplasms (IPMNs) of the pancreas (main duct type).

a Tortuous dilation of the main pancreatic duct in the pancreatic neck.

b Cystic spaces with incompletely anechoic luminal contents in the pancreatic body.

c The orifice of the main pancreatic duct is wide open.

d There is also dilation of the accessory pancreatic duct, viewed from the minor papilla.

e, f The corresponding endoscopic retrograde cholangiopancreatography (ERCP) images show tortuous dilation and cystic cavities in the pancreatic head and neck, as well as dilation of the main pancreatic duct in the body and tail of the pancreas: opacification from the major (**e**) and from the minor (**f**) papilla.

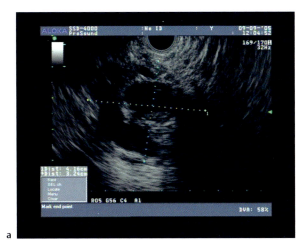
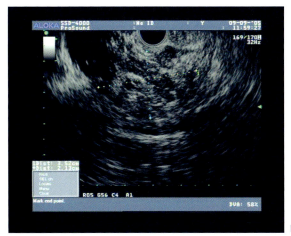
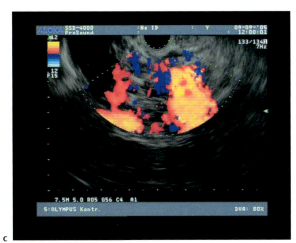
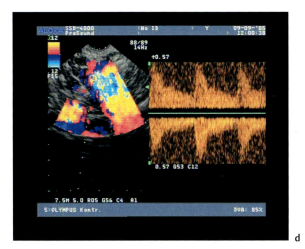

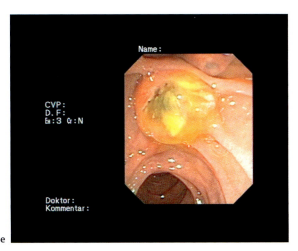

Fig. 18.6a–e Intraductal papillary mucinous neoplasms (IPMNs) of the pancreas (courtesy of M. Hocke, Meiningen, Germany).
a, b B-mode.
c Color Doppler imaging.
d Spectral analysis.
e Endoscopic image.

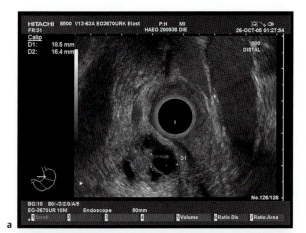

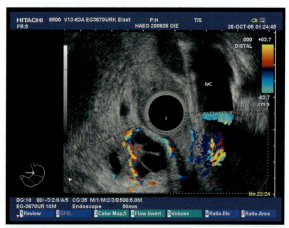

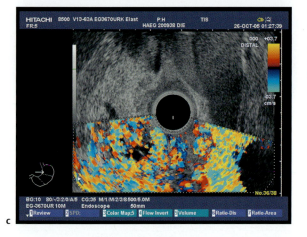

Fig. 18.7a–c Serous cystadenoma (▶ Videos 18.1–3)

a Serous cystadenomas of the pancreas appear as inhomogeneous masses with multiple small hypoechoic or anechoic lesions and hyperechoic septa (honeycomb pattern), demonstrated using B-mode.

b A central vessel (also known as focal nodular hyperplasia of the pancreas) can be identified with color duplex sonography (spectral analysis revealed a low-resistance index with a high diastolic flow; not shown). IVC, inferior vena cava.

c Contrast-enhanced imaging with SonoVue revealed numerous vessels within the tiny hyperechoic septa, indicating a hypervascularized pancreatic tumor.

ing the tumor type. In patients with suspected serous cystadenomas, core biopsies for histology are therefore required if the lesion appears solid, in order to avoid surgery. The results of a recent pilot study suggested that EUS-guided Tru-Cut biopsy (EUS-TCB) is capable of collecting sufficient tissue in cases of serous cystadenoma.[21] In a patient with a definitive diagnosis of a serous cystadenoma, the management is determined by age, comorbidity, symptoms, progression, and lesion location. Symptomatic or enlarging serous cystadenomas in healthy young patients should be resected. Lesions in the body or tail of the pancreas require distal pancreatectomy, while those in the head of the gland are enucleated or resected with pancreaticoduodenectomy. Small, asymptomatic, and nonenlarging serous cystadenomas can be monitored, as the risk of malignant change is very low. The optimal interval for repeating imaging examinations in such patients is not known, but should be not longer than 12 months.

Solid Pseudopapillary Neoplasm

Solid pseudopapillary neoplasms (also known as papillary cystic neoplasm, pseudopapillary neoplasms, solid pseudopapillary tumor, or Frantz–Gruber tumor) usually occur in young women, have a low malignant potential, and are most commonly found in the tail or body of the pancreas. EUS shows a mixed solid and cystic encapsulated tumor with distinct margins (**Fig. 18.8**). There are sometimes a few calcifications. The tumors are often very large. EUS-FNA shows very distinctive cytopathological features, which make it possible to distinguish this type from other pancreatic neoplasms. Cytopathological slides show branching papillae with myxoid and fibrovascular stroma. The tumor cells are monomorphic, with round nuclei and an eosinophilic, foamy cytoplasm. The cystic components contain bloody fluid, sometimes with necrotic debris. Immunoreactivity for vimentin, α_1-antitrypsin, neuron-specific enolase, and progesterone receptor is typical of this rare type of pancreatic tumor.[31,32] Patients with solid pseudopapillary tumors of the pancreas have a very good prognosis if the tumor is resected completely. However, recurrences and even metastases may occur in a small number

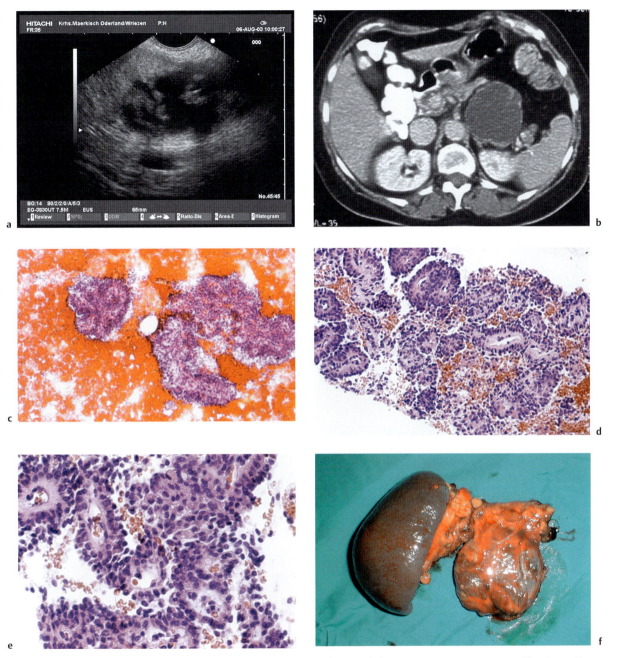

Fig. 18.8a–f Solid pseudopapillary neoplasm of the pancreas: cystic tumor of the pancreatic tail in a 45-year-old asymptomatic woman. The tumor is predominantly cystic, with some solid parts (**a** EUS; **b** CT). EUS-FNA shows the characteristic branching papillae with myxoid and fibrovascular stroma. Tumor cells are isomorphic. The prominent nuclei are rounded, slightly hyperchromatic, and show no mitotic activity. Tumor cells stained positive for vimentin, NSE, and progesterone receptor. Staining for CA 19–9, CEA, MFN 116, synaptophysin, and chromogranin A was negative. Proliferative activity (Ki-67 labeling index: 1%) was low (**c** cell smears, hematoxylin–eosin, original magnification × 100; **d, e** core biopsy, hematoxylin–eosin, original magnifications × 200 and × 400, courtesy of Dr. B. Fiedler, Berlin, Germany). **f** Resection of the pancreatic tail, the tumor, and the spleen was carried out (courtesy of Dr. G. Reiche, Strausberg, Germany).

of cases. Histological prediction of the malignant potential is not yet possible. The most important differential diagnosis to consider is neuroendocrine tumor of the pancreas.[33] The type of resection depends on the location of the tumor.

■ Teratoma of the Pancreas

Teratoma of the pancreas is mentioned in the WHO classification and represents a very rare entity (**Fig. 18.9**).

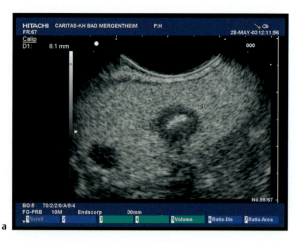

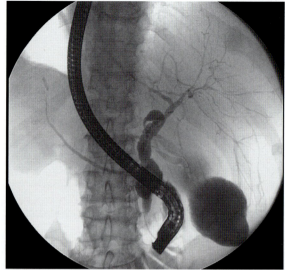

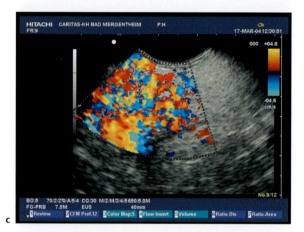

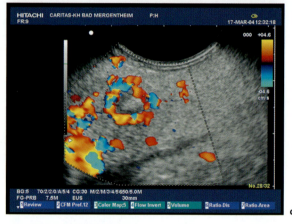

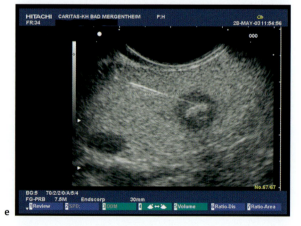

Fig. 18.9a–l Mature pancreatic teratoma

a B-mode sonography shows a weakly echogenic mass with central calcification (8 × 6 mm in size).

b Endoscopic retrograde cholangiopancreatography shows blockage of the distally positioned part of the pancreatic duct, raising a suspicion of pancreatic carcinoma.

c, d Contrast-enhanced endoscopic ultrasonography proved useful for characterization, as the vessels are visible and only the central part is not seen.

e The diagnosis was only reached histologically; EUS-guided aspiration was not completely unambiguous.

Fig. 18.9f–l ▷

■ Rare Cystic Neoplasms and Miscellaneous Pancreatic Lesions Mimicking Cystic Neoplasms

A wide variety of cystic pancreatic lesions should be considered in the differential diagnosis—for example, lymphoepithelial cysts, cystic neuroendocrine tumors, the cystic form of acinar cell carcinoma (**Fig. 18.10**), mucin-producing ductal adenocarcinomas (**Figs. 18.11** and **18.12**),[34] primary pancreatic lymphomas (**Fig. 18.13**), which are much more rare than the involvement in systemic disease, and cystic metastatic disease. Interobserver variability has been reported to be high for many aspects of the EUS assessment[35] (**Fig. 18.14**).

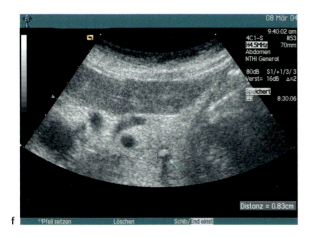
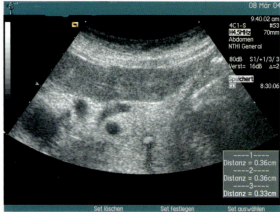

f

g

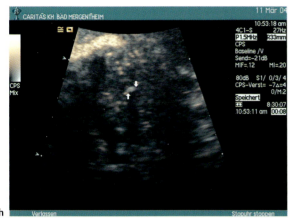
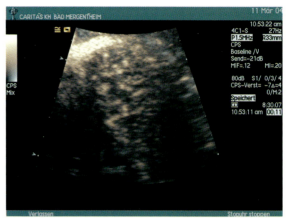

h

i

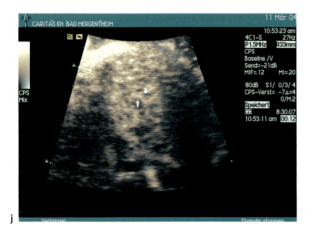
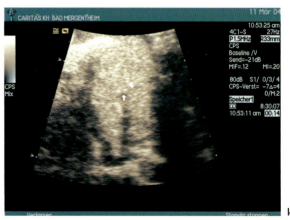

j

k

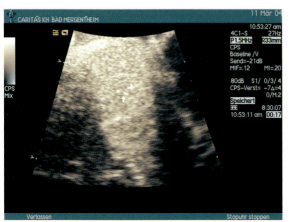

l

Fig. 18.9f–l (continued)

f, g The transabdominal findings were compared side by side. With the ductal blockage, these were primarily interpreted as signs of pancreatitis.

h–l After contrast enhancement, the color power method showed concentration in the tumor tissue, ruling out a single calcified structure and allowing a diagnosis of neoplasia.

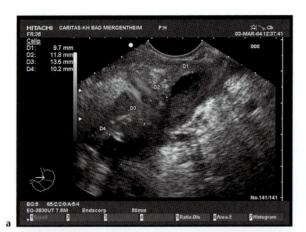
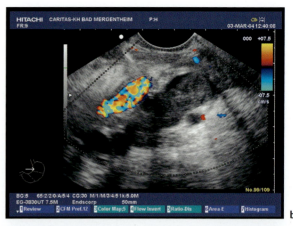
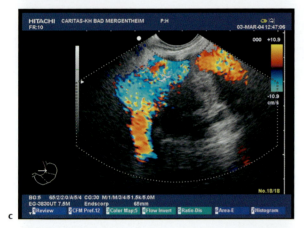
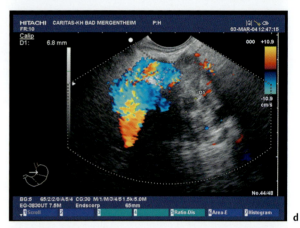
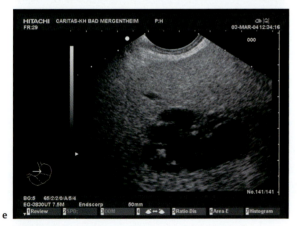
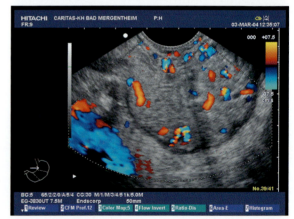

Fig. 18.10a–f Acinar cell carcinoma

a Conventional B-mode image of a portal vein thrombosis, with varying stages of development between the markers.

b On color duplex ultrasonography, there are no signs of flow in the portal vein, although the splenic artery is visible.

c, d Contrast enhancement with SonoVue shows that the tumor areas are barely supplied with blood, which can be taken as an indication of malignancy.

e, f In the same examination, it was possible to identify metastases in the liver (**e**), as well as extended circulation surrounding the gastric fundus region (varices, **f**). The diagnosis of the rare condition of acinar cell carcinoma was confirmed histologically.

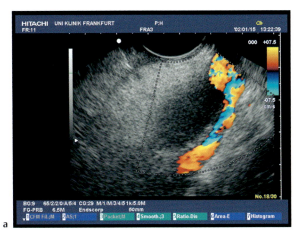
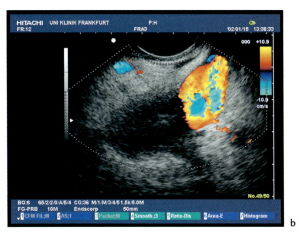

a b

Fig. 18.11a, b Differential diagnosis of cystic lesions. Ductal adenocarcinoma of the pancreas infiltrating the portal vein, revealed by color Doppler imaging demonstrating turbulence, may rarely create the impression of a pseudocystic lesion.[34]

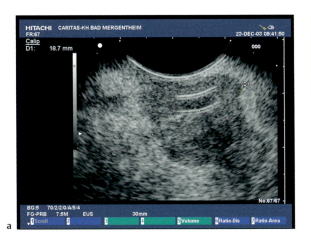
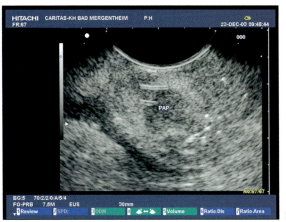

a b

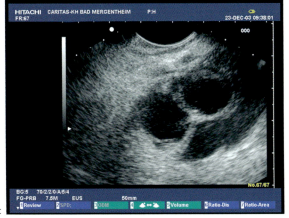
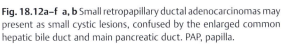
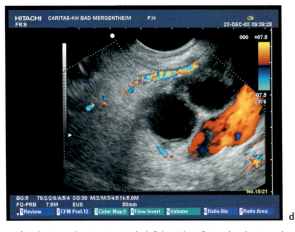

c d

Fig. 18.12a–f a, b Small retropapillary ductal adenocarcinomas may present as small cystic lesions, confused by the enlarged common hepatic bile duct and main pancreatic duct. PAP, papilla.

c, d Color Doppler imaging is helpful in identifying the ducts and vessels.

Fig. 18.12e, f ▷

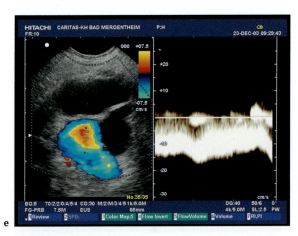

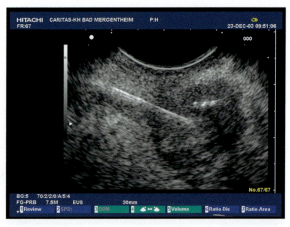

Fig. 18.12e, f (continued)
e Color Doppler imaging can also identify the tumor.

f The final diagnosis can be confirmed using EUS-guided fine-needle aspiration.

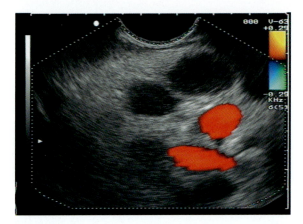

Fig. 18.13 An isolated non-Hodgkin lymphoma (NHL) in the pancreas. Non-Hodgkin lymphoma of the pancreas is a rare lesion, but it may be seen particularly in patients with acquired immune deficiency syndrome (AIDS) and may present in the form of cystic-type lesions. Color Doppler imaging is helpful in differentiating the infiltration from the vessel.

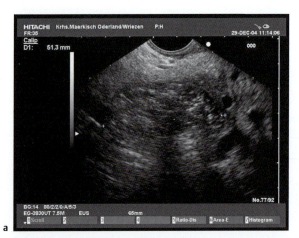

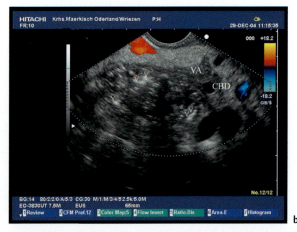

Fig. 18.14a–d A possible pitfall in the diagnosis of cystic pancreatic tumors.
a EUS shows a large, well-delineated, heterogeneous mass in the pancreatic head, with a honeycomb pattern, resembling a microcystic serous adenoma.

b Color-coded duplex imaging does not show any vascular signals inside the lesion, but after air insufflation into the duodenum, a few hyperechoic mobile reflexes (arrowheads) were seen inside the lesion, representing a very large duodenal diverticulum displacing the pancreatic head (hypoechoic ventral anlage, VA, and common bile duct, CBD, on the right side of the image).

Fig. 18.14c, d ▷

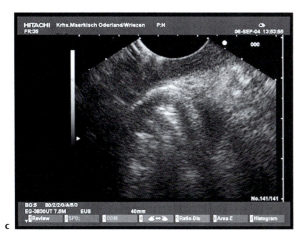
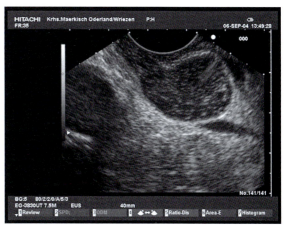

c

d

Fig. 18.14c, d (continued)
c, d For comparison, these images show a typical example of a duodenal diverticulum. At the beginning of the examination, after air insufflation, there are hyperechoic peripancreatic and periduodenal reflexes (**c**); water filling allows the diagnosis of a periduodenal diverticulum (**d**).

Neuroendocrine Tumors (Table 18.3)

Definition and epidemiology. Neuroendocrine pancreatic tumors are considered to be rare tumors in the pancreas or peripancreatic region (stomach or duodenal wall). More than 50% of these tumors (up to 85%) secrete biologically active hormones or demonstrate biochemical abnormalities, resulting in specific clinical syndromes. Although the tumors have a similar histological appearance, they can be distinguished by the use of immunostaining for the hormone being secreted.

Pancreatic endocrine tumors are named after the predominant hormone that they secrete. Insulinomas are reported to be the most common type of tumor, accounting for 60% of pancreatic endocrine tumors. Gastrinomas are the second most common type, occurring in ≈ 20% of cases. Glucagonomas, somatostatinomas, and tumors secreting vasoactive intestinal peptide (VIPomas) are much rarer. The 15–40% of tumors that are nonfunctional do not become apparent clinically until they are large enough to impinge on adjacent structures and cause symptoms due to mass effects. We have diagnosed the latter form much more commonly than has recently been reported, and in our own series they are the most frequently encountered entity.

Biological behavior. The clinical behavior of pancreatic endocrine tumors can be benign or malignant, and it is difficult to assess the malignant potential on the basis of the histological appearance. Since benign and malignant pancreatic endocrine tumors are not distinguishable histologically, the absence or presence of metastases (either nodal or distant) has been used to make this distinction. However, this criterion alone is not an ideal indicator of the prognosis, since some benign tumors recur.

Symptoms. Pancreatic endocrine tumors—most often insulinomas or gastrinomas—become clinically apparent in approximately half of the patients with this disorder. However, subclinical involvement is more common.

Diagnosis. Once a diagnosis is made, the primary tumor has to be localized and the presence of metastases has to be assessed. EUS is also used to evaluate the response to chemotherapy. Pancreatic endocrine tumors are often small and hard to detect with radiographic techniques. Since these tumors are rare, it is difficult to compare the accuracy of the various imaging tests.

Endoscopic ultrasound provides the highest resolution of the pancreas and can distinguish structures as small as < 2–3 mm. EUS has also proved to be a useful tool for identifying tumors in the duodenal wall and peripancreatic lymph nodes. EUS-guided fine-needle aspiration biopsy may help identify the type of tumor, but may not be sufficiently accurate to exclude the diagnosis in all cases. In one early report in patients who had negative ultrasound and computed tomography (CT) scans, EUS detected endocrine tumors in the pancreas with a high level of sensitivity (82%) and specificity (95%).[36] The excellent results of this initial study were confirmed in several other studies including some 300 patients. In comparison with abdominal ultrasound, CT, magnetic resonance imaging, angiography, and somatostatin-receptor scintigraphy, endoscopic ultrasound is clearly superior for localizing endocrine pancreatic tumors preoperatively. The sensitivity of EUS in detecting pancreatic gastrinomas and insulinomas has been reported to be in the range of 79–100%. EUS can therefore be regarded as the method of choice for localizing pancreatic neuroendocrine tumors.

EUS-FNA may be of value in particular for differentiating between nonfunctioning pancreatic neuroendocrine

III Gastrointestinal Tract

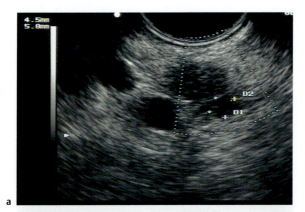

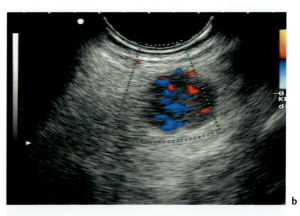

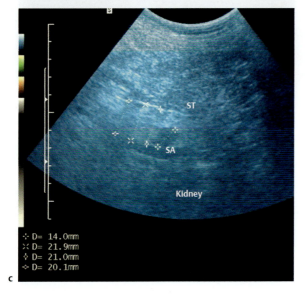

Fig. 18.15a–c Neuroendocrine tumor: insulinoma. A small cyst is delineated next to a small lesion in the pancreatic tail.
a B-mode.
b Color Doppler imaging.
c Transabdominal imaging. SA, splenic artery; ST, stomach.

tumors and other pancreatic neoplasms, to avoid extended pancreatic surgery. EUS-FNA is also effective and accurate in establishing the diagnosis of functioning pancreatic neuroendocrine tumors.[37,38]

Preliminary experience with intraductal techniques has suggested that these may be helpful in a few cases. However, experience is limited, and the technique is not widely available.

Typically, neuroendocrine tumors are hypoechoic, well-circumscribed, and hypervascularized in comparison with the surrounding tissue (**Figs. 18.15, 18.16, 18.17, 18.18,** and **18.19**). Some tumors may resemble peripancreatic lymph nodes, as they may be connected to the pancreas by a small vascular stalk. Cystic degeneration can typically be observed mainly in larger tumors and in up to 50% of liver metastases (data not yet published).

Other imaging techniques. *Somatostatin-receptor scintigraphy.* Neuroendocrine tumors may have high concentrations of somatostatin receptors and can therefore sometimes be imaged with a radiolabeled form of the somatostatin analogue. Somatostatin-receptor scintigraphy has proved particularly effective for visualizing gastrinomas and glucagonomas, as well as nonfunctioning pancreatic tumors. As somatostatin-receptor scintigraphy fails to identify most insulinomas, it should not be used as a primary imaging test.

Intraoperative localization. Intraoperative ultrasonography (IOUS) has been used in combination with palpation of the pancreas with promising results, with a sensitivity for tumor detection of up to 83–100%. IOUS is not so far capable of replacing preoperative imaging.

Prognosis. The prognostic impact of hormone secretion is unclear. Although several studies have suggested that the survival in patients with nonfunctional tumors is poorer than in those with functional lesions, others have found no differences in the survival.

Therapy. Curative surgical resection can be attempted if there is no metastatic disease. If metastatic disease is present, its extent has to be determined so that optimal treatment can be instituted (e.g., cytoreductive surgery or chemotherapy).

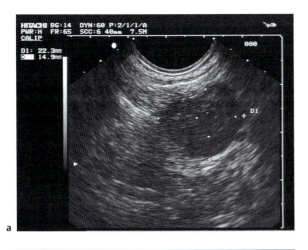

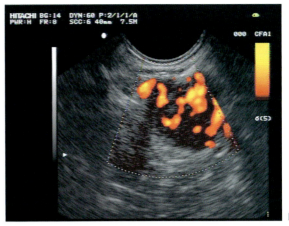

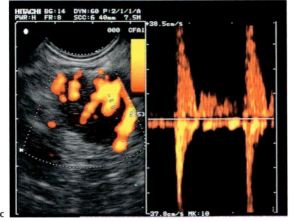

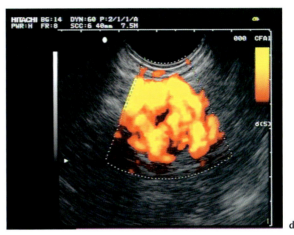

Fig. 18.16a–d Insulinoma
a B-mode.
b Color Doppler imaging.

c Fast Fourier transform (FFT) analysis.
d Contrast-enhanced ultrasonography.

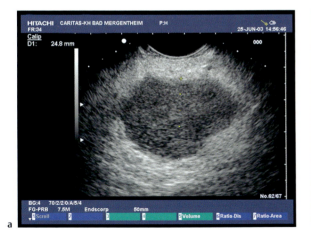

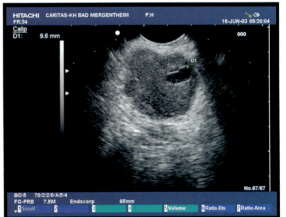

Fig. 18.17a–e Semimalignant neuroendocrine tumor of the pancreas.
a A 36-year-old patient presented with a clearly defined localized pancreatic mass.

b Minor cystic changes; color duplex sonography shows no blood supply—typical of neuroendocrine tumors.

Fig. 18.17c–e ▷

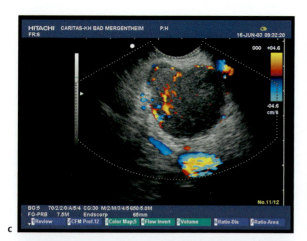

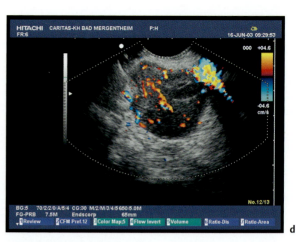

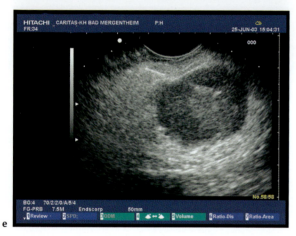

Fig. 18.17c–e (continued)
c, d After contrast enhancement with SonoVue, vascularization becomes clearly visible on the edges of the tumor.
e EUS-guided aspiration and removal of potentially malignant cells. Histological assessment of the surgical specimen confirmed a neuroendocrine tumor with malignant transformation.

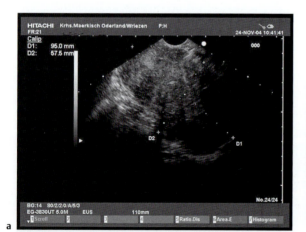

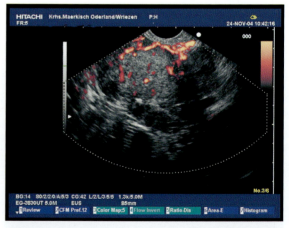

Fig. 18.18a–k A large, nonfunctioning pancreatic neuroendocrine tumor in an asymptomatic 68-year-old woman. The tumor was identified on transabdominal ultrasonography.
a Endoscopic ultrasound showed a very large, inhomogeneous and hypoechoic tumor in the pancreatic body and tail, infiltrating and totally occluding the splenic vein.

b Color-coded duplex imaging shows vascular signals inside the tumor.

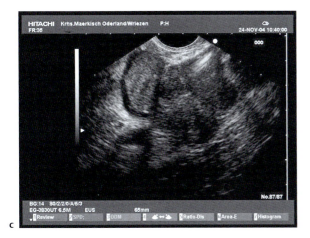

c

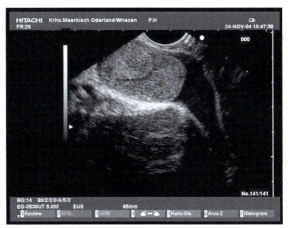

d

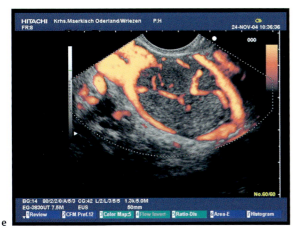

e

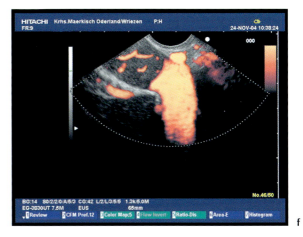

f

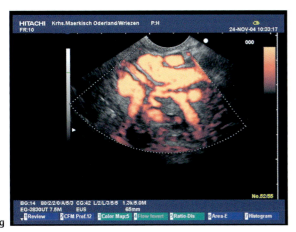

g

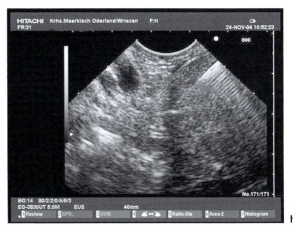

h

Fig. 18.18c–h (continued) **c, d** The tumor is infiltrating the portal vein, forming a tumor thrombus (**c**) that extends into the porta hepatis (**d**).
e, f Color-coded duplex imaging shows vascular signals within the tumor thrombus, so that it can be distinguished from an appositional fibrin thrombus.

g, h Despite considerable numbers of peripancreatic portoportal collaterals (**g**), transgastric EUS-guided fine-needle aspiration was performed using a 22-gauge aspiration needle, without any complications (**h**).

Fig. 18.18i–k ▷

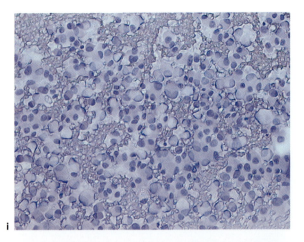

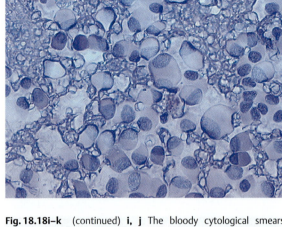

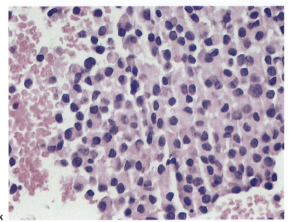

Fig. 18.18i–k   (continued) **i, j** The bloody cytological smears showed numerous ovoid large cells, with bright cytoplasm. The variably large nuclei are located eccentrically, some of them containing nucleoli. A few of the tumor cells contain giant or double nuclei (Papanicolaou, original magnifications × 200 and × 400).
k Histological examination of a few small cylinders was possible and showed tumor cells with enlarged hyperchromatic nuclei and perinuclear brightening of the cytoplasm (hematoxylin–eosin, original magnification × 200; courtesy of Dr. Wagner, Königswusterhausen, Germany). Immunohistochemical staining was positive for chromogranin A and synaptophysin.

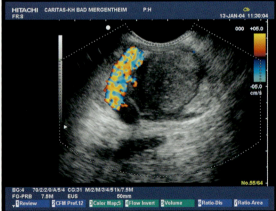

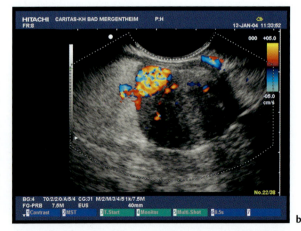

Fig. 18.19a–e Suspected carcinoma of the pancreas. The patient presented with a 1-year history of weight loss. Computed tomography showed tumorlike changes, which improved during the course of the illness.
a Using color duplex ultrasound, it was not possible to confirm the classification of the mass located next to the splenic artery.

b–e Contrast enhancement was seen after administration of Sono-Vue. A ductal pancreatic adenocarcinoma was excluded at surgery (with a histological diagnosis of chronic pancreatitis).

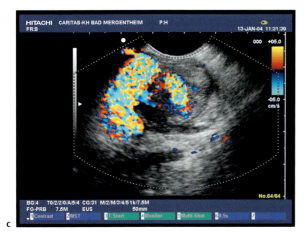

c

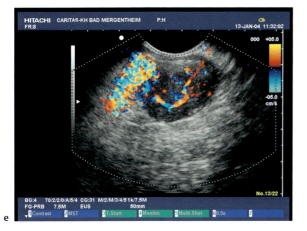

e

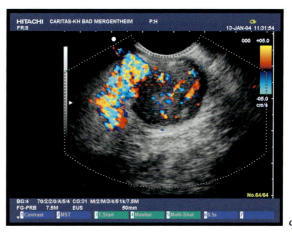

d

Fig. 18.19c–e (continued)

Differential Diagnosis of Pancreatic Lesions

Most solid pancreatic tumors are reported to be ductal adenocarcinomas. Pancreatic lesions other than ductal adenocarcinomas represent a heterogeneous group of tumors with regard to their clinical presentation, biologic behavior, prognosis, and imaging features.

Incidental pancreatic tumors are found in autopsy series in up to 1.5% of unselected cases. It is important to distinguish between nonductal adenocarcinomas and ductal adenocarcinomas, which are much more commonly reported neoplasms of the exocrine pancreas, as most neuroendocrine tumors progress only slowly and imply different treatment approaches from those used with ductal adenocarcinoma. Serous microcystic adenomas of the pancreas are rarely malignant and therefore do not generally require surgery. Other forms of solid tumor are rare. Differential diagnosis has been reported to be difficult. An ideal imaging method for differentiating between pancreatic tumors has not previously been available, but contrast-enhanced ultrasound using the endoscopic technique

(EUS) and contrast-enhanced ultrasound (CEUS) with the transabdominal route appear to be promising.

The vascular pattern of pancreatic tumors has been examined in a few studies, mainly using the transabdominal approach, but the patient groups, examination techniques used and tumor characteristics varied. Pancreatic metastases, for example, are usually not clinically challenging, as they correspond to the underlying disease and often present as multiple pancreatic nodules. Primary lymphoma of the pancreas is a very rare disease. Ductal adenocarcinomas are rarely cystic, and most cystic lesions behave in a biologically different way from pancreatic adenocarcinomas.

The aim of two recently published studies was to analyze the vascular pattern of solitary solid pancreatic tumors in comparison with the surrounding parenchyma, using contrast-enhanced endoscopic ultrasound[39] and contrast-enhanced transabdominal ultrasound.[40]

Contrast-enhanced endoscopic ultrasound.[39] Endoscopic ultrasonography was carried out using an electronic linear ultrasound probe. Levovist was administered as the contrast agent in all patients (4 g, 400 mg/dL, bolus injection).

In contrast to first-generation microbubble echo enhancers with air bubbles developed for Doppler imaging purposes (e.g., Levovist) second-generation microbubble echo enhancers contain gas and are mainly used with resonating low mechanical index techniques. The aim of the study was to compare air-derived Levovist with newer second-generation contrast agents containing gas in relation to their Doppler enhancement properties. When SonoVue and Levovist were compared in 10 consecutive patients, similar results for imaging the pancreatic vascular pattern were obtained with Levovist 4 g 10 mL (400 mg/dL) and SonoVue 4.8 mL. Vascularity was measured in all of the lesions in comparison with the surrounding pancreatic tissue and classified as hypovascular, isovascular, or hypervascular using conventional and contrast-enhanced Doppler imaging. For analysis, isovascular and hypervascular lesions were compared jointly with hypovascular lesions.

The criterion for inclusion in the study was an indeterminate, solitary, predominantly solid lesion ≤40 mm in size, with a histologically confirmed diagnosis. The lesions had been detected by transabdominal ultrasound, computed tomography, or magnetic resonance imaging.

The exclusion criteria were as follows:

- *Metastases.* Ductal adenocarcinomas of the pancreas with metastases to the liver, lung, or any other organ were not examined on endoscopic ultrasound, as the metastases determined the clinical work-up (e.g., liver biopsy) and prognosis for the patients.
- *Tumor size.* The EUS range of high-quality images is restricted to ≈50 mm. Lesions larger than 40 mm were therefore excluded from the analysis, so that the outer edge of a pancreatic lesion was within a range of 50 mm of the surrounding stomach or duodenum on at least one side of the probe. The measurement was made using transabdominal ultrasound or computed tomography and endoscopic ultrasound; the latter was decisive in patients in whom there were discrepancies between the findings.
- *Multiple lesions.* Only patients with solitary lesions were included in the study. Patients with multiple lesions were excluded from the study, as these lesions are mostly secondary (metastases or lymphomas) or are caused by functional (hormone-producing) neuroendocrine tumors.
- *Predominantly solid lesions.* Predominantly solid lesions were defined as those with cysts <20 mm or with a cystic area or areas representing less than 50% of the total tumor volume.
- *Chronic pancreatitis.* Patients with chronic pancreatitis were excluded from the study, as the contrast enhancement pattern was being compared with the surrounding pancreatic parenchyma. Chronic pancreatitis was assumed if any imaging modality revealed inflammatory changes in the surrounding pancreatic parenchyma. Two patients with suspected ductal adenocarcinoma of the pancreas on computed tomography were found to have thrombosed aneurysms of the gastroduodenal ar-

tery (28 mm) and splenic artery (25 mm), neither of which was histologically confirmed, and were therefore also excluded from the study.

- *Autoimmune pancreatitis.* Patients with a definite diagnosis of autoimmune pancreatitis and lesion size >40 mm were excluded from the study.
- *Neuroendocrine tumors in hormone-derived syndromes.* Neuroendocrine tumors with hormone-derived syndromes (e.g., insulinoma, glucagonoma, gastrinoma) were excluded from the study, as pancreatic tumors in patients with a clinically defined syndrome do not present problems in the differential diagnosis of pancreatic tumor lesions.
- *Pancreatic metastases.* Patients with a final diagnosis of pancreatic metastases with no clinical relevance for the course of the disease were excluded from the study.

The final diagnosis in a total of 93 tumors was always established histologically on the basis of the surgical specimen (n = 83), transabdominal/percutaneous guided puncture (n = 35), or EUS-guided 22-G fine-needle aspiration cytology (n = 22; overlapping was possible). The results are summarized in **Tables 18.4, 18.5, 18.6,** and **18.7.**

Contrast-enhanced transabdominal ultrasound. The use of transabdominal contrast-enhanced ultrasound to characterize pancreatic tumors has also recently been reported.[40] Several limitations with the transabdominal route have to be taken into account. Transabdominal ultrasound penetration may be limited by meteorism or other causes. In larger tumors, heterogeneity is more prominent and typical tumor features may be obscured by regressive changes. As in the EUS study, the criterion for inclusion in the study was an indeterminate solitary pancreatic solid lesion of any size suspected on transabdominal ultrasound, computed tomography, or magnetic resonance imaging, with a definite and histologically confirmed diagnosis.

The exclusion criteria were as follows:

- *Inadequate visualization.* Adequate visualization of the pancreas was not achieved with CEUS in 9% of patients, a figure that is in accordance with published data for visualization of the peripancreatic region and hepatoduodenal ligament.
- *Chronic pancreatitis.* Patients with a history of chronic pancreatitis, with or without circumscribed lesions, were not examined using CEUS and/or were excluded from the study, as the contrast enhancement pattern of pancreatic tumors was being compared with the surrounding pancreatic parenchyma on the assumption that it was normal.
- *Cystic lesions.* Cystic lesions with cysts larger than 20 mm were excluded from the study as well, as the aim of the study was to differentiate between ductal adenocarcinomas (which rarely show cystic elements) and solid nodules with other causes. Patients with pancreatic cysts (n = 22, mainly in patients with polycystic

Table 18.4 Inclusion and exclusion criteria for patients with ductal adenocarcinoma, neuroendocrine tumors, and serous microcystic pancreatic adenoma. The inclusion criteria for the study were mainly solid tumors, tumor size ≤ 40 mm, and a solitary nodule. The exclusion criteria were tumor size > 40 mm, multiple lesions, hormone-producing syndromes, and metastases

	Patients examined to identify exclusion criteria	Included in the study
Ductal adenocarcinoma	212	62
Excluded	114 (liver metastases with or without chronic pancreatitis)	
Excluded	52 (lesion size > 40 mm with or without chronic pancreatitis)	
Neuroendocrine tumors	76	20
Excluded	26 (liver metastases)	
Excluded	25 (hormone-producing syndromes)	
Excluded	5 (lesion size > 40 mm)	
Serous microcystic pancreatic adenoma	12	10
Excluded	2 (lesion size > 40 mm)	
Teratoma	1	1

Table 18.5 Contrast-enhanced color Doppler ultrasound in 93 patients was used to analyze inclusion and exclusion criteria. The inclusion criteria for the study were mainly solid lesions, tumor size ≤ 40 mm, and solitary nodule. The exclusion criteria were tumor size > 40 mm, multiple lesions, hormone-producing lesions, and metastases

Entity	No.	Hypovascular (marginal tumor vessels)	Isovascular/hypervascular
Ductal adenocarcinoma of the pancreas	62	57 (92%)	5 (8%)
Pancreatic tumors of other origin:			
Neuroendocrine tumor	20	0 (0%)	20 (100%)
Microcystic serous pancreatic adenoma	10	0 (0%)	10 (100%)
Teratoma	1	0 (0%)	1 (100%)

Table 18.6 Sensitivity, specificity, positive predictive value, negative predictive value, and accuracy for characterizing pancreatic tumors (hypovascularity as a sign of ductal adenocarcinoma versus hypervascularity as a sign of tumors of other origin) using contrast-enhanced endoscopic ultrasound (CEUS) or color Doppler imaging (CDI)

	Sensitivity (%)	Specificity (%)	Positive predictive value (%)	Negative predictive value (%)	Accuracy (%)
Hypovascularity as a sign of ductal adenocarcinoma using CEUS	92% (82% to 97%)	100% (89% to 100%)	100% (94% to 100%)	86% (71% to 95%)	95% (88% to 98%)
Hypervascularity as a sign of tumors of other origin using CEUS	100% (89% to 100%)	92% (82% to 97%)	86% (71% to 95%)	100% (94% to 100%)	95% (88% to 98%)
Hypervascularity as a sign of tumors of other origin using CDI	61% (42% to 78%)	100% (94% to 100%)	100% (82% to 100%)	84% (73% to 91%)	87% (79% to 93%)

95% confidence intervals are shown in parentheses. NB: It should be noted that hypovascularity could not be assessed using conventional color Doppler imaging, as the normal pancreatic parenchyma did not show any reproducible vascularity at all with the instruments used.

disease) and adult patients with cystic fibrosis and pancreatic cysts (n = 27) were excluded, as ductal adenocarcinomas are rarely cystic.

- *Hormone-producing tumors.* Patients with diseases involving hormone-producing tumors were excluded from the study, as detecting a pancreatic tumor in these patients implies that the tumor is a neuroendocrine one.
- *Multiple lesions.* Only patients with solitary lesions were included in the study. Patients with multiple lesions were excluded, as these lesions are mostly secondary

(metastases or lymphomas) or are caused by functional (hormone-producing) neuroendocrine tumors.

- *Metastases.* Patients with pancreatic nodules and metastatic disease (e.g., liver, lung) were excluded from the study, as the diagnosis was usually achieved by biopsying the metastatic site.
- *Pancreatic metastases and lymphomas.* Patients with a final diagnosis of pancreatic metastases without clinical relevance (no impact on treatment, prognosis, or clinical work-up) were excluded from the study.

Table 18.7 Contrast-enhanced color Doppler ultrasound in 118 patients not included in the study due to cystic origin, lesion size > 40 mm, and multiple lesions and signs of chronic pancreatitis. The final diagnosis was obtained with surgery or fine-needle aspiration cytology (with additional follow-up in nonsurgical patients)

	n	Explanations
Intraductal papillary mucinous neoplasia	6	Contrast-enhancing neoplastic nodules were identified in all six patients, independently of the type and malignant status of the lesion,
Mucinous cystadenoma / cystadenocarcinoma	19	Contrast-enhancing neoplastic nodules were identified in 15 of the 19 patients (79%), while four patients showed hypovascularity (all benign lesions with small neoplastic nodules difficult to identify).
Acinar cell carcinoma	2	Contrast-enhancing neoplastic nodules were identified in both patients
Solid pseudopapillary neoplasia	1	Contrast-enhancing vessels were identified
Pseudocysts	90	Contrast-enhancing vessels traversing the pseudocyst were identified in eight of the 90 patients

Table 18.8 Patients who were included or excluded relative to the final diagnosis. Exclusion criteria were: no sign of chronic pancreatitis, cystic lesion > 20 mm, no active hormone production by the tumor, multiple lesions, metastasis, allergic reaction to SonoVue

Final diagnosis	CEUS performed	Excluded from study evaluation	Included in study evaluation
Pancreatic cancer	224	154	70 (31%)
Neuroendocrine tumor	107	82	25 (23%)
Serous microcystic adenoma	30	16	14 (47%)
Lymphoma	8	8	0 (0%)
Acinar cell carcinoma	3	3	0 (0%)
Mucinous cystadenoma or cystadenocarcinoma	16	16	0 (0%)
Intraductal papillary mucinous neoplasia	5	5	0 (0%)
Autoimmune pancreatitis	6	3	3 (50%)
Total	399	287	112 (28%)

Table 18.9 Isovascularity/hypervascularity as a sign of nonductal adenocarcinoma showed a sensitivity of 100%, a specificity of 90%, and an accuracy of 93.8%. Hypovascularity as a sign of ductal adenocarcinoma showed a sensitivity of 90%, a specificity of 100%, and an accuracy of 93.8%

	Sensitivity (%)	Specificity (%)	Positive predictive value (%)	Negative predictive value (%)	Accuracy (%)
Hypovascularity as a sign of ductal adenocarcinoma	90.0 (80.5–95.9)	100 (91.6–100)	100 (94.3–100)	85.7 (72.8–94.1)	93.8 (87.6–97.5)
Hypervascularity as a sign of non-ductal adenocarcinoma	100 (91.6–100)	90.0 (80.5–95.9)	85.7 (72.8–94.1)	100 (94.3–100)	93.8 (87.6–97.5)

NB: Test characteristics for predicting the benign or malignant status of the pancreatic lesion are given in **Table 18.6**, including 95% confidence intervals.

A total of 112 solitary indeterminate pancreatic masses (70 ductal adenocarcinomas and 42 neoplastic nodules of other origin) were thus prospectively examined using transabdominal ultrasound in patients without metastatic disease. Tumor-enhancing features were analyzed in comparison with the surrounding pancreatic parenchyma in patients in whom adequate visualization was achieved. The results are summarized in **Tables 18.8** and **18.9**. The findings have been reproduced in a multicenter trial, the Pancreatic Multicenter Ultrasound Study (PAMUS) including more than 1000 patients in Italy, Japan, and Germany (data not yet published).

Conclusions

Successful management and treatment of pancreatic tumors require highly sensitive and specific imaging techniques. Endoscopic or transabdominal contrast-enhanced ultrasonography can effectively differentiate between solid pancreatic tumors in many cases. Histology is still the reference standard for differentiating pancreatic lesions, although it can produce false-negative results if the specimens obtained are not representative.

When there is definitive proof of a *hypovascular* pancreatic tumor and a strong suspicion of a ductal adenocarcinoma without distant metastases in which curative surgery is possible, there is a primary indication for surgery, and puncture to obtain a histological sample is not necessary. This does not imply that every patient with a pancreatic mass should undergo surgery without further consideration, however, but rather that all options for preoperative diagnosis (in particular imaging methods) must have been exhausted. In contrast to the earlier view that 95% of all pancreatic tumors are ductal adenocarcinomas, it can be shown that up to 50% of these lesions examined in specialized centers are in fact other tumor entities. It is therefore crucially important to clarify the malignant status of these lesions preoperatively, as the significant level of perioperative mortality needs to be taken into account. The quality of the preoperative diagnostic work-up at an interdisciplinary center can therefore also be rated on the basis of preoperatively correctly identified diagnoses—for example, avoidance of modified Whipple–Kausch operations (pancreatoduodenectomies).

In patients who are not candidates for surgery, it is mandatory to carry out biopsy sampling to provide at least a cytological finding before palliative chemotherapy is started. Most other very rare entities are also hypervascular, and biopsy sampling to provide a histological diagnosis (not cytology!) is mandatory for individual therapeutic strategies, which mostly result in resection.

In summary, biopsy is important, since isovascular and hypervascular lesions imply different therapeutic approaches in comparison with ductal adenocarcinomas of the pancreas, which are usually hypovascular. It should be taken into account that histology is mandatory for definitive diagnosis of serous microcystic pancreatic adenomas (to determine the vascular nature and architecture of this type of lesion, which cannot be determined by cytology), autoimmune pancreatitis (to determine periductal inflammation and fibrosis, which cannot be determined by cytology), and neuroendocrine neoplasia (to yield at least 50 high-power fields, to determine whether the lesion is benign or malignant). In patients with serous cystadenomas, follow-up may be recommended, whereas patients with nonfunctional neuroendocrine tumors will undergo surgery due to the malignant potential of the lesions. Differentiated neuroendocrine tumors should be enucleated (if possible), preserving pancreatic tissue

Table 18.10 Indication for fine-needle aspiration cytology

Documentation of malignancy in patients with unresectable pancreatic tumor before palliative therapy
To exclude other malignant tumor entities
In patients who are hesitant to undergo radical surgery due to a relatively high associated mortality rate
To document benign status when there is a low pretest probability of a malignant mass

(and observing the appropriate criteria—for example, a margin between the tumor and the main pancreatic duct of >5 mm/10 mm, etc.) and should not undergo radical surgery. Patients with hypovascular pancreatic lesions and no contraindications (such as liver metastases or peritoneal metastases) should primarily undergo surgery without biopsy, as the findings are indicative of ductal adenocarcinoma.

The indications for fine-needle aspiration cytology are listed in **Table 18.10**.

Elastography

The value of elastography in the differential diagnosis of pancreatic lesions is discussed in Chapter 8.

Autoimmune pancreatitis. A recently published prospective evaluation aimed to investigate the role of real-time EUS elastography in the diagnosis of autoimmune pancreatitis (AIP). The patterns of elastographic images were compared with conventional EUS aspects and with histological findings obtained by transabdominal needle biopsy.

We recently evaluated the indications and possible limitations of tissue real-time elastography using EUS in patients with focal pancreatic disease. It was shown that adequate and reproducible elastographic imaging of focal pancreatic disease is confined to lesions less than 30 mm in diameter. In larger lesions, elastographic delineation was incomplete. It is also important to note that adequate acquisition of elastographic images depends on examining the surrounding pancreatic parenchyma. For optimal elastographic image acquisition, the density of the region of interest needs to be compared with the surrounding tissue as the reference standard, with a ratio of displayed target tissue to the surrounding parenchyma of ≈ 1 : 1.

In contrast to the initially disappointing data on the differential diagnosis of benign and malignant pancreatic disease using elastography, the results are much more promising with AIP. The most important implication of optimized diagnostic imaging is that surgery can be avoided. This was demonstrated in a study with a long follow-up period. AIP was not diagnosed at surgery in any of the patients examined during the study period, between 2005 and 2009; the condition was identified in all of the patients using real-time tissue elastography[41]. These findings are in contrast to recently published studies showing that ≈ 5% of patients with a final diagnosis of AIP underwent surgery. Kajiwara and co-workers reported on ≈ 160 patients with suspected pancreatic adenocarcinomas, 15 of whom (9%) proved to have nonneoplastic pancreatic changes, seven of them (4%) with AIP.[42] Other publications have reported a rate of 10% benign findings and 3–5% with AIP at surgery.[42–47]

On elastographic imaging, most pancreatic tumors have a monotonous appearance, largely dominated by blue (stiff) planes or strands with only minor heterogeneity, including softer tissue colors, but with a normal elastographic pattern in the remaining pancreatic parenchyma if no calcifications or duct enlargement appear as signs of chronic obstructive pancreatic disease. Patients with AIP do not show any calcifications or pancreatic duct enlargement. In contrast, all five patients with histologically confirmed AIP presented with a unique pattern of small, spotted, mainly blue (stiff) color signals that were evenly spread over the head and body of the pancreas. The elastographic pattern of AIP was characteristic enough to distinguish it from all other disease entities and normal pancreatic tissue that were evaluated in this recently published study, and it can be concluded elastography may be helpful in identifying patients with AIP.[41]

Jansen et al. recently investigated the clinical application of sonoelastography in patients with inflammatory pancreatic disease and in patients presenting with and without pancreatic lesions.[48] In agreement with our own recently published findings,[49] the elastographic patterns for chronic pancreatitis and most pancreatic tumors were described as monotonous, with a blue/green honeycomb pattern. Patients with the classical form of chronic obstructive calcified pancreatitis and mass lesions in the pancreatic head typically show duct enlargement and/or parenchymal calcification and fibrous strands, an appearance that is different from the echo-rich parenchyma in patients with AIP without ductal enlargement.

EUS-guided real-time elastography of the pancreas may therefore provide complementary information for improved tissue characterization and thereby avoid the need for surgery, particularly when it is used to characterize AIP. A final diagnosis of AIP should be obtained with transcutaneous transabdominal biopsy and histological analysis, showing the typical signs of periductal inflammation and fibrosis that cannot be demonstrated with fine-needle aspiration cytology. However, this hypothesis still requires further confirmation in prospective and controlled studies.

References

1. Dietrich CF, Chichakli M, Hirche TO, et al. Sonographic findings of the hepatobiliary-pancreatic system in adult patients with cystic fibrosis. J Ultrasound Med 2002; 21(4):409–416, quiz 417.
2. Seifert H. Endoscopic treatment of chronic pancreatitis. [Article in German] Praxis (Bern 1994) 2005;94(22): 911–923.
3. Seifert H, Faust D, Schmitt T, Dietrich C, Caspary W, Wehrmann T. Transmural drainage of cystic peripancreatic lesions with a new large-channel echo endoscope. Endoscopy 2001;33(12):1022–1026.
4. Seifert H, Wehrmann T, Schmitt T, Zeuzem S, Caspary WF. Retroperitoneal endoscopic debridement for infected peripancreatic necrosis. Lancet 2000;356(9230):653–655.
5. Seifert H, Dietrich C, Schmitt T, Caspary W, Wehrmann T. Endoscopic ultrasound-guided one-step transmural drainage of cystic abdominal lesions with a large-channel echo endoscope. Endoscopy 2000;32(3):255–259.
6. Jenssen C, Dietrich CF. Endoscopic ultrasound in chronic pancreatitis. [Article in German] Z Gastroenterol 2005; 43(8):737–749.
7. François E, Kahaleh M, Giovannini M, Matos C, Devière J. EUS-guided pancreaticogastrostomy. Gastrointest Endosc 2002;56(1):128–133.
8. Giovannini M, Moutardier V, Pesenti C, Bories E, Lelong B, Delpero JR. Endoscopic ultrasound-guided bilioduodenal anastomosis: a new technique for biliary drainage. Endoscopy 2001;33(10):898–900.
9. Giovannini M, Pesenti C, Rolland AL, Moutardier V, Delpero JR. Endoscopic ultrasound-guided drainage of pancreatic pseudocysts or pancreatic abscesses using a therapeutic echo endoscope. Endoscopy 2001;33(6):473–477.
10. Giovannini M, Bernardini D, Seitz JF. Cystogastrotomy entirely performed under endosonography guidance for pancreatic pseudocyst: results in six patients. Gastrointest Endosc 1998;48(2):200–203.
11. Volkan Adsay N. Cystic lesions of the pancreas. Mod Pathol 2007;20(Suppl 1):S71–S93.
12. Kosmahl M, Pauser U, Peters K, et al. Cystic neoplasms of the pancreas and tumor-like lesions with cystic features: a review of 418 cases and a classification proposal. Virchows Arch 2004;445(2):168–178.
13. Compagno J, Oertel JE. Mucinous cystic neoplasms of the pancreas with overt and latent malignancy (cystadenocarcinoma and cystadenoma). A clinicopathologic study of 41 cases. Am J Clin Pathol 1978;69(6):573–580.
14. Compagno J, Oertel JE. Microcystic adenomas of the pancreas (glycogen-rich cystadenomas): a clinicopathologic study of 34 cases. Am J Clin Pathol 1978;69(3):289–298.
15. Frossard JL, Amouyal P, Amouyal G, et al. Performance of endosonography-guided fine needle aspiration and biopsy in the diagnosis of pancreatic cystic lesions. Am J Gastroenterol 2003;98(7):1516–1524.
16. Brugge WR. The use of EUS to diagnose cystic neoplasms of the pancreas. Gastrointest Endosc 2009; 69(2, Suppl): S203–S209.
17. Dietrich CF, Jenssen C, Allescher H-D, Hocke M, Barreiros AP, Ignee A. Differential diagnosis of pancreatic lesions using endoscopic ultrasound. [Article in German] Z Gastroenterol 2008;46(6):601–617.
18. Palazzo L, O'Toole D, Hammel P. Technique of pancreatic cyst aspiration. Gastrointest Endosc 2009; 69(2, Suppl): S146–S151.

19. Brugge WR, Lewandrowski K, Lee-Lewandrowski E, et al. Diagnosis of pancreatic cystic neoplasms: a report of the cooperative pancreatic cyst study. Gastroenterology 2004;126(5):1330–1336.
20. Brugge WR. Evaluation of pancreatic cystic lesions with EUS. Gastrointest Endosc 2004;59(6):698–707.
21. Levy MJ, Smyrk TC, Reddy RP, et al. Endoscopic ultrasound-guided trucut biopsy of the cyst wall for diagnosing cystic pancreatic tumors. Clin Gastroenterol Hepatol 2005;3(10):974–979.
22. Scheiman JM. Management of cystic lesions of the pancreas. J Gastrointest Surg 2008;12(3):405–407.
23. Fasanella KE, McGrath K. Cystic lesions and intraductal neoplasms of the pancreas. Best Pract Res Clin Gastroenterol 2009;23(1):35–48.
24. Le Borgne J, de Calan L, Partensky C; French Surgical Association. Cystadenomas and cystadenocarcinomas of the pancreas: a multiinstitutional retrospective study of 398 cases. Ann Surg 1999;230(2):152–161.
25. DeWitt J, McGreevy K, Schmidt CM, Brugge WR. EUS-guided ethanol versus saline solution lavage for pancreatic cysts: a randomized, double-blind study. Gastrointest Endosc 2009;70(4):710–723.
26. Farrell JJ, Brugge WR. Intraductal papillary mucinous tumor of the pancreas. Gastrointest Endosc 2002;55(6):701–714.
27. Furukawa T, Klöppel G, Volkan Adsay N, et al. Classification of types of intraductal papillary-mucinous neoplasm of the pancreas: a consensus study. Virchows Arch 2005;447(5):794–799.
28. Andrejevic-Blant S, Kosmahl M, Sipos B, Klöppel G. Pancreatic intraductal papillary-mucinous neoplasms: a new and evolving entity. Virchows Arch 2007;451(5):863–869.
29. Maire F, Couvelard A, Hammel P, et al. Intraductal papillary mucinous tumors of the pancreas: the preoperative value of cytologic and histopathologic diagnosis. Gastrointest Endosc 2003;58(5):701–706.
30. Kobayashi G, Fujita N, Noda Y, et al. Mode of progression of intraductal papillary-mucinous tumor of the pancreas: analysis of patients with follow-up by EUS. J Gastroenterol 2005;40(7):744–751.
31. Bardales RH, Centeno B, Mallery JS, et al. Endoscopic ultrasound-guided fine-needle aspiration cytology diagnosis of solid-pseudopapillary tumor of the pancreas: a rare neoplasm of elusive origin but characteristic cytomorphologic features. Am J Clin Pathol 2004;121(5):654–662.
32. Master SS, Savides TJ. Diagnosis of solid-pseudopapillary neoplasm of the pancreas by EUS-guided FNA. Gastrointest Endosc 2003;57(7):965–968.
33. Kosmahl M, Peters K, Anlauf M, et al. Solid pseudopapillary neoplasms. Enigmatic entity with female preponderance. [Article in German] Pathologe 2005;26(1):41–45.
34. Bunk A, Pistorius S, Konopke R, Ockert D, Kuhlisch E, Saeger HD. The value of colour duplex sonography in the assessment of surgical resectability of pancreatic tumors. [Article in German] Ultraschall Med 2001;22(6):265–273.
35. Meining A, Dittler HJ, Wolf A, et al. You get what you expect? A critical appraisal of imaging methodology in endosonographic cancer staging. Gut 2002;50(5):599–603.
36. Rösch T, Lightdale CJ, Botet JF, et al. Localization of pancreatic endocrine tumors by endoscopic ultrasonography. N Engl J Med 1992;326(26):1721–1726.
37. Fritscher-Ravens A, Sriram PV, Krause C, et al. Detection of pancreatic metastases by EUS-guided fine-needle aspiration. Gastrointest Endosc 2001;53(1):65–70.
38. Fritscher-Ravens A. Endoscopic ultrasound and neuroendocrine tumours of the pancreas. JOP 2004;5(4):273–281.
39. Dietrich CF, Ignee A, Braden B, Barreiros AP, Ott M, Hocke M. Improved differentiation of pancreatic tumors using contrast-enhanced endoscopic ultrasound. Clin Gastroenterol Hepatol 2008;6(5):590–597, e1.
40. Dietrich CF, Braden B, Hocke M, Ott M, Ignee A. Improved characterisation of solitary solid pancreatic tumours using contrast enhanced transabdominal ultrasound. J Cancer Res Clin Oncol 2008;134(6):635–643.
41. Dietrich CF, Hirche TO, Ott M, Ignee A. Real-time tissue elastography in the diagnosis of autoimmune pancreatitis. Endoscopy 2009;41(8):718–720.
42. Kajiwara M, Gotohda N, Konishi M, et al. Incidence of the focal type of autoimmune pancreatitis in chronic pancreatitis suspected to be pancreatic carcinoma: experience of a single tertiary cancer center. Scand J Gastroenterol 2008;43(1):110–116.
43. Abraham SC, Wilentz RE, Yeo CJ, et al. Pancreaticoduodenectomy (Whipple resections) in patients without malignancy: are they all 'chronic pancreatitis'? Am J Surg Pathol 2003;27(1):110–120.
44. Hardacre JM, Iacobuzio-Donahue CA, Sohn TA, et al. Results of pancreaticoduodenectomy for lymphoplasmacytic sclerosing pancreatitis. Ann Surg 2003;237(6):853–858; discussion 58–59.
45. Kennedy T, Preczewski L, Stocker SJ, et al. Incidence of benign inflammatory disease in patients undergoing Whipple procedure for clinically suspected carcinoma: a single-institution experience. Am J Surg 2006;191(3):437–441.
46. Sasson AR, Gulizia JM, Galva A, Anderson J, Thompson J. Pancreaticoduodenectomy for suspected malignancy: have advancements in radiographic imaging improved results? Am J Surg 2006;192(6):888–893.
47. Weber SM, Cubukcu-Dimopulo O, Palesty JA, et al. Lymphoplasmacytic sclerosing pancreatitis: inflammatory mimic of pancreatic carcinoma. J Gastrointest Surg 2003;7(1):129–137; discussion 37–39.
48. Janssen J, Schlorer E, Greiner L. EUS elastography of the pancreas: feasibility and pattern description of the normal pancreas, chronic pancreatitis, and focal pancreatic lesions. Gastrointest Endosc 2007;65(7):971–978.
49. Hirche TO, Ignee A, Barreiros AP, et al. Indications and limitations of endoscopic ultrasound elastography for evaluation of focal pancreatic lesions. Endoscopy 2008;40(11):910–917.

19 Pancreatic Interventions

H. Seifert, C.F. Dietrich

Due to its retroperitoneal position, the pancreas is difficult to reach using all of the conventional surgical techniques, including open or laparoscopic surgery. From the endosonographic point of view, however, it is only a few millimeters from the transducer—a distance corresponding to the thickness of the duodenal or gastric wall. The development of endoscopic ultrasound (EUS) therefore led to the development of EUS-guided interventions in the pancreas. These interventions almost always relate to peripancreatic fluid collections, usually resulting from acute or chronic pancreatitis.

In the early 1980s, for patients with chronic pancreatitis, the alternatives to letting the process run its spontaneous course, on the one hand, and carrying out pancreatectomy with unsatisfactory results on the other, included surgical drainage procedures with dilation of the pancreatic duct in cases of obstruction. At about the same time, alternative techniques were developed, with the objective of making the resection less radical and the drainage less invasive: resection of the head of the pancreas, preserving the duodenum, and endoscopic decompression using pancreatic papillotomy, extraction of stones, and stent placement. At the same time, as part of the new endoscopic treatments for chronic pancreatitis, the first endoscopic transpapillary and transmural drainage procedures were carried out in pancreatic pseudocysts. These endoscopic techniques have been found to be technically successful, with low complication rates, and not just in individual cases. It has also been established that successful puncture and drainage can at least reduce the often considerable symptoms. This form of treatment has developed substantially, particularly with the aid of endosonography.

Cystic Pancreatic Lesions: Definition and Classification

Pathological cavities in the region of the pancreas can be classified using a wide variety of characteristics. In clinical practice, lesions can be described from various points of view (**Table 19.1**),[1–4] although the characteristics of one category (e.g., size) do not necessarily allow conclusions to be drawn about another category (such as the prognosis).

This situation has led to some uncertainty regarding the classification and definition of cystic lesions of this type. The most important questions in clinical practice are answered by simple sonomorphological characterization of the lesions with regard to shape, size, position, and echo pattern. This applies in particular when the technique also provides information about the topographical and pathological anatomy of the vessels and of the pancreatic and bile ducts, and when information about the development of the cysts can be obtained over a period of a few weeks. Information of similar value to that provided by ultrasound can also be obtained with magnetic resonance imaging (MRI) and computed tomography (CT).

A second classification according to etiology and pathogenesis can be made on the basis of the sonomorphology and medical history, but sometimes not until endoscopic retrograde cholangiopancreatography (ERCP) or histological assessment have been carried out (**Table 19.2**).

Awareness of these differential-diagnostic alternatives is important during the endoscopic drainage of cystic lesions. In particular, cystic neoplasias must not be over-

Table 19.1 Normal methods of clinical description of peripancreatic fluid collections

Criteria	Terms used
Medical history, age	Acute/chronic, mature/immature
Underlying illness	Post-pancreatitis, idiopathic, neoplastic
Symptoms	Symptomatic/asymptomatic
Size	Microcystic, large (>6 cm), small (≤6 cm)
Shape	Monocystic/polycystic, causing bulging/no bulging, septate/nonseptate
Image of contents	Anechoic/hypoechoic/echogenic
Content as aspirate	Serous, liquid, mucinous, putrid, hemorrhagic ("chocolate cyst"), solid, infected/sterile, amylase present/absent
Boundaries	With/without wall, sharply/poorly delineated, arched–round, complex/branched
Connections	With/without fistula to: pancreatic duct, stomach, ascites, retroperitoneum, pleura, mediastinum, other cysts
Position	Intrapancreatic/extrapancreatic, head–body–tail
Malignancy	Benign/malignant

Table 19.2 Classification of cystic peripancreatic lesions in relation to etiology and pathogenesis

Diagnosis	Comments
Result of pancreatitis	Pseudocysts and other lesions (see the Atlanta classification, **Table 19.3**)
Duodenal wall cysts	Intramural. Genesis unclear; caused by ectopic pancreas or inflammation of the head of the pancreas?
Idiopathic pancreatic cysts	Rare, sporadic, or in polycystic disease
Cystic pancreatic tumors	Microcystic or macrocystic, serous or mucinous. Malignancy in principle unclear
Genuine pancreatic cysts	Rare, probably mostly IPMN
Pancreas duplication cysts	Rare, benign[1]
Lymphocele	Benign, rare, in parenchyma; the surroundings are normal, the edges smooth and very delicate, no wall[2]
Hydatid disease	Rare[3,4]
Wall abscess	Rare; endoscopic ultrasound demonstrates the position in the wall of the stomach

looked. Even acute or chronic pancreatitis can cause or possibly be the consequence of a pancreatic carcinoma.

Malignant pancreatic tumors, the prevalence of which among cystic pancreatic processes is estimated to be ≈ 5–10%, are the most important differential diagnosis. Detailed descriptions of the classification and diagnosis of cystic pancreatic tumors have recently been published.[5–7] Serous or mucinous neoplasia should always be considered; they cannot always be recognized by the typical microcystic or polycystic shape or by mucous filling of the duct (**Figs. 19.1, 19.2, 19.3,** and **19.4**).[8]

The most accurate method of imaging various cystic lesions is endosonography. By far the majority of peripancreatic fluid collections are the result of episodes of pancreatitis. Following less convincing attempts to classify pseudocysts systematically, the classification shown in **Table 19.3**[9] was finally proposed for fluid collections caused by pancreatitis, as part of the Atlanta classification of acute pancreatitis. The Atlanta classification includes the common *postacute fluid collections,* which are not sharply delimited and often resolve spontaneously, and are filled with clear (anechoic) fluid; *pseudocysts* surrounded by a fibrous wall; and *necroses*—three findings that can also be differentiated very easily on a clinical basis. In practice, however, such pure findings are the exception, and transitional states are the norm. If it is difficult even to draw a clear line between acute pancreatitis and acute episodes of chronic pancreatitis, it is certainly difficult and unreliable to attempt a clear clinical classification of their "cystic" complications, with superimposition of older and more recent findings, liquid and solid, echogenic and hypoechoic, sterile, contaminated and infected (purulent) cysts with more or less well-defined walls (and anatomic delimitation). Despite these limitations, the Atlanta classification is currently the best and only clinically useful classification of pancreatogenic cysts, precisely because it bows to practice and attempts to use different categories to do justice to the characteristics of quite different types of cyst.

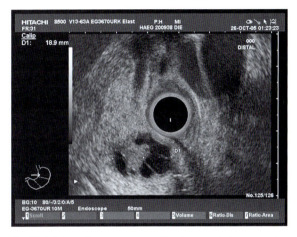

Fig. 19.1 Polycystic serous pancreatic adenoma. Endosonography, radial scanner (3670 UR). The tumor as a whole has a roundish border. It displays larger cysts, but also honeycombed, microcystic areas. The surrounding pancreatic parenchyma is normal.

The classification proposed by Nealon and Walser in 2002[10] is based solely on the anatomy of the pancreatic duct:

- Type I: normal duct, no communication with the pseudocyst
- Type II: normal duct, communication with the pseudocyst
- Type III: otherwise normal duct with stricture, no communication with the pseudocyst
- Type IV: otherwise normal duct with stricture, communication with the pseudocyst
- Type VI: otherwise normal duct with complete cut-off
- Type VII: chronic pancreatitis, no duct–pseudocyst communication
- Type VIII: chronic pancreatitis, duct–pseudocyst communication

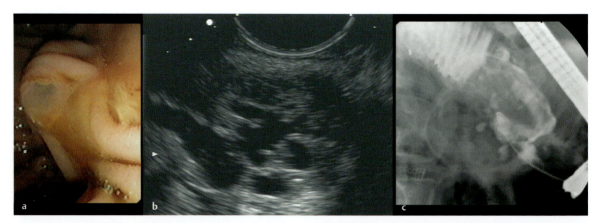

Fig. 19.2a–c A mucus-producing pancreatic tumor.
a The tumor was revealed by a fishmouth papilla. The viscous mucus forced the pancreatic ostium wide open.

b The mucus filled the pancreatic duct system, which had a cystically dilated appearance on EUS (longitudinal scanner, 7.5 MHz, Pentax FG38-UX, Pentax, Hamburg, Germany).
c The corresponding endoscopic retrograde cholangiogram.

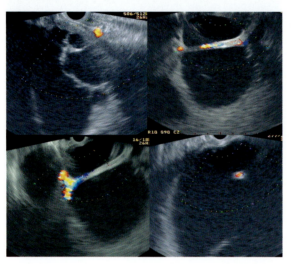

Fig. 19.3 A huge cystic retroperitoneal finding dorsal to the stomach, with anechoic contents, delicate septa, and unusually with arteries flowing through the lumen. There was no definite pancreatitis in the medical history, and no changes in the pancreatic parenchyma as found in chronic pancreatitis. Transmural drainage was not performed due to the suspect finding, and open surgery was performed instead. Histological analysis showed that the lesion was a benign pseudocyst.

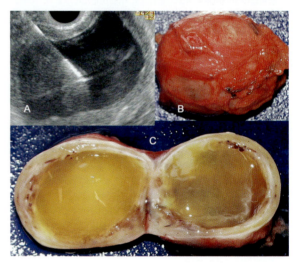

Fig. 19.4a–c a A cystic lesion in the body of the pancreas with a strong wall, thickened dorsally, and anechoic contents, in a 46-year-old patient with no signs of acute or chronic pancreatitis in the medical history or abdominal ultrasound findings. The symptoms included a slight pulling sensation during vigorous movement.
b, c Surgically, a previously unreported type of pancreatic ganglioneuroma was enucleated.[8] EUS-guided fine-needle aspiration revealed highly viscous mucus. The course was uncomplicated. This example shows how difficult it can be to distinguish between cystic lesions following pancreatitis and neoplastic lesions.

This classification addresses the important and previously unclear issue of the influence of communications between the pancreatic duct and the fluid collection on the treatment strategy and its chances of success. Using their own retrospective data, the authors show that percutaneous drainage has little chance of success when a communication is present.

The present authors have not found that it is beneficial to make the treatment procedure dependent on the existence of this type of communication, particularly since the

existence of a fistula of this type is often difficult to establish and even more difficult to rule out. This fact is also reflected in the large differences between the values for the prevalence of such fistulas reported by different authors. The values vary between 6%, cited by Neoptolemos,[11] 20% by Barthet et al.,[12] and up to 60% by Nealon et al.[13] Large pseudocysts or necrotic cavities, inflammatory swelling of the head of the pancreas or of the duodenal wall, or scarring and calcification in chronic pancreatitis can change the normal anatomy to such an extent that

Table 19.3 Clinical classification of peripancreatic fluid collections in accordance with the 1992 Atlanta classification[9]

Description	Definition	Clinical manifestation	Pathology	Comments
Acute fluid collections	Fluid collections in or on the pancreas, occurring early in the course of acute pancreatitis and lacking a wall	Occurs in 30–50%; spontaneous regression in approx. 50%. Most easily detected by sonography	Sometimes contaminated with bacteria, composition variable, fluid	Can develop into pseudo-cysts or abscesses. Course cannot be predicted
Pancreatic necrosis	Diffuse or focal tissue necrosis, typically together with peripancreatic fatty tissue necrosis	Detection by sonography, dynamic computed tomography or MRI	The necroses can involve fatty tissue and all parts of the pancreas. Sometimes with hemorrhage.	Can become infected, and is then life-threatening (fine-needle biopsy, bacteriography of the aspirate)
Infected necrosis			Contains pus and necrotic tissue	Life-threatening, indication for surgical treatment
Acute pseudocyst	Fluid collection present more than 4 weeks after acute pancreatitis, with a wall of fibrous or granulation tissue	Clinical symptoms depend on position and size; most easily detected by sonography with CT	Usually contains pancreatic juice with high enzyme concentration; is (initially) sterile, sometimes contaminated with bacteria	Often has fistula connecting to pancreatic duct. Danger of infection
Chronic pseudocyst	Fluid collection with a wall of fibrous or granulation tissue in chronic pancreatitis, without previous episodes of acute pancreatitis	Clinical symptoms depend on position and size, most easily detected by sonography or CT	Usually contains pancreatic juice with high enzyme concentrations, is (initially) sterile, sometimes contaminated with bacteria	Often has fistula connecting to pancreatic duct. Danger of infection
Pancreatic or peri-pancreatic abscess	Circumscribed peri-pancreatic putrid abscess that occurs as a result of acute pancreatitis or pancreatic trauma	Symptoms variable, as for pseudocyst; in addition, occasionally clinical picture of sepsis	Contains pus, no or very little necrosis, synonymous with infected pseudocyst, but also with liquefied and infected circumscribed necrosis	Less threatening than infected necrosis, easier to treat

CT, computed tomography; MRI, magnetic resonance imaging.

endoscopic retrograde pancreatography (ERP) is impossible or very difficult. Even if the pancreatic duct can be examined, fistulas often cannot be clearly identified due to compression caused by the cystic lesions and calcification. In addition, a high level of injection pressure is often required, and—especially for very large pseudocysts—large quantities of contrast agent are needed to clearly identify the communication between the pancreatic duct and pseudocyst, necrotic cavity, or even stomach, mediastinum, abdominal cavity, or bile duct. We avoid this sort of procedure, which involves a substantial risk of introducing bacterial contamination (almost always) or manifest septic complications. In addition, the anatomy can often be imaged without any problems following decompression of the pseudocyst or necrotic cavity. Magnetic resonance cholangiopancreatography (MRCP) is not capable of detecting narrow fistulas in complex anatomy either, so it is not an alternative to ERCP. On the other hand, if the latter is easy to do and shows a clear communication between the duct and the pseudocyst, transpapillary drainage is often successful on its own. It has not been demonstrated whether, in such cases, it is better to fit the pancreatic duct with a stent to bridge the fistula (our preference, which we like to combine with transmural drainage) or to drain the cyst directly through the fistula.

None of the classifications of cystic lesions mentioned is suitable for stratifying patients according to the severity of the condition. In clinical practice, an overview of aspects covered by the individual classifications, the serum C-reactive protein (CRP) level, and symptoms during the course of the illness provide a tried-and-tested basis for the treatment strategy.

Epidemiology

Pseudocysts are typical complications of chronic pancreatitis. They are found in up to 60% of surgical specimens from patients with chronic pancreatitis, and, according to Stolte,[14] more often in preparations with segmental (48%) than with nonsegmental (23%) chronic pancreatitis. In large clinically recorded populations with chronic pancreatitis, pseudocysts have been described in 23% of patients (56 of 245).[15] These data relate to a symptomatic and consequently treated population (usually treated surgically). The actual prevalence of pancreatic pseudocysts and other cystic lesions in chronic pancreatitis, including uncomplicated courses, is presumably substantially lower.

Values cited for the incidence of peripancreatic fluid accumulations in acute pancreatitis lie between 14%[16] and (when detected with CT) over 50%.[17]

Pancreatic necroses develop in ≈ 5% (17 of 348)[18] to 20% (38 of 194)[19] of patients with acute pancreatitis. Up to 70% of them have primary infection. In recent publications, the mortality rate due to infected necroses has been reported to be 10–35%.

In 100 patients included in a study in Glasgow,[20] the mortality rate due to pseudocysts of biliary origin, at 22%, was distinctly higher than for pseudocysts of alcoholic origin, at 5%. The overall figure was 12%; only patients with postacute pseudocysts who had undergone surgery were included. In most cases, the cause of death was sepsis or hemorrhage. All patients with chronic pseudocysts survived. A mortality rate of 5–15% has generally been reported for cystic lesions following pancreatitis. However, it is scarcely possible to give a figure for the spontaneous course, as the patients detected epidemiologically have usually been treated and thus represent a selection.

With very few exceptions, the data shown here apply to "publication-relevant" groups of patients in fairly large centers—i.e., only to the more severe courses of the clinical pictures concerned. The incidence and prevalence of problems and complications may therefore have been overestimated. However, selection of this sort also applies in general to patients, including those undergoing interventional treatment.

Etiopathogenesis

Peripancreatic or intrapancreatic fluid collections can have various origins and are probably often the result of several pathological mechanisms working together.

Severe acute pancreatitis gives rise to peripancreatic fatty tissue necroses, occasionally with large fields of necrosis surrounding the pancreas like a coat and spreading along the fibrous tissue septa to the intrapancreatic fatty tissue, on the one hand, and to the more distant extrapancreatic fatty tissue (mesentery, omental bursa, retroperitoneum) on the other. Pseudocysts containing hemorrhagic and necrotic material develop from the larger necrosis fields within 7–30 days of the acute necrosis. With time, they separate themselves more clearly from their surroundings through the formation of granulation tissue. In most cases, they communicate with the pancreatic duct. Confluent intrapancreatic fatty tissue necroses are usually replaced by sclerotic tissue. This fibrotic process can involve the interlobular pancreatic ducts and encourage the development of chronic pancreatitis. Intrapancreatic pseudocysts can also persist due to communication with the ductal system and lead to local complications due to compression of the environment. In dogs, it has been shown that a pseudocyst takes ≈ 6 weeks to develop a "mature" fibrous wall.

Post-traumatic pancreatic pseudocysts are not common; in large populations, they represent a maximum of 5%. In children, they mainly occur after pancreatic rupture due to car accidents or due to trauma from bicycle handlebars. If the pancreatic duct remains continuous, spontaneous regression is possible.

Despite important recent evidence concerning the genetic and autoimmune pathogenesis of acute and chronic pancreatitis, the concept of more or less mechanical development is still the most important idea guiding the therapeutic procedure and the patient's well-being. Stolte's discussion of this subject from 1984,[14] based on thorough morphometric investigations, remains valid: whatever the nature of the etiology or course of the pancreatitis, "in the end, there is always an area of scar tissue. So the various subdivisions of chronic pancreatitis, with their histological types and duct patterns only appear to be snapshots of a continuous, progressive process ... There is a vicious circle of self-perpetuation in chronic pancreatitis. " The fact that a persistent fistula, traumatic rupture of the duct, and pancreas divisum are established causes or contributing factors in the formation of pseudocysts supports the view that the impaired flow is at least partly mechanical in origin.

Therapeutic Approaches

Any therapeutic intervention has to be weighed up in comparison with alternative treatments. Surgical or endoscopic interventions are only justified if their risk is lower than that of the spontaneous course or of noninvasive approaches. Different therapeutic strategies, including open surgery, have to be discussed with the patient to provide a basis for informed consent to any therapy. These alternatives are therefore considered here.

■ Objectives of Treatment

As in the treatment of chronic pancreatitis in general, a treatment strategy for pancreatogenic cystic lesions can serve very different purposes. As emergency treatment in acute complications such as rupture or hemorrhage, the objective is to avert the immediate danger, which is almost always achieved by surgery and does not require any discussion. In the case of infected pseudocysts or necroses, the prevention of life-threatening septic complications is without question an absolute indication for therapeutic intervention. The situation is similar for compression stenoses of the bile duct, duodenum, or stomach, which require surgery.

The most common reason for surgical treatment of pseudocysts is severe pain, followed by nausea and vomiting (as a consequence of the above-mentioned compression of the gastric and intestinal lumen), loss of weight, and jaundice. However, in the surgical literature, clear reference to the indications or the objectives of the intervention is not always made.

In asymptomatic or oligosymptomatic patients with large or persistent cysts, the prevention of likely complications of the spontaneous course (see below) always influences the therapeutic objectives, although there are no reliable data regarding the incidence of these. The complications can also be considered to include loss of the endocrine or exocrine function of the pancreas. In this case, maintaining the function of the organ (or preventing its loss in the "natural" course of the disease) would be the therapeutic objective. In the context of organ conservation, the treatment of cystic lesions—which is justified even for isolated lesions for improvement of symptoms—should be understood as only part of the decompressive and drainage treatment of the chronic pancreatitis. In this way, surgery has achieved encouraging results.[21–23] Endoscopic interventions are generally based on the hypothesis that reconstructing the normal anatomy, usually by drainage of congested regions, and restoring the normal flow of pancreatic juice can lead to an improvement in the symptoms and sometimes of the entire clinical course. In a multicenter retrospective analysis of more than 1000 patients with chronic pancreatitis, the symptoms improved in the long term in 65% of patients and in the short term in 85%.[24]

■ Spontaneous Course

The expected spontaneous course of a pancreatic pseudocyst depends on the time of observation. If a iquid lesion develops during the acute phase of pancreatitis, it is very probably peripancreatic edema with a good chance of spontaneous regression. Clinically, acute fluid collections of this type can correspond to a pseudocyst.

Spontaneous regression rates of 7%,[8] 12%,[25] 28%,[26] and 60%[27,28] have been reported, sometimes depending on the size of the cyst. According to some authors, spontaneous regression of pseudocysts is unlikely after more than 6 weeks. On the other hand, Vitas and Sarr, who retrospectively analyzed patients with pancreatic pseudocysts who were treated at the Mayo Clinic in the years 1980–85, came to a different conclusion.[29] Of 114 patients, 46 were given primary treatment by surgery. Only six (9%) of the remaining 68 patients, who were treated conservatively, had serious complications during a mean observation period of 46 months; 19 of them ultimately underwent elective surgery. Overall, the pseudocyst regressed spontaneously in 57% of the patients treated conservatively, in 38% of them more than 6 months after the diagnosis. Among these, seven patients had cysts more than 10 cm in diameter which regressed without complications. The authors conclude that, contrary to the earlier view, even older and very large pseudocysts can regress spontaneously; that a "wait-and-see" approach is therefore justified in most patients.

Relevant complications of the spontaneous course include hemorrhage, rupture, and infection. The incidence of these is difficult to specify, as it is normal to try to avoid such complications using surgical treatment. No reports on the spontaneous course in large populations of patients over prolonged observation periods are available.

Hemorrhagic complications—which can manifest as hemosuccus pancreaticus, and also as fulminant hemorrhage into a pseudocyst or as a consequence of cyst rupture—mostly arise from the splenic artery. The artery is affected by local reactions resulting from pancreatitis and can develop pseudoaneurysms as a typical complication in ≈3% of patients. Rupture of the pseudoaneurysm then leads to arterial bleeding. Major arteries originating from the celiac trunk, and not infrequently the splenic artery or hepatic artery, often pass directly by the walls of cystic lesions. They can be clearly seen there using ultrasonography even without Doppler imaging, whereas smaller vessels can only be seen with EUS. The splenic vein lies in the immediate vicinity in most cases of pancreatitis and pseudocysts. If it is affected by the inflammatory process, the typical complication is splenic vein thrombosis. This is apparent from the almost pathognomonic endoscopic picture of isolated gastric varices (without esophageal varices), sometimes together with duodenal varices. Bleeding varices can develop as life-threatening sequelae. The literature contains a large number of case studies on this topic, but there is no reliable information on the incidence of such vascular and hemorrhagic complications.

The same applies to spontaneous rupture of pseudocysts. Sankaran and Walt[30] observed spontaneous rupture in 19 of 131 pseudocysts (15%), with hemorrhage in four cases. Because of the high rate of spontaneous complications (33%), the authors advocate surgical drainage. Such a high rate of spontaneous complications has not been confirmed in the few other papers on the spontaneous course. Nevertheless, Seiler et al.,[31] on the basis of 154 patients with complicated chronic pancreatitis, describe the formation of pseudocysts as the most important prognostic risk factor, correlating highly significantly not only with pain but also with a higher incidence of vascular complications and a significantly higher risk of mortality (7.1%) than for patients without pseudocysts (1.8%).

There have been isolated reports of fistulas to the stomach, and of the spread of pseudocysts into the mediastinum with rupture or fistula into the esophagus, pseudoachalasia, or cardiac compression.

There is no reliable information on the incidence of spontaneous infection of initially sterile pseudocysts. Kolars et al.[32] found bacterial infection in 17 of 51 (33%) pseudocysts, although this was in a group of hospitalized patients who later underwent surgery—i.e., certainly not a representative population.

Imrie et al.[20] reported a mortality rate of 22% for patients with pancreatic pseudocysts of biliary origin (27% of the group), significantly higher than the mortality rate of 5% for pseudocysts of alcohol-induced origin (59% of the patients). In 1979, Bradley et al.[33] recommended that pseudocysts should not be kept under observation for long, as 41% of 54 patients with pancreatic cysts developed complications after an observation period of 2–4 months, with a mortality rate of 14%—higher than with surgical intervention.

Conservative Treatment

Patients with symptomatic cystic lesions have generally already undergone weeks or months of conservative treatment by various hospitals and doctors, require high doses of analgesics, and have undergone prolonged hospital stays and periods of fasting, often with parenteral feeding. They are referred because of the failure of these treatments. For most of the patients encountered here, conservative treatment is no longer a genuine alternative; instead, they specifically represent "the failures of the waiting game."[34]

Although treatment with somatostatin analogues has been repeatedly suggested for chronic pancreatitis, the usefulness of these agents has at best been demonstrated in combination with surgical treatment. They are of doubtful efficacy in conservative treatment regimens, at least in relation to pain.

Parenteral nutrition is at best of limited use in the treatment of symptomatic pseudocysts. In addition, it is not a low-risk therapy; potentially severe complications should be taken into consideration.

Interventional Treatment

Surgical Procedures

The objective of surgical treatment has been defined for decades. It consists of avoiding the various complications by removing necrotic and infected material and through drainage and lavage of existing cavities. The first successful treatment of a pancreatic pseudocyst by excision was performed in 1882 by Bozeman.[35] The first external drainage by marsupialization was described the following year by Gussenbauer,[36] a method that was still being practiced in recent times. Resection is now avoided. The objectives are to relieve cystic cavities and to carry out gentle (manual) removal of easily mobilized necrotic tissue. Cystic processes are opened and either drained externally or into the stomach (the first pseudocystogastrostomy was carried out in 1921 by Jedlica[37]), the duodenum (the first pseudocystoduodenostomy was performed in 1928 by

Hahn[38]), or the jejunum (the first pseudocystojejunostomy was carried out in 1931 by Jurasz[39]). In the last two cases, surgical anastomoses are established between the pseudocysts and the intestinal lumen and, in the case of the jejunum, Roux-en-Y anastomoses as well. The prerequisite for this type of cystointestostomy is that the cyst must have a wall that can be sutured. For this reason, the surgical literature often recommends waiting 5–6 weeks after the acute attack or the development of the cystic lesion before surgery, to provide sufficient time for a fibrous wall to form.

In the case of surgery, as for any other form of treatment, the question arises of whether different cystic lesions require specific therapeutic strategies. The procedure may depend on the clinical picture, the presence of infection, the pathogenesis, the morphology, etc. Infected and uninfected lesions should in principle be treated differently, with classical pseudocysts on the one hand and infected necroses on the other representing two very different clinical extremes in peripancreatic fluid collections. The most important aspects of these from a surgical viewpoint are therefore described in brief below.

The best surgical technique is a matter of dispute and may perhaps be a question both of the anatomical circumstances in the individual case and the surgeon's experience. Longitudinal opening and anastomosis of the pancreatic duct (Partington–Rochelle pancreaticojejunostomy) is favored by many, but—like endoscopic techniques—only secures drainage without reliably removing the chronic inflammatory foci frequently present in the head of the pancreas. In addition, the main problem of a pancreatogenic distal bile duct stenosis remains untreated. Whether resection of the head of the pancreas conserving the duodenum or a modified Whipple procedure with pancreaticoduodenectomy (whether or not conserving the pylorus) should be preferred in this case is still a matter of debate even among specialists. Jimenez et al. were unable to identify any advantage of pylorus-conserving pancreaticoduodenectomy over the classical Whipple procedure.[40]

In a randomized study, Izbicki et al. found that a combination of a drainage operation and local resection of the pancreatic head was slightly better than pylorus-conserving resection of the pancreatic head,[22] and a recent randomized study showed that the duodenum-conserving technique was clearly better than the classical Kausch–Whipple procedure in terms of pain, quality of life, and the patient's nutritional status.[41] As a rule of thumb, it may be stated that classical procedures for the treatment of the complications of chronic pancreatitis should solve all anatomical problems as rigorously as possible, so that further regular endoscopic treatment efforts after surgery can be expected to be unnecessary. A severely inflamed and often stenotic duodenum, a fibrotic bile duct that is stenotic over a long distance, and a long-standing "pseudotumor" in the head of the pancreas should be removed, and drainage secured. The outcome is considered to depend on the size of the inflamed head of the pancreas. In rare cases, a splenectomy may also be indicated. However, left subphrenic abscesses penetrating the spleen can also be successfully treated endoscopically.[42] Nealon and Walser found that, in the presence of ductal changes and pseudocysts, surgical drainage of the pancreatic duct without drainage of the cyst itself was adequate.[43]

In a prospective and randomized study comparing endoscopic and surgical treatment, 35% of the surgically treated and 15% of the endoscopically treated patients were pain-free after 5 years, and approximately half showed improvement in each case. Thus, if the less invasive endoscopic technique does not lead to success as the primary therapy, surgery is a good alternative.[44] Left resection of the pancreas has led to unsatisfactory results and should at best be considered in exceptional cases.

Data on intraportal autologous islet transplantation after pancreatectomy provide hope that more than half of those affected may be able to remain independent of insulin treatment.

Pseudocysts. Once CT and sonography in particular allowed precise morphological description of cystic lesions in the course of their development, the question of the correct time for surgical intervention became more urgent. Warshaw encouraged a waiting period of 6 weeks for spontaneous regression of pseudocysts after acute pancreatitis or an acute episode of chronic pancreatitis;[34] in chronic pancreatitis without an acute episode, persistence of cystic lesions for more than 4–6 weeks, and presence of thick walls and cicatricial ductal changes, regression was however considered unlikely. The author regarded a connection between the cyst and the pancreatic duct as a precondition for spontaneous regression. The specified minimum age of 4–6 weeks was calculated from the time of diagnosis, so it can only be regarded as reliable if the cyst was observed at the time it developed—i.e., in the course of acute pancreatitis. This "maturation period," which is still often considered to be necessary even today, originated in a number of papers by surgeons and does not appear to be essential from the endoscopic point of view.

Because of the realistic chance of spontaneous regression, treatment is usually regarded as indicated only in the case of symptomatic, infected, or very large pseudocysts.

Multiple pancreatic pseudocysts, which are reported in ≈ 10% of the affected patients, place particular demands on surgical drainage. In a recently published study,[45] pseudocysts were the most common indication for surgery in 231 patients with chronic pancreatitis.

Necroses. Up to 20% of patients with acute pancreatitis develop pancreatic necrosis. A secondary infection can be expected in more than 50% of these cases; this is regarded as an indication for an open drainage operation and is associated with a mortality rate of 10–15%. There is wide agreement on the indication for surgical or interventional treatment of infected necroses. The mortality rate is given as 10–35%.

Conservative treatment of sterile necroses is increasingly being advocated. According to this view, careful necrosectomy should be reserved for patients with extensive necroses, a clinical picture of sepsis, and multiple-organ failure. Every resection in acute pancreatitis becomes excessive treatment if vital tissue capable of recovery is removed as well. Bradley considers that surgical debridement of sterile necroses is not indicated, as it does not improve the course of the disease and leads to secondary infection in 25% of cases. For infected necroses, he believes that surgery is the treatment of choice, although the optimal drainage technique needs to be discussed, "despite occasional anecdotal reports of successful management by transcutaneous or endoscopic means."[46] Other centers recommend removal of sterile necroses as well[47] and report a mortality rate of less than 10% after surgical debridement.[48] The debridement has to be as complete as possible, as residual infected necrotic material adversely affects the prognosis. Recently, in a prospective trial, a minimally invasive "step-up" approach has been shown to be superior to open surgery in terms of morbidity.[70]

Percutaneous Drainage

Percutaneous drainage of uncomplicated pancreatic pseudocysts is a low-risk procedure when appropriate sonographic techniques are used, and it can produce good results, at least in the short term. It can be controlled by CT or sonography.[49,50]

Adams and Anderson[51] reported retrospectively on 52 CT-controlled punctures of pancreatic pseudocysts. The mortality rate was 0%, but the rate of infection in the puncture channel was 48%. The advantage of this method in comparison with surgery is the lower mortality rate (0% versus 7%), the lack of surgical trauma, and the fact that surgical treatment remains an option.

Some authors consider that percutaneous drainage is promising in normal ductal anatomy but is not indicated in chronically altered ductal anatomy with fistulas or strictures.

Van Sonnenberg et al. reported success rates of more than 90% after percutaneous puncture and drainage, despite 51% (of 101) pseudocysts having a primary infection.[50] The authors emphasized that large-caliber catheters and patience (average duration of drainage 33 days, maximum 119 days) are decisive for success; the mortality rate in patients with infected cysts was 8%.[52]

Percutaneous debridement of pancreatic necroses with special catheters has also been reported; this requires very long examination and exposure times.

Endoscopic Transmural Drainage

Intrapancreatic or peripancreatic fluid collections can be treated endoscopically using transpapillary drainage or transmural puncture and drainage. The transmural procedure should always be carried out under endosonographic guidance, as hemorrhagic complications can be avoided and complex anatomical situations can be mastered in this manner. This view can only be based on one comparative study,[53] which reported a significantly higher technical success rate for transmural puncture and drainage with EUS (100%) in comparison with no EUS (33%), as well as two bleeding complications (one fatal) without EUS, in comparison with no complications with EUS. In another comparative study, all patients were initially examined with EUS, and after futile conventional puncture it was considered logical to cross the patients over to the EUS-guided arm.[54] Today, an experienced investigator who had access to EUS would not perform transmural punctures without EUS due to immediate practical evidence.

The first transmural cyst puncture, reported in 1975 by Rogers et al.,[55] was only successful in the short term, as a relapse occurred. After only one further case report on the endoscopic transgastric method had been published, the technique of internal gastrocystic drainage, established percutaneously with ultrasound guidance and gastroscopic control, was developed by Hancke, Henriksen, and others. This technique produced promising results. Recently, there have been occasional reports of good results with combined percutaneous–endoscopic transgastric cyst drainage with ultrasound guidance.

However, the more rigorous procedure using gastroscopy was direct endoscopic puncture, favorable results with which in somewhat larger numbers of patients were then published.[56] Sahel et al. reported on 19 patients who underwent endoscopic cystoduodenostomy.[57] Eleven of the patients had communications between the cyst and the ductal system, which had no discernible effect on the clinical outcome. The complications that occurred were two cases of hemorrhage, one of which was fatal, and two perforations in patients without visible compression of the intestinal wall by the pseudocyst. Cremer et al. reported good success rates over 7 years, with only one hemorrhage as a complication, in 22 patients who underwent cystogastrostomy via a nasocystic catheter.[58] They mention the presence of an impression on the enteric wall by the cyst as a prerequisite for this procedure. In suitable cases, they regarded surgical treatment as the option of second choice after endoscopy. This report was followed by publications on the successful treatment of pancreatic pseudocysts, and also of abscesses by transpapillary drainage. Various instruments have been developed for endoscopic cyst drainage.

In 1999, Terblanche's group published their technical success rate, complication rate, and relapse rate for endoscopic drainage of pancreatic pseudocysts.[59] Among 66 pancreatic pseudocysts, 34 (52%) were suitable for endoscopic treatment, namely when they caused bulging of the stomach or duodenal wall. Endoscopic drainage was successful in 24 cases (71%), and the success rate with a follow-up period of 46 months was 62%, with a relapse rate of 7%. The factors held responsible for failure were a thick cyst wall, unfavorable position, and association with necrotizing pancreatitis.

Endoscopic transmural puncture was initially restricted to lesions with clear bulging of the gastric or duodenal wall caused by the cyst, as reliable hits could not otherwise be achieved and substantial complications such as puncture of the gallbladder, and hemorrhage in particular, were to be feared. In addition, the proportion of cystic lesions accessible to endoscopic treatment in these conditions was distinctly limited. Even large pseudocysts or abscesses do not necessarily cause bulging in adjacent sections of the intestine. Infected necroses are not normally clearly visible with endoscopy. Although conventional sonography provides more or less reliable preliminary information about the topography of the possible puncture site in this situation, no exact statements can be made about the vascular situation, and the combined endoscopic–sonographic procedure proved to be very complex and difficult. The unavoidable insufflation of air through the endoscope led to loss of the transgastric sonographic image. With the development of endosonography, the almost ideal method became available. The anatomical situation in the pancreas and surrounding structures, and their positions relative to the intestinal wall, could now be imaged precisely from the stomach and duodenum. Longitudinal scanners also provided reliable identification of larger vessels close to the point of puncture so that they could be avoided.

Baron et al. reported a long-term success rate for endoscopic treatment of chronic pseudocysts (according to the Atlanta classification) of 92%, and for acute pseudocysts and necroses of 70–75%. The rate of complications for pseudocysts was barely 20%, for necroses almost twice as high.[60]

Even extensive, solid, and infected retroperitoneal necroses can be successfully treated endoscopically using the transmural procedure and direct debridement.[61,62] In a recent multicenter study, transluminal endoscopic therapy of infected pancreatic necrosis in 93 patients had a technical success rate of 80%, with a complication rate of 26% and a 30-day mortality rate of 7.5%.[63] The seven fatal outcomes were due to bleeding and air embolism (in one case each) and septic complications in five patients.

Preliminary anatomical remarks. For endoscopic therapy, the entire expanse of a cyst has to be accessible from the stomach or duodenum, whether via a transpapillary route through the pancreatic duct or by transmural puncture. What this means in concrete terms, and the method to be used to establish the prerequisites for endoscopic treatment, are matters of controversy. The question of which pathoanatomical conditions favor the endoscopic procedure and which argue for surgical treatment is also open.

For this reason, some preliminary remarks concerning the anatomy of pancreatogenic fluid collections are given here. This will certainly not include anything new to abdominal surgeons, but may include some aspects that are not so familiar to internal-medicine specialists. It is essential to be aware of the mesenteric relationships and retroperitoneal connections when carrying out endoscopic surgery.

The retroperitoneal position of the pancreas determines the spread, as well as the limits, of pancreatogenic cystic lesions. The pancreas extends retroperitoneally between the duodenum and the splenic hilum. Anteriorly, it is only separated from the stomach by the omental bursa, so that it is directly next to it. The omental bursa is normally only a gap between two peritoneal membranes and cannot be seen directly with imaging methods. However, if it is filled with fluid and prevented by adhesions from draining into the free abdominal cavity through the omental foramen, it appears as a cystic structure between the pancreas and stomach. Intact or even necrotic peripancreatic or pancreatic tissue can thus be found dorsal to this "pseudocyst," or in its lumen. Fluid collections in the omental bursa may be adjacent to the stomach or duodenum. Their greatest extent generally follows the transverse pancreas, and they can normally be drained completely from a single point. Usually, the best opportunity for puncture is from the body of the stomach.

During endoscopic puncture, particular attention has to be paid to the splenic artery and the dorsal pancreatic artery, which usually emerges from it close to the celiac trunk. In typical anatomy, the latter has two branches—one to the arteries of the head of the pancreas to the right and the other (in this connection the important one) to the left, often strong and passing into the parenchyma (or necrosis) in the direction of the splenic hilum. Along with the pancreatic branches of the splenic artery, there are arteries supplying the stomach in the region of the puncture.

On transduodenal puncture, attention has to be paid to the artery in the duodenal concavity, which is fed by the hepatic artery and the superior mesenteric artery. The superior pancreaticoduodenal artery (from the gastroduodenal artery) and the inferior pancreaticoduodenal artery (from the superior mesenteric artery) communicate at the back of the head of the pancreas at about the level of the major duodenal papilla.

Veins can also lead to hemorrhage following transmural puncture; the veins concerned are almost always collateral veins in splenic vein thrombosis or portal hypertension, in the context of cirrhosis of the liver. Splenic vein thrombosis is a common and typical complication of inflammatory or compressive processes in the pancreatic capsule. Endoscopically, and especially endosonographically, there is a typical pattern of gastric varices, especially in the fundus, without esophageal varices (hepatopetal flow, if cirrhosis of the liver is absent), with major veins in the splenic hilum, and dorsal of the stomach wall. Not infrequently, the vessels are precisely in the area of the optimal transmural puncture point.

Indications. Interventional treatment is always indicated in patients with pseudocysts or peripancreatic necroses with septic complications. However, the situation is usually much less clear in clinical practice. Cystic bodies containing purulent matter are often oligosymptomatic or asymptomatic. Large pseudocysts, and especially extensive necrosis, can persist for weeks or even months, during antibiotic treatment sometimes with CRP declining or remaining in the moderately increased pathological range and stable. If the symptoms do not require surgical intervention, only involving persistent nausea, a more or less troublesome lack of appetite, and a feeling of pressure of varying severity, it is not easy to decide on whether to carry out endoscopic or surgical intervention. In some patients with extensive necroses, we have successfully waited until the lesions had finally consolidated. A procedure of this type requires patience (2–3 months) and involves a risk of septic complications. If the intervention is delayed until septic complications absolutely require it, the success of treatment appears impressive, but the risks increase. There are no reliable data on the best time for an intervention. It may be that, because of its minimal tissue trauma, endoscopic EUS-guided retroperitoneal decompression or debridement is justified earlier than the surgical procedure. There are no comparative prospective data on this issue.

Urgent indications for interventional therapy in pseudocysts or retroperitoneal necroses include:
- Obstruction of the stomach or duodenum
- Pain
- Vomiting
- Hemorrhage
- Septic complications (fever, increase in CRP)

Uncertain indications include:
- Feeling of fullness
- Loss of appetite
- Weight loss
- Persistence or increase in size
- Influence on vessels, close to vessels
- Bacterial contamination (positive aspirate without symptoms)

When there are no urgent indications for surgery—which include a request for treatment by the patient after receiving detailed information—we always monitor the course for 2–6 weeks. If there is no improvement during this period, we tend to operate even when the indication is not fully clear. If CRP is normal and there is no sign of bacterial infection, prophylactic antibiotic treatment is not generally indicated, as recently shown by the German ASAP Study Group.[64]

Practical procedure for endoscopic treatment of cystic peripancreatic lesions. Although liquid cyst contents can be drained through conventional plastic stents, solid necroses require a more aggressive procedure. The retroperitoneal space is punctured directly from the stomach or duodenum with a suitable EUS endoscope.[8,42,65–67] A transmural window is created using through-the-scope balloon dilation with an 8-mm balloon (Max-Force, Microvasive Inc., Boston, Massachusetts, USA), followed by an 18-mm or 20-mm balloon. Direct endoscopic debridement of the necrotic material is performed through this window, and is initially repeated every 2–3 days. In some cases, the necrotic cavity is not restricted to the omental bursa, but has wide-ranging retroperitoneal branches, which have to be conscientiously drained.

The most important *principles of the endoscopic strategy* are:

- Firstly, reconstruction of the normal flow of pancreatic juice, transpapillary drainage of the *entire* pancreatic duct (no "uncoupled" areas should be allowed). Special catheters and wires are often required to do this. The duct has to be cleaned (with extraction of stones) and defects have to be reconstructed along its entire length (with plastic stents).
- Secondly, transmural decompression, drainage, and lavage of cystic lesions. The window has to be large enough: if necessary, necroses should be debrided endoscopically. No infected necroses should be left behind. EUS is essential; large vessels are associated with a high risk in larger interventions. No undrained lacunae should be left behind; if necessary, percutaneous puncture of perforating abscesses in the pelvis should be carried out.

If these two principles are successfully observed, even extensive fluid collections (ascites, pleural effusions, large abscesses) disappear rapidly and fistulas dry up (**Fig. 19.5**). Endoscopic sealing of fistulas with tissue glue is rarely necessary.

Endoscopic treatment requires patience and experience, and it is best for it to be administered by a combined gastroenterology and abdominal surgery team.

There are strong arguments for the view that mobile patients should be able to eat immediately after surgery, and thus against the use of nasocystic drains (which are very irritating and easily dislodged).

Preinterventional Diagnosis

Patient information and consent. The patient should be briefed on the day before the procedure regarding alternative techniques (see above) and their risks, and in particular the risks of endoscopic transmural fenestration—hemorrhage, incorrect puncture (gallbladder), infections, and septic complications, surgery, low mortality rate. In addition, the typical risks of endoscopy (aspiration, dental damage, pancreatitis) and sedation should be mentioned.

Laboratory tests. Coagulation, cholestasis, raised CRP (procalcitonin is probably not better than CRP as a marker of bacterial infection in this context), kidney function, cancer (hyperparathyroidism as a possible cause of pancreatitis of "unclear origin").

Doppler sonography. Recent imaging findings for the abdominal organs, their relative positions, vascularity, exclusion of anatomical details likely to lead to complications (pseudoaneurysms, varices, kidney and liver cysts, large gallbladder, extended branched systems, possible tumors) as close as possible to the time of surgery.

CT with contrast agents or MRI. Anatomic overview of the abdomen (considerable overlap with the ultrasound examination) and mediastinum, objectively evaluable images (which the radiographer interprets and the surgeon accepts, and which can later confirm the correct diagnosis) (**Fig. 19.6**).

EUS (potentially in preparation for puncture). An EUS information briefing should be provided about possible interventions (green light for surgery even before the first intervention). Precise imaging (**Fig. 19.7**)[62] of the relative positions of the target structure and its surroundings, the best puncture position (vascularity), the pancreatic parenchyma (possible tumors, chronic pancreatitis, calcification), multiple cystic lesions, communications, imaging of pancreatic duct (occlusions by strictures or intraductal stones, possible prestenotic dilation, maintained or interrupted continuity, possible blockage in the necrosis).

ERCP. An information briefing should be provided regarding possible interventions. ERCP should *not* be performed if the papilla is difficult to access, or if very large compressive processes are causing displacement and affect the anatomy, when surgical treatment is likely anyway in conditions that are still sterile (contamination of the ducts almost always occurs when contrast agents are used). An initial ERP is helpful for the intervention. If technically feasible, reconstruction of the pancreatic duct in the presence of occlusions, diagnosis of a pancreas divisum, bile duct stenosis, or detection of a ductal injury can indicate the appropriate form of treatment. In some cases, even endoscopic treatment of abscesses or infected necroses using an exclusively transpapillary technique is successful.

Reconstruction of the pancreatic duct, ensuring transpapillary flow and as far as possible maintaining continuity into the tail must *always* be attempted. If dominant stenoses persist, then prestenotic congestion and resulting recurrence of the cyst is inevitable. For diagnostic purposes, magnetic resonance imaging of the pancreas (MRCP) gives excellent information on the anatomy of the pancreatic duct.

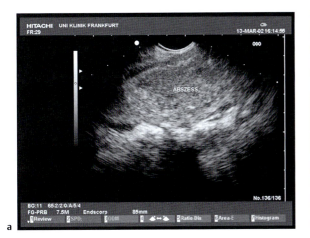

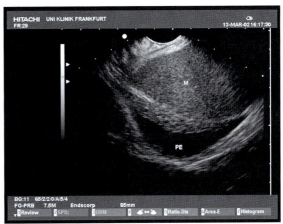

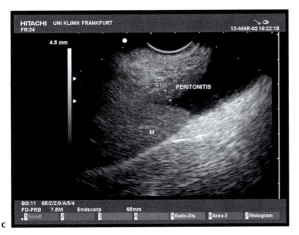

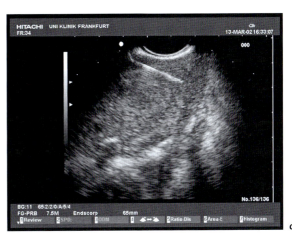

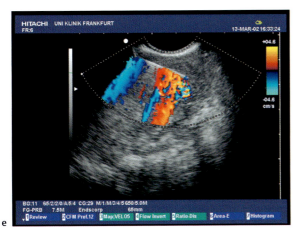

Fig. 19.5a–e An older and thus atypical pancreatic abscess with inflammatory changes in the surrounding tissues (**a**) in a patient who also had pleural thickening and effusion (**b**) and local peritonitis next to the spleen (**c**). M, spleen; PE, pleural effusion.
d, e After transmural drainage, the pleural effusion also cleared up.

Transmural Intervention

Position. The standard position is on the left side (with the least risk of aspiration).

Sedation. The authors have found that sedation with propofol is optimal.

Preliminary endoscopy. Before the transmural puncture, one should "sound out the terrain" using a large-diameter endoscope (normally a gastroscope). If necessary, the stomach should be emptied and one should identify or exclude abnormalities (stenoses, scars, ulcers, anatomical variants).

EUS-guided transmural drainage, debridement of necroses. In principle, two different puncture techniques are available:

- Sharp puncture with a needle and without diathermy
- Passage into the cavity with diathermy current

Without diathermy. Stiff, large-diameter needles should be used (Echo-19, Wilson-Cook, Winston-Salem, North Carolina, USA). Large-diameter stiff needles are usually easily visualized endosonographically. They maintain their direction relatively reliably, and even fix the transducer to the puncture point. They almost always allow diagnostic aspiration of material for bacteriology and pathology (with the exception of solid necroses). In particular, the risk of

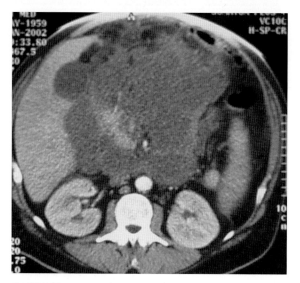

Fig. 19.6 The computed tomogram shows an extensive retroperitoneal necrosis. After transmural fenestration, ≈ 1500 mL of pus and solid necroses was drained, followed by notable clinical improvement.

hemorrhage is low, as the procedure only leads to puncture on the axis of the defined channel, rather than a cut to the side of it. Large-diameter needles can be used with a guide wire passing through the needle. Alternatively, a 1-mm needle with a fitted Teflon dilator or pusher–stent combination has proved successful for puncture and drainage in one step.[42] Unfortunately, only prototypes of such combinations are so far available.

With regard to guide wires, either easily bent pure steel wires have to be used, or the fundamental principle of never passing coated wires through sharp needles has to be breached. When advancing the needle or retracting the wire, the coating may be peeled off, or the tip of the wire could even be cut off. Thus, if one is using bend-resistant wires with hydrophilic and atraumatic radiopaque ends, which are otherwise very suitable, after stable placement of the wire in the punctured cavity (if possible with several turns), the needle must always be drawn back and removed. The guide wire can then be used either (when using echoendoscopes with narrow working channels) to replace the echoendoscope with a therapeutic gastroscope or duodenoscope (depending on availability and the anatomical situation), or drainage can be carried out directly. The use of puncture needles for complex interventions always involves the risk of damaging the working channel of the endoscope (with extremely expensive repairs). This usually happens when drawing back and then advancing the needle again, so that the fundamental rule is: if the situation is unclear, it is better to start in an orderly way from the beginning (perhaps with diathermy) rather than to try to "rescue" an attempt that has already been started.

The procedure without diathermy reaches its limits when the very tough wall of the retroperitoneal cavity is in the way of the needle. If forced puncture is attempted, the endosonographic image goes out of control, the tip of the needle departs from the plane of the image, and the transducer becomes uncoupled from the wall. With mod-

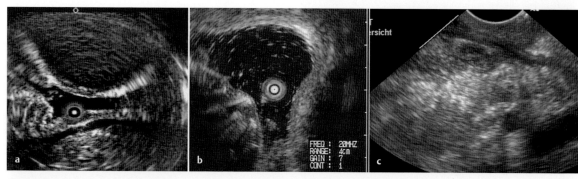

Fig. 19.7a–c Even at the first endoscopic examination, the miniprobe showed the most important features in this case.

a At the bottom of the image, there is a normal stomach wall with typical stratification; behind that, there is pancreatic tissue, and at the top only the mucosal layer; and behind that, there is no pseudocyst but an abscess in the gastric wall.

b This image shows a preserved anterior gastric wall on the right, while on the left the gastric wall is no longer present and there is only

an amorphous boundary layer (complete necrosis of the posterior gastric wall); behind that, there is hypoechoic tissue with gas bubbles.

c The longitudinal scanner shows extensive infected necroses in the same patient. Successful treatment was administered with transmural debridement, with resection of large necrotic masses and the ischemic–necrotic spleen.[62]

ern endoscopes, which produce excellent endoscopic images, the operation can then sometimes be completed under endoscopic guidance. In such cases, diathermy-assisted methods have advantages.

With diathermy current. This technique uses needle-knife papillotomes with a cutting wire (rather than a blade) and an extra lumen for aspiration and the guide wire (e.g., Triple-Lumen Needle-Knife, Boston Scientific, Natick, Massachusetts, USA). The puncture point has to be selected particularly carefully in this technique, since unlike stiff needles, the needle-knife is not capable of fixing the transducer in position. With the position stable, the needle is advanced into the mucous membrane and then advanced along the axis with diathermy current (e.g., Endo-Cut). The puncture channel is burnt free. *Caution:* if the position is unstable, sideways cutting into the stomach wall (with major arteries) or tissue outside the EUS plane is possible. The diathermy effect can be visualized very well with endosonography. It clearly shows the position of the needle-knife (which is otherwise often difficult to see) and produces impressive effects at this point on reaching the cyst lumen. At that point, the guide wire and/or catheter has to be advanced further into the punctured lumen (*caution:* only the thin cutting wire should be in the lumen; the guide wire should be outside, between the layers).

As an alternative to the needle-knife, specially developed puncture sets provided by several suppliers can be used. The Giovannini needle wire (Wilson-Cook) has a special guide wire with a diathermy tip inside a catheter and, over it, an 8.5-Fr stent, which is placed in one step. The cystotome (Wilson-Cook) combines a needle-knife with a ring-shaped 10-Fr electrocauterizer. It is not always easy to maintain a stable position with these instruments during cautery.

Irrespective of the technique used, the following principles and prerequisites apply:

- Experienced endoscopist (better: two physicians) and two experienced endoscopy assistants

- Potent suction (massive releases of pus or bleeding is possible after puncture), Hemoclips to stop bleeding, epinephrine, collection containers for aspirate for diagnosis (particularly bacteriology, also amylase, carcinoembryonic antigen, cytology, possibly hematocrit); photodocumentation if available
- Puncture equipment
- Catheter, stents, balloons
- Prograde endoscope
- Possibly nasocystic catheter or percutaneous endoscopic gastrostomy (PEG; a matter of preference)
- Preoperative antibiotic prophylaxis with sulbactam and ampicillin (Unacid), ciprofloxacin
- In very large lesions, tracheal intubation or an esophageal protective overtube are recommended to prevent aspiration.

The intervention

- The best position for puncture has to be established.
  - There should be intimate contact between the cavity to be punctured and the intestinal wall. The optimal puncture point is typically transgastric, just below the cardia, at ≈ 41–45 cm from the incisors (tail, body, spleen abscesses, infradiaphragmatic spread, to splenic hilum) or oral to the angular notch of the stomach, 45–50 cm from the incisors (pancreatic head region, extension to the porta hepatis, bile duct, retrocecal) through the posterior gastric wall to the omental bursa, or the descending duodenum back toward the pancreatic head region, slightly above the major duodenal papilla.
  - Arteries should be avoided, especially when using diathermy (**Fig. 19.8**). Are any vessels interposed along the puncture route? Is there a perfused solid "necrotic area"? Are any vessels in the cyst wall, especially dorsal? Are gastric wall arteries or varices present? (Searching should be carried out with *minimal* pressure from the transducer and compression.) Retracting the instrument from the wall is possible, with optical inspection of the puncture site (**Fig. 19.9**).

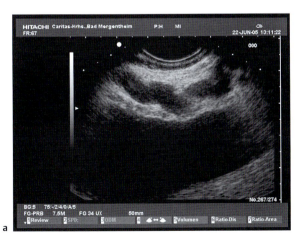
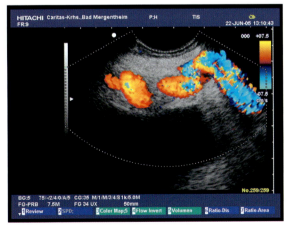

Fig. 19.8a–e There is always a danger of injuring blood vessels during puncture.

a B-mode.
b Color Doppler imaging.

Fig. 19.8c–e ▷

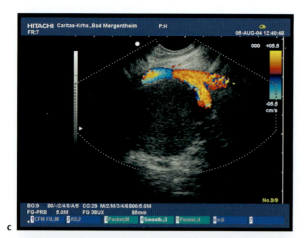

c

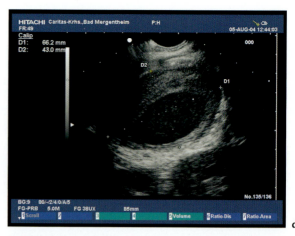

d

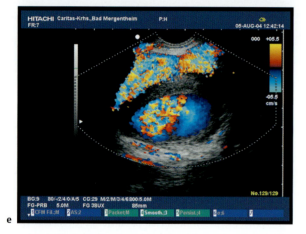

e

Fig. 19.8c–e (continued)
c–e In this patient with intramural and perigastric varices, this sequence shows a pseudocystic lesion of the pancreas that was referred for drainage. Evidence of an arterial pseudoaneurysm changed the treatment options to surgery or embolization of the afferent vessels. (▶ Video 19.1.)

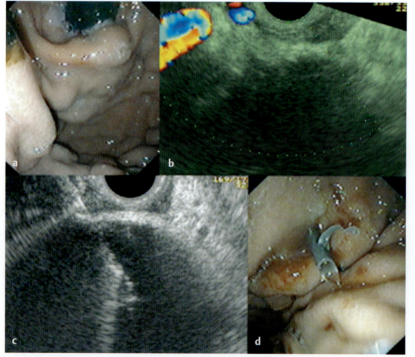

Fig. 19.9a–d a Pronounced fundic varices in splenic vein thrombosis.
b, c The Doppler image helps the varices to be avoided during EUS-guided puncture (**c**) and drainage of the large pseudocyst.
d Placement of a plastic stent, with no hemorrhage.

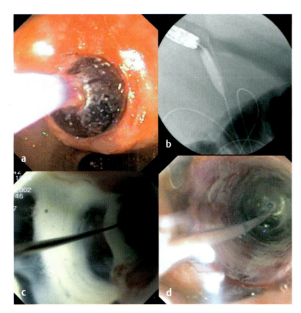

Fig. 19.10a–d Various aspects of transmural balloon dilation. Balloon filling, either pneumatic or with a diluted contrast agent, makes the air easier to draw out. Direct endoscopic guidance means that radiographic support is not necessarily required.

– The minimum possible bending of the instrument should be used (often difficult).
- Puncture of the cyst with a 19-G aspiration biopsy needle.
- Aspiration of cyst fluid in a stable position:
  – Bacteriology (blood culture bottles)
  – Laboratory tests (amylase, lipase, leukocyte count, carcinoembryonic antigen)
  – Cytology
- Introduction of an appropriate (e.g., 0.018-inch or 0.025-inch) guide wire with a flexible tip (which should be advanced as far as possible, until two or three loops form in the cyst, to ensure that the wire is in a stable position)
- Withdrawal of the puncture needle and bougienage of the access route with a 7-Fr or 8.5-Fr dilator.

Options after successful puncture, with the wire or catheter in place:
- Insertion of a plastic transmural stent (such as a double-pigtail stent or a U-shaped, suspended stent), which is often sufficient for uncomplicated pseudocysts. It is sometimes sensible to use several stents.
- A nasocystic irrigation catheter allows regular irrigation and radiographic monitoring, especially of infected cysts. However, these are easily dislocated and are very troublesome for the patient. Combination with a transmural stent is useful.
- Balloon dilation of the transmural window with an 8-mm balloon through the endoscope (up to 20 mm) (**Fig. 19.10**). This step is essential for infected necroses

with solid contents. Dilation to the desired diameter can be performed in steps over several days, or immediately at the first step (as the authors prefer). With large windows, no additional plastic drain is required.
- Insertion of the endoscope through the 15–20-mm window into the retroperitoneal cyst and endoscopic debridement of demarcated necroses. Any endoscope can be used; large-channel therapeutic gastroscopes have proved successful, as have side-viewing instruments in special cases or thin 6-mm gastroscopes for the irrigation of a narrow recessus.

After the intervention. There are even fewer standards for the procedure after successful drainage than for the puncture technique itself. The procedure is determined to a large extent by the peculiarities of the individual case, but also by the technical facilities available and, not least, the investigator's experience. For this reason, no treatment instructions can be given here, and only the most important comments on the endoscopic treatment of cystic retroperitoneal lesions can be offered.
- Initially, after major interventions (debridement of infected necroses, retroperitoneal endoscopy), there is often a *transient increase in CRP.* Clinically, patients improve immediately after decompression of large cysts or abscesses, and even after debridement clinical improvement usually starts at the latest on day 2.
- Infected cavities have to be cleaned up as soon as possible. In the case of abscesses, this means systematic irrigation; in the case of infected necroses, repeated debridement with careful (often very difficult) visits to the retroperitoneal recesses, which typically lie in the region to the left of the splenic hilum and retrocecally on the right (**Fig. 19.11**). At present, inadequate instruments still have to be used (baskets, balloons, irrigation catheters with atraumatic wires). *It is essential to avoid damage to blood vessels.* Puncture of large veins involves a risk of *fatal air embolisms,* and *arterial hemorrhages* have to be treated surgically. Vessels with patent lumens (often thrombosed in necrotic zones) can be identified with EUS miniprobes (**Fig. 19.12**).
- Initially, it is better for irrigation to be too frequent rather than not frequent enough. It should be carried out with nasocystic or transmural access (PEG with a long section in the cavity), preferably several times daily, endoscopically every 2–3 days. There are no data regarding the best irrigation solution. We have used taurine in necrotic cavities, but this did not have any particularly impressive effects. For endoscopic irrigation, we otherwise use saline containing gentamicin (80 mg/500 mL) and, if necessary, a little contrast agent. Most of the solution is reaspirated. Instilling large volumes of physiological saline via nasogastric irrigation tubes leads to nausea and symptoms due to the volume, so that it has limitations.
- The *transmural window* in the stomach is usually unproblematic; it closes spontaneously so quickly that it is

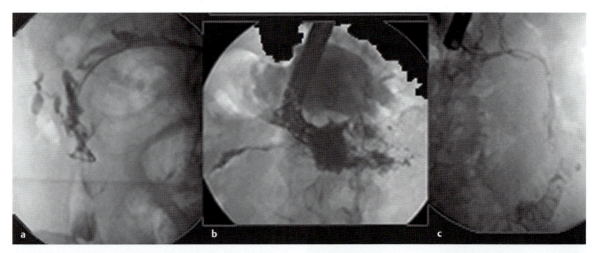

Fig. 19.11a–c From the retroperitoneal cavity (**b**; stomach with air and contrast, with the endoscope in the transmural window), it is possible to reach extensive recesses that need to be irrigated and cleaned. **a** Retrocecal. **c** With spontaneous connection and drainage into a sigmoid anastomosis.

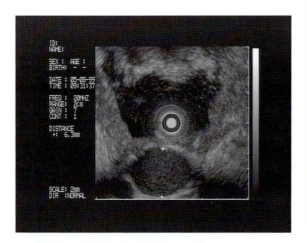

Fig. 19.12 The miniprobe inside the retroperitoneal necrotic cavity (through a therapeutic gastroscope). A large artery (the splenic artery) is seen immediately next to the cavity.

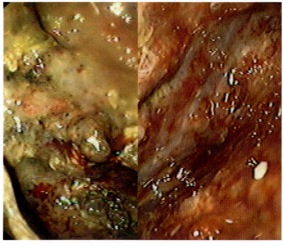

Fig. 19.13 The transmural window in the stomach, with a suspended U stent (10-Fr Teflon, bent with hot air) in place to keep it open.

often difficult to locate after a few days and needs to be dilated again. The wall of the duodenum is thinner and closes somewhat more slowly. The window should be kept open until the lumen of the cavity only has a minimal image (and only on EUS or with direct contrast). If the wall of the cavity is clean and greasy coatings have been replaced by granulation tissue, retroperitoneal endoscopic procedures are no longer required (**Fig. 19.13**). The window can be kept open for irrigation and drainage with a 10-Fr stent.

- The right time to consider that the treatment is complete and to remove all transmural place-holders is often difficult, and always has to be decided on a case-by-case basis. Sometimes the decision takes place automatically, if the cavity becomes granulated and the last

place-holder detaches itself (this is not possible with the classic double-pigtail stents; we use U-shaped Teflon stents ≈ 6 cm long or soft silicone drains). Treatment of uncomplicated pseudocysts is usually complete after 4 weeks.

- If the window closes earlier than expected, we wait to see what will happen even in the presence of a residual cyst. If it becomes larger and leads to symptoms and a relapse, we puncture it again.
- Patients can resume eating on the first day, even if they have large transmural windows of 2 cm. They should be rapidly mobilized and treated as outpatients as soon as possible. When pulmonary complications occur, or intensive treatment or comorbidities make the patient

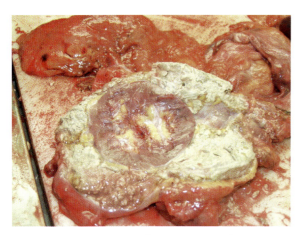

Fig. 19.14 Autopsy specimen. There is suppurating fatty tissue necrosis in the entire left kidney position. Extensive findings such as these cannot be successfully treated endoscopically.

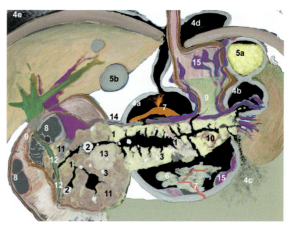

Fig. 19.15 Morphological complications of acute and chronic pancreatitis and differential diagnoses are best assessed by endosonography (key: see **Table 19.4**).

bedridden and immobilized, we have observed very slow and difficult courses.

- Perioperative antibiotic prophylaxis is always administered—the duration of this can be left to the clinician's judgment. We have often found *Candida* infection in large necrotic cavities, and generally do not treat this systemically. The infection disappears with the appearance of granulation tissue.
- Perhaps the most important point is that treatment must always be administered as part of an overall plan to restore normal pancreatic flow. The endoscopy team need to have mastered all the methods of interventional endoscopy in the pancreas. Transpapillary therapy can be performed before or after transmural puncture, but to be successful, there has to be free transpapillary flow, as otherwise pseudocysts and fistulas will persist. It is always necessary to weigh up whether the intended drainage effect could also be achieved, or could exclusively be achieved, with the transpapillary route alone.
- Minor injuries to the bile duct with escape of bile into the retroperitoneal cavity can be treated with transpapillary stents.
- Constructive cooperation with an experienced abdominal surgeon is always required. Pancreatic surgery is a typical field for an abdominal surgery center. Collaboration should be ensured even from the planning stage.
- If an unfavorable course starts to develop, usually because of extensive fatty tissue necroses that cannot all be reached by endoscopy (**Fig. 19.14**), with septic complications, an increase in CRP after initial improvement, and failure to improve despite technically successful drainage, one should move to an early open surgical procedure rather than defending the endoscopic approach.

Complications. Fatal complications of endoscopic retroperitoneal procedures reported in a recent multicenter study consisted of bleeding, air embolism, and sepsis.

While fatal outcomes in septic patients with multiple organ failure are not endoscopy-specific and sometimes cannot be prevented, in some instances they may be due to the endoscopic procedure itself. Deep introduction of the endoscope is necessary in order to reach all purulent retentions. However, the scope should be introduced with extreme care to ensure that the infected retroperitoneal space is not connected with sterile regions, especially the abdominal cavity; otherwise septic shock may ensue. Bleeding from arteries in the gastric wall can usually be stopped by inflating the dilator balloon in the gastric window for a few minutes, and/or with endoscopic clip application. We have also used Hemoclips for bleeding vessels in the retroperitoneal cavity without complications. Bleeding from major arteries should be avoided and may require emergency surgery. Air embolism occurred in two of our patients, with one fatality, probably due to minor lesions in low-pressure vessels. No further complications have been observed since we switched from air to carbon dioxide for endoscopic insufflation.

Summary and Prospects

EUS with modern, Doppler-enabled, large-channel longitudinal scanners has opened up new dimensions in interventional endoscopy that have not yet been exhausted by a long way. In the field of abdominal surgery, and laparoscopic surgery in particular, there are exciting prospects especially for interventions in the retroperitoneal cavity, particularly in the pancreas and its surroundings. EUS-supported interventions, along with other endoscopic procedures, have the most important role in the treatment of the complications of acute and chronic pancreatitis. EUS is superior to all other imaging procedures in the diagnosis of

Table 19.4 Complications of pancreatitis (key to Fig. 19.15)

No.	Complication	Symptoms	Diagnosis	Treatment of choice
1	Stricture	Pain	ERP, EUS, US, MRCP	Stent, drainage surgery
2	Stone in duct	Pain	US, EUS, ERP, MRCP	EPT, extraction, lithotripsy, ESWL, surgery
3	Stone (calcification) in parenchyma	Pain	US, EUS, radiography	ESWL, surgery
4	Fistula to:			
4a	Bursa (pseudocyst)	Size-dependent sensation of fullness, loss of appetite, pressure	US, EUS, ERP	Always secure transpapillary flow. Endoscopic drainage transpapillary and/or transmural. Possibly percutaneous puncture. Any extrapancreatic juice can lead to tissue necroses
4b	Pseudocyst in splenic hilum	Sensation of pressure	US, EUS, ERP	
4c	Ascites	Sensation of fullness, weight gain	US, EUS, ERP	
4d	Mediastinum	None	US, EUS, ERP	
4e	Pleural effusion (usually on the left)	Dyspnea	US, radiography, EUS, ERP	
5	Abscess	Fever, malaise	US, EUS, ERP, CT	Endoscopic drainage transpapillary and/or transmural
5a	Infradiaphragmatic/ intrasplenic	Often with few symptoms	US, EUS, ERP, CT	
5b	Intrahepatic		US, EUS, ERP, CT	
6	Necrosis	Variable (in infection fever, loss of appetite)	US, EUS, CT	In infection, transmural debridement or surgery
7	Arteries in the necrosis (pseudoaneurysm)	Only on hemorrhage	US, EUS + Doppler	Angiography, embolization
8	Duodenal wall cysts	Usually none	Endoscopy, EUS	None, possibly incision or puncture
9	Compression of pylorus/duodenum with retention	Nausea, loss of appetite, pain	US, EGD	Cyst drainage, pancreatic head resection
10	Focal inflammations	Pain	? EUS	Duct decompression? Elimination of the noxa?
11	Inflammatory pseudotumor of the head of the pancreas	Pain, nausea	US, EUS, CT, MRI	Pancreatic head resection
12	Bile duct stenosis by compression and fibrosis	Jaundice, pruritus, fever	US, EUS, ERC	Cyst drainage, duct stent (short term), pancreatic head resection, choledochojejunostomy
13	Pancreatic carcinoma	Nonspecific	(EUS + FNAC?)	Resection
14	Occlusion of the splenic vein by compression/ thrombosis	None	US/EUS + Doppler, MRI	Cyst drainage
15	Fundic varices, collateral circulation	None, hemorrhage	EGD	Histoacryl obliteration in hemorrhage, splenectomy

CT, computed tomography; EGD, esophagogastroduodenoscopy; EPT, endoscopic papillotomy; ERP, endoscopic retrograde pancreatography; ESWL, extracorporeal shock-wave lithotripsy; EUS, endoscopic ultrasonography; FNAC, fine-needle aspiration cytology; MRCP, magnetic resonance cholangiopancreatography; MRI, magnetic resonance imaging; US, ultrasonography.

the numerous possible pathoanatomical changes (**Fig. 19.15**; **Table 19.4**).

Endoscopic transmural drainage of pseudocysts is a long-established standard practice, and endoscopic debridement of even very large necroses[63]—in one case with resection of an ischemic spleen[62]—and direct transmural puncture of a pancreatic duct not accessible by the transpapillary route[68,69] illustrate the possibilities that are available here. Suitable specialized instruments now need to be developed for these methods, and prospective treatment protocols are even more urgently required. If possible, the techniques should be used in centers with appropriate endoscopic and open surgical expertise and collaboration. Appropriate staffing and technical resources are required for such centers, and in particular, appropriate recognition of these complex procedures within the framework of therapeutic procedures in hospitals is needed.

References

1. Black PR, Welch KJ, Eraklis AJ. Juxtapancreatic intestinal duplications with pancreatic ductal communication: a cause of pancreatitis and recurrent abdominal pain in childhood. J Pediatr Surg 1986;21(3):257–261.
2. Kazumori H, Sizuku T, Ueki T, Uchida Y, Yamamoto S. Lymphoepithelial cyst of the pancreas. J Gastroenterol 1997;32(5):700–703.
3. Papadimitriou J. Pancreatic abscess due to infected hydatid disease. Surgery 1987;102(5):880–882.
4. Regan JK, Brown RD, Marrero JA, Malik P, Rosenberg F, Venu RP. Chronic pancreatitis resulting from primary hydatid disease of the pancreas: a case report and review of the literature. Gastrointest Endosc 1999;49(6):791–793.
5. Brugge WR, Lauwers GY, Sahani D, Fernandez-del Castillo C, Warshaw AL. Cystic neoplasms of the pancreas. N Engl J Med 2004;351(12):1218–1226.
6. Kosmahl M, Pauser U, Peters K, et al. Cystic neoplasms of the pancreas and tumor-like lesions with cystic features: a review of 418 cases and a classification proposal. Virchows Arch 2004;445(2):168–178.
7. Levy MJ, Clain JE. Evaluation and management of cystic pancreatic tumors: emphasis on the role of EUS FNA. Clin Gastroenterol Hepatol 2004;2(8):639–653.
8. Seifert H, Faust D, Schmitt T, Dietrich C, Caspary W, Wehrmann T. Transmural drainage of cystic peripancreatic lesions with a new large-channel echo endoscope. Endoscopy 2001;33(12):1022–1026.
9. Bradley EL III. A clinically based classification system for acute pancreatitis. Summary of the International Symposium on Acute Pancreatitis, Atlanta, Ga, September 11 through 13, 1992. Arch Surg 1993;128(5):586–590.
10. Nealon WH, Walser E. Main pancreatic ductal anatomy can direct choice of modality for treating pancreatic pseudocysts (surgery versus percutaneous drainage). Ann Surg 2002;235(6):751–758.
11. Neoptolemos JP. Endoscopic sphincterotomy in acute gallstone pancreatitis. Br J Surg 1993;80(5):547–549.
12. Barthet M, Bugallo M, Moreira LS, Bastid C, Sastre B, Sahel J. Management of cysts and pseudocysts complicating chronic pancreatitis. A retrospective study of 143 patients. Gastroenterol Clin Biol 1993;17(4):270–276.
13. Nealon WH, Townsend CM Jr, Thompson JC. Preoperative endoscopic retrograde cholangiopancreatography (ERCP) in patients with pancreatic pseudocyst associated with resolving acute and chronic pancreatitis. Ann Surg 1989;209(5):532–538, discussion 538–540.
14. Stolte M. Chronische Pankreatitis. Erlangen, Germany: Perimed; 1984.
15. Ammann RW, Akovbiantz A, Largiader F, Schueler G. Course and outcome of chronic pancreatitis. Longitudinal study of a mixed medical-surgical series of 245 patients. Gastroenterology 1984;86(5 Pt 1):820–828.
16. Lankisch PG, Burchard-Reckert S, Petersen M, et al. Morbidity and mortality in 602 patients with acute pancreatitis seen between the years 1980-1994. Z Gastroenterol 1996;34(6):371–377.
17. Siegelman SS, Copeland BE, Saba GP, Cameron JL, Sanders RC, Zerhouni EA. CT of fluid collections associated with pancreatitis. AJR Am J Roentgenol 1980;134(6):1121–1132.
18. Allardyce DB. Incidence of necrotizing pancreatitis and factors related to mortality. Am J Surg 1987;154(3):295–299.
19. Bradley EL III, Allen K. A prospective longitudinal study of observation versus surgical intervention in the management of necrotizing pancreatitis. Am J Surg 1991;161(1):19–24, discussion 24–25.
20. Imrie CW, Buist LJ, Shearer MG. Importance of cause in the outcome of pancreatic pseudocysts. Am J Surg 1988;156(3 Pt 1):159–162.
21. Beger HG, Schlosser W, Siech M, Poch B. The surgical management of chronic pancreatitis: duodenum-preserving pancreatectomy. Adv Surg 1999;32:87–104.
22. Izbicki JR, Bloechle C, Broering DC, Knoefel WT, Kuechler T, Broelsch CE. Extended drainage versus resection in surgery for chronic pancreatitis: a prospective randomized trial comparing the longitudinal pancreaticojejunostomy combined with local pancreatic head excision with the pylorus-preserving pancreatoduodenectomy. Ann Surg 1998;228(6):771–779.
23. Nealon WH, Thompson JC. Progressive loss of pancreatic function in chronic pancreatitis is delayed by main pancreatic duct decompression. A longitudinal prospective analysis of the modified Puestow procedure. Ann Surg 1993;217(5):458–466, discussion 466–468.
24. Rösch T, Daniel S, Scholz M, et al; European Society of Gastrointestinal Endoscopy Research Group. Endoscopic treatment of chronic pancreatitis: a multicenter study of 1000 patients with long-term follow-up. Endoscopy 2002;34(10):765–771.
25. Andersson R, Janzon M, Sundberg I, Bengmark S. Management of pancreatic pseudocysts. Br J Surg 1989;76(6):550–552.
26. Aranha GV, Prinz RA, Esguerra AC, Greenlee HB. The nature and course of cystic pancreatic lesions diagnosed by ultrasound. Arch Surg 1983;118(4):486–488.
27. Czaja AJ, Fisher M, Marin GA. Spontaneous resolution of pancreatic masses (pseudocysts?)—Development and disappearance after acute alcoholic pancreatitis. Arch Intern Med 1975;135(4):558–562.
28. Yeo CJ, Bastidas JA, Lynch-Nyhan A, Fishman EK, Zinner MJ, Cameron JL. The natural history of pancreatic pseudocysts documented by computed tomography. Surg Gynecol Obstet 1990;170(5):411–417.
29. Vitas GJ, Sarr MG. Selected management of pancreatic pseudocysts: operative versus expectant management. Surgery 1992;111(2):123–130.
30. Sankaran S, Walt AJ. The natural and unnatural history of pancreatic pseudocysts. Br J Surg 1975;62(1):37–44.
31. Seiler CA, Boss MA, Czerniak A, Gertsch P, Berne TV, Blumgart L. Complications of chronic pancreatitis. Dig Surg 1997;14:540–545.
32. Kolars JC, Allen MO, Ansel H, Silvis SE, Vennes JA. Pancreatic pseudocysts: clinical and endoscopic experience. Am J Gastroenterol 1989;84(3):259–264.
33. Bradley EL, Clements JL Jr, Gonzalez AC. The natural history of pancreatic pseudocysts: a unified concept of management. Am J Surg 1979;137(1):135–141.
34. Warshaw AL. Pain in chronic pancreatitis. Patients, patience, and the impatient surgeon. [editorial] Gastroenterology 1984;86(5 Pt 1):987–989.
35. Bozeman N. Removal of a cyst of the pancreas weighing twenty and one-half pounds. Med Rec 1882;21:46–47.
36. Gussenbauer C. Zur operativen Behandlung der Pankreas-Cysten. [Article in German] Arch Klin Chir 1883;29:355–364.

37. Jedlica R. Eine neue Operationsmethode der Pankreascys-ten (Pancreatogastrostomie). [Article in German] Zentralbl Chir 1923;50:132.

38. Hahn O. Beitrag zur Behandlung der Pankreasfisteln. [Article in German] Klin Chir 1928;143(73):73.

39. Jurasz A. Zur Frage der operativen Behandlung der Pan-kreascysten. [Article in German] Arch Klin Chir 1931; 164:272–279.

40. Jimenez RE, Fernandez-Del Castillo C, Rattner DW, War-shaw AL. Pylorus-preserving pancreaticoduodenectomy in the treatment of chronic pancreatitis. World J Surg 2003;27(11):1211–1216.

41. Witzigmann H, Max D, Uhlmann D, et al. Outcome after duodenum-preserving pancreatic head resection is im-proved compared with classic Whipple procedure in the treatment of chronic pancreatitis. Surgery 2003;134(1): 53–62.

42. Seifert H, Dietrich C, Schmitt T, Caspary W, Wehrmann T. Endoscopic ultrasound-guided one-step transmural drain-age of cystic abdominal lesions with a large-channel echo endoscope. Endoscopy 2000;32(3):255–259.

43. Nealon WH, Walser E. Duct drainage alone is sufficient in the operative management of pancreatic pseudocyst in patients with chronic pancreatitis. Ann Surg 2003;237(5): 614–620, discussion 620–622.

44. Díte P, Ruzicka M, Zboril V, Novotný I. A prospective, randomized trial comparing endoscopic and surgical ther-apy for chronic pancreatitis. Endoscopy 2003;35(7): 553–558.

45. Malka D, Hammel P, Sauvanet A, et al. Risk factors for diabetes mellitus in chronic pancreatitis. Gastroenterol-ogy 2000;119(5):1324–1332.

46. Bradley EL III. Operative vs non-operative management in sterile necrotizing pancreatitis. HPB Surg 1997;10(3): 188–191.

47. Rattner DW, Legermate DA, Lee MJ, Mueller PR, Warshaw AL. Early surgical debridement of symptomatic pancreatic necrosis is beneficial irrespective of infection. Am J Surg 1992;163(1):105–109, discussion 109–110.

48. Fernández-del Castillo C, Rattner DW, Makary MA, Mosta-favi A, McGrath D, Warshaw AL. Debridement and closed packing for the treatment of necrotizing pancreatitis. Ann Surg 1998;228(5):676–684.

49. Hancke S, Pedersen JF. Percutaneous puncture of pancreatic cysts guided by ultrasound. Surg Gynecol Obstet 1976; 142(4):551–552.

50. van Sonnenberg E, Wittich GR, Casola G, et al. Percutaneous drainage of infected and noninfected pancreatic pseudo-cysts: experience in 101 cases. Radiology 1989;170(3 Pt 1): 757–761.

51. Adams DB, Anderson MC. Percutaneous catheter drainage compared with internal drainage in the management of pancreatic pseudocyst. Ann Surg 1992;215(6):571–576, discussion 576–578.

52. van Sonnenberg E, Wittich GR, Chon KS, et al. Percutaneous radiologic drainage of pancreatic abscesses. AJR Am J Roentgenol 1997;168(4):979–984.

53. Varadarajulu S, Christein JD, Tamhane A, Drelichman ER, Wilcox CM. Prospective randomized trial comparing EUS and EGD for transmural drainage of pancreatic pseudocysts (with videos). Gastrointest Endosc 2008;68(6):1102–1111.

54. Park DH, Lee SS, Moon SH, et al. Endoscopic ultrasound-guided versus conventional transmural drainage for pan-creatic pseudocysts: a prospective randomized trial. Endo-scopy 2009;41(10):842–848.

55. Rogers BH, Cicurel NJ, Seed RW. Transgastric needle aspira-tion of pancreatic pseudocyst through an endoscope. Gastrointest Endosc 1975;21(3):133–134.

56. Kozarek RA, Brayko CM, Harlan J, Sanowski RA, Cintora I, Kovac A. Endoscopic drainage of pancreatic pseudocysts. Gastrointest Endosc 1985;31(5):322–327.

57. Sahel J, Bastid C, Pellat B, Schurgers P, Sarles H. Endoscopic cystoduodenostomy of cysts of chronic calcifying pancrea-titis: a report of 20 cases. Pancreas 1987;2(4):447–453.

58. Cremer M, Devière J, Engelholm L. Endoscopic management of cysts and pseudocysts in chronic pancreatitis: long-term follow-up after 7 years of experience. Gastrointest Endosc 1989;35(1):1–9.

59. Beckingham IJ, Krige JE, Bornman PC, Terblanche J. Long term outcome of endoscopic drainage of pancreatic pseu-docysts. Am J Gastroenterol 1999;94(1):71–74.

60. Baron TH, Harewood GC, Morgan DE, Yates MR. Outcome differences after endoscopic drainage of pancreatic ne-crosis, acute pancreatic pseudocysts, and chronic pancre-atic pseudocysts. Gastrointest Endosc 2002;56(1):7–17.

61. Seewald S, Groth S, Omar S, et al. Aggressive endoscopic therapy for pancreatic necrosis and pancreatic abscess: a new safe and effective treatment algorithm (videos). Gastrointest Endosc 2005;62(1):92–100.

62. Seifert H, Wehrmann T, Schmitt T, Zeuzem S, Caspary WF. Retroperitoneal endoscopic debridement for infected peri-pancreatic necrosis. Lancet 2000;356(9230):653–655.

63. Seifert H, Biermer M, Schmitt W, et al. Transluminal endo-scopic necrosectomy after acute pancreatitis: a multicentre study with long-term follow-up (the GEPARD Study). Gut 2009;58(9):1260–1266.

64. Isenmann R, Rünzi M, Kron M, et al; German Antibiotics in Severe Acute Pancreatitis Study Group. Prophylactic anti-biotic treatment in patients with predicted severe acute pancreatitis: a placebo-controlled, double-blind trial. Gastroenterology 2004;126(4):997–1004.

65. Giovannini M, Bernardini D, Seitz JF. Cystogastrotomy en-tirely performed under endosonography guidance for pan-creatic pseudocyst: results in six patients. Gastrointest Endosc 1998;48(2):200–203.

66. Giovannini M, Pesenti C, Rolland AL, Moutardier V, Delpero JR. Endoscopic ultrasound-guided drainage of pancreatic pseudocysts or pancreatic abscesses using a therapeutic echo endoscope. Endoscopy 2001;33(6):473–477.

67. Vilmann P, Hancke S, Pless T, Schell-Hincke JD, Henriksen FW. One-step endosonography-guided drainage of a pan-creatic pseudocyst: a new technique of stent delivery through the echo endoscope. Endoscopy 1998;30(8): 730–733.

68. Burmester E, Niehaus J, Leineweber T, Huetteroth T. EUS-cholangio-drainage of the bile duct: report of 4 cases. Gastrointest Endosc 2003;57(2):246–251.

69. Mallery S, Matlock J, Freeman ML. EUS-guided rendezvous drainage of obstructed biliary and pancreatic ducts: Report of 6 cases. Gastrointest Endosc 2004;59(1):100–107.

20 Endosonography of the Hepatobiliary System

C.F. Dietrich, M. Hocke, H. Seifert

Definitions

The term "cholelithiasis" refers to the presence of gallstones in the extrahepatic biliary tract. Depending on the location of the concrement, a further distinction is made between cholecystolithiasis and choledocholithiasis. A combination of the two conditions can be expected in 15% of patients.

Reliability of Examination Methods for Detecting Gallstones

The reported accuracy of examination methods is measured using four indices: sensitivity, specificity, and positive and negative predictive values (**Table 20.1**). Cholecystolithiasis can be detected by transabdominal ultrasound with a high level of sensitivity (**Fig. 20.1**, **Table 20.2**),[1-7] but choledocholithiasis is more difficult do diagnose transabdominally (**Table 20.3**).[8-16] **Tables 20.4, 20.5, 20.6, 20.7, 20.8,** and **20.9**[8,9,11-13,16-44] present a review of the literature for the different methods used.

Choledocholithiasis can be detected with conventional endoscopic ultrasonography (EUS), which is routinely used as a diagnostic procedure. Endoscopic retrograde cholangiopancreatography (ERCP) is currently regarded as the diagnostic gold standard, with a reported success rate of 90–96%. However, the value of diagnostic ERCP

Table 20.1 Definition of terms used in assessing the accuracy of diagnostic tests

Term	Definition
Sensitivity (%)	True positives/(true-positives + false-negatives)
Specificity (%)	True-negatives/(true-negatives + false-positives)
Positive predictive value (PPV) (%)	True-positives/total positives
Negative predictive value NPV (%)	True-negatives/total negatives
Accuracy (%)	True-positives + true-negatives)/total number
Youden index (%)	Sensitivity + specificity – 1

Table 20.2 Reported detection rates for cholecystolithiasis using transabdominal ultrasonography

Ref.	Sensitivity (%)	Specificity (%)
1	98	94–98
2	70	100
3	97	92
4	91	99
5	98	–
6	91	100
7	87	93

Table 20.3 Detection of choledocholithiasis using transabdominal ultrasonography: review of the literature

Ref.	Patients (n)	Sensitivity (%)	Specificity (%)	NPV (%)	PPV (%)	Gold standard
8	62	25	100	56	100	ERCP with or without EST or IOC
9	52	80	94	–	–	ERCP/EST or surgical exploration
10	–	38	100	–	–	No results
11	35	47	90	–	–	ERCP/EST
12	142	63	95	–	–	ERCP with or without EST or surgical exploration
13	36	50	100	74	100	ERCP/EST
14	50	100	97	92	100	ERCP/PTC
15	132	68	–	–	–	ERCP/EST
16	29	38	100	–	–	ERCP

ERCP, endoscopic retrograde cholangiopancreatography; EST, endoscopic sphincterotomy; IOC, intraoperative cholangiography, NPV, negative predictive value; PPV, positive predictive value; PTC, percutaneous transhepatic cholangiography.

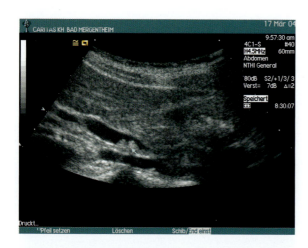

Fig. 20.1 Transabdominal imaging of choledocholithiasis. The lack of acoustic shadowing is a typical phenomenon in primary choledocholithiasis.

Table 20.4 Detection of choledocholithiasis with computed tomography: review of the literature

Ref.	Patients (n)	Sensitivity (%)	Specificity (%)	Gold standard
12	155	71	97	ERCP and EST
17	220	23–37	–	ERCP
18	82	86	98	ERCP
19	101	96	–	Direct cholangiography
19	101	60	–	Direct cholangiography
20	40	80	100	ERCP
21	80	89	98	CT cholangiography
22	51	88	97	ERCP
23	52	85	88	ERCP
11	35	47	95	ERCP with or without EST

Helical CT cholangiography. CT, computed tomography; ERCP, endoscopic retrograde cholangiopancreatography; EST, endoscopic sphincterotomy.

Table 20.5 Detection of choledocholithiasis using endoscopic ultrasonography: review of the literature

Ref.	Patients (n)	Sensitivity (%)	Specificity (%)	NPV (%)	PPV (%)	Gold standard
8	62	97	100	97	100	ERCP with or without EST
9	52	100	100	–	–	ERCP and EST or surgical exploration
24	50	100	97	100	92	Surgical exploration
25	32	100	95	100	91	ERCP and EST
26	20	75	100	–	–	Surgical exploration
27	50	97	77	–	–	ERCP with or without EST
28	240	85	93	96	75	Surgical exploration
29	422	95	96	96	95	Surgical exploration
23	52	91	100	–	–	ERCP with or without EST
30	119	93	97	88	98	ERCP and EST
11	35	100	100	–	–	ERCP and EST
12	155	96	100	–	–	ERCP with or without EST or surgical exploration
31	100	97	98	–	–	ERCP and EST
13	36	91	100	95	100	ERCP and EST
32	50	88	96	–	–	ERCP and EST

ERCP, endoscopic retrograde cholangiopancreatography; EST, endoscopic sphincterotomy; NPV, negative predictive value; PPV, positive predictive value.

Table 20.6 Detection of choledocholithiasis using magnetic resonance cholangiopancreatography (MRCP): review of the literature

Ref.	Patients (n)	Sensitivity (%)	Specificity (%)	NPV (%)	PPV (%)	Gold standard
25	43	100	73	100	63	ERCP and EST
33	146	98	89	99	84	ERCP or surgical exploration
34	28	40	96	88	66	ERCP
35	74	100	97	–	–	ERCP
36	35	100	50	100	87	ERCP and EST
37	50	95	96	–	–	ERCP, IOC, or surgical exploration
38	133	84	96	93	91	ERCP
16	29	91	98	–	–	ERCP

ERCP, endoscopic retrograde cholangiopancreatography; EST, endoscopic sphincterotomy; IOC, intraoperative cholangiography; NPV, negative predictive value; PPV, positive predictive value.

Table 20.7 Detection of choledocholithiasis using intraductal ultrasonography (IDUS)

Ref.	Patients (n)	Accuracy (%)	Sensitivity (%)	Specificity (%)	NPV (%)	PPV (%)	Gold standard
39	31	97	–	–	–	–	EST [c] or surgical exploration
40	81	95	–	–	–	–	EST [c]
41	65	97	100	67	–	–	EST [c]
42	62	97[a]/87[b]	–	–	–	–	EST [c]

EST, endoscopic sphincterotomy; NPV, negative predictive value; PPV, positive predictive value.
[a] ERCP with IDUS.
[b] ERCP without IDUS.
[c] Endoscopic sphincterotomy.

Table 20.8 Comparison of the diagnostic accuracy of endoscopic ultrasonography and other imaging techniques in relation to the detection of choledocholithiasis

Ref.	Patients (n)	EUS (%)	US (%)	CT (%)	ERCP (%)	MRCP (%)
9	52	100	80	83	–	–
25	43	97	–	–	–	82
34	30	89	–	–	–	61
23	52	94	–	86	–	–
13	36	97	83	–	89	–
41	65	97	–	–	94	–
31	100	98	–	–	96	–

CT, computed tomography; ERCP, endoscopic retrograde cholangiopancreatography; EUS, endoscopic ultrasonography; MRCP, magnetic resonance cholangiopancreatography; US, ultrasonography.

Table 20.9 Detection of choledocholithiasis using endoscopic retrograde cholangiopancreatography (ERCP). Endoscopic sphincterotomy (EST) was used as the gold standard

Ref.	Patients (n)	Sensitivity (%)	Specificity (%)	NPV (%)	PPV (%)
30	119	89	100	83	100
43	–	84–89	97–100	88	100
11	35	100	–	–	–
41	65	100	67	–	–
17	220	67–81	–	–	–
31	100	97	–	–	–
44 *	72	90	98	–	–
13	36	92	–	–	–

NPV, negative predictive value; PPV, positive predictive value. * The gold standard used was intraoperative cholangiography.

Table 20.10 Incidence of complications in endoscopic retrograde cholangiopancreatography (ERCP) and endoscopic sphincterotomy (EST)

Ref.	Procedures (n)	Total complication rate (%)	Pancreatitis (%)	Cholangitis (%)	Bacterial complications (%)
[45]	2444	5	2	1	–
[46]	590	2–9	2–4	1	–
[47]	118	5	3	–	3
[48]	2769	4	1	1	–
[49]	51	16	4	–	–
[50]	32	30	12	3	–
[51]	50	4	2	–	–
[52]	80	6	–	–	–
[53]	238	7	3	1	–
[54]	2347	10	5	–	–
[55]	180	12	8	1	–

All of the studies included diagnostic and therapeutic ERCP procedures.

Table 20.11 Incidence of complications in endoscopic retrograde cholangiopancreatography (ERCP) and endoscopic sphincterotomy (EST)

Ref.	Procedures (n)	Bleeding (%)	Perforation (%)	Death (%)	Other (%)
[45]	2444	1	1	0	1
[46]	590	0–3	1–2	0–1	–
[47]	118	–	–	–	–
[48]	2769	1	1	0	1
[49]	51	4	8	–	–
[50]	32	9	6	–	–
[51]	50	2	–	–	–
[52]	80	–	–	–	–
[53]	238	2	1	–	–
[54]	2347	2	–	0.5	–
[55]	180	–	1	–	–

All of the studies included diagnostic and therapeutic ERCP procedures.

may have been considerably overestimated, as the rate of correctly diagnosed choledocholithiasis appears to be much lower—particularly since small gallstones (<3 mm in diameter) with normal or even dilated bile ducts are easily overlooked even in ERCP.

A combination of ERCP with endoscopic sphincterotomy (EST) is the treatment of choice in patients with choledocholithiasis, but this is an invasive technique with a significant risk of early and late complications. Typical early complications include pancreatitis, cholangitis, cholecystitis, bleeding, and perforation. In addition, EST leads to permanent dysfunction of the sphincter of Oddi. Late complications include recurrent gallstones (3–20%) and papillary stenosis (2–6%). The total rate of complications is reported to be in the range of 2–30%. A review of the

literature on the incidence of various complications in ERCP and EST is presented in **Tables 20.10** and **20.11**.[45–55]

In conditions with equivocal signs or symptoms suggesting choledocholithiasis, EUS is a reliable low risk-method to establish a correct diagnosis and indication for EST. **Table 20.12** presents a review of the literature.[8,9,11–13,23–25,27–32]

EUS provides excellent visualization of the proximal and distal common bile duct (**Fig. 20.2**), and of the ampulla and left intrahepatic bile ducts, with a very high sensitivity for even very small stones. In 96% of patients, the entire length of the common bile duct can be visualized, but imaging of the bile ducts of the right lobe of the liver and the hepatic hilum is more difficult. The results of endosonography have been shown to be independent of the size of the

III Gastrointestinal Tract

Table 20.12 Diagnosis of choledocholithiasis by endosonography

Ref.	Patients (n)	Sensitivity (%)	Specificity (%)	NPV (%)	PPV (%)	Gold standard
8	62	97	100	97	100	ERCP with or without EST
9	52	100	100	–	–	ERCP and EST or surgical exploration
24	50	100	97	100	92	Surgical exploration
25	32	100	95	100	91	ERCP and EST
27	50	97	77	–	–	ERCP with or without EST
28	240	85	93	96	75	Surgical exploration
29	422	95	96	96	95	Surgical exploration
23	52	91	100	–	–	ERCP with or without EST
30	119	93	97	88	98	ERCP and EST
11	35	100	100	–	–	ERCP and EST
12	155	96	100	–	–	ERCP with or without EST or surgical exploration
31	100	97	98	–	–	ERCP and EST
13	36	91	100	95	100	ERCP and EST
32	50	88	96	–	–	ERCP and EST

ERCP, endoscopic retrograde cholangiopancreatography; EST, endoscopic sphincterotomy; NPV, negative predictive value; PPV, positive predictive value.

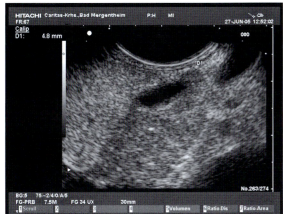

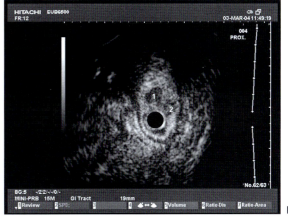

Fig. 20.2a, b a A normal duodenal papilla (between the markers) in routine conditions.

b In a few patients, the orifices of the common hepatic bile duct and pancreatic duct can be imaged separately. The common bile duct orifice (1) and the pancreatic duct orifice (2) are indicated here. (▶ Videos 20.1–4.)

concrement or the diameter of the bile duct, and gallstones smaller than 2 mm have been detected even in dilated bile ducts. Another major advantage of endosonography is the very low rate of morbidity, mortality, and severe complications associated with the procedure. In summary, conventional EUS is a safe, reliable, and minimally invasive method of detecting choledocholithiasis.

The relevance of endosonography for diagnosing cholecystolithiasis before cholecystectomy has yet to be examined and can only be determined in large prospective studies including sufficient numbers of patients with and without cholecystolithiasis. Unexpected diagnostic results, such as benign papillary stenosis and anatomic variations in the bile duct system, need to be taken into account in advance.

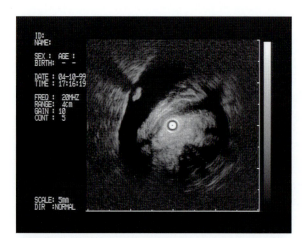

Fig. 20.3 Imaging of choledocholithiasis using extraductal ultrasound (EDUS). Ideally, minuscule concrements only a few millimeters in size (microlithiasis) can be identified even in bile ducts of normal width. Concrements of this type may not be visible on endoscopic retrograde cholangiopancreatography.

Miniprobe EUS and Extraductal Ultrasound

EUS miniprobes introduced through the working channel of a regular endoscope can be used in the same way as ordinary endoscopy accessories such as biopsy forceps. With a penetration depth of ≈ 2 cm, they allow visualization of considerable areas of important anatomy around the upper gastrointestinal tract. Catheter probes may be able to cover most of the indications for conventional diagnostic EUS; this would certainly apply to pathological structures in the intestinal wall. Interventional procedures may be reserved for longitudinal scanners with stiff shafts and wide working channels.

The distal common bile duct (CBD), running from the major duodenal papilla up to the liver just behind the duodenal wall, is certainly within the reach of diagnostic miniprobe EUS. Extraductal ultrasonography (EDUS) of the distal CBD for the detection of choledocholithiasis, with the miniprobe in a duodenal position, was investigated in a prospective study including 119 patients with suspected choledocholithiasis.[30] The probe was introduced through a duodenoscope and first placed on the duodenal papilla to image the sphincter, and then moved slightly more cranially to scan the distal CBD and pancreatic duct. A diagnosis of choledocholithiasis was made when hyperechoic structures not adherent to the ductal wall were detected, with or without acoustic shadowing (**Fig. 20.3**). ERCP with EST and pull-through of a Dormia basket were used as the gold standard. The EDUS diagnosis of choledocholithiasis was confirmed in 33 of 34 patients (97%). As expected, EDUS failed to detect peripheral lesions. The study shows that EDUS can reliably detect pathological lesions in the distal

common bile duct, particularly small concrements, and can therefore avoid the need for sphincterotomy with the associated complications.

Additional diagnostic applications of EDUS for the duodenal papilla were evaluated in another prospective study including 150 patients with similar diagnostic issues and methods. It was shown that in addition to choledocholithiasis, chronic pancreatitis, adenomas of the papilla, adenomas of the bile duct, and primary sclerosing cholangitis (PSC) were capable of being detected reliably using this method.[56] In summary, EUS or EDUS is indicated before cholecystectomy, especially in patients who are at intermediate risk, and these techniques appear to be superior to other diagnostic methods. In addition, EUS is definitely indicated for staging of carcinoma of the ampulla of Vater. EUS is less important in the staging of cholangiocellular carcinoma than it is for pathologic processes in the papilla. Intraductal ultrasonography (IDUS) has diagnostic value particularly in stenoses of unknown origin in the common bile duct.

When evaluating tumors of the bile ducts, it needs to be borne in mind that tumors in the immediate vicinity of the papilla are much easier to diagnose and classify than intrahepatic tumors. Klatskin tumors that are located more peripherally can often not be classified adequately with endosonography. In the case of bile duct carcinoma, lymph-node metastases are not associated with the T stage in the TNM classification, and the accuracy of diagnosis of lymph-node infiltration is reported to be 50–60%. Adequate comparisons between conventional endosonography and intraductal ultrasound have not yet been reported, although several case reports are available. What is known as the "common channel" can be visualized well with endosonography.

Adenoma and Carcinoma of the Papilla of Vater

In the same way as carcinomas of the pancreas, tumors of the papilla of Vater are classified using the TNM staging system. T1 tumors are confined to the papilla, without infiltration of the duodenal wall. T2 is characterized by invasion of the duodenal wall no deeper than the duodenal muscularis propria. T3 means that invasion of the pancreas is less than 2 cm; T4 includes tumors invading the pancreas by more than 2 cm or invading neighboring vessels or organs. The N classification categorizes the presence (N1) or absence (N0) of pathological lymph nodes. More sophisticated and differentiated staging systems have not proved helpful. It is not possible to distinguish between a T1 papillary carcinoma and an adenoma using endosonography (**Figs. 20.4** and **20.5**); histological assessment is required for this crucial differentiation. Multiloculated tumors have to be taken into account. It is also difficult with

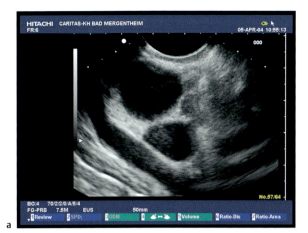

a

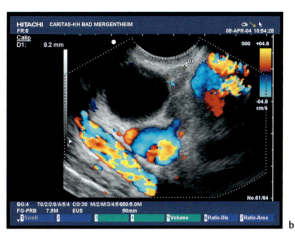

b

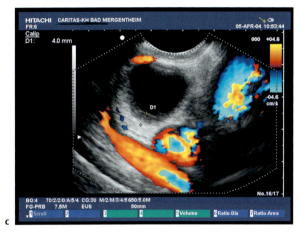

c

Fig. 20.4a–c a Conventional endosonographic imaging of an adenoma in the papilla of Vater.
b The use of color duplex ultrasonography has been shown to facilitate correct detection of ductal structures. Blood vessels are detected within the adenoma here (between the markers).
c It is important to remember that adenomas can develop multilocularly, especially in the extrahepatic bile ducts (between the markers here).

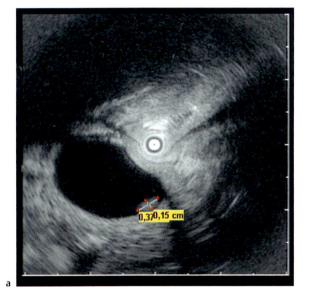

a

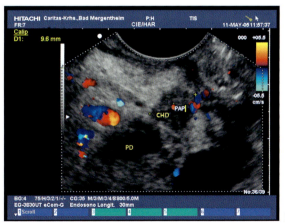

b

Fig. 20.5a, b Adenoma of the papilla, visualized with EUS. In contrast to miniprobe ultrasonography, the conventional technique allows imaging of blood vessels with color duplex ultrasonography.

The beginning of the common hepatic duct (CHD) and pancreatic duct (PD) are also shown. PAP, papilla.

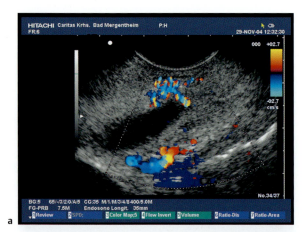

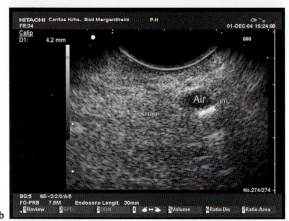

Fig. 20.6a, b Rare pathological conditions in the papilla.
a Color Doppler imaging showing the papilla of Vater with inflammation (papillitis).
b Aerobilia after endoscopic retrograde cholangiopancreatography.

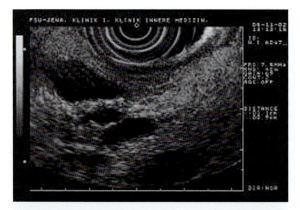

Fig. 20.7 Adenomyomatosis of the papilla, with funnel-shaped narrowing of the common bile duct.

Table 20.13 The Milwaukee classification of sphincter of Oddi dysfunction

Stage	Biliary pain	Elevated liver function tests	Bile duct dilation > 12 mm
I	+	+	+
II	+	–	+
III	+	–	–

EUS to distinguish between inflammatory alterations after the expulsion of gallstones or after endoscopic sphincterotomy and malignant processes. The differential diagnosis of papillitis or adenomyomatosis of the bile duct with EDUS is equally difficult.

EUS of the Papillary Region, Adenomyomatosis

The papilla of Vater is a smooth muscle containing an outlet system for the common bile duct and the main pancreatic duct, which frequently (but not always) join to form a single orifice. Specifically, the papilla consists of the circular muscle of the common bile duct and an additional circular muscle that encloses the two ducts. The normal size of the major duodenal papilla is 10 × 5 mm. It can be visualized endosonographically (**Figs. 20.2** and **20.6**).

There can be many causes of dilation of the common bile duct as a sign of biliary obstruction. In addition to cholangiolithiasis, benign and malignant neoplasms such as adenomas, neuroendocrine tumors, or adenocarcinomas of the papilla are possible causes. A less well known, but in our experience not uncommon, condition is what is known as stenotic papillitis or adenomyomatosis of the papilla (**Fig. 20.7**). The prevalence of this condition is frequently underestimated and was ≈ 50% in older autopsy studies. In a more recent study, Elek and colleagues[57] describe an inflammatory alteration of the papilla as the reason for biliary obstruction in 36% of their patients. Adenomatous hyperplasia and adenomyomatosis were observed in 5% and 7% of examinations, respectively. The clinical symptoms of these conditions are reflected in the Milwaukee classification of sphincter of Oddi dysfunction (**Table 20.13**).

Clinical experience shows that adenomyomatosis is more often seen in elderly women with a history of cholecystectomy, but may also be seen in any patient with increasing age. Pathomorphology shows an increase in the musculature of the sphincter apparatus, with or without a simultaneous inflammatory reaction. Since muscular hypertrophy in biopsies is not necessarily regarded as abnormal by pathologists, close collaboration between the endoscopist and pathologist is required.

At present, the only reliable imaging method for identifying adenomyomatosis of the papilla of Vater is endosonography. Only endosonography allows visualization of the papillary region with sufficient magnification for alterations in the sphincter apparatus to be diagnosed. In Dietrich et al[58], according to Will et al., pathological findings were observed in the papillary region in 311 of 4832 endosonographic examinations. Of these, 183 were further confirmed by biopsy or surgery, showing that EUS has a sensitivity of 92.3% and a specificity of 75.3% for detecting

Table 20.14 Criteria for adenomyomatosis

Concentric thickening of the papillary region
Mixed echogenic, predominantly echodense alterations in the papilla
Smooth borders of the tumor
Preserved layers of the duodenal wall
Convex growth of the tumor
As the most important criterion, a funnel-shaped narrowing and filiform discharge of the common bile duct into the papilla. Typical findings are illustrated in **Fig. 20.7**

Table 20.15 Criteria for noninvasive neoplasm of the papilla (e.g., adenoma, neuroendocrine tumor)

Intraluminal growth
Preserved duodenal wall layers
Homogeneous structure
Narrowing of the common bile duct due to compression
Proximal ductal dilation
Size frequently > 1 cm

Table 20.16 Criteria for a malignant tumor of the papilla of Vater

Irregular borders
Heterogeneous, predominantly poorly echogenic structure
Disruption of duodenal wall layering
Invasion of the duodenal wall, pancreas, ducts, and blood vessels
Suspicious lymph nodes

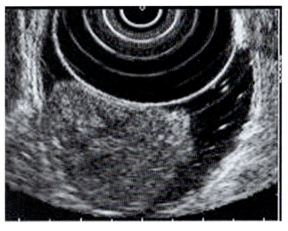

Fig. 20.8 A neuroendocrine tumor of the papilla of Vater, with a homogeneous structure and preserved duodenal wall layers.

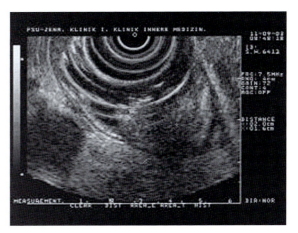

Fig. 20.9 Carcinoma of the papilla of Vater with invasive growth. The duodenal wall layering is disrupted, and the lesion is poorly echogenic, with an irregular base.

papillary carcinoma, with an accuracy of 82%. The criteria used in the study are listed in **Table 20.14**. Criteria for a noninvasive neoplasia of the papilla (e.g., adenomas, neuroendocrine tumors) are listed in **Table 20.15**.

It should be emphasized that it is not possible to distinguish between extensive adenomyomatosis and adenoma (or carcinoid) of the papilla of Vater using endosonographic criteria alone. Further histological examination and verification are required in these cases. An example of a neuroendocrine tumor is shown in **Fig. 20.8**. Criteria for the differential diagnosis of a malignant tumor of the papilla of Vater are listed in **Table 20.16**; a typical example is shown in **Fig. 20.9**.

The detailed diagnosis of papillary lesions is therefore an important area of application for endosonography before further diagnostic or therapeutic procedures such as sphincterotomy, papillectomy, or surgical intervention are carried out.

Cholangiocellular Carcinomas

Carcinomas of the bile duct are classified using the TNM system. T1 is defined as tumor growth within the ductal wall while the outer border is still smooth. T2 tumors invade the periductal connective tissue, resulting in an irregular border. T3 is characterized by invasion of neighboring organs or vessels. As in carcinoma of the pancreas, invasion into the portal vein is the decisive prognostic marker. The N classification designates the presence (N1) or absence (N0) of pathological lymph nodes.

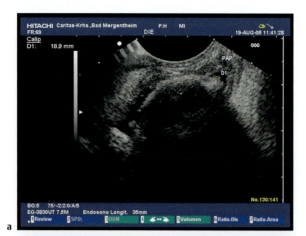

a

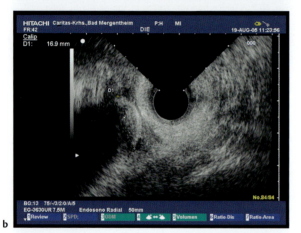

b

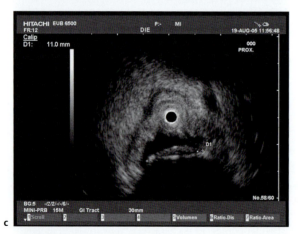

c

Fig. 20.10a–c Choledocholithiasis
a Longitudinal scanning. PAP, papilla.
b Radial scanning.
c Miniprobe imaging. It can be seen that longitudinal scanning, radial EUS, and miniprobe ultrasonography provide similarly good imaging results.

Carcinomas of the Gallbladder

Carcinomas of the gallbladder are also classified using the TNM system. T1 shows invasion no deeper than the muscularis propria, with a smooth border. T2 shows invasion of the gallbladder serosa, but the tumor is still contained in the gallbladder and does not invade the liver. In T3, there is invasion of the liver no deeper than 2 cm and in T4, the tumor is invading the liver by more than 2 cm or penetrating into adjacent organs. The N classification categorizes the presence (N1) or absence (N0) of pathological lymph nodes. As with other tumors of the upper gastrointestinal tract, definitive distinction between inflammatory and neoplastic alterations or changes in the connective tissue is not possible with EUS. In some cases, an endosonographic diagnosis of adenomyomatosis, cholesterol polyps, and other forms of gallbladder pathology (e.g., cholecystolithiasis) can be made, although there is no indication for endosonography in these differential diagnoses. The relevance of endosonography for the diagnosis of invasive tumor growth in primary sclerosing cholangitis is unknown. As with the findings in examinations of the esophagus, stomach, and duodenum, inflammatory alterations can lead to narrowing of the bile duct, which can mimic an invasive tumor in the ductal wall.

Conclusions

EUS (or EDUS) may be indicated before cholecystectomy, particularly in patients with an intermediate risk of choledocholithiasis. EUS appears to be more sensitive for choledocholithiasis than other diagnostic methods, particularly in patients with microlithiasis. It has been shown that longitudinal scanning, radial EUS, or miniprobe ultrasonography are of similar value in the detection of choledocholithiasis (**Figs. 20.10, 20.11,** and **20.12**). Periductal changes in elasticity are illustrated in **Fig. 20.13**. In addition, EUS is indicated for staging of carcinoma of the ampulla of Vater. EUS is less important for the staging of cholangiocellular carcinoma.

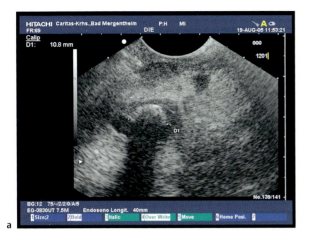

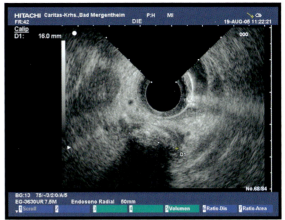

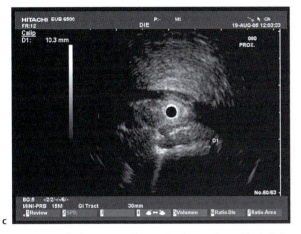

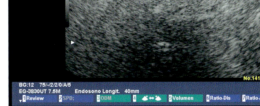

Fig. 20.11a–d The retropapillary region in a patient with choledocholithiasis.
a Longitudinal scanning.
b Radial scanning.

c Miniprobe imaging. PAP, papilla.
d The miniprobe (MP) is also shown with the longitudinal echoendoscope.

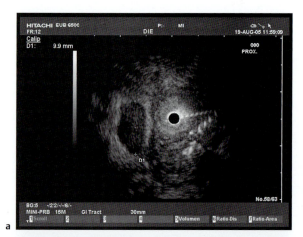

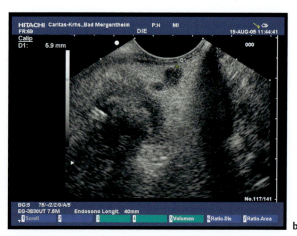

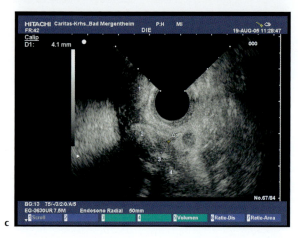

Fig. 20.12a–c Cystic duct lymph node. Close to the aperture of the cystic duct, lymph nodes within the dorsal hepatoduodenal ligament can usually be seen, as shown here in a patient with choledocholithiasis.

a This is best displayed using high-resolution miniprobe technology.

b, c However, it is also visible with longitudinal scanning (**b**) and radial scanning (**c**). Radial scanning shows 4 gallstones (1–4).

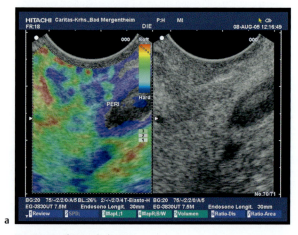

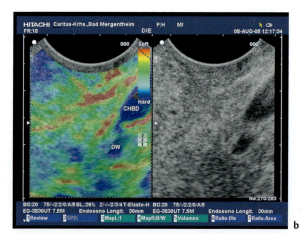

Fig. 20.13a, b Pericholangitis

a Periductal fibrosis (PERI) in a patient with chronic cholangitis, reproducibly demonstrated with elastography (blue indicates harder elasticity here).

b CHBD, common hepatic bile duct; DW, duct of Wirsung (pancreatic duct).

References

1. Cooperberg PL, Burhenne HJ. Real-time ultrasonography. Diagnostic technique of choice in calculous gallbladder disease. N Engl J Med 1980;302(23):1277–1279.
2. Di Nardo R, Urbano D, Drudi FM, et al. Ultrasonography in the preoperative assessment of candidates for laparoscopic cholecystectomy: examination technique and results. [Article in German] Radiol Med (Torino) 1996;92(5): 605–609.
3. Fang R, Pilcher JA, Putnam AT, Smith T, Smith DL. Accuracy of surgeon-performed gallbladder ultrasound. Am J Surg 1999;178(6):475–479.
4. Krook PM, Allen FH, Bush WH Jr, Malmer G, MacLean MD. Comparison of real-time cholecystosonography and oral cholecystography. Radiology 1980;135(1):145–148.
5. Seitz K, Hege-Blank U, Holzinger H. 10 years of sonographic diagnosis of gallstones—what do surgical statistics tell us about its reliability? [Article in German] Ultraschall Med 1987;8(3):121–125.
6. Silidker MS, Cronan JJ, Scola FH, et al. Ultrasound evaluation of cholelithiasis in the morbidly obese. Gastrointest Radiol 1988;13(4):345–346.
7. Goodman AJ, Neoptolemos JP, Carr-Locke DL, Finlay DB, Fossard DP. Detection of gall stones after acute pancreatitis. Gut 1985;26(2):125–132.
8. Amouyal P, Amouyal G, Lévy P, et al. Diagnosis of choledocholithiasis by endoscopic ultrasonography. Gastroenterology 1994;106(4):1062–1067.
9. Amouyal P, Palazzo L, Amouyal G, et al. Endosonography: promising method for diagnosis of extrahepatic cholestasis. Lancet 1989;2(8673):1195–1198.
10. Scientific Committee of the European Association for Endoscopic Surgery (E.A.E.S.). Diagnosis and treatment of common bile duct stones (CBDS). Results of a consensus development conference. Surg Endosc 1998;12(6):856–864.
11. Sugiyama M, Atomi Y. Acute biliary pancreatitis: the roles of endoscopic ultrasonography and endoscopic retrograde cholangiopancreatography. Surgery 1998;124(1):14–21.
12. Sugiyama M, Atomi Y. Endoscopic ultrasonography for diagnosing choledocholithiasis: a prospective comparative study with ultrasonography and computed tomography. Gastrointest Endosc 1997;45(2):143–146.
13. Chak A, Hawes RH, Cooper GS, et al. Prospective assessment of the utility of EUS in the evaluation of gallstone pancreatitis. Gastrointest Endosc 1999;49(5):599–604.
14. Kumar M, Prashad R, Kumar A, Sharma R, Acharya SK, Chattopadhyay TK. Relative merits of ultrasonography, computed tomography and cholangiography in patients of surgical obstructive jaundice. Hepatogastroenterology 1998;45(24):2027–2032.
15. Shim CS, Joo JH, Park CW, et al. Effectiveness of endoscopic ultrasonography in the diagnosis of choledocholithiasis prior to laparoscopic cholecystectomy. Endoscopy 1995; 27(6): 428–432.
16. Varghese JC, Liddell RP, Farrell MA, Murray FE, Osborne H, Lee MJ. The diagnostic accuracy of magnetic resonance cholangiopancreatography and ultrasound compared with direct cholangiography in the detection of choledocholithiasis. Clin Radiol 1999;54(9):604–614.
17. Pasanen P, Partanen K, Pikkarainen P, Alhava E, Pirinen A, Janatuinen E. Ultrasonography, CT, and ERCP in the diagnosis of choledochal stones. Acta Radiol 1992;33(1):53–56.
18. Pickuth D, Spielmann RP. Detection of choledocholithiasis: comparison of unenhanced spiral CT, US, and ERCP. Hepatogastroenterology 2000;47(36):1514–1517.
19. Cabada Giadás T, Sarría Octavio de Toledo L, Martínez-Berganza Asensio MT, et al. Helical CT cholangiography in the evaluation of the biliary tract: application to the diagnosis of choledocholithiasis. Abdom Imaging 2002;27(1):61–70.
20. Jiménez Cuenca I, del Olmo Martínez L, Pérez Homs M. Helical CT without contrast in choledocholithiasis diagnosis. Eur Radiol 2001;11(2):197–201.
21. Takahashi M, Saida Y, Itai Y, Gunji N, Orii K, Watanabe Y. Reevaluation of spiral CT cholangiography: basic considerations and reliability for detecting choledocholithiasis in 80 patients. J Comput Assist Tomogr 2000;24(6):859–865.
22. Neitlich JD, Topazian M, Smith RC, Gupta A, Burrell MI, Rosenfield AT. Detection of choledocholithiasis: comparison of unenhanced helical CT and endoscopic retrograde cholangiopancreatography. Radiology 1997;203(3): 753–757.
23. Polkowski M, Palucki J, Regula J, Tilszer A, Butruk E. Helical computed tomographic cholangiography versus endosonography for suspected bile duct stones: a prospective blinded study in non-jaundiced patients. Gut 1999;45(5): 744–749.
24. Aubertin JM, Levoir D, Bouillot JL, et al. Endoscopic ultrasonography immediately prior to laparoscopic cholecystectomy: a prospective evaluation. Endoscopy 1996;28(8): 667–673.
25. de Lédinghen V, Lecesne R, Raymond JM, et al. Diagnosis of choledocholithiasis: EUS or magnetic resonance cholangiography? A prospective controlled study. Gastrointest Endosc 1999;49(1):26–31.
26. Edmundowicz SA, Aliperti G, Middleton WD. Preliminary experience using endoscopic ultrasonography in the diagnosis of choledocholithiasis. Endoscopy 1992;24(9): 774–778.
27. Lachter J, Rubin A, Shiller M, et al. Linear EUS for bile duct stones. Gastrointest Endosc 2000;51(1):51–54.
28. Montariol T, Msika S, Charlier A, et al; French Associations for Surgical Research. Diagnosis of asymptomatic common bile duct stones: preoperative endoscopic ultrasonography versus intraoperative cholangiography—a multicenter, prospective controlled study. Surgery 1998;124(1):6–13.
29. Palazzo L, Girollet PP, Salmeron M, et al. Value of endoscopic ultrasonography in the diagnosis of common bile duct stones: comparison with surgical exploration and ERCP. Gastrointest Endosc 1995;42(3):225–231.
30. Seifert H, Wehrmann T, Hilgers R, Gouder S, Braden B, Dietrich CF. Catheter probe extraductal EUS reliably detects distal common bile duct abnormalities. Gastrointest Endosc 2004;60(1):61–67.
31. Liu CL, Lo CM, Chan JK, et al. Detection of choledocholithiasis by EUS in acute pancreatitis: a prospective evaluation in 100 consecutive patients. Gastrointest Endosc 2001;54(3): 325–330.
32. Norton SA, Alderson D. Prospective comparison of endoscopic ultrasonography and endoscopic retrograde cholangiopancreatography in the detection of bile duct stones. Br J Surg 1997;84(10):1366–1369.
33. Taylor AC, Little AF, Hennessy OF, Banting SW, Smith PJ, Desmond PV. Prospective assessment of magnetic resonance cholangiopancreatography for noninvasive imaging of the biliary tree. Gastrointest Endosc 2002;55(1):17–22.
34. Scheiman JM, Carlos RC, Barnett JL, et al. Can endoscopic ultrasound or magnetic resonance cholangiopancreatogra-

phy replace ERCP in patients with suspected biliary disease? A prospective trial and cost analysis. Am J Gastroenterol 2001;96(10):2900–2904.

35. Lomas DJ, Bearcroft PW, Gimson AE. MR cholangiopancreatography: prospective comparison of a breath-hold 2D projection technique with diagnostic ERCP. Eur Radiol 1999;9(7):1411–1417.

36. Linares Torres P, Vivas Alegre S, Espinel Díez J, et al. Current status of endoscopic retrograde cholangiopancreatography. What is the effect of the introduction of magnetic resonance cholangiography? [Article in German] Gastroenterol Hepatol 2001;24(10):483–488.

37. Hussein FM, Alsumait B, Aman S, et al. Diagnosis of choledocholithiasis and bile duct stenosis by magnetic resonance cholangiogram. Australas Radiol 2002;46(1):41–46.

38. Griffin N, Wastle ML, Dunn WK, Ryder SD, Beckingham IJ. Magnetic resonance cholangiopancreatography versus endoscopic retrograde cholangiopancreatography in the diagnosis of choledocholithiasis. Eur J Gastroenterol Hepatol 2003;15(7):809–813.

39. Ueno N, Nishizono T, Tamada K, et al. Diagnosing extrahepatic bile duct stones using intraductal ultrasonography: a case series. Endoscopy 1997;29(5):356–360.

40. Ohashi A, Ueno N, Tamada K, et al. Assessment of residual bile duct stones with use of intraductal US during endoscopic balloon sphincteroplasty: comparison with balloon cholangiography. Gastrointest Endosc 1999;49(3 Pt 1):328–333.

41. Tseng LJ, Jao YT, Mo LR, Lin RC. Over-the-wire US catheter probe as an adjunct to ERCP in the detection of choledocholithiasis. Gastrointest Endosc 2001;54(6):720–723.

42. Das A, Isenberg G, Wong RC, Sivak MV Jr, Chak A. Wire-guided intraductal US: an adjunct to ERCP in the management of bile duct stones. Gastrointest Endosc 2001;54(1):31–36.

43. Berthou JC, Drouard F, Charbonneau P, Moussalier K. Evaluation of laparoscopic management of common bile duct stones in 220 patients. Surg Endosc 1998;12(1):16–22.

44. Frey CF, Burbige EJ, Meinke WB, et al. Endoscopic retrograde cholangiopancreatography. Am J Surg 1982;144(1):109–114.

45. Masci E, Toti G, Mariani A, et al. Complications of diagnostic and therapeutic ERCP: a prospective multicenter study. Am J Gastroenterol 2001;96(2):417–423.

46. Halme L, Doepel M, von Numers H, Edgren J, Ahonen J. Complications of diagnostic and therapeutic ERCP. Ann Chir Gynaecol 1999;88(2):127–131.

47. Brandes JW, Scheffer B, Lorenz-Meyer H, Körst HA, Littmann KP. ERCP: Complications and prophylaxis a controlled study. Endoscopy 1981;13(1):27–30.

48. Loperfido S, Angelini G, Benedetti G, et al. Major early complications from diagnostic and therapeutic ERCP: a prospective multicenter study. Gastrointest Endosc 1998;48(1):1–10.

49. Thatcher BS, Sivak MV Jr, Tedesco FJ, Vennes JA, Hutton SW, Achkar EA. Endoscopic sphincterotomy for suspected dysfunction of the sphincter of Oddi. Gastrointest Endosc 1987;33(2):91–95.

50. Neoptolemos JP, Bailey IS, Carr-Locke DL. Sphincter of Oddi dysfunction: results of treatment by endoscopic sphincterotomy. Br J Surg 1988;75(5):454–459.

51. Roberts-Thomson IC, Toouli J. Is endoscopic sphincterotomy for disabling biliary-type pain after cholecystectomy effective? Gastrointest Endosc 1985;31(6):370–373.

52. Geenen JE, Hogan WJ, Dodds WJ, Toouli J, Venu RP. The efficacy of endoscopic sphincterotomy after cholecystectomy in patients with sphincter-of-Oddi dysfunction. N Engl J Med 1989;320(2):82–87.

53. Wojtun S, Gil M, Gil J. Recognition of ERC-induced pancreatitis in patients with choledocholithiasis by an analysis of laboratory findings. Hepatogastroenterology 2000;47(32):550–553.

54. Freeman ML, Nelson DB, Sherman S, et al. Complications of endoscopic biliary sphincterotomy. N Engl J Med 1996;335(13):909–918.

55. Sharma SK, Larson KA, Adler Z, Goldfarb MA. Role of endoscopic retrograde cholangiopancreatography in the management of suspected choledocholithiasis. Surg Endosc 2003;17(6):868–871.

56. Seifert H, Wehrmann T, Hilgers R, Gouder S, Braden B, Dietrich CF. Catheter probe extraductal EUS reliably detects distal common bile duct abnormalities. Gastrointest Endosc 2004;60:61–67 and unpublished data.

57. Elek G, Gyôri S, Tóth B, Pap A. Histological evaluation of preoperative biopsies from ampulla vateri. Pathol Oncol Res 2003;9(1):32–41.

58. Dietrich CF, Seifert H, Gouder S, Hocke M. Endosonographie des hepatobiliären Systems. Endoskopischer Ultraschall, eine Einführung. Constance, Germany: Schnetztor; 2005:254–271.

21 Endoscopic Ultrasound Imaging of the Adrenals

C.F. Dietrich, P.H. Kann

Endosonographic imaging of the adrenal glands, and the systematic use of the method in diagnostic procedures for adrenal diseases, have been reported for over 15 years. Endosonographic imaging of the left adrenal gland was first described by Chang et al.[1] In a small group of 31 patients, the normal left adrenal gland was delineated using endoscopic ultrasonography (EUS) in 97% of cases; detection of the right adrenal gland was only reported in one patient, with a J-shaped stomach. Imaging of the right adrenal gland was therefore initially found to be more problematic.

In the meantime, a great deal of experience has been gained in carrying out endosonographic imaging of the adrenal glands and in assessing the value of this diagnostic technique.[2–18] Both the imaging quality and precise identification of healthy—i.e., morphologically normal—tissue in the adrenals have markedly improved. In particular, modifying the imaging technique for the right adrenal gland made a substantial contribution to progress in this area. It is now possible to distinguish between the medulla and cortex in both adrenals, very small tumors can be identified, and in particular, atrophic adrenals can be demonstrated as a manifestation of autoimmune Addison disease.

Examination Technique

Due to the complementary role of transabdominal and endoscopic ultrasound for examining the adrenal glands, both methods are described here.

■ Transabdominal Examination Technique

Cadaver studies. The transabdominal and endoscopic examination technique has recently been validated in corpses. To establish the correct identification and echo pattern of the adrenal glands, the sonographic appearance was documented.

Right adrenal gland. The right adrenal gland is examined in a slightly left lateral position, with the patient's right arm raised above the head to widen the intercostal space. The right adrenal gland is located using the upper pole of the kidney, the inferior vena cava, the crus of the dia-

phragm, and the margin of the liver as guiding structures. The inferior vena cava, as the medial border, can always be delineated, as well the crus of the diaphragm. For correct identification, the typical echo pattern (bright, dark, bright, dark, and bright echo lines), defined by the pathological anatomical study, has to be visualized. The thickness was measured as $5 \pm 1\,mm$ (range 4–8 mm). The thickness of the adrenal wings, measured in their middle representative symmetrical portion in healthy control individuals, was comparable to the EUS findings. Both were slightly larger than the documented diameters in the cadavers. This may have been due to pressure from the directly applied transducer on the adrenal gland, or differences in blood filling.

Left adrenal gland. The left adrenal gland can be examined with the patient in a supine or slightly (right) oblique position, with the left hand raised above the head to widen the intercostal space. Typically, it is seen between the upper pole of the left kidney, pancreatic tail, spleen, crus of the diaphragm, and aorta. In some cases, better visualization is achieved by applying the transducer ventrally, documenting the celiac trunk, splenic and left renal vessels, pancreas, aorta, and left kidney.

Identification of normal adrenal glands, and particularly the right adrenal gland, is possible with transabdominal ultrasonography in most healthy individuals. Reported differences in the detection rate of the adrenal glands may also be due to differences in the equipment used. However, EUS is capable of detecting almost all left and most right adrenal glands, if required.

■ Endoscopic Ultrasound Examination Technique

Endosonographic imaging of the adrenals is easier with a longitudinal echoendoscope, but is also possible with radial transducers. Using these instruments, the adrenal glands can be visualized best by sector scanning; switching the frequency from 7.5 to 5.0 MHz is sometimes useful, as it improves the imaging of the right adrenal gland, which is frequently further away from the transducer than the left adrenal gland, within a range of < 30 mm. In addition, the device also provides the option of carrying out EUS-guided fine-needle aspiration biopsy of adrenal masses in patients who may benefit from cytological and histological assessment.

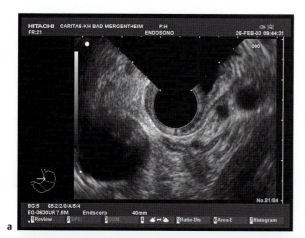

a

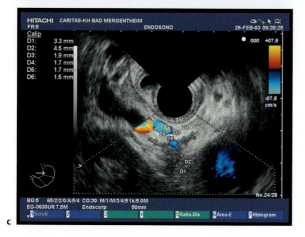

c

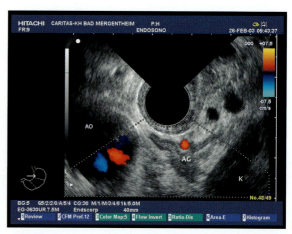

b

Fig. 21.1a–e a A normal left adrenal gland imaged using conventional B-mode.
b, c Color Doppler imaging, showing the hilum with the afferent artery (**b**) and efferent vein (**c**). AG, adrenal; AO, aorta; K, kidney.

Fig. 21.1d, e ▷

Sedation. The echoendoscope is inserted with the patient lying on the left side. Since imaging of the adrenals often involves detection or exclusion of very small morphological changes, sufficient sedation is mandatory. The authors use different approaches to sedation. One author (C.F.D.) always uses propofol sedation without local anesthesia; the other (P.H.K.) prefers the following approach: after administering local anesthesia of the pharynx with a spray, and an intravenous injection of atropine (0.25 mg), premedication is administered with pentazocine (30 mg) and diazepam (10–20 mg).

Left adrenal gland. Landmarks for correct identification of the left adrenal are the cranial pole of the left kidney, the distal pancreatic tail, and the splenic vessels. Typically, after entering the stomach the transducer is kept toward the left posterior gastric wall and shows a variable section of the abdominal aorta at 45 cm; a little more caudally, the upper pole of the left kidney is seen. The transducer should be angulated slightly medially and retracted. The adrenal gland is seen on the way between the upper pole of the left kidney and the aorta, just below the splenic vein. The fact that it typically overlaps the aorta ventromedially by ≈ 0.5 cm is very helpful in finding the correct position. In

some cases, the left adrenal gland can also be seen with the transducer in the ascending part of the duodenum. For correct identification, the typical sonographic echo pattern (bright, dark, bright, dark, and bright echo lines) has to be documented. The mean EUS examination time for the left adrenal gland has been reported to be 2 ± 1 minutes, starting on entry into the stomach, demonstrating that the procedure is not time-consuming (**Fig. 21.1**).

Due to its proximity to the posterior gastric wall, miniprobe ultrasonography of the left adrenal gland is also possible (**Fig. 21.2**).

Right adrenal gland. Imaging of the right adrenal gland is easiest to carry out when the transducer is placed in the antrum, just in front of the pylorus, after which the patient should lie on the right side. The transducer is now flexed fully toward the right, so that the tip of the echoendoscope is behind the angular notch. With the transducer in this position, the echoendoscope is carefully retracted until the landmarks (the cranial pole of the right kidney, inferior vena cava, caudal parts of the liver, and the portal vein) can be identified. After this, the right adrenal gland can be imaged behind the inferior vena cava. As in the transabdominal examination, this technique makes it possible to

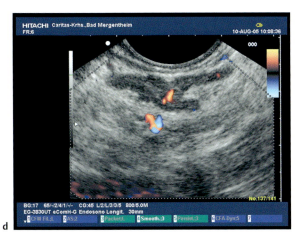

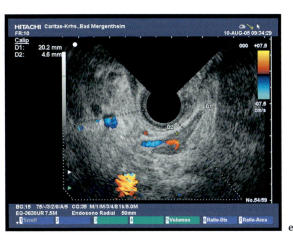

Fig. 21.1d, e (continued)
d Longitudinal scanning.

e Radial scanning. The adrenal hilum and adrenal vessels can be delineated with both methods. Miniprobe ultrasound with longitudinal scanning is of no value (not shown).

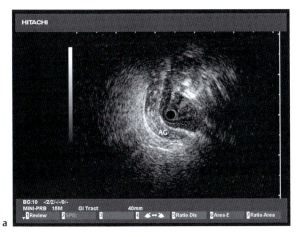

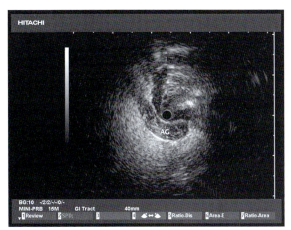

Fig. 21.2a–c Imaging of a normal left adrenal gland (AG) using miniprobe technology next to the pancreas.

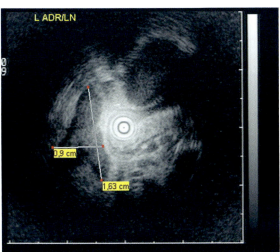

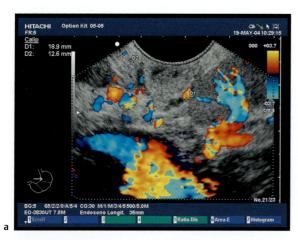

Fig. 21.3a, b a The right adrenal gland, between the markers.   **b** Color Doppler imaging demonstrates the hilum as well.

distinguish between the echoes generated by the adrenal medulla and those generated by the cortex (**Fig. 21.3**).

Adrenal gland morphology. It is possible to visualize abnormalities in the structure of the adrenal glands, although the relevance of these has not yet been fully assessed. For example, in patients with genetic disorders such as multiple endocrine neoplasia types 2a and 2b and von Hippel–Lindau disease, it is now possible to identify clear hyperplasia of the adrenal medulla. Further studies are needed in order to clarify whether this is a preliminary stage in the development of manifest pheochromocytoma, in the same way that there is a progression from C cell hyperplasia to medullary thyroid carcinoma.

Indications for EUS of the Adrenal Glands

On this basis of the information currently available, the following can be regarded as valid indications for endosonography of the adrenal glands:

- Detection of small adrenal tumors
- Characterization of adrenal tumors
- Assessing criteria of malignancy in adrenal tumors
- Early detection of recurrences of malignant adrenal tumors
- Preoperative identification of morphologically healthy parts of the adrenals
- Detection of extra-adrenal/ectopic tumors (pheochromocytomas)
- Differentiation between different entities in adrenal insufficiency
- EUS-guided fine-needle aspiration biopsy

Pathological Findings

Detection of small adrenal tumors. Endosonography of the adrenal glands makes it possible to detect morphological abnormalities such as nodular formations in the adrenals, down to a diameter of ≈ 3 mm (**Fig. 21.4**). In addition, nodular hyperplasia occurring in multiple endocrine neoplasia type 1 can be identified. There is some evidence that endosonography of the adrenal glands may be superior to magnetic resonance imaging and/or computed tomography (CT) in relation to small adrenal tumors, with postoperative histological assessment as the gold standard.

Incidentalomas. Incidentally found adrenal tumors without hormone production are known as incidentalomas. These can be found in up to 5% of transabdominal examinations, as well as CT and EUS examinations, in unselected populations. Surgery is recommended in patients with

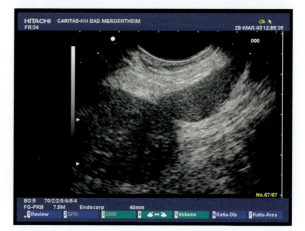

Fig. 21.4 Diffuse enlargement of the left adrenal gland, often observed as a nonspecific finding in elderly patients.

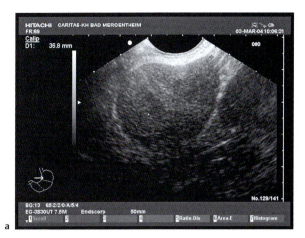

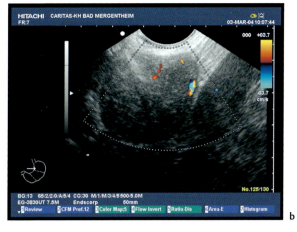

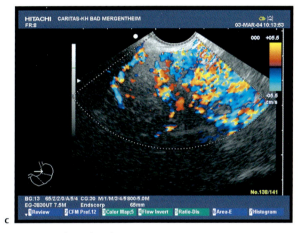

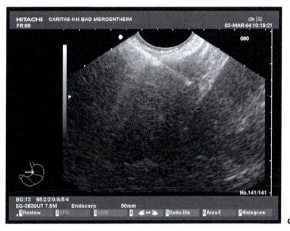

Fig. 21.5a–d Incidentaloma
a B-mode.
b Color duplex scanning.

c Contrast-enhanced ultrasound using SonoVue.
d Puncture.

tumors 4–6 cm in size and/or tumor growth. Fine-needle aspiration cytology is helpful in the diagnosis of lymphoma and metastases (**Fig. 21.5**).

In the case of enlarged adrenals, it is also possible to identify lipid-containing tumors such as myelolipoma, due to their high echogenicity. Adrenal cysts are rare and have the typical features known from conventional sonography in other organs (**Fig. 21.6**).

Characterization of adrenal tumors. Micronodular hyperplasia of the adrenal glands can be identified by EUS as a rare morphological substrate of Cushing syndrome independent of adrenocorticotropic hormone (ACTH). It is easily distinguished from unilateral, solitary adenoma of one adrenal gland.

In the differential diagnosis of primary hyperaldosteronism, endosonography allows the identification of unilateral adenoma. Important criteria for this appear to be a round or oval shape of the tumor and detection of the border of the normal adrenal tissue. Bilateral adrenal hyperplasia can also be imaged and differentiation between a

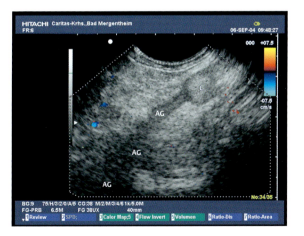

Fig. 21.6 A small hyperechoic tumor in the left adrenal gland (AG): a typical lipid-containing myelolipoma (L).

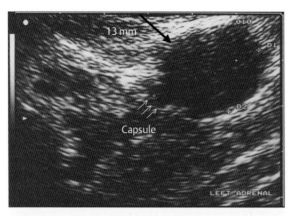

Fig. 21.7 A solitary adenoma (arrow) in the left adrenal gland (lateral limb) in a patient with Conn syndrome (primary aldosteronism).

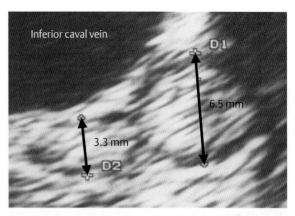

Fig. 21.8 Nodular transformation (assessed histologically as nodular hyperplasia) in the body of the right adrenal gland in a patient with rapidly progressive virilization.

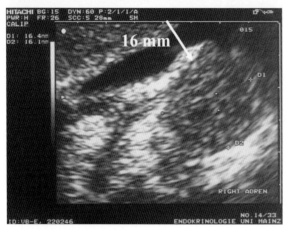

Fig. 21.9 A solitary adenoma (arrow) in the right adrenal gland (lateral limb) in a patient with Cushing syndrome independent of adrenocorticotropic hormone (ACTH).

diffuse type or nodular morphology is possible. The precise differential diagnosis is very important clinically, since in the first case surgery is indicated, while in the second case medical treatment is mandatory.

Figures 21.7, 21.8, 21.9, 21.10, and **21.11** show examples of various hormone-producing tumors and hyperplasia. **Figures 21.12** and **21.13** show examples of atrophy in patients with insufficiency.

Assessment criteria for malignancy in adrenal tumors.
Preoperative detection of criteria for malignancy is very important during the planning of the surgical strategy for adrenal masses. Endocrinologists and endocrine surgeons may consider endoscopic resection to be the wrong approach in such cases.

Adrenocortical carcinomas are generally heterogeneous and have a complex echo pattern, but malignant and be-

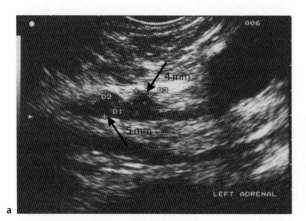

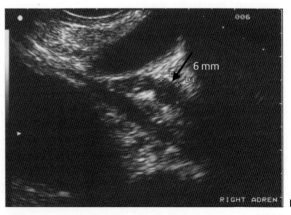

Fig. 21.10a, b Hyperplasia of the adrenal glands (arrows; morphologically nodular) in idiopathic hyperaldosteronism.

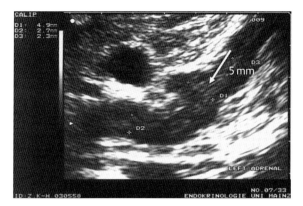

Fig. 21.11 Hyperplasia of the adrenal medulla in a patient with multiple endocrine neoplasia (MEN) type 2a.

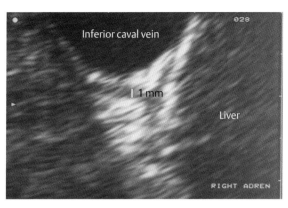

Fig. 21.12 Marked atrophy of the adrenal glands (the right adrenal is shown here) in a patient with autoimmune Addison disease.

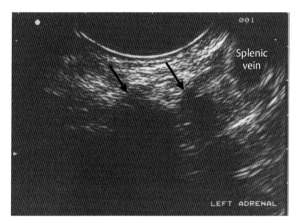

Fig. 21.13 Calcification of the left adrenal gland in a patient with adrenal tuberculosis and primary adrenal insufficiency.

nign pheochromocytomas can also have the same characteristics. Heterogeneity of an adrenal tumor is therefore not a clear criterion for malignancy (**Fig. 21.14**). The value of endosonography is that it can demonstrate or exclude infiltration of neighboring organs as a valid criterion for malignancy. In addition, the detection of effusion is suggestive of malignancy. Detection of local or regional lymph-node metastases and vascular invasion is a clear criterion for malignancy.

Early detection of recurrences of malignant adrenal tumors. In the postoperative care of adrenocortical carcinomas and pheochromocytomas, endosonography allows detection of small recurrences in the tumor area and in neighboring regions earlier than with other techniques.

Preoperative identification of morphologically normal parts of the adrenals. Bilateral adrenal masses are detected in some cases, particularly in diseases with genetic causes such as multiple endocrine neoplasia types 2a and 2b and von Hippel–Lindau disease. The patients affected

are often young. It is very important to know preoperatively whether there are morphologically completely normal parts of an adrenal gland that can be left in situ in order to avoid the need for lifelong substitution treatment with adrenal steroid hormones in these patients.

Detection of extra-adrenal/ectopic masses (pheochromocytomas). The typical symptoms and hormonal findings of a pheochromocytoma are the principal reason for conducting morphological diagnostic procedures in the adrenals. However, some of these tumors are ectopic, either para-adrenal or in other regions of the body. In these circumstances, endosonography allows detection of ectopic tumors (**Fig. 21.15**).

Differentiation of different causes of adrenal insufficiency. Different diseases causing adrenocortical insufficiency have typical morphologies, which can be detected using endosonography. Autoimmune Addison disease is associated with marked atrophy of the adrenal glands. Calcifications in the organs are suggestive of adrenal insufficiency following adrenal tuberculosis. Adrenal metastases are typically large and hypoechoic, and clear identification and histopathological differentiation can be achieved with EUS-guided fine-needle aspiration biopsy.

EUS-guided fine-needle aspiration biopsy. Endosonography allows guided fine-needle aspiration biopsies of the adrenal glands. In most cases, this makes a definitive diagnosis possible. The following points apply to the indication for fine-needle aspiration biopsy of the adrenal glands:

• Biopsy of an adrenal mass makes it possible to differentiate between adrenal tissue and nonadrenal tissue— i.e., in particular, detection of metastases and/or lymphomas.
• Differentiation between adrenocortical adenoma and adrenocortical carcinoma is not possible with fine-needle aspiration biopsy. This is therefore not an indication for biopsy.

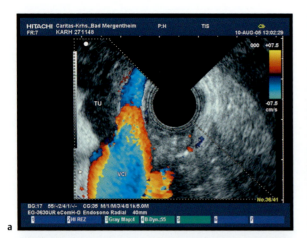

a

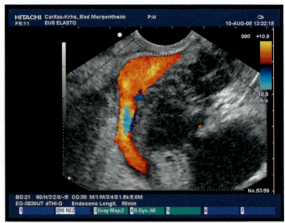

b

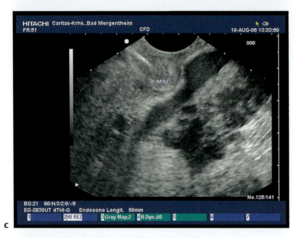

c

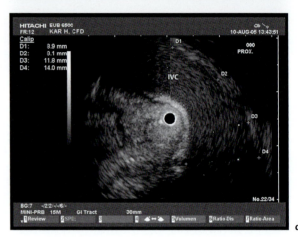

d

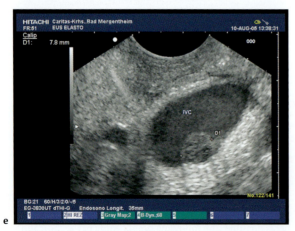

e

Fig. 21.14a–e A right adrenal gland tumor (TU) infiltrating the inferior vena cava (IVC).

a, b While visualization was comparable with the radial (**a**) and longitudinal (**b**) systems, tumor puncture is only possible with the longitudinal scanner.

c Miniprobe ultrasound (MINI) was not helpful in delineating tumor infiltration. The miniprobe position is shown here with the longitudinal scanner.

d The corresponding miniprobe image, showing the inferior vena cava.

e Infiltration of the lumen of the inferior vena cava (IVC) was only visualized using the longitudinal probe.

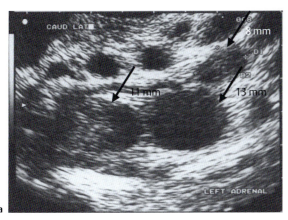

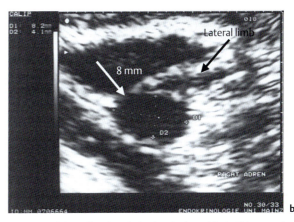

Fig. 21.15a, b Pheochromocytomas in both adrenal glands (**a**, three on the left; **b**, one on the right) in a patient with multiple endocrine neoplasia type 2a, with clear identification of morphologically nor-mal parts of the right adrenal gland in the lateral limb. This part of the organ was left in situ during surgery, allowing the patient to avoid lifelong substitution treatment with steroid hormones.

- Due to complications reported in the literature resulting from mechanical manipulations of pheochromocytomas, fine-needle aspiration biopsy of adrenal masses should not be performed unless pheochromocytoma has been excluded.

Contrast enhanced (endoscopic) ultrasound. Contrast enhanced (endoscopic) ultrasound (CEUS) is helpful in delineating atypical cysts, abscesses, and hemorrhage in the adrenal glands as described for example for the liver and other organs. It was also shown that CEUS is not helpful in differentiating malignant and benign adrenal tumors[19] but controversely discussed findings have also been published.[20] Myelolipoma (and lipoma) are often less enhancing than other tumors.

Conclusion and Summary

Endosonographic imaging of the adrenal glands has developed from an experimental procedure into an established diagnostic method. Endosonography conducted by an experienced investigator in patients who have received sufficient premedication is a harmless procedure for the patient. The complication rate is comparable to that with conventional gastroscopy, there is no radiation exposure, the diagnostic value and clinical impact are high, and the procedure is inexpensive. The technique is therefore an advantageous one in the diagnosis and differentiation of adrenal diseases.

References

1. Chang KJ, Erickson RA, Nguyen P. Endoscopic ultrasound (EUS) and EUS-guided fine-needle aspiration of the left adrenal gland. Gastrointest Endosc 1996;44(5):568–572.
2. Chhieng DC, Jhala D, Jhala N, et al. Endoscopic ultrasound-guided fine-needle aspiration biopsy: a study of 103 cases. Cancer 2002;96(4):232–239.
3. Dietrich CF, Wehrmann T, Hoffmann C, Herrmann G, Caspary WF, Seifert H. Detection of the adrenal glands by endoscopic or transabdominal ultrasound. Endoscopy 1997; 29(9):859–864.
4. Heinz-Peer G, Hönigschnabl S, Schneider B, Niederle B, Kaserer K, Lechner G. Characterization of adrenal masses using MR imaging with histopathologic correlation. AJR Am J Roentgenol 1999;173(1):15–22.
5. Kann P, Bittinger F, Hengstermann C, Engelbach M, Beyer J. Endosonographic imaging of the adrenal glands: a new method. [Article in German] Ultraschall Med 1998;19(1): 4–9.
6. Kann P, Hengstermann C, Heussel CP, Bittinger F, Engelbach M, Beyer J. Endosonography of the adrenal glands: normal size—pathological findings. Exp Clin Endocrinol Diabetes 1998;106(2):123–129.
7. Kann P, Heintz A, Bittinger F, Herber S, Kunt T, Beyer J. Endosonographie bei kleinen Nebennierenraumforderungen: Morphologischer Nachweis der mikro- und makronodulären Nebennierenrindenhyperplasie in vivo als Ursache einer autonomen Sekretion von Steroidhormonen. [Article in German] Tumordiagn Ther 1999;20:135–143.
8. Kann P, Heintz A, Bittinger F, et al. Bildgebende Diagnostik der Nebennieren: neue Aspekte durch die Einführung der Endosonographie. [Article in German] Minimal Inv Chir 2000;9:58–61.
9. Kann PH, Wirkus B, Behr T, Klose KJ, Meyer S. Endosonographic imaging of benign and malignant pheochromocytomas. J Clin Endocrinol Metab 2004;89(4):1694–1697.
10. Kann PH. Endoscopic ultrasound imaging of the adrenals. Endoscopy 2005;37(3):244–253.
11. Korobkin M, Brodeur FJ, Francis IR, Quint LE, Dunnick NR, Londy F. CT time-attenuation washout curves of adrenal adenomas and nonadenomas. AJR Am J Roentgenol 1998; 170(3):747–752.

12. Langer P, Bartsch DK, Fendrich V, Kann PH, Rothmund M, Zielke A. Minimal-invasive operative treatment of organic hyperinsulinism. [Article in German] Dtsch Med Wochenschr 2005;130(10):514–518.

13. Meyer S, Bittinger F, Keth A, Von Mach MA, Kann PH. Endosonographically controlled transluminal fine needle aspiration biopsy: diagnostic quality by cytologic and histopathologic classification. [Article in German] Dtsch Med Wochenschr 2003;128(30):1585–1591.

14. Müller MF, Meyenberger C, Bertschinger P, Schaer R, Marincek B. Pancreatic tumors: evaluation with endoscopic US, CT, and MR imaging. Radiology 1994;190(3):745–751.

15. Reincke M, Allolio B. Das Nebenniereninzidentalom. [Article in German] Dt Aerztebl 1995;92:A764–A770.

16. Sample WF. A new technique for the evaluation of the adrenal gland with gray scale ultrasonography. Radiology 1977;124(2):463–469.

17. Trojan J, Schwarz W, Sarrazin CM, Thalhammer A, Vogl TJ, Dietrich CF. Role of ultrasonography in the detection of small adrenal masses. Ultraschall Med 2002;23(2):96–100.

18. Vilmann P. Endoscopic ultrasound-guided fine-needle biopsy in Europe. Endoscopy 1998;30(Suppl 1):A161–A162.

19. Dietrich CF, Ignee A, Barreiros AP, et al. Contrast-enhanced ultrasound for imaging of adrenal masses. [Article in German] Ultraschall Med 2010;31(2):163–168.

20. Friedrich-Rust M, Schneider G, Bohle RM, et al. Contrast-enhanced sonography of adrenal masses: differentiation of adenomas and nonadenomatous lesions. AJR Am J Roentgenol 2008;191(6):1852–1860.

22 Contrast-Enhanced EUS

M. Hocke, C.F. Dietrich

Detection

The potential of contrast-enhanced endoscopic ultrasound (EUS) to detect pancreatic lesions that are not identified with conventional endoscopic ultrasound is limited. This situation is also unlikely to change, since it is difficult to improve the local resolution of endoscopic ultrasound, and with correct positioning of the scope and mastery of the examination technique, even structures only a few millimeters in size can be clearly recognized.

Characterization of Malignancy

The primary aim in using contrast enhancement in endoscopic ultrasound, therefore, is to improve the assessment of malignancy in pathological changes by optimizing the

imaging of vessel distribution. Endoscopic ultrasound with amplified echo signals has been found helpful in differentiating between benign and malignant pancreatic tumors, although a definitive conclusion cannot be reached in every case. Initial attempts to diagnose malignant areas in cases of chronic pancreatitis have been very promising. Above and beyond this, however, it has become apparent that with improved equipment and classification of the pancreatic vascular structures, the quality of malignancy assessment in pancreatic tumors can be greatly improved. The examination of patients with undiagnosed pancreatic masses has shown that pancreatic adenocarcinomas have a few arteries with an irregular configuration and that focal pancreatitis demonstrates both veins and arteries with a regular treelike distribution (**Figs. 22.1** and **22.2**).

Endoscopic ultrasound is also useful for clarifying less common localized pancreatic growths. It is particularly valuable in cases of hypervascularization of microcystic pancreatic adenomas or neuroendocrine tumors, as well as macrocystic ones, although these are less well

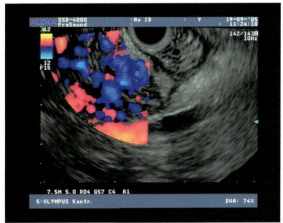

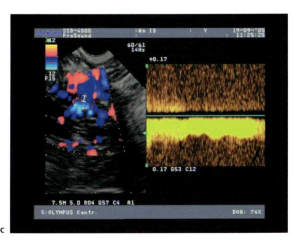

Fig. 22.1a–c Chronic pancreatitis
a No evidence of vascularization on color Doppler imaging before contrast administration.
b Evidence of long, regular blood vessels, homogeneously distributed, after contrast administration.
c Evidence of arterial and venous signals on Doppler imaging.

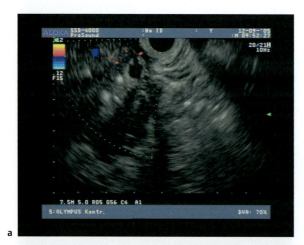

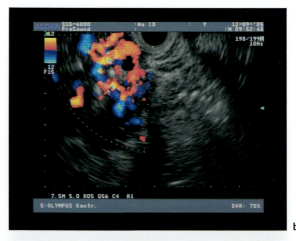

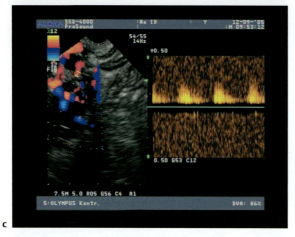

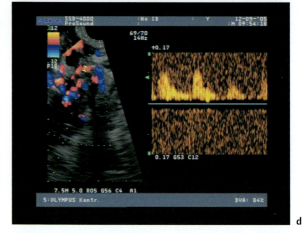

Fig. 22.2a–d Pancreatic carcinoma
a No evidence of vessels on color Doppler imaging before contrast administration.

b Evidence of short, irregular vessels with an inhomogeneous distribution after contrast administration.
c, d Evidence of exclusively arterial signals on Doppler imaging.

delineated (**Figs. 22.3** and **22.4**). The lesions can be diagnosed relatively reliably using color duplex endoscopic ultrasound and contrast-enhanced sonography. It is essential to make a differentiated diagnosis when there are mixed pancreatic tumors with different degrees of malignancy and in cases of hypervascularized pancreatic metastases, which are relatively often diagnosed using modern imaging, but which play a lesser role in determining the prognosis. In cases of hypervascularized pancreatic metastases, it is also important to take into consideration the possibility that they are metastases from renal adenocarcinoma, melanoma, small cell bronchial carcinoma, or mammary carcinoma.[1]

With the help of EUS-guided fine-needle aspiration, endoscopic ultrasound represents an important tool in the diagnosis of pancreatic tumors. Preliminary data indicate that it is already possible today to do without histological specimens and rely on cytological specimens. This hypothesis is currently being tested—for example, at Topalidis's cytology laboratory in Hanover, Germany (who kindly provided the images for **Fig. 22.4**).

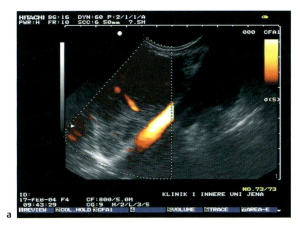

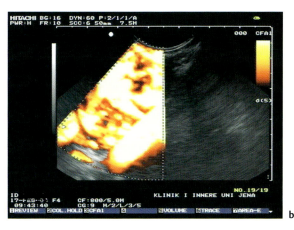

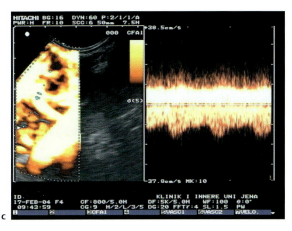

Fig. 22.3a–c Neuroendocrine tumor
a Evidence of vessels on power Doppler imaging, even before contrast administration.
b Evidence of a long, regular vessel structure after contrast administration.
c Evidence of both arterial and venous signals on Doppler imaging.

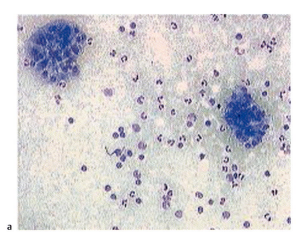

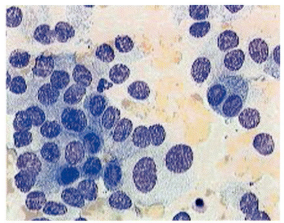

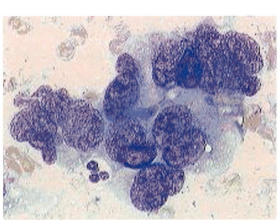

Fig. 22.4a–c Cytological images (courtesy of T. Topalidis, Hanover).
a Chronic pancreatitis.
b Undifferentiated pancreatic carcinoma.
c Neuroendocrine carcinoma.

Review of the Literature[2]

Contrast-enhanced transabdominal ultrasound techniques were recently introduced. Administration of liver-specific microbubbles using Levovist makes it possible to detect metastases smaller than 1 cm and improves the ability to differentiate between benign and malignant lesions.[3–5] Due to the complexity of the (intermittent) examination technique, with a high mechanical index and bubble destruction, the method was found to be difficult to use routinely. More recent advances with SonoVue combined with low mechanical index techniques have improved the transabdominal use of contrast-enhanced techniques, allowing real-time imaging with or without three-dimensional reconstruction.[6]

Several studies have been carried out to assess the potential role of contrast-enhanced endoscopic ultrasonography. Initial data on the practicality of using first-generation contrast agents were published by Bhutani et al.,[7] who were able to demonstrate better imaging of vessels in swine after administration of Levovist. It should be noted that only one study has been conducted to date using second-generation contrast agents, and no research has yet been published on contrast-specific software.

Recognizing malignant neoplasia in chronic pancreatitis has always been difficult. The gold standard is still surgery. Although the introduction of EUS-guided fine-needle aspiration has made this easier, an improved noninvasive method of detecting malignant tissue would be preferable. In a recently published study, contrast-enhanced EUS was used to distinguish between benign and malignant pancreatic lesions. High sensitivity and specificity rates are possible when strong inclusion criteria are used. Isovascularity or hypervascularity as a sign of nonductal adenocarcinoma showed a sensitivity of 100%, a specificity of 90%, and an accuracy rate of 93.8%. Hypovascularity as a sign of ductal adenocarcinoma showed a sensitivity of 90%, a specificity of 100%, and an accuracy rate of 93.8%. Using this method, there is no real difference between endoscopic and transabdominal ultrasound. The only difference that needs to be taken into account is that the transabdominal approach is limited due to poor visibility of the lesion in ≈ 9% of patients. The main factor limiting differentiation using the global contrast-enhancing effect is that patients with chronic pancreatitis have to be excluded.[8] This topic is further discussed in Chapters 8 and 18.

When not only global enhancement effects of the contrast agent but also advanced vessel analysis are used for differentiation, it is possible to obtain reliable results even when patients with chronic pancreatitis are included. In patients with pancreatic cancer, contrast enhancement only shows arterial microvessels, whereas both venous and arterial microvessels are displayed after contrast enhancement in patients with chronic pancreatitis. We have used this effect in a study which produced the best differentiation results currently available. The study compared conventional EUS with contrast-enhanced EUS plus advanced microvessel analysis. Using conventional EUS criteria, the sensitivity for pancreatic cancer was 73% and the specificity was 83%. With contrast-enhanced EUS, the sensitivity increased to 91%, identifying 51 of 56 patients with malignant pancreatic lesions. In 28 of 30 patients with chronic inflammatory pancreatic disease, the diagnosis was correctly recognized, giving a specificity value of 93.3%.[9] These figures remained the same in a second study including 194 patients.[10]

As the method relies on the current resolution available with color Doppler, it is possible that improved equipment might in the future lead to uncertainties, with a few venous microvessels also becoming visible in patients with pancreatic cancer.

To obtain a second criterion for distinguishing between focal pancreatitis and pancreatic carcinoma, we investigated the resistance index of the arterial microvessels shown on contrast enhancement. The study identified a cut-off point for the arterial resistance index of 0.7 in pancreatic cancer. A resistance index of more than 0.7 indicates pancreatic cancer, whereas a figure below 0.7 indicates chronic pancreatitis.[11]

As in studies using contrast-enhanced transabdominal ultrasound,[12–15] ductal adenocarcinoma of the pancreas was found to be hypoenhancing in an EUS study by Hirooka et al.[16] using Albunex. The authors found that Albunex improved the endoscopic ultrasound diagnosis in examinations of the gallbladder and pancreas. They were able to show enhancement in the various layers of tissue and an absence of it in pancreatic carcinoma. However, it should be noted that all of the investigations were based on contrast differences that could be detected using a mechanical radial scanner.

Optison was also used in a small study by Becker et al.[17] to differentiate ductal adenocarcinoma from focal chronic pancreatitis, with a sensitivity of 94% and a specificity of 100%. Interestingly, neuroendocrine tumors were not distinguishable from inflammation. This is the only report in the current literature describing the use of second-generation ultrasound contrast agents with electronic scanners.

In a case report, insulinoma was found to be distinguishable from the main pancreatic duct, with a separation of 3 mm, so that enucleation instead of pancreatectomy was considered preoperatively.[18]

Bile duct carcinoma at the hepatic bifurcation was differentiated from primary and secondary sclerosing cholangitis by analyzing the enhancement pattern of the wall of the bile ducts; hypoenhancement was found to be a typical sign of malignancy.[19] In five patients with autoimmune pancreatitis, strong enhancement of the thickened wall of the common bile duct after injection of Levovist was able to rule out pancreatic-obiliary malignancy.[20] The accuracy of predicting the T staging of malignancies of the gallbladder using contrast-enhanced endoscopic ultrasound with Albunex was better than with conventional EUS, improving from 79% to 93%.[21]

Contrast-enhanced endoscopic ultrasound was also used in patients with gastric and esophageal cancer, and improved the accuracy of T staging from 77% to 90%. Most malignant lesions showed no enhancement.[21]

The detection of perforating veins in patients with esophageal varices due to portal hypertension as a predictive sign of recurrence was improved by the use of Levovist-enhanced Doppler techniques. Using unenhanced endoscopic ultrasonography, 31% of patients with recurrent esophageal varices, and none of the patients without recurrences, were shown to have perforating veins. Using contrast-enhanced EUS, 76% of patients with recurrences were found to have perforating veins. Again, none of the patients who had no recurrences showed this sign.

A summary of the literature is given in **Table 22.1**.[2]

Wide-Band Harmonic Imaging

Although EUS has become an established procedure during the last 20 years, real-time contrast applications using a low mechanical index (MI) have been limited to the transabdominal approach.[22,23] Recent advances in tech-

Table 22.1 Findings in contrast-enhanced endoscopic ultrasound techniques, as reported in the literature[1]

Criteria evaluated	Lesions	Patients (n)	Method	Conclusion	Reference
To detect perforating veins as a criterion for recurrence of esophageal varices	Esophageal varices	29	CE-EUS, Levovist, color/power Doppler	Detection of perforating veins in patients with vs. without recurrence of varices in EUS: 31% vs. 0%; in CE-EUS: 76% vs. 0%	[26]
To describe esophageal varices	Esophageal varices	62	CE-EUS, Levovist, color/power Doppler	Levovist improves the diagnostic quality of EUS, providing improved images	[27]
Concentric wall thickening of the common bile duct	Common bile duct	5	CE-EUS, EUS, IDUS, Levovist	Strong enhancement after Levovist rules out pancreatic-obiliary malignancy in auto-immune-related pancreatitis	[20]
Enhancement of bile duct wall	Primary (2) and secondary sclerosing cholangitis (1), bile duct carcinoma of the hepatic bifurcation (4)	7	CE-IDUS, Levovist, quantitative assessment	The wall of the bile duct is not enhanced in bile duct carcinoma but is enhanced in sclerosing cholangitis	[19]
Hypoperfusion as a criterion for malignancy	Solid pancreatic masses	23	CE-EUS, Optison, color/power Doppler	Sensitivity 94%, specificity 100% for malignancy	[17]
Negative enhancement as a criterion for malignancy	Esophageal (4), gastric carcinoma (30), gastric myogenic tumors (5), gastric ulcers (3)	42	CE-EUS, Albunex, high MI B-mode	In gastric cancer, improved accuracy of T staging from 77% to 90%; sharper delineation of tumors	[25]
To evaluate pancreas-saving operability	Insulinoma of the pancreas, detected by CT	Case study	CE-EUS Levovist	Enhancement, distance to pancreatic duct was 3 mm so enucleation was possible	[17]
Enhancement in ductal adenocarcinoma and pseudocysts	Ductal adeno-carcinoma (11), mucin-producing tumors (10), pseudocysts (5), islet cell tumors (4), chronic pancreatitis (4), serous cystadenoma (3)	37	CE-EUS, Albunex	Combined evaluation of fundamental and contrast enhanced images of EUS useful for diagnosis of pancreatic diseases	[15]
To differentiate different lesions of the gallbladder	Adenocarcinoma of the gallbladder (12), adeno-squamous carcinoma (2), cholesterol polyp (6), cholecystitis (10), adenomyomatosis (8)	38	CE-EUS, Albunex	No enhancement in adeno-squamous carcinomas and cholesterol polyps; accuracy for detection of tumor invasion using CE-EUS improved from 79 to 93%	[20]

CE, contrast-enhanced; CT, computed tomography; EUS, endoscopic ultrasonography; IDUS, intraductal ultrasonography; MI, mechanical index.

nology have allowed the development of new endoscopic systems, making it possible to use low MI contrast-enhanced imaging techniques (wide-band harmonic imaging) in endoscopic ultrasonography, with encouraging preliminary results.[2,24]

During the arterial phase of ≈ 10–20 seconds, it is possible to characterize the celiac trunk, common hepatic artery, and splenic artery as arterial target vessels. It is also possible to demonstrate the portal vein and its branches, as well as collaterals, in patients with portal vein thrombosis. In contrast to angiographic imaging, parenchymal enhancement was only possible in patients who did not have underlying liver disease. The enhancement was strongest and homogeneous in a band of ≈ 2–4 cm around the level of the focal zone. No significant bubble destruction was visualized. This method is limited by a depth of penetration of just over 50 mm, due to the higher har-

monic frequency ranges used. As with all new methods, a learning curve needs to be taken into account, since steady and targeted transducer manipulation is a prerequisite for optimal image documentation[2] (**Fig. 22.5**).

Lymph Nodes

Contrast-enhanced endoscopic ultrasound is particularly important for assessing malignancy in mediastinal or abdominal lymph nodes (**Figs. 22.6, 22.7,** and **22.8**). It has been shown in case reports that malignant infiltration of regional lymph nodes can be better imaged and aspirated with guidance from endoscopic ultrasound. Analysis of the vascular structure has proved to be useful here, as lymph

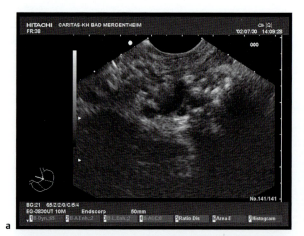

a

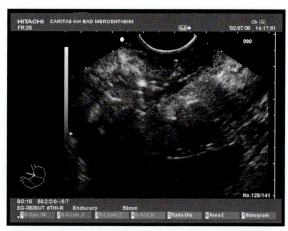

b

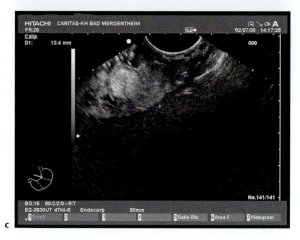

c

Fig. 22.5a–c Wide-band harmonic imaging. The first images using contrast-enhanced low mechanical index wide-band harmonic imaging equipment produced very promising results. The circulation surrounding a portal vein thrombosis is visible in a contrasted image.

nodes are normally fed by arteries through their sinus and drained correspondingly by veins. These changes can also be corroborated by the histopathology. When the vessel invasion extends beyond the capsule, it should be assumed that the infiltration of the lymph node is malignant, although this criterion has not yet been sufficiently evaluated in the current literature. The criteria for size, shape, and echo pattern analysis that have been described are ambiguous in many cases. Unfortunately, research to date has not yet demonstrated any clear superiority for contrast-enhanced analysis of the vascular distribution in determining whether the enlargement of lymph nodes is benign or malignant. A study on this issue analyzed the vascularization tendencies in various lymph nodes before and after contrast administration and verified the results by carrying out fine-needle aspiration immediately after the examination. A total of 122 patients were included in the study. Using normal endoscopic ultrasound diagnosis, 64 of 74 cases of benign lymph-node enlargement were correctly identified (specificity 86%); after contrast administration, this increased to 68 of the 74 cases (a specificity of 91%). Thirty-three of 48 malignant lymph nodes were correctly diagnosed with normal endoscopic ultrasound (sensitivity 68%). However, when the criteria for vascula-

rization assessment after contrast administration were taken into account, the results deteriorated to 29 of 48 cases (sensitivity 60%). The majority of false-positive findings with contrast-enhanced endosonography were malignant lymphomas (n = 10). Using this technique, no differences were observed in the vascular lymph-node pattern between benign lymph nodes and lymph-node enlargements caused by malignant lymphomas, and this was the problem that mainly led to the poor results. These data suggest that contrast-enhanced assessment of lymph nodes is not capable of improving visual differentiation between malignant and benign lymph-node enlargements.[28] However, further trials would be useful in order to define the criteria for differentiation more precisely.

Prospects

Ultrasonography is currently the most commonly used imaging modality in many countries. The advantages of endoscopic ultrasonography (e.g., lack of radiation exposure and relatively low cost) are limited by its operator-

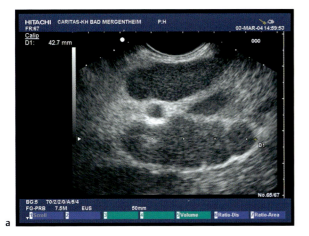
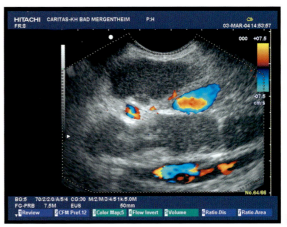

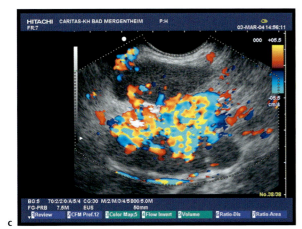
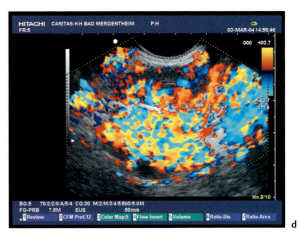

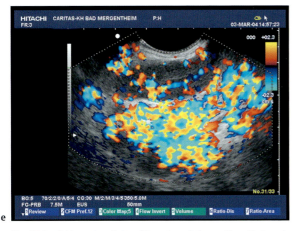
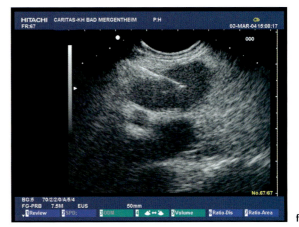

Fig. 22.6a–f Ventral and dorsal imaging of the perihepatic lymph-node group in the hepatoduodenal ligament in a patient with suspected lymphoma.

a B-mode sonography showed lymph nodes enlarged to 43 mm in the direct vicinity of the common hepatic artery and portal vein.

b No relevant vessels were identified on color duplex sonography.

c–e After administration of the contrast agent SonoVue, the lymph-node sinus is clearly recognizable both ventrally and dorsally in the hepatoduodenal ligament, with no damaged vascular structure or localized infiltration.

f Endoscopic ultrasound-guided fine-needle aspiration demonstrated granulomatous inflammation qualified by a hepatic manifestation of sarcoidosis.

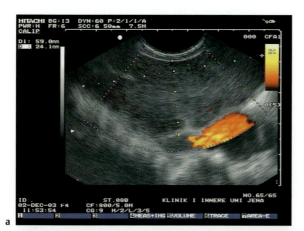

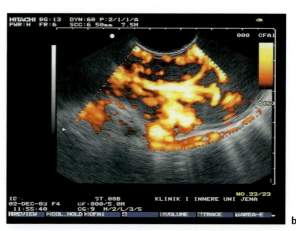

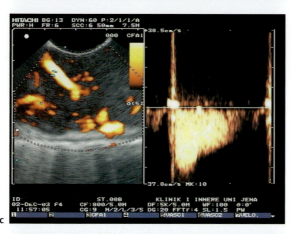

Fig. 22.7a–c Another example of sarcoidosis before and after contrast administration. Note the preserved lymph node architecture.

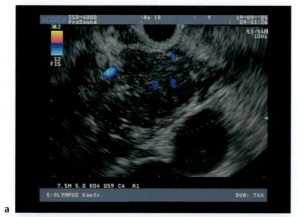

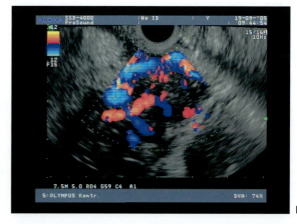

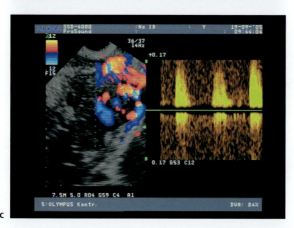

Fig. 22.8a–c A malignant lymph node before and after contrast administration. The vascular distribution is not regular, and only arterial vessels are seen.

dependency. EUS using contrast-enhancing agents might improve our understanding of the morphological imaging methods by allowing additional analysis of functional criteria such as with perfusion, with better characterization of tumors, lymph-node staging, and organ infiltration, for example. Improved imaging documentation of this type would improve confidence in the sonographic method. Other possible new applications might be lymph-node biopsies guided by contrast-enhanced imaging, with demarcation of the infiltrated site even in small lymph nodes. It is even possible to use US contrast enhancement outside the blood vessel system to guide biliary endoscopic interventions.[29,30] The potential future scope of contrast-enhanced endosonography is therefore virtually unlimited.[31]

Addendum

The ultrasound systems Hitachi HI VISION Avius, HI VISION Preirus and HI VISION Ascendus are equipped with two contrast specific software modes using multi pulse technology to perform contrast enhanced EUS (CE-EUS) at low mechanical indices (MI of 0.08–0.15).

The conventional method of "dynamic Contrast Harmonic Imaging" (dCHI) utilizes a wideband pulse inversion technique providing low MI contrast imaging. However, with dCHI, tissue harmonic signals are not completely eliminated even at very low US power levels. Therefore in situations where strong tissue signals occur such as with fatty changes of organs, or calcifications, the contrast-to-tissue noise ratio (CTR) could be suboptimal, hindering the correct interpretation of the image.

To obtain high CTR (HCTR) an improved advanced method "Color Wideband Pulse Inversion" (CWPI) has been developed. The received signals from both tissue and contrast agent consist of two frequency components, a harmonic part and a fundamental part of the frequency spectrum. To remove both components of the tissue signal (fundamental and harmonic) this algorithm uses a combination of phase inversion and amplitude modulation. The result is a much better CTR (HCTR), reducing the risk of misinterpretation (**Fig. 22.9**). In addition, CWPI provides the option to display the contrast image as an overlay

Table 22.2 Settings recommended for CWPI-Imaging

Frequency	CWPI-R (or CWPI-P)	Smoothing	3
Color Map	Map 5	Line density	2
MI	0.10	Persistence	2
DR	50	Receiving Filter	C

Table 22.3 Settings Recommended for dCHI

Frequency	dCHI-R (or dCHI-P)*	Gray Map	4
Mechanical Index	0.10	Receiving Filter	C
Scan Line Density	2	Persistence	2
Initial Gain	**5**	Dynamic Range	50
HI REZ "On"	**2**	B-Color	21

* Depending on patient

mode on the low MI fundamental image as one single image.

To optimize visualization and trace the path of microbubbles in the microvasculature, a peak hold method called Microbubble Trace Imaging (MTI) is available.

■ Parameters and Settings for Contrast Harmonic Imaging

The MI should be set at a range of 0.09–0.12 depending on the method (CWPI, d-CHI-W) and patient habitus, however a base setting of MI 0.10 is recommended. At higher values (> MI: 0.12) there may be stronger enhancement of the bubble signal, however some bubble destruction will occur and stronger tissue harmonic signals will be generated (**Tables 22.2** and **22.3**).

- **Dynamic Range (DR):** Distribution of echo amplitudes over a certain number of gray levels. DR has an influence on the display of gray levels available and thus on the signal brightness of the highest echo signals. High DR produces a softer image but reduces overall signal brightness and vice versa. A lower DR between 45–55 is recommended for the base contrast setting.
- **Gamma curve:** Linear curve is recommended for contrast imaging.
- **Persistence:** As persistence is increased, noise is reduced, less "real-time" character

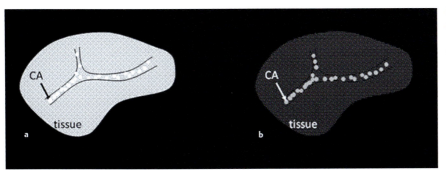

Fig. 22.9a, b
a Conventional pulse inversion method—some background tissue harmonic signal is present.
b CWPI mode—tissue signal is eliminated and CTR significantly improved.

- **Line density:** Increasing line density results in higher spatial resolution, lower frame rate
- **HI REZ:** Noise and speckle reduction and edge enhancement. Low HI REZ results in noise; too high a HI REZ setting might cause suppression of low contrast signals.

References

1. Dietrich CF, Jenssen C, Allescher HD, Hocke M, Barreiros AP, Ignee A. Differential diagnosis of pancreatic lesions using endoscopic ultrasound. [Article in German] Z Gastroenterol 2008;46(6):601–617.
2. Dietrich CF, Ignee A, Frey H. Contrast-enhanced endoscopic ultrasound with low mechanical index: a new technique. Z Gastroenterol 2005;43(11):1219–1223.
3. Harvey CJ, Blomley MJ, Eckersley RJ, Heckemann RA, Butler-Barnes J, Cosgrove DO. Pulse-inversion mode imaging of liver specific microbubbles: improved detection of subcentimetre metastases. Lancet 2000;355(9206):807–808.
4. Blomley M, Albrecht T, Cosgrove D, et al. Stimulated acoustic emission imaging ("sono-scintigraphy") with the ultrasound contrast agent Levovist: a reproducible Doppler ultrasound effect with potential clinical utility. Acad Radiol 1998;5(Suppl 1):S236–S239, discussion S252–S253.
5. Dietrich CF, Ignee A, Trojan J, Fellbaum C, Schuessler G. Improved characterisation of histologically proven liver tumours by contrast enhanced ultrasonography during the portal venous and specific late phase of SHU 508A. Gut 2004;53(3):401–405.
6. Dietrich CF. 3D real time contrast enhanced ultrasonography, a new technique. [Article in German] Rofo 2002; 174(2):160–163.
7. Bhutani MS, Hoffman BJ, van Velse A, Hawes RH. Contrast-enhanced endoscopic ultrasonography with galactose microparticles: SHU508 A (Levovist). Endoscopy 1997;29(7): 635–639.
8. Dietrich CF, Ignee A, Braden B, Barreiros AP, Ott M, Hocke M. Improved differentiation of pancreatic tumors using contrast-enhanced endoscopic ultrasound. Clin Gastroenterol Hepatol 2008;6(5):590–597, e1.
9. Hocke M, Schulze E, Gottschalk P, Topalidis T, Dietrich CF. Contrast-enhanced endoscopic ultrasound in discrimination between focal pancreatitis and pancreatic cancer. World J Gastroenterol 2006;12(2):246–250.
10. Hocke M, Schmidt C, Zimmer B, Topalidis T, Dietrich CF, Stallmach A. Contrast enhanced endosonography for improving differential diagnosis between chronic pancreatitis and pancreatic cancer. [Article in German] Dtsch Med Wochenschr 2008;133(38):1888–1892.
11. Hocke M, Ignee A, Topalidis T, Stallmach A, Dietrich CF. Contrast-enhanced endosonographic Doppler spectrum analysis is helpful in discrimination between focal chronic pancreatitis and pancreatic cancer. Pancreas 2007;35(3): 286–288.
12. Rickes S, Unkrodt K, Ocran K, Neye H, Lochs H, Wermke W. Evaluation of Doppler ultrasonography criteria for the differential diagnosis of pancreatic tumors. [Article in German] Ultraschall Med 2000;21(6):253–258.
13. Rickes S, Unkrodt K, Neye H, Ocran KW, Wermke W. Differentiation of pancreatic tumours by conventional ultrasound, unenhanced and echo-enhanced power Doppler sonography. Scand J Gastroenterol 2002;37(11):1313–1320.
14. Ding H, Kudo M, Onda H, Nomura H, Haji S. Sonographic diagnosis of pancreatic islet cell tumor: value of intermittent harmonic imaging. J Clin Ultrasound 2001;29(7): 411–416.
15. Kitano M, Kudo M, Maekawa K, et al. Dynamic imaging of pancreatic diseases by contrast enhanced coded phase inversion harmonic ultrasonography. Gut 2004;53(6): 854–859.
16. Hirooka Y, Goto H, Ito A, et al. Contrast-enhanced endoscopic ultrasonography in pancreatic diseases: a preliminary study. Am J Gastroenterol 1998;93(4):632–635.
17. Becker D, Strobel D, Bernatik T, Hahn EG. Echo-enhanced color- and power-Doppler EUS for the discrimination between focal pancreatitis and pancreatic carcinoma. Gastrointest Endosc 2001;53(7):784–789.
18. Kasono K, Hyodo T, Suminaga Y, et al. Contrast-enhanced endoscopic ultrasonography improves the preoperative localization of insulinomas. Endocr J 2002;49(4):517–522.
19. Hyodo T, Hyodo N, Yamanaka T, Imawari M. Contrast-enhanced intraductal ultrasonography for thickened bile duct wall. J Gastroenterol 2001;36(8):557–559.
20. Hyodo N, Hyodo T. Ultrasonographic evaluation in patients with autoimmune-related pancreatitis. J Gastroenterol 2003;38(12):1155–1161.
21. Hirooka Y, Naitoh Y, Goto H, et al. Contrast-enhanced endoscopic ultrasonography in gallbladder diseases. Gastrointest Endosc 1998;48(4):406–410.
22. Dietrich CF, Braden B, Hocke M, Ott M, Ignee A. Improved characterisation of solitary solid pancreatic tumours using contrast enhanced transabdominal ultrasound. J Cancer Res Clin Oncol 2008;134(6):635–643.
23. Claudon M, Cosgrove D, Albrecht T, et al. Guidelines and good clinical practice recommendations for contrast enhanced ultrasound (CEUS) - update 2008. Ultraschall Med 2008;29(1):28–44.
24. Dietrich CF. Contrast-enhanced low mechanical index endoscopic ultrasound (CELMI-EUS). Endoscopy 2009; 41(Suppl 2):E43–E44.
25. Nomura N, Goto H, Niwa Y, Arisawa T, Hirooka Y, Hayakawa T . Usefulness of contrast-enhanced EUS in the diagnosis of upper GI tract diseases. Gastrointest Endosc 1999; 50(4):555–560.
26. Sato T, Yamazaki K, Toyota J, et al. Perforating veins in recurrent esophageal varices evaluated by endoscopic color Doppler ultrasonography with a galactose-based contrast agent. J Gastroenterol 2004;39(5):422–428.
27. Sato T, Yamazaki K, Toyota J, Karino Y, Ohmura T, Suga T. Evaluation of hemodynamics in esophageal varices. Value of endoscopic color Doppler ultrasonography with a galactose-based contrast agent. Hepatol Res 2003;25(1):55–61.
28. Hocke M, Menges M, Topalidis T, Dietrich CF, Stallmach A. Contrast-enhanced endoscopic ultrasound in discrimination between benign and malignant mediastinal and abdominal lymph nodes. J Cancer Res Clin Oncol 2008; 134(4):473–480.
29. Ignee A, Baum U, Schuessler G, Dietrich CF. Contrast-enhanced ultrasound-guided percutaneous cholangiography and cholangiodrainage (CEUS-PTCD). Endoscopy 2009; 41(8):725–726.
30. Dietrich CF, Hocke M, Jenssen C. Interventional Endosonography. Ultraschall in Med 2011;32:8–25 [to be verified since in press] .
31. Hocke M, Ignee A, Dietrich CF. Contrast-enhanced endoscopic ultrasound in the diagnosis of autoimmune pancreatitis. Endoscopy 2010.

23 Incidental Findings in the Surrounding Organs (Miscellaneous)

C.F. Dietrich

Common Incidental Findings

The term "incidental findings" refers to unexpected findings in the surrounding organs that are not within the typical indications for routine endoscopic ultrasonography (EUS). They are much more common than expected. This chapter discusses incidental findings reported in the author's own publications on transabdominal ultrasonography. I would be most grateful if readers were willing to contribute further case reports on incidental findings for future editions of this book.

Thyroid. The thyroid can be routinely imaged with EUS. Thoracic goiter can be found in many patients with EUS, but parathyroid tumors may be diagnosed in only a few selected patients.

Lung parenchyma. Pleural effusion and lung infarction can be seen using endoscopic ultrasound if the defects are close to the esophagus, or next to the spleen or left liver lobe.[1,2] Changes in the lung parenchyma should be noted even if a systematic examination of the parenchyma does not appear worthwhile (**Fig. 23.1**).

Heart. In individual cases, the potential of EUS can extend much further; we have been able to assess cardiac masses using fine-needle aspiration in two patients, without complications (**Fig. 23.2**). In one of these cases, a paracardiac lipoma with an impression on the left atrium was diagnosed, and in the other an extremely malignant angiomyosarcoma of the left atrium was confirmed, allowing appropriate therapy to be started.

Liver (left liver lobe). The left liver lobe can always be examined (at least in part), whereas only parts of the right liver lobe can be visualized.

Focal hepatic lesions. Typical focal liver lesions seen with endoscopic ultrasound are small subcapsularly located cholangiofibromas and hemangiomas (**Figs. 23.3** and **23.4**). Liver tumors have the same B-mode and color Doppler imaging characteristics as in transabdominal imaging[3,4] (**Figs. 23.5, 23.6,** and **23.7**).

Diffuse liver disease. Diffuse liver disease—for example, fatty liver with areas of different fatty infiltration around the liver veins, as well as next to the round ligament—can often be displayed in patients who have lost weight due to malignancies, as well as in those receiving corticosteroid treatment and patients with diabetes and many other diseases[5,6] (**Fig. 23.8**).

Perihepatic lymphadenopathy is a typical sign of inflammatory parenchymal liver disease and can be seen in chronic virus hepatitis, primary biliary cirrhosis, and primary sclerosing cholangitis, as well as in malignant liver disease. It is important to be aware of this in the differential diagnosis.[7–10] Normal perihepatic lymph nodes <20 mm in size can be demonstrated in up to 75% of healthy individuals (**Fig. 23.9**).

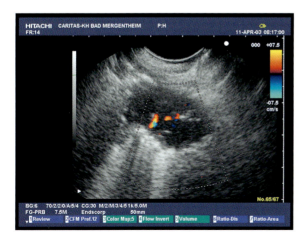

Fig. 23.1 Lung embolism with infarction, discovered incidentally in a patient being examined to exclude a pancreatic mass.

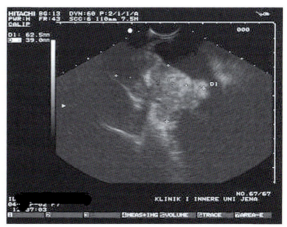

Fig. 23.2 Angiomyosarcoma of the left atrium, diagnosed by endoscopic ultrasound-guided fine-needle aspiration. (Courtesy of M. Hocke).

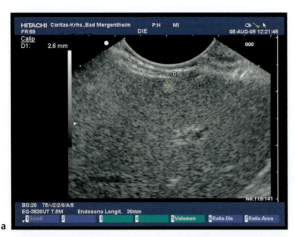
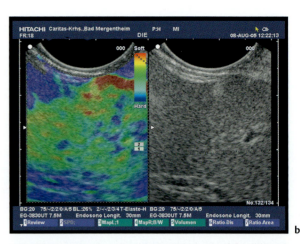

Fig. 23.3a, b a Cholangiofibromas (between the markers) are typically found in a subcapsular location and are less than 10 mm in diameter.

b On elastography, they show similar elasticity to that of the surrounding liver tissue.

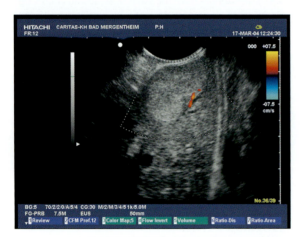

Fig. 23.4 Hemangioma. Typical hemangiomas (in this case confirmed histologically, due to a suspected pancreatic malignancy) are found to have afferent vessels on power Doppler sonography.

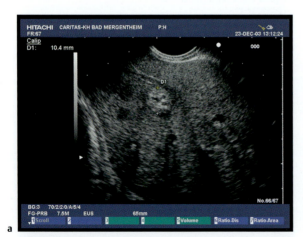
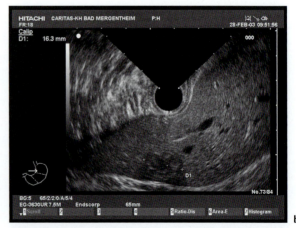

Fig. 23.5a–d Liver metastases

a Small liver metastases may only be visible with EUS, particularly in patients with pancreatic cancer who are being examined for staging purposes.

b Lesions in a subdiaphragmatic location are particularly difficult to identify with computed tomography and magnetic resonance imaging.

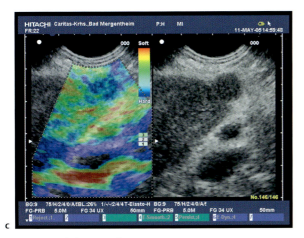

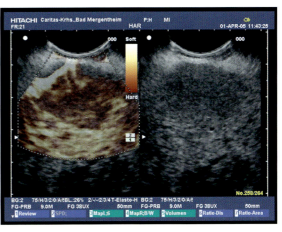

Fig. 23.5c, d (continued)
c The differences in elasticity displayed with elastography in a small exophytic metastasis should be noted.

d Diffuse malignant infiltration can be demarcated using elastography.

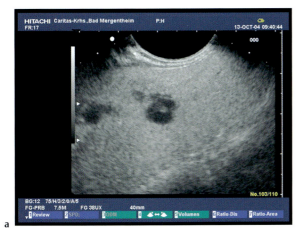

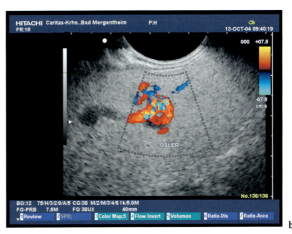

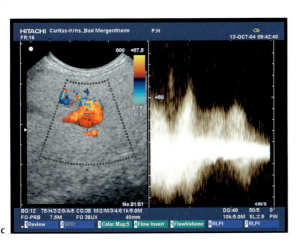

Fig. 23.6a–c a Osler disease should be suspected in patients with atypical cysts.
b, c Color Doppler imaging (**b**) and continuous duplex scanning (**c**) are helpful in the diagnosis.

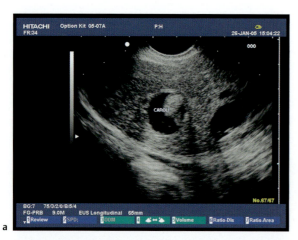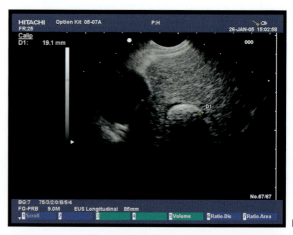

Fig. 23.7a, b Caroli disease. The differential diagnosis of cystic lesions with debridement (**a**) and calcifications (**b**) includes Caroli disease.

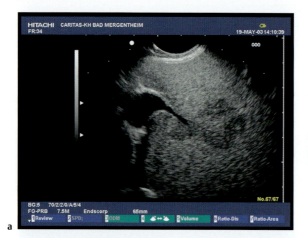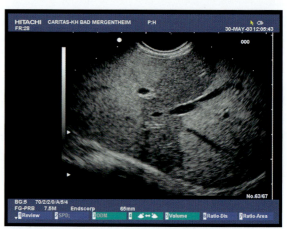

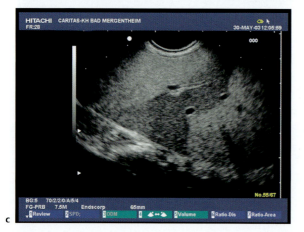

Fig. 23.8a–c a Fatty liver with areas of different fatty infiltration can mimic liver tumors.
b, c Typically, the hepatic architecture is not destroyed.

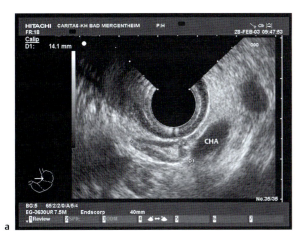

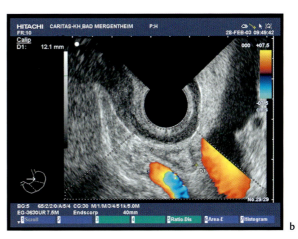

Fig. 23.9a, b Normal perihepatic lymph nodes < 20 mm in size can be demonstrated in up to 75% of healthy individuals. The regular architecture of the lymph-node sinus next to the common hepatic artery (CHA) should be noted.

a B-mode.
b Color Doppler imaging.

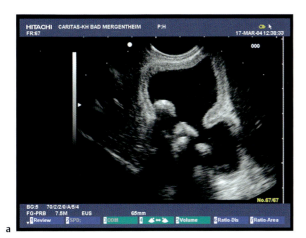

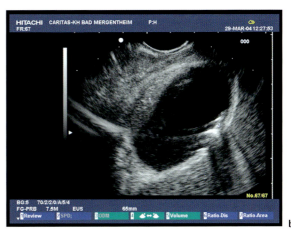

Fig. 23.10a, b a Cholecystolithiasis is easily demonstrated using EUS, particularly in patients with microlithiasis (see also Chapter 20).
b More confusing images result in patients with aerobilia.

Gallbladder. The gallbladder can be examined from the duodenal bulb in most cases. Carcinomas of the gallbladder are discussed in Chapter 20. In some cases, an endosonographic diagnosis of adenomyomatosis, cholesterol polyps, microgallbladder,[11] and other forms of gallbladder pathology (e.g., cholecystolithiasis) can be made, although there is no indication for endosonography in these differential diagnoses (**Figs. 23.10** and **23.11**). As in other tumors of the upper gastrointestinal tract, a definite endosonographic distinction between inflammatory and neoplastic alterations or changes in connective tissue is not possible.

Kidney, urogenital system. The upper pole of the left kidney can be visualized in almost all patients (see Chapter 21). Landmarks for correct identification of the cranial pole of the left kidney are the aorta, the pancreatic tail, the splenic vessels, and the left adrenal gland. Typically, after

entering the stomach, the transducer should be kept toward the left posterior gastric wall, showing a variable section of the abdominal aorta at 45 cm; slightly more caudally, the upper pole of the left kidney is seen. In some cases, the kidney and ureter can also be seen by positioning the transducer in the ascending part of the duodenum—a route that is used in only a few patients (**Figs. 23.12, 23.13,** and **23.14**).

Retroperitoneum. Incidental findings of enlarged retroperitoneal lymph nodes may be found in particular in patients with asymptomatic lymphoma, tuberculosis, and many other diseases (**Fig. 23.15**).

Spleen. The spleen can be visualized by identifying the aorta, pancreatic tail, splenic vessels, cranial pole of the left kidney, and left adrenal gland (**Figs. 23.16** and **23.17**).

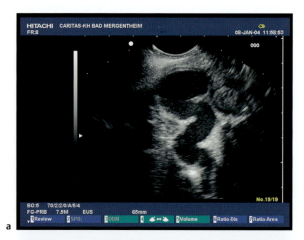

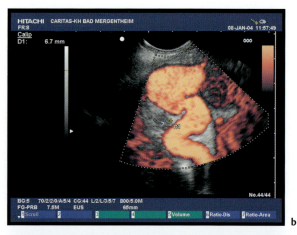

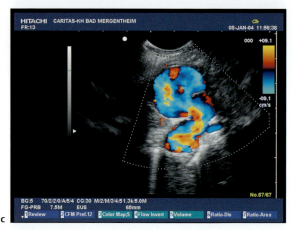

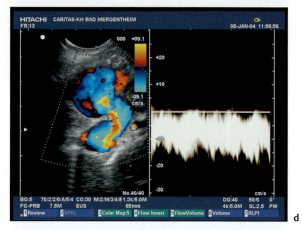

Fig. 23.11a–d Perihepatic varices
a Large varices and Cruveilhier–Baumgarten syndrome produce confusing images when B-mode imaging is used.

b–d Power Doppler (**b**), color Doppler (**c**), and coded duplex scanning (**d**) are helpful for defining the underlying vessels.

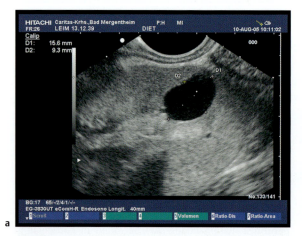

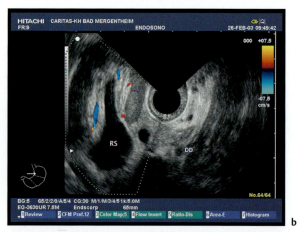

Fig. 23.12a, b The most common findings in the kidney are parenchymal cysts (**a**) and physiological sinus pyelectasia (**b**). RS, renal sinus; DD, small intestine.

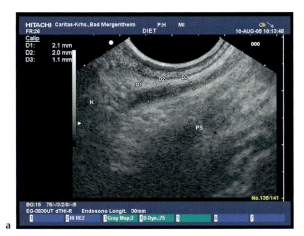

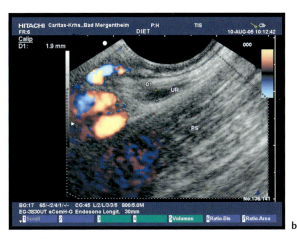

Fig. 23.13a, b Ureter. The normal ureter (between the markers), next to the retroperitoneal muscles (iliopsoas, PS), is best imaged from the ascending duodenum.

a B-mode imaging.
b Color Doppler imaging. K, kidney; UR, ureter.

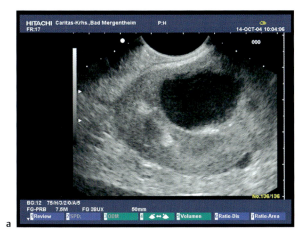

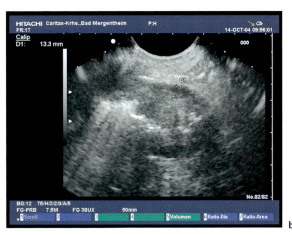

Fig. 23.14a, b a An incidental finding of hydronephrosis.

b This was misinterpreted as a centrally located cyst, due to colorectal carcinoma in the left colon. In a few patients, incidental EUS findings may be diagnostic.

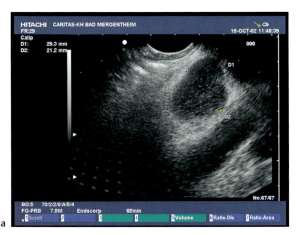

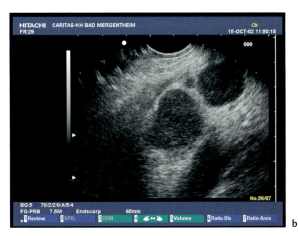

Fig. 23.15a, b An incidental finding of non-Hodgkin lymphoma.

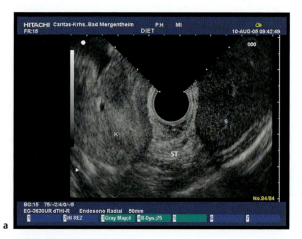
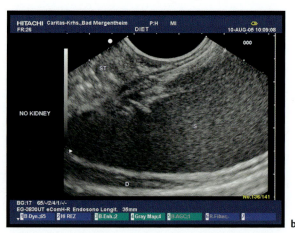

Fig. 23.16a, b Normal spleen.
a Using radial scanning techniques, the spleen (S) can be demonstrated with the kidney (K) in the same image, separated by the stomach (ST).

b The image obtained with the longitudinal technique differs. D, diaphragm; ST, stomach; S, spleen.

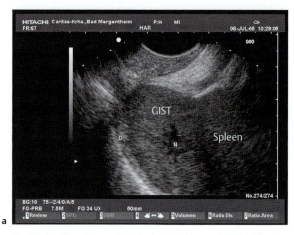
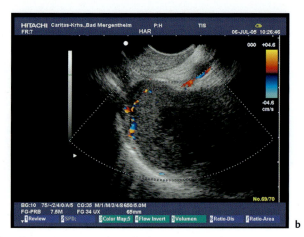

Fig. 23.17a, b a A gastrointestinal stromal tumor (GIST) infiltrating the spleen is seen in B-mode. D, diaphragm; N, central necrosis.
b Infiltration of the diaphragm is visible with color Doppler imaging.

Typically, after entering the stomach, the transducer should be kept toward the left posterior gastric wall, showing a variable section of the abdominal aorta at 45 cm; slightly more caudally, the upper pole of the left kidney is seen. In this partly inverted position, the endoscope has to be pushed forward into the gastric fundus.

Peritoneum. Peritoneal carcinosis can be visualized using EUS, but the clinical value of this has not been determined. EUS-guided fine-needle aspiration is helpful in the final diagnosis (**Fig. 23.18**).

Small intestine. The same principles as in EUS of the esophagus and stomach are applied in the small bowel. Due to the difficult diagnosis of diseases of the small intestine, the value of EUS is variable. Examples (e.g., Osler disease of the small intestine) are discussed in Chapter 20 (**Fig. 23.19**).[12–14]

A variety of incidental findings using sonoelastography have recently been published.[15]

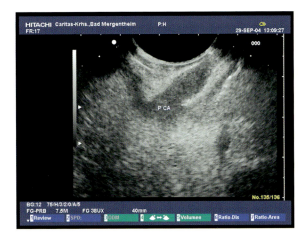

Fig. 23.18 Peritoneal carcinosis (PCA) can be visualized using EUS.

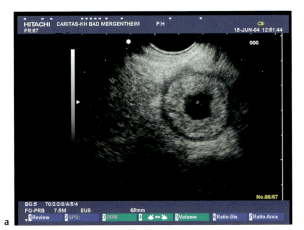

a

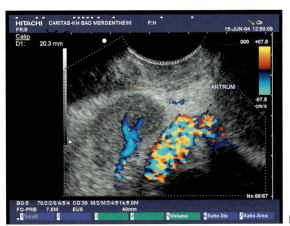

b

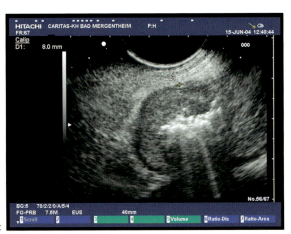

c

Fig. 23.19a–c a Vasculitis of the small intestine is typically diagnosed due to edema of the circular folds of the small intestine (Kerckring folds).[12–14]
b It may also be evident from enlarged peri-intestinal lymph nodes, with a normal architecture.
c However, it can also present in the form of tumorlike lesions due to necrosis.

References

1. Dietrich CF, Hirche TO, Schreiber D, Wagner TO. Sonographie von pleura und lunge. [Article in German] Ultraschall Med 2003;24(5):303–311.
2. Hirche TO, Wagner TO, Dietrich CF. Mediastinal ultrasound: technique and possible applications. [Article in German] Med Klin (Munich) 2002;97(8):472–479.
3. Dietrich CF, Ignee A, Trojan J, Fellbaum C, Schuessler G. Improved characterisation of histologically proven liver tumours by contrast enhanced ultrasonography during the portal venous and specific late phase of SHU 508A. Gut 2004;53(3):401–405.
4. Dietrich CF. Characterisation of focal liver lesions with contrast enhanced ultrasonography. Eur J Radiol 2004; 51(Suppl):S9–S17.
5. Dietrich CF, Wehrmann T, Zeuzem S, Braden B, Caspary WF, Lembcke B. Analysis of hepatic echo patterns in chronic hepatitis C. [Article in German] Ultraschall Med 1999; 20(1):9–14.
6. Dietrich CF, Schall H, Kirchner J, et al. Sonographic detection of focal changes in the liver hilus in patients receiving corticosteroid therapy. Z Gastroenterol 1997;35(12): 1051–1057.
7. Dietrich CF, Stryjek-Kaminska D, Teuber G, Lee JH, Caspary WF, Zeuzem S. Perihepatic lymph nodes as a marker of antiviral response in patients with chronic hepatitis C infection. AJR Am J Roentgenol 2000;174(3):699–704.
8. Dietrich CF, Zeuzem S. Sonographic detection of perihepatic lymph nodes: technique and clinical value. [Article in German] Z Gastroenterol 1999;37(2):141–151.
9. Dietrich CF, Lee JH, Herrmann G, et al. Enlargement of perihepatic lymph nodes in relation to liver histology and viremia in patients with chronic hepatitis C. Hepatology 1997;26(2):467–472.
10. Hirche TO, Russler J, Braden B, et al. Sonographic detection of perihepatic lymphadenopathy is an indicator for primary sclerosing cholangitis in patients with inflammatory bowel disease. Int J Colorectal Dis 2004;19(6):586–594.
11. Dietrich CF, Chichakli M, Hirche TO, et al. Sonographic findings of the hepatobiliary-pancreatic system in adult patients with cystic fibrosis. J Ultrasound Med 2002; 21(4):409–416, quiz 417.
12. Dietrich CF, Lembcke B, Seifert H, Caspary WF, Wehrmann T. Ultrasound diagnosis of penicillin-induced segmental hemorrhagic colitis. [Article in German] Dtsch Med Wochenschr 2000;125(24):755–760.
13. Dietrich CF, Brunner V, Seifert H, Schreiber-Dietrich D, Caspary WF, Lembcke B. Intestinal B-mode sonography in patients with endemic sprue. Intestinal sonography in endemic sprue. [Article in German] Ultraschall Med 1999; 20(6):242–247.
14. Dietrich CF, Brunner V, Lembcke B. Intestinal ultrasound in rare small and large intestinal diseases. [Article in German] Z Gastroenterol 1998;36(11):955–970.
15. Dietrich CF. Echtzeit-Gewebeelastographie. Anwendungsmöglichkeiten nicht nur im Gastrointestinaltrakt..Endoskopie Heute 2010;23:177–212.

III Gastrointestinal Tract

24 Endoanal and Endorectal Sonography

M. Sailer, H. Allgayer, C.F. Dietrich

Sonographic examination of the perineum, anus, and rectum, including the surrounding structures, using intraluminal transducers with transanal/rectal imaging—i.e., endoscopic ultrasonography (EUS)—has become increasingly important in clinical practice during the last 10 to 15 years.[1–3] Anal and rectal EUS have been shown to be useful tools in evaluating colorectal, anal, and pelvic disorders, due to the high resolution provided, with clearly distinguishable tissue-dependent echo signals.[4,5] The use of anal and endorectal ultrasonography is now recommended for a wide variety of indications, on the basis of the diagnostic and therapeutic guidelines published by technical review groups in various societies representing specialties and/or subspecialties.[6]

Normal Anatomy

EUS is able to image the rectal wall layers and adjacent structures, including the pelvic organs, with a high degree of precision. Detailed knowledge of the anatomy and morphology is needed for correct interpretation of the images provided. Modern intraluminal ultrasound probes make it possible to image the anal and pelvic structures in multiple planes relative to the body-axis, providing sagittal, frontal, transverse, and longitudinal sections.

■ Anatomy of the Perineum and Anus

The anal mucosa and internal anal sphincter (IAS) muscle are considered to represent the continuation of the inner rectal ring muscle. They form the innermost structures and can be visualized from the anal lumen. The hyperechoic longitudinal fibers of the corrugator ani muscle are regarded as an extension of the exterior rectal longitudinal muscle. The levator ani muscle is located at the cranial edge of the external anal sphincter (EAS) muscle, which has a funnellike shape and forms the muscular floor of the pelvis. The funnellike structure of the levator ani separates the extraperitoneal pelvis from the infraperitoneal and the pelvirectal space. The lateral region corresponds to the obturator internus muscle. The deep transverse perineal muscle and superficial transverse perineal muscle, as well as the ischiocavernous muscle, can also be imaged with EUS. The transverse orientation is the one most commonly used, and it can be varied depending on the height and angle of the corresponding sections (**Figs. 24.1, 24.2, 24.3, 24.4, 24.5, 24.6, 24.7, 24.8, 24.9, 24.10,** and **24.11**).

Anal canal. The echogenicity of the various mural layers in the anal canal is very similar to that in the rest of the gastrointestinal tract and is characterized by various well-distinguishable bands when imaged from the lumen. The anal canal is covered with columnar epithelium below the anal crypts. The mucosa is a transitional cell epithelium

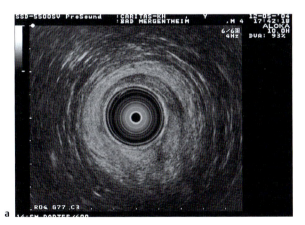

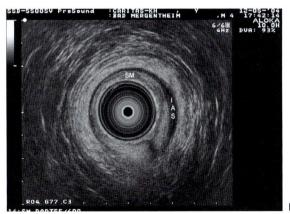

Fig. 24.1a–f Views of the internal anal sphincter (IAS) as the principal structure at the first level from anal to oral, with six horizontal sections (**a–f**) a few millimeters long, which should be seen as a continuum. **a** The subcutaneous part of the external anal sphincter muscle is seen as a strong hyperechoic ring. At this level, the IAS is not visible. **b–d** A hypoechoic inner ring (the IAS) is seen, accompanied by an outer hyperechoic ring representing the external anal sphincter (EAS), with the superficial part initially and the deep part following. LM, longitudinal muscle (the corrugator cutis muscle of the anus); RVP, rectal venous plexus; SM, submucosa.

Fig. 24.1c–f ▷

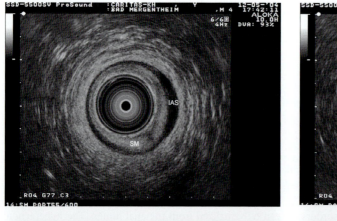

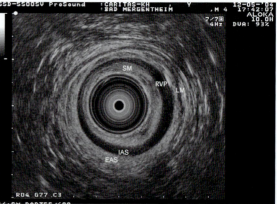

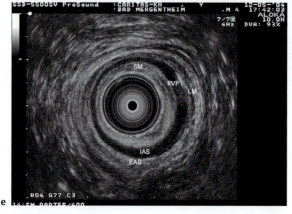

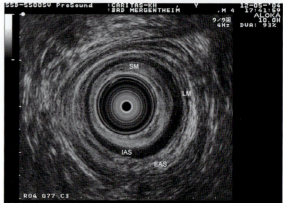

Fig. 24.1c–f (continued)

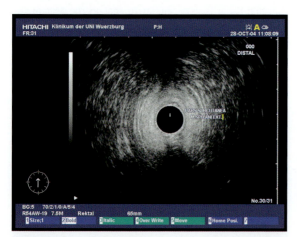

Fig. 24.2 The subcutaneous part of the external anal sphincter muscle, seen as a strong hyperechoic ring. The internal anal sphincter is not visible at this level.

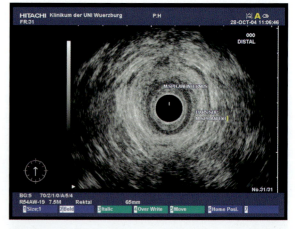

Fig. 24.3 A hypoechoic inner ring (the internal anal sphincter), accompanied by the superficial part of the external anal sphincter (the outer hyperechoic ring).

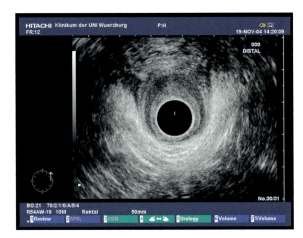

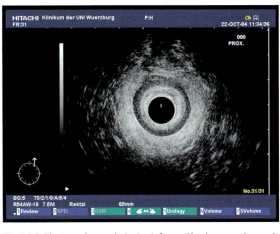

Fig. 24.4 A strong puborectal sling is seen here, which is hyper-echoic like all the striated muscles in the external anal sphincter, in contrast to the internal anal sphincter, which is seen as a hypoechoic ring internal to the puborectal sling.

Fig. 24.5 The inner hypoechoic ring is formed by the smooth muscle of the internal anal sphincter. There is also an outer hyperechoic ring, representing the strong and circumferentially intact external anal sphincter (striated muscle).

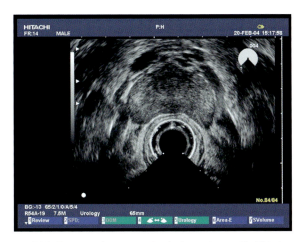

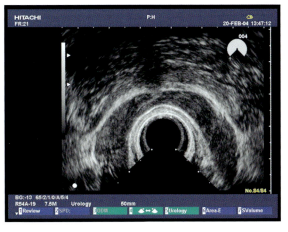

Fig. 24.6 The normal prostate gland, situated ventrally. This is a useful landmark during routine endorectal ultrasound examinations.

Fig. 24.7 Normal seminal vesicles, situated cranial to the prostate gland. The moustache shape and symmetry of the structure should be noted.

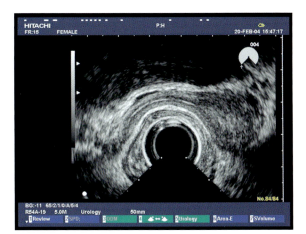

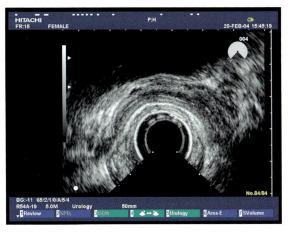

Fig. 24.8 A normal pear-shaped uterus, with slight deviation to the left. This is a useful landmark during routine endorectal ultrasound examinations in female patients.

Fig. 24.9 The normal vagina, situated ventrally between the bladder (the echo-free urine-filled structure above the vagina) and the rectum. Typically, a three-layer morphology is seen, with a fine hyper-echoic inner layer.

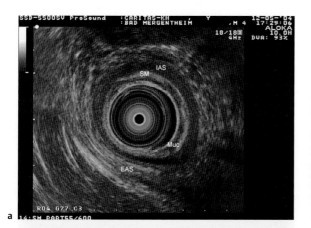

a

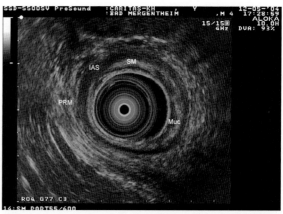

b

Fig. 24.10a–c Views of the external anal sphincter (EAS) at the second level from anal to oral, in three sections at very short distances from each other. IAS, internal anal sphincter (seen less prominently); Muc, mucosa; PRM, puborectal muscle and perirectal fatty and connective tissue (i.e., mesorectum); SM, submucosa.

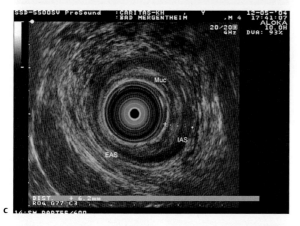

c

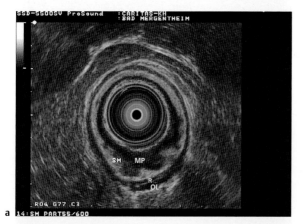

a

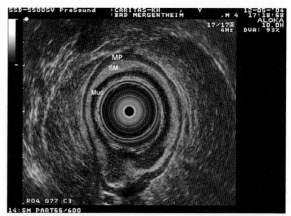

b

Fig. 24.11a–e View at the third level from anal to oral in five sections, with the rectal ampulla as the principal structure, in a patient with proctitis. MP, muscularis propria, with the inner ring (R) and outer (longitudinal) layer (OL), including the perirectal fatty and connective tissue structures; SM, submucosa; Muc, mucosa. Perirectally, a lymph node is visible between the markers in **d**.

Fig. 24.11c–e ▷

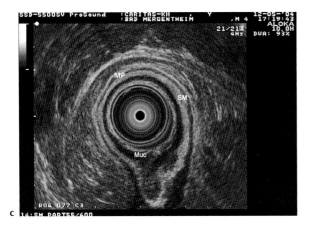

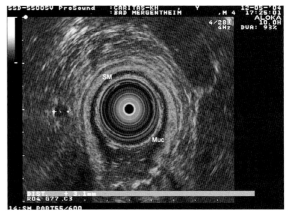

Fig. 24.11c–e   (continued)

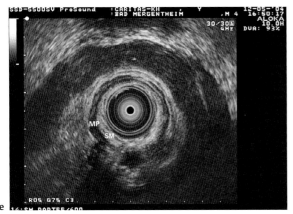

and starts at the level of the anal crypts; however, it can only be visualized irregularly as a faintly dark layer with scattered echoes of medium density. The transitional epithelium disappears in the first echodense border area, depending on the type of ultrasound probe used and the frequency being used.

The pectinate line and the crypts are often not visible, mainly due to compression of the anal canal by the endorectal probe. The submucosa and subcutaneous connective tissue appear as a homogeneous echogenic layer, increasing in thickness from the superior to the inferior margin of the anal canal. The rectal venous plexus is normally almost invisible unless very thin probes are used. The IAS can regularly be seen as a homogeneous hypoechoic layer with a thickness of 2–4 mm, with no significant sex-dependent differences. However, the thickness measured depends on the probes used, as larger probe diameters lead to thinning of the surrounding structures.[7] The echodensity and thickness of the IAS tend to increase with age. However, the normal thickness does not exceed 4 mm even in the elderly. The intersphincteral space, with fibers of the corrugator muscle as a continuation of the rectal longitudinal muscle, is seen endosonographically as a thin hypoechoic layer containing hyperechoic connective-tissue septa, representing the border areas of the hypoechoic IAS and the first less echogenic layer in the EAS. It can be

identified at ≈ 2 cm from the anocutaneous line. At this level, the ischioanal fossa, anococcygeal ligament, and coccyx can be visualized, provided that appropriate acoustic penetration is produced.

Adequate differentiation is possible in the hyperechoic border area between the ultrasound probe and the mucosa (or the anal cutis): the hypoechoic, extremely thin mucosa, which often cannot be recognized as a defined layer, due to a lack of the muscularis and its very thin diameter; the hyperechoic submucosa (and subcutis); and the hypoechoic IAS, with the adjacent partly hypoechoic and partly hyperechoic intersphincteral space corresponding to the corrugator ani muscle.

The EAS contains connective-tissue fibers in increasing amounts toward its distal section and appears as a layer 5–10 mm wide with irregular echo patterns and a series of concentrically bright and gray echo lines, depending on the ultrasound resolution power and, in relation to the thickness, the probe diameter. The EAS continues into the puborectalis muscle at the cranial margin of the anal canal. This part of the puborectalis muscle, with its more echogenic patterns, is only identifiable by its course. More orally, the muscular structures are no longer imaged vertically, so that this part of the muscle produces a weaker and less defined image. Ventrally, this broad muscle layer reaches the inferior part of the pubic bone, with inclusion of the urethra and the inferior part of the prostate or vagina. This typical configuration can be seen in the transverse section at 3 cm from the anocutaneous line between the 10-o'clock and 2-o'clock positions, with visualization of the urethra, prostate, inferior pubic ramus, levator ani muscle (puborectalis muscle), EAS, and ischioanal fossa and pelvirectal fossa.

The EAS consists of three more or less separate parts: the subcutaneous part, the superficial part, and the deep part. It is of great importance to understand that the shape and configuration of the EAS differs significantly between males and females. The anal canal is generally 0.5–1.0 cm longer in males, and the three different parts of the EAS are configured cylindrically around the anus, which means that the muscle shape and length are roughly the same ventrally and dorsally. In contrast, the three sections of the EAS are fused into a narrow band ventrally at the level of the superficial part in females.[8,9] Awareness of this anatomical difference is very important in order not to misinterpret normal anatomical findings.

The subperitoneal/pelvirectal layer and the subcutaneous and ischiorectal space are confluent relative to each other. The remaining muscles forming the levator ani muscle (the coccygeus muscle, iliococcygeus muscle, and pubococcygeus muscle) are identifiable with EUS only to a limited extent, but can be seen as an inhomogeneous, mostly hyperechoic layer with increasing cranial distance to the rectal wall.

It is important to appreciate that the hyperechoic structures are not directly imaged, but instead represent ultrasound artifacts indicating borderline areas behind which the real anatomical structures are imaged, such as the mucosa and muscularis propria—especially when older ultrasound equipment is used. In addition, it is also clinically relevant to note that these two hypoechoic structures are important in the staging of rectal cancers in accordance with the TNM classification.

Endosonographic Imaging at Different Anatomical Levels

The anatomical relationship between the IAS, levator ani, and ischioanal/iliorectal fossa can only be reconstructed if the operator is sufficiently familiar with the anatomy and has a good spatial imagination. Reproducible documentation and visualization in a single image are only possible with the aid of longitudinal sonographic sections through the anal canal. Systematic and comprehensive categorization can be achieved formally by producing corresponding sections at a superficial level at 0–2 cm, at a second level at 2–4 cm, and at a deeper level >4 cm above the anocutaneous line. For learning purposes, a step-by-step approach centimeter by centimeter appears helpful.

Table 24.1 Endoscopic ultrasound delineation of anorectal muscles

| Internal anal sphincter muscle |
| External anal sphincter muscle
• Subcutaneous part
• Superficial part
• Deep part |
| Levator ani muscle |
| Obturator internus muscle |
| Deep and superficial transverse perineal muscle |
| Ischiocavernous muscle |

Table 24.2 Normal sphincter values (highly dependent on age, sex, and probe diameter)

Muscle	Depth
Internal anal sphincter	1.5–4.0 mm
External anal sphincter	5–10 mm

Internal anal sphincter level. The first section shows the cutis, the transitional epithelium, and the subcutis with the transition to the submucosa, and more orally the IAS surrounded by the transverse perineal muscle and the ischioanal fossa. At this level, the corrugator ani (or longitudinal) muscle, containing hyperechoic connective-tissue fibers, can be distinguished from the IAS, which has weaker echogenicity (i.e., a hypoechoic pattern). Additional points of orientation at this level are the root of the penis with the ischiocavernous muscle and the ramus of the ischium.

External anal sphincter level. The second section shows the less pronounced hypoechoic IAS, and as the principal structure the more prominent EAS with inhomogeneous echo patterns (with a series of concentrically bright and gray areas or lines); more in the distance and posteriorly, the coccyx and coccygeal ligament (the dural part of the filum terminale) are seen. The anorectal muscles delineated with ultrasound are listed in **Table 24.1**, and normal sphincter values are listed in **Table 24.2**.

Rectal wall. The third section is at the level of the prostate gland with the urethra; the inferior pubic ramus yields images of the lumen and the variably hyperechoic EAS at an increasing distance, and the transition into the levator ani muscle forming the pelvic floor. The funnel of the levator ani separates the extraperitoneal pelvis into an infraperitoneal or pelvirectal space and a subcutaneous or ischiorectal space. The lateral border corresponds to the obturator internus muscle, with the obturator foramen. At this point, which is distinctly marked by the U-shaped puborectalis, the anal canal terminates and the rectum begins.

The typical ultrasound features of the rectal wall are found above this transition zone. These structures, which appear to have five layers with less sophisticated equipment, consist of the hyperechoic borderline between the probe and the mucosa, the hypoechoic mucosa, the hyperechoic submucosa, the hypoechoic muscularis propria, the hyperechoic serosa, and the border area to the perirectal fat tissue. More differentiated views are possible with the higher resolution power provided by more advanced equipment. With high-resolution probes, the two parts of the muscularis propria can be differentiated, with a circular layer (inner ring layer) and a longitudinal layer (outer ring layer) separated by a connective tissuelike septum. Further differentiation yields additional layers, such as a superficial layer of the muscularis propria and a deeper one, with a total of up to nine separate ultrasonographically discernible structures.

Instruments and Equipment

A transverse section with a 360° transducer is helpful for examining the anal canal, whereas for examining more orally located structures, radial as well as sector scanners can be used. Most modern probes, however, provide 360° transducers, which makes orientation much easier.

Patient preparation. Before rectal/anal EUS is performed, the patient's history should be carefully noted, with subsequent digital examination, and sigmoidoscopy (rectoscopy, colonoscopy) should be carried out to evaluate potential obstacles (contraindications) and obtain important additional information. No special bowel lavage is needed, except for the application of a cleansing enema 10–20 minutes before a rectal examination. An enema is not required if only the anal canal is examined (e.g., sphincter evaluation in incontinent patients or patients with anal fistulas). The patient is examined either in the left lateral or the lithotomy position, depending on the examiner's preference. However, reporting of the findings should always use clock points for reference (the pubic symphysis is always at the 12-o'clock position).

Introducing the transducer. Before the ultrasound probe is introduced, a thin layer of jelly is applied to the transducer's outer protective latex cover. The probe itself can either be introduced "blindly," or with the palpating finger, or using a rectoscope (rarely performed). Optimal viewing of the perianal and perirectal processes is achieved when the transducer is directed toward the umbilical region. When lower frequencies are used, a filling balloon may be helpful, but in this case it has to be taken into account that the degree of filling of the water balloon may affect the imaging of the rectal wall and/or pathological processes. Water filling is not required if only the anal region is

examined. The rectal wall may be stretched, depending on the extent of the filling, resulting in compression of the single wall layers. Even a tumor can then be overlooked if inappropriate pressure is applied. As in rigid rectoscopy, problems may arise starting at 15 cm above the anocutaneous line. However, there are cases in which viewing with the rigid instrument is already hampered at a level at or just above 10 cm, particularly when the examination is being conducted to search for a tumor. In normal circumstances, the rigid probe can be advanced up to 20 cm above the anocutaneous line.

Examination. It should be emphasized that EUS is not an appropriate screening test in the way that endoscopy is—for example, for detecting hitherto unknown tumors or other types of pathology. EUS is a supplementary examination intended to provide additional clinical information in a patient's diagnostic work-up. In the case of a rectal tumor, for instance, EUS serves as a staging tool; in a patient with fecal incontinence, it is used to examine the sphincter morphology, and so forth. The ultrasound examination is carried out during slow, step-by-step withdrawal of the transducer into the anal canal. Orientation is achieved by identifying the principal surrounding structures (bladder, prostate, vagina, puborectal muscle, etc.); details are best seen with appropriate focusing and adjustment of the instrument.

Clinical Indications for Endorectal Ultrasound Techniques

Whereas rectal EUS primarily visualizes the rectal wall layers and their surroundings, the purpose of anal EUS examinations is to investigate the sphincter muscles and pelvic floor. Due to the variability of the organ structures and the complex conditions affecting the precise location of the organs, detailed anatomical knowledge and precise orientation are mandatory for correct interpretation of EUS images. Starting from the lumen, a thin hypoechoic circular structure and a thicker hyperechoic circular structure are seen, which are interpreted as border echoes and subepithelial tissue, respectively, followed by a hypoechoic homogeneous ring pattern, which corresponds to the IAS. This muscle is usually thickest at the level of the pectinate line, with the diameter decreasing in the oral direction. The superposed longitudinal muscle is not always clearly visible with relatively hypoechoic fibers. The EAS consists of horizontally oriented (striated) fibers with complex, mainly hyperechoic structures (see **Fig. 24.3**). At the outermost level—i.e., immediately at the anocutaneous junction—the IAS is not visible. Only the subcutaneous portion of the EAS forms the sphincter apparatus at this level, which is recognized by a strong circular band with the typical hyperechoic pattern of striated muscle. More

Table 24.3 Indications for anorectal ultrasonography (ARUS) and endorectal ultrasonography (ERUS)

Anal carcinoma	T and N staging
Rectal carcinoma	T and N staging
Tumor follow-up	Submucosal and extrarectal tumor recurrence
Incontinence	Assessment of sphincter morphology
Extrarectal pathology	Abscess, fistula

orally, the structures of the levator ani and puborectalis muscle can be seen, the latter passing the rectum dorsally in a U-shaped loop and continuing ventrally as two lateral crura to the pubic bone. Sonomorphologically, these structures are represented by inhomogeneous longitudinal echo patterns lateral to the sphincter organ (see **Fig. 24.4**). At this level, the adjacent organs (prostate, seminal glands, urethra, vagina, uterus, and bladder) are also visualized. The indications for anorectal ultrasonography (ARUS) and endorectal ultrasonography (ERUS) are listed in **Table 24.3**.

■ Rectal Cancer

Clinically, rectal cancer is regarded a separate entity, which can be distinguished from colon cancer on the basis of the surrounding anatomy, despite a similar pathogenesis. The treatment options also vary distinctly between rectal and colon cancers—including local excision and neoadjuvant chemoradiotherapy, for example. Accurate preoperative staging using EUS is therefore mandatory in order to allow an individualized approach to treatment in rectal cancer patients.

■ Tumor Staging

T and N staging. Precise preoperative assessment of the tumor's penetration depth (T staging) is possible with EUS; the endosonographically assessed tumor stage is labeled with the prefix "u" for ultrasound (**Figs. 24.12, 24.13, 24.14, 24.15, 24.16, 24.17, 24.18, 24.19, 24.20, 24.21,**

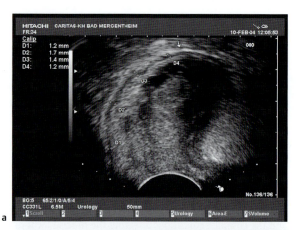

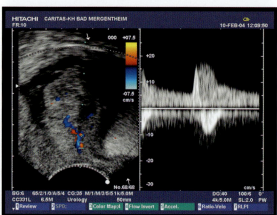

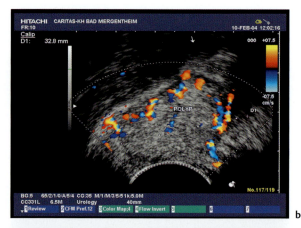

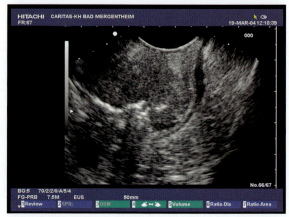

Fig. 24.12a–d uT1 carcinoma of the rectum in two patients (patient A in **a–c**, patient B in **d**).

a Infiltration of the tumor does not reach the muscularis propria (seen between the markers).

b At the transition to the muscularis, vessels can be misinterpreted as infiltration.

c Color Doppler and spectral analysis can be helpful for identifying blood vessels (arterial flow spectrum).

d The muscularis should be visualized in all sections, but this is not always possible at one level.

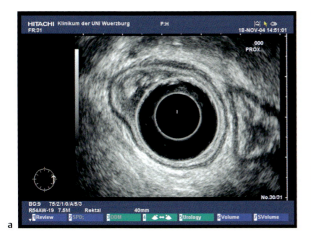

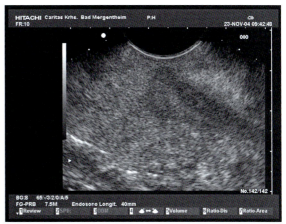

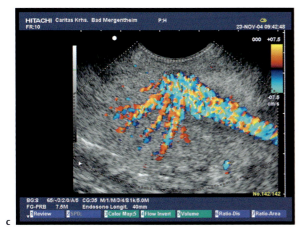

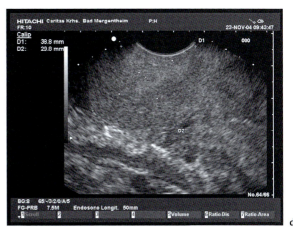

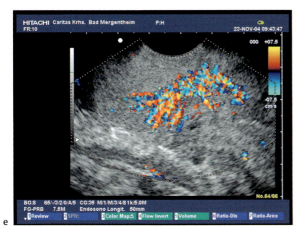

Fig. 24.13a–e Large adenoma (uT0/1)

a Note that the hyperechoic layer between the tumor and the muscularis propria remains fully intact.

b–e A sequence in a patient with benign adenoma, demonstrating the usefulness of color Doppler imaging. (▶ Video 24.1.)

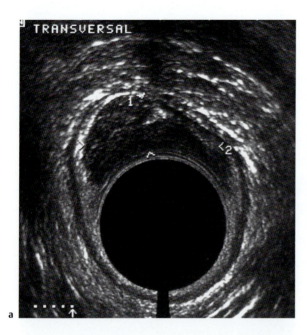

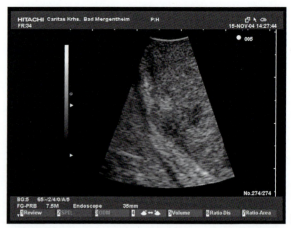

Fig. 24.14a, b a uT1 and pT1 carcinoma between the 11-o'clock and 1-o'clock positions.
b Note the intact muscularis propria layer.

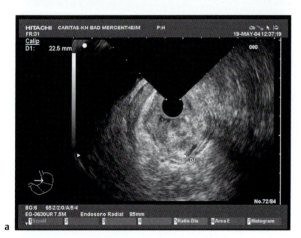

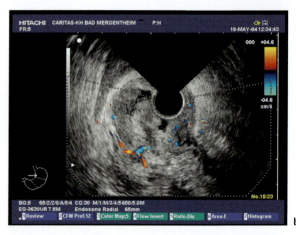

Fig. 24.15a, b uT2 Carcinoma of the rectum.
a Stage T2 is characterized by infiltration of the muscularis, which can be seen on the left lower side of the image.

b Color duplex imaging, here showing an afferent vessel, may be helpful to provide a better grasp of the architecture.

Fig. 24.16 uT2 carcinoma

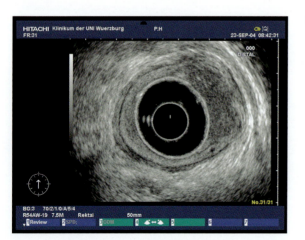

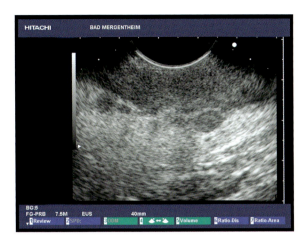

Fig. 24.17 uT3 carcinoma of the rectum. Stage T3 is characterized by infiltration into the perirectal connective tissue, seen at the lower left side of the image.

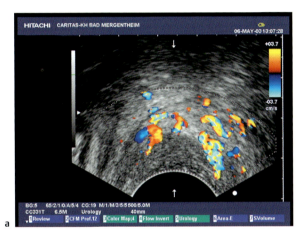

a

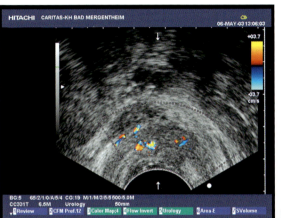

b

Fig. 24.18a, b uT3 carcinoma of the rectum. Stage T3 is characterized by infiltration into the perirectal connective tissue. An inflammatory peritumoral tissue reaction can lead to misinterpretation

(overstaging). After radiotherapy, no tumor tissue can be visualized in many cases either endoscopically or endosonographically.

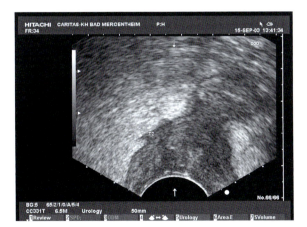

Fig. 24.19 uT3 carcinoma of the rectum. Stage T3 is characterized by infiltration into the perirectal connective tissue, as seen at the left margin here.

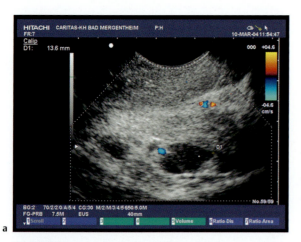

a

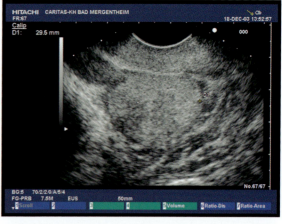

b

Fig. 24.20a, b uT3, uN+ carcinoma of the rectum.
a As a rule, lymph nodes with malignant infiltration (between the markers) are less echogenic.

b However, when there are also mixed inflammatory signs, it is not possible to assess the benign or malignant status of the lymph node (between the markers) clearly. The echogenicity of this lymph node corresponds to that of the underlying tumor.

Fig. 24.21 A large uT3 uN+ carcinoma, with a small lymph node at the 8-o'clock position.

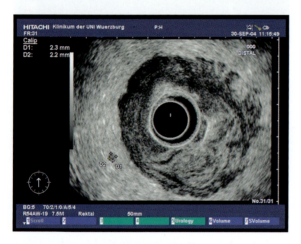

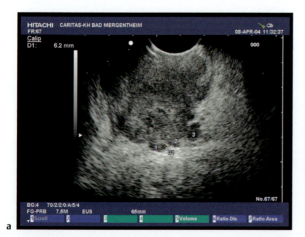

a

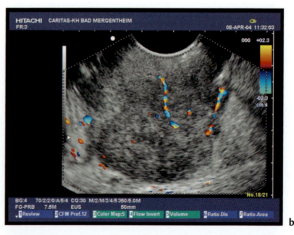

b

Fig. 24.22a, b uT4 carcinoma of the rectum.
a Stage T4 is characterized by infiltration into adjacent organs, as seen here in a patient with infiltration into the uterus. The infiltration extends beyond the borders of the organ (marked with 1–3).

b Color duplex imaging is helpful to provide a better grasp of the architecture.

24.22, and **24.23**). uT1 carcinomas are present when the mucosa/submucosa is involved, the second layer (hypoechoic) is often thickened, and the subsequent hyperechoic layer (layer III) is still intact. In uT2 tumors, the fourth (hypoechoic) layer, corresponding to the muscularis propria, is enlarged, with interruption of the layer located immediately below (III) and hypoechoic thickening of the mucosa (layer II); the outermost layer (V) remains intact. In uT3 tumors, each of the wall layers is involved, including layer V, with extension into the hyperechoic perirectal fat tissue. The continuity of layer V is disrupted. In stage T4, the tumor infiltrates either neighboring organs (such as the prostate, vagina, or bladder), which can be visualized easily with EUS, or the visceral peritoneum, although the latter is not distinguishable as a separate layer. Other malignant and nonmalignant processes can be examined with EUS and provide important additional information. Tumor recurrences (at the anastomosis or perirectal), recurrences in the pelvic floor, tumors in the lower pelvis (e.g., uterus, vagina, or bladder), transmural inflammatory processes (Crohn disease of the colon) and/or fistulas are also accessible to EUS, as well as other forms of disease (**Figs. 24.24, 24.25, 24.26,** and **24.27**).[10]

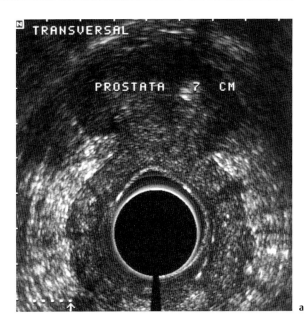

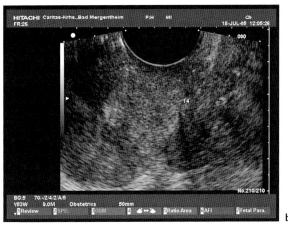

Fig. 24.23a , b A circular uT4 carcinoma with broad infiltration into the prostate (pT4).

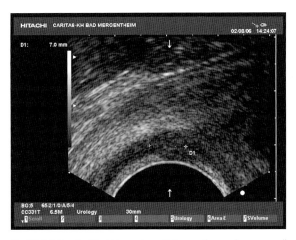

Fig. 24.24 Carcinoid of the rectum. Between the markers, a small carcinoid is seen infiltrating the muscularis propria. Local excision is therefore not an option.

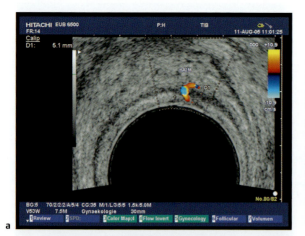

a

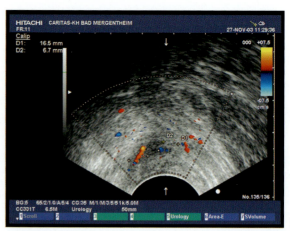

b

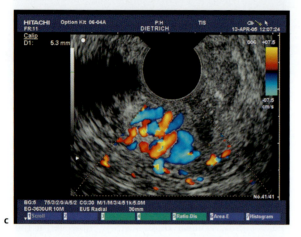

c

Fig. 24.25a–c
a Rectal venous plexus.
b A thrombosed node.
c A hemangioma. With arterially perfused hemangiomas, hemangiosarcoma has to be considered in the differential diagnosis.

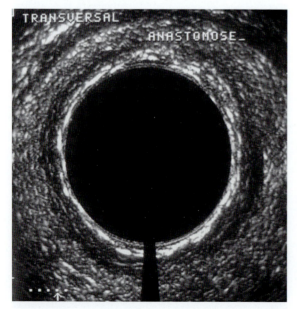

Fig. 24.26 A normal anastomosis, showing the metal clips from the circular stapler.

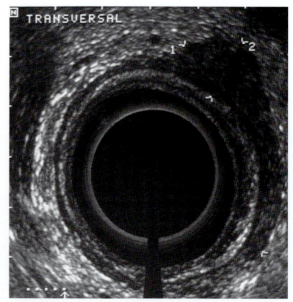

Fig. 24.27 An extramucosal recurrence at the 1-o'clock position. The rectal wall is intact, and the growth is therefore not detectable endoscopically.

Table 24.4 T staging (primary tumor) of rectal tumors with endorectal ultrasonography

First author (ref.)	Year	Patients (n)	Accuracy (%)	Sensitivity (%)	Specificity (%)	PPV (%)	NPV (%)
Akahoshi[14]	2000	39	82	83	65	59	87
Akasu[15]	1997	150	89	96	78	88	91
Beynon[16]	1989	99	93	99	91	97	95
Fedyaev[17]	1995	109	95	97	91	96	94
Garcia-Aguilar[18]	2002	545	69	–	–	72	93
Glaser[11]	1990	110	94	96	91	92	96
Herzog[19]	1993	118	93	98	75	90	95
Katsura[20]	1992	112	97	96	100	100	94
Nielsen[13]	1996	100	94	96	87	96	87
Rafaelsen[21]	1994	107	89	96	77	88	91
Rifkin[22]	1989	101	72	67	77	73	72
Sailer[23]	1997	162	89	97	81	83	97
Santoro[24]	2001	–	89	82	93	89	94
Yamashita[25]	1988	122	86	96	52	88	78

NPV, negative predictive value; PPV, positive predictive value.

Preoperative Diagnosis of Rectal Carcinomas

In the preoperative diagnostic work-up of rectal carcinoma, rectoscopy and/or colonoscopy with biopsies and an abdominal ultrasound examination are mandatory. Computed tomography (CT) is also necessary if abdominal ultrasonography does not provide satisfactory information. EUS imaging is a useful tool for the further evaluation of these tumors, due to its high sensitivity for T staging in particular, which lies in the range of 80–90%—so that this technique can define the tumor location precisely within the rectal wall (**Tables 24.4** and **24.5**).[1,11–29] Recent reviews and meta-analyses have confirmed the high degree of accuracy of EUS rectal cancer staging, further supporting previous recommendations that EUS should be used as the investigation of choice in these patients.[30–32]

In addition, pathological conditions in the pararectal area also can be visualized, particularly lymph nodes. However, the sensitivity and specificity of ultrasound for lymph-node staging is somewhat lower, in the range of 70–80% (**Table 24.5**).[1,33] The T stage may be overestimated in individual cases, particularly if a hypoechoic peritumoral inflammatory reaction is present. It should be noted that biopsies taken before the EUS examination can lead to significant mis-staging (usually involving overstaging) of cancers. This was confirmed in a large study of 333 tumors, which showed that staging is most accurate if biopsies are taken after the EUS examination.[34] Again, the explanation for this phenomenon is the inflammatory reaction caused by the biopsy trauma, which in turn leads to blurring and/or pseudoinfiltration of layers that are not primarily involved.

In comparison with T staging, evaluation of the lymph nodes is fraught with a greater possibility of errors involving overstaging and understaging, as hypoechoic lymph-node structures can be found in inflammatory as well as in malignant processes. The probability of malignancy increases with increasing diameter of the lymph nodes. In unclear cases, EUS-guided fine-needle biopsy can be carried out using a linear transducer.[33,35] However, if the histology is negative, a metastasis can still not be ruled out, as the biopsy needle may have missed the lymph node or malignant tissue within it. It is therefore the authors' practice to classify all visible lymph nodes as N+, while being fully aware that some tumors may be overstaged in this way.

When T1 tumors are suspected, with histomorphological signs of low-grade carcinoma, and local excision is planned, EUS is considered to be mandatory.[36] New studies focusing on the usefulness of EUS in the decision-making process for local versus transabdominal resection of rectal tumors have confirmed the important role of EUS imaging.[37,38] With the growing acceptance of neoadjuvant approaches, reliable preoperative staging of rectal cancers is mandatory. Studies have shown that tumors that penetrate through the rectal wall—i.e., T3 cancers and all node-positive tumors—have a better outcome when preoperative radiotherapy or chemotherapy is administered.[39,40] The German Rectal Cancer Trial in particular demonstrated a clear advantage for preoperative treatment in contrast to a postoperative setting.[41] Of course, as has already been common practice for many years, all T4 carcinomas require neoadjuvant chemoradiotherapy. The modern differentiated approach to rectal tumor treatment, ranging from transanal excision to neoadjuvant chemoradiotherapy with subsequent surgery, requires an equally differ-

Table 24.5 N staging (lymph nodes) of rectal tumors with endorectal ultrasonography

First author (ref.)	Year	Patients (n)	Accuracy (%)	Sensitivity (%)	Specificity (%)	PPV (%)	NPV (%)
Akasu[15]	1997	164	76	77	74	79	72
Beynon[16]	1989	95	83	88	79	78	89
Fedyaev[17]	1995	109	72	94	55	61	92
Frascio[26]	2001	–	75	74	73	–	–
Garcia-Aguilar[18]	2002	238	64	33	64	52	68
Glaser[11]	1990	97	80	80	81	78	82
Herzog[19]	1993	111	80	89	73	71	90
Hildebrandt[27]	1990	113	79	72	83	72	83
Katsura[20]	1992	98	68	80	62	54	85
Kim[28]	2000	–	64	53	75	71	59
Nielsen[13]	1996	81	67	79	56	61	75
Rafaelsen[21]	1994	53	70	58	76	58	76
Rifkin[22]	1989	102	81	50	92	68	84
Saitoh[29]	1986	88	75	73	82	95	42
Santoro[24]	2001	–	74	70	79	72	84

NPV, negative predictive value; PPV, positive predictive value.

entiated and precise staging instrument. At present, EUS appears to be the most accurate imaging method in comparison with other techniques such as CT and magnetic resonance imaging (MRI).[30–32,42,43]

Tumor Follow-Up

EUS is of clinical importance in the follow-up of colorectal carcinoma and is recommended by interdisciplinary guidelines published in 2000, particularly for rectal tumors staged as UICC II or III.[6] The advantage is that pathological submucosal and pararectal (extrarectal) conditions can be detected that normally escape rectal digital and endoscopic examination due to their extraluminal location. In a comparative study, Giovannini found that the additional diagnostic value of this method is due to its ability to detect locoregional recurrences in patients who have undergone surgery and/or radiotherapy in 10–25% of cases, in comparison with more conventional methods such as digital examination, rectoscopy, and/or CT.[44] Endorectal ultrasound is also of considerable value in the follow-up of patients who have undergone transanal resection. It has been shown that EUS can identify one-third of asymptomatic recurrences that have been missed on digital or proctoscopic examinations.[45]

Recurrences characteristically have a hypoechoic appearance, similar to primary tumors. As with other imaging techniques, it is not possible to distinguish between scarring and malignant tissue solely on the basis of imaging criteria. Increasing growth over time and/or an irreg-

ular appearance constitute typical signs of malignancy. However, if there is any doubt, EUS-guided biopsies can be taken, and this is certainly an additional advantage of this technique.[10,46,47] A detailed description of three-dimensional endorectal ultrasonography is provided in Chapter 25.

Anorectal Endosonography in Fecal Incontinence

An essential precondition for rational treatment of fecal incontinence is detailed knowledge of individual anatomical and functional defects in the sphincter system and the adjacent structures. Anorectal EUS plays an important role in the evaluation of fecal incontinence and is used as a valuable and noninvasive imaging tool.[5,48,49] In particular, small disruptions or scars in the anal sphincter complex can escape clinical examination. Anal inspection and a digital rectal examination can provide accurate information about internal and external anal sphincter function, but are inaccurate for assessing external anal sphincter defects <90°. Adequate diagnostic work-up therefore needs to include at least a rectal examination, anal inspection, and also endoanal ultrasonography, as was shown in a Dutch study including 312 patients with incontinence.[50] On the basis of the combined methods of EUS and rectal perfusion manometry, four major types of fecal incontinence can be distinguished:
- A predominantly sensory form
- A mainly muscular form

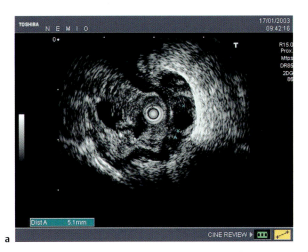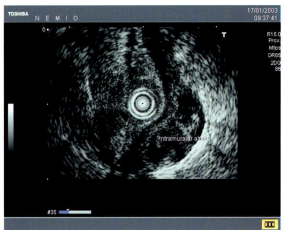

Fig. 24.28a, b Crohn disease with intramural abscess formation, seen between the markers.

- A form with both sensory and muscular components
- A form with predominantly decreased rectal compliance and impaired reservoir function

Each of these requires different therapeutic approaches.[51] Interestingly, when EUS was introduced into the diagnostic work-up for incontinent patients, it was noticed that the vast majority of patients who had previously had conditions described as "idiopathic" did in fact have morphological changes in the sphincter.[52,53] The principal cause of incontinence is obstetric trauma,[54] and sphincter disruption is therefore mainly seen at the level of the EAS, somewhere between the 10-o'clock and 2-o'clock positions (i.e., ventrally, between the vagina and anus). With more excessive forces, such as a complete perineal tear in situations with an uncontrolled third stage at birth or instrumental (forceps) delivery, injury even to the IAS can be encountered.[55] Scars in the hyperechoic EAS are usually hypoechoic on EUS imaging, whereas injuries to the hypoechoic IAS result in hyperechoic scar tissue.

The predominantly sensory form is characterized by normal EUS morphology and manometry; the second is characterized by normal endosonographic structures, including the IAS and EAS, the levator ani, and the puborectalis muscle, but shows pathological sphincter pressure (resting and/or squeeze pressure); in the third form, both pathological morphology and manometry are usually present; and in the last form, EUS and manometry may or may not be pathological. Endosonographically, the IAS may be found to be thickened, or its contour may be disrupted, as may also be the case in patients with solitary rectal ulcer and/or after hemorrhoidal surgery.[56,57]

Various degrees of interruption of the continuity of the EAS are mainly observed in elderly patients with anal incontinence and a history of gynecological/obstetric trauma.[58] Endosonographic features such as structural gaps appear to be clinically relevant when corresponding correlations with clinical and/or functional parameters are present—for example, decreased sphincter pressure.

It should be mentioned that such disturbances may not always be observed in these patients. In a study including more than 100 patients with different degrees of fecal incontinence, a weak but significant correlation was observed between the diameter of the EAS and the maximal squeeze pressure.[59,60] However, these data need further confirmation, as others have not found such a correlation.

■ Anal Fistula

EUS can be a valuable tool in the evaluation of anal fistulas, particularly in patients with complex and/or recurrent fistulas, as in Crohn disease.[61] Precise imaging of the puborectalis loop with the levator ani muscle is mandatory to help in surgical decision-making regarding this region (**Figs. 24.28, 24.29, 24.30, 24.31, 24.32,** and **24.33**). The levator ani extends continuously into the EAS, with a laterocranial continuation to the obturator muscle. Above this strong musculature lies the pelvirectal fossa, below the ischioanal fossa. Familiarity with the anatomy enables the examiner to distinguish between pelvirectal (suprasphincteral) and ischiorectal (infrasphincteral) abscesses and fistulas.[5] Instillation of hydrogen peroxide or even simple mineral water through the external orifice of the fistula allows even better examination of the structures involved. The contrast medium helps delineate side tracks and fistula extensions that may escape notice in the unenhanced state.[62] EUS examination of complex fistulas is mainly helpful if it is carried out by the operating surgeon himself, as it can help decisively in the planning of the surgical procedure.[63] In acute situations with pain and discomfort, EUS, like any other clinical or instrumental examination, should be performed with the patient under general anesthesia.

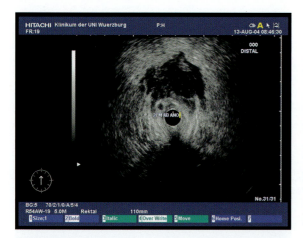

Fig. 24.29 A large abscess in a 31-year-old patient with Crohn disease.

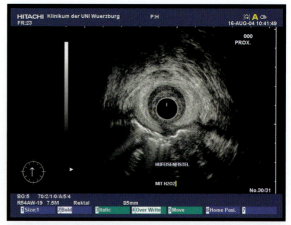

Fig. 24.30 A dorsal horseshoe fistula, enhanced with hydrogen peroxide through the external opening.

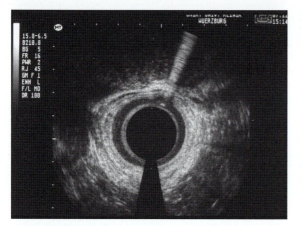

Fig. 24.31 Echoes from a metal probe in a trans-sphincteral fistula, indicating the internal opening at the 1-o'clock position.

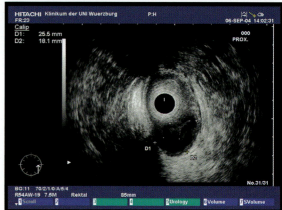

Fig. 24.32 A large presacral abscess.

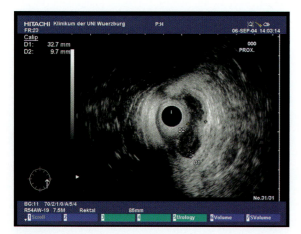

Fig. 24.33 A pararectal abscess in a patient with Crohn disease.

Interventional Procedures with Endoscopic Anorectal Ultrasound

■ EUS-Guided Transrectal Biopsies of Pelvic Tumors

The diagnostic work-up of pelvic tumors can occasionally be laborious. Using imaging techniques such as CT or MRI, or both, in patients with a history of a pelvic malignancy (e.g., rectal, prostate, or cervical cancer), it is often difficult to differentiate between scar tissue and recurrent tumor, particularly if the space-occupying lesion is small and tumor markers are not raised, or raised only slightly. Positron-emission tomography (PET) allows further classification of these lesions into those that do or do not show uptake of the marker, which is usually fluorodeoxyglucose.[64] However, a definitive histological diagnosis needs to be established in order to decide conclusively on further therapeutic strategies, which may range from palliative conservative measures to major surgery such as multi-visceral resection. The same applies to patients with no previous history who either present with a symptomatic or incidental pelvic tumor that cannot be clearly classified using imaging, laboratory investigations, or follow-up examinations by the respective specialists—i.e., the urologist, gynecologist, or colorectal surgeon.

Percutaneous biopsies assisted either by CT or by abdominal ultrasonography have several limitations. The distance from the surface to the lesion can be considerable, making it difficult if not impossible to achieve precise aspiration. Tumors can be obscured by anatomical structures such as the uterus, adnexa, or bowel. In addition, patient discomfort and the risk of intraperitoneal infection should also be borne in mind when this type of approach is used. Transrectal EUS overcomes most of these limitations, and most importantly, its spatial resolution is considerably better than that of any of the other imaging techniques, including PET. EUS is therefore potentially capable of detecting lesions at a stage at which conventional diagnostic tools would fail to do so.[65]

We have reported our results with EUS-guided biopsies in a total of 48 patients.[10] Apart from one post-biopsy hemorrhage, which was managed conservatively, no other complications were encountered. Sufficient tissue was removed to allow histological examination in all cases. A wide range of diagnoses, including primary and secondary malignancies (n = 25) and benign lesions (n = 23) were established. There were no false-positive cases, but three false-negative histological diagnoses in patients in whom local recurrence of a malignant tumor was confirmed during the follow-up period. This represents a sensitivity of 88%, a specificity of 100%, a positive predictive value of 100%, and a negative predictive value of 89%. Only 13 tumors (27%) in the series were easily palpable by rectal examination. Theoretically, these tumors could have been approached using simple digitally guided transrectal needle biopsy. However, EUS provides biplanar imaging with very precise target localization and needle monitoring. Lesions can be biopsied under visual guidance, rendering the procedure more controlled and consequently safer.

EUS-guided biopsy of the prostate gland is a well-established method in the field of urology and has gained widespread acceptance in routine practice. Well-documented studies including several thousand patients have shown that the procedure is safe and effective, with little patient discomfort and very low morbidity rates.[66] Infection, although a rare event, is probably the most serious complication, and administration of a prophylactic antibiotic is generally recommended. As the perirectal tissue is not as well vascularized and contained as the prostate, we consider that more thorough preparation, including complete bowel lavage and single-shot antibiotics, is warranted. As with any other invasive procedure, it appears prudent not to carry out EUS-guided transrectal biopsy in patients receiving anticoagulant or thrombolytic medication. If a biopsy is nevertheless needed, medication should either be discontinued if possible, or else the patient should be monitored on an in-patient basis.

Only a few studies have been published in the nonurological and nongynecological literature on transrectal biopsy of pelvic masses. Apart from anecdotal reports including small numbers of patients, two articles described transrectal ultrasound-guided biopsies in larger series of patients with suspected recurrences of rectal carcinoma. Hünerbein et al.[46] report 30 patients who underwent transrectal ERUS-guided biopsies during tumor follow-up. They found 10 patients with malignant histological findings, while the remaining patients had no evidence of recurrent disease during a follow-up period of 7 months. No complications were encountered. Löhnert and colleagues[47] used a transperineal approach under local anesthesia in 111 patients with suspicious masses following low anterior resection for rectal cancer. Local recurrences were demonstrated histologically in 52 patients. Potentially curative salvage surgery was possible in 31 patients, 25 of whom had been diagnosed by EUS alone (81% of all curatively resected patients with local recurrences). There were no false-positive or false-negative results. The total numbers of biopsy samples retrieved in each patient are not mentioned in either of these papers. However, taking into consideration our own three cases of false-negative histology, all of which occurred in the early period of the study in which only one or two aspirations were performed, we would now recommend obtaining at least five tissue samples per patient. Using this policy, we increased the sensitivity of the method to 100%.

According to the urology literature, transrectal ultrasound-guided needle biopsy is generally considered to cause no discomfort or only minimal discomfort and it has therefore been common practice to carry out this procedure without anesthesia or analgesia. We can confirm that the vast majority of patients have no pain, or only insignificant pain. We used a sedative drug in only three patients who expressed anxiety before the biopsy. It appears from the literature that younger patients (i.e., those under 60 years of age) experience more discomfort, so that this subgroup may benefit from analgesia and/or sedation.[66]

◼ EUS-Guided Transrectal Aspiration of Pelvic Fluid Collections

As the resolution of EUS is less than 1 mm, even very small lesions that might otherwise evade detection on clinical examination or conventional imaging such as CT can be visualized with great accuracy. In addition, their location and relationship with neighboring structures can be precisely outlined, which greatly increases the safety of any interventional procedures such as endorectal ultrasound-guided biopsies or aspiration of abscesses. We have recently reported our experience in 29 patients who under-

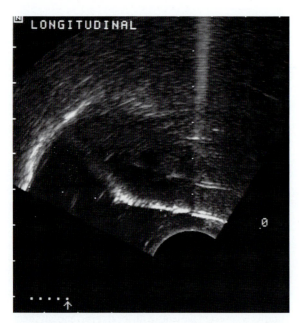

Fig. 24.34 Ultrasound-guided biopsy or aspiration. The needle tip can be seen precisely along the dotted line (the distance between two dots equals 1 cm).

went a total of 33 EUS-guided aspiration procedures.[67] No procedure-related complications were encountered. In 22 cases (76%), the lesions were identified following a surgical procedure. Amounts of fluid varied between 5 and 750 mL. The fluids were sterile in 14 cases (42%). The fluid collections consisted of hematomas, seromas, peritoneal cysts, and a mucocele. Microorganisms were found in the remaining 19 aspirations (58%), with lesions consisting of abscesses (n = 16) and infected hematomas (n = 3). A transrectal (n = 14) or transvaginal (n = 2) drainage catheter was placed in 16 patients under endosonographic guidance using the Seldinger technique. Only two patients required a subsequent laparotomy for definitive treatment of the septic focus, while the remaining patients were all treated successfully using this conservative approach. It was demonstrated that transrectal drainage of pelvic fluid collections can be carried out with no morbidity, or only insignificant morbidity, in carefully selected patients. Most cases involve patients with postoperative complications, particularly pelvic abscesses or hematomas with or without anastomotic dehiscence. Transrectal EUS-guided drainage in these circumstances is a comparatively minor intervention, causing only little discomfort to the patient. This report shows that the procedure can be performed safely and that it avoids the need for further surgery in the great majority of patients. This is not surprising, as interventional drainage of infectious foci is a well-known and widely applied principle. Other investigators have also recently confirmed that ultrasound-guided transvaginal or transrectal drainage of pelvic abscesses is safe and technically practicable.[68]

Since no radiation exposure is involved, EUS is also useful in the follow-up of these patients. In cases of abscesses, the cavities can be easily visualized by instilling a few milliliters of hydrogen peroxide through the draining catheter. This allows evaluation of the cavity size and its configuration. Cystic structures need to be reviewed thoroughly to rule out infection or malignancy. However, benign peritoneal cysts are occasionally encountered after pelvic operations, typically following hysterectomies. In suitable patients who present with cyst-related symptoms, obliteration therapy can be attempted. Following the principles of pleurodesis, a sealant such as doxycycline or fibrin glue can be injected into the cyst.

In conclusion, endorectal ultrasound is a useful and complementary imaging technique in the assessment of pelvic pathology. The major advantage of EUS, however, is that it makes it possible to carry out ultrasound-guided punctures and aspirations of extrarectal fluid collections and biopsies of solid lesions. Microbiological, cytological, and/or histological examination of the specimens allows accurate diagnosis. In cases of abscess formation or infected hematoma, a drain can be placed at the same time, avoiding the need for surgery in the majority of patients. EUS-guided interventions are safe and cost-effective and cause minimal discomfort to the patient (**Fig. 24.34**).

■ Anal Cancer

Whereas surgical excision used to be the standard method in the treatment of anal malignancies, most tumors are nowadays treated using combined chemoradiotherapy. Only very small cancers of the anal margin can safely be excised without compromising the anal sphincter. Very advanced tumors causing obstruction and/or bleeding or cancers that have failed to respond to chemoradiotherapy also need to be treated surgically, usually with an abdominoperineal resection.

Anal cancers are classified according to their size (T stage). However, with regard to lymph-node metastases, two distinctly different classifications are applied, depending on the precise location of the malignancy (**Table 24.6**). While tumors located at the anal margin tend to involve inguinal lymph nodes as the principal metastatic route, cancers in the anal canal primarily metastasize to the perirectal nodes. The ultrasound appearance of squamous cell cancers of the anus is typically that of a hypoechoic lesion.

Anal ultrasound is useful for determining not only the precise depth of infiltration, but also for delineating sphincter involvement.[69] Bartram and Burnett proposed a new classification for the endoanal ultrasound staging of anal cancers.[70] They suggest that the T level should not be determined according to the size of the lesion, but according to the anatomical structures involved (**Table 24.7**). In

Table 24.6 TNM classification of cancers in the anal margin and anal canal. The differences in the N staging should be noted

Stage	Anal canal	Anal margin
Tis	Carcinoma in situ	Carcinoma in situ
T1	Tumor < 2 cm	Tumor < 2 cm
T2	Tumor > 2 and < 5 cm	Tumor > 2 and < 5 cm
T3	Tumor > 5 cm	Tumor > 5 cm
T4	Tumor infiltrates neighboring organs[a]	Tumor infiltrates extradermal structures (e.g., cartilage, muscle)
N0	No regional lymph nodes involved	No regional lymph nodes involved
N1	Perirectal lymph nodes	Ipsilateral inguinal lymph nodes
N2	Inguinal and/or iliac lymph nodes on one side	
N3	Bilateral and/or perirectal and inguinal lymph nodes on one side	
M0	No distant metastases	No distant metastases
M1	Distant metastases	Distant metastases

[a] The anal sphincter is not a neighboring organ.

Table 24.7 Endosonographic staging of anal cancers proposed by Bartram and Burnett (1991)[70]

Stage	Depth of infiltration
T1	Infiltration into the internal anal sphincter
T2	Infiltration into the external anal sphincter (EAS)
T3	Tumor penetrates through the EAS
T4	Infiltration into neighboring organs

addition, anal ultrasound can be used to monitor the treatment response and for follow-up examinations in these patients.[71] If complete regression is achieved, the ultrasound morphology of the anatomic area involved may revert to normal. However, in most cases some echo patterns differing from the neighboring healthy tissue are seen representing the residual scar.

There have been reports that three-dimensional (3D) anal ultrasonography may be able to improve the accuracy of staging further.[72] Löhnert and co-workers describe an interesting new application of 3D ultrasound in the treatment of anal tumors.[73] They used 3D reconstructions for radiotherapy simulation to improve the radiation dose to the target field. They also implanted afterloading needles using endosonographic transperineal guidance. They concluded that this new technique is capable of minimizing radiation-induced damage to adjacent organs and/or healthy tissue (**Fig. 24.35**). A recent study comparing normal EUS with 3D EUS in the evaluation of recurrent anal cancer reported significantly better interobserver and intraobserver agreement with the 3D technique.[74] However, the number of patients included was fairly small—36 patients with anal cancer, seven of whom developed recurrent disease during a follow-up period of 5 years.

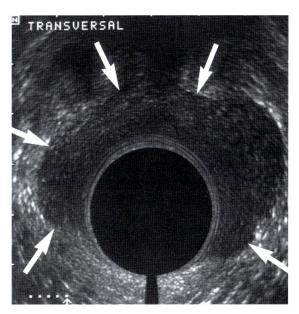

Fig. 24.35 A large carcinoma at the anal margin (arrows), infiltrating the subcutaneous part of the external anal sphincter.

■ **Perineal Transcutaneous Ultrasound**

Perineal transcutaneous ultrasound (PTUS) is very effective, but is rarely considered in the imaging work-up for perianal inflammatory lesions—for example, in patients with Crohn disease. In contrast to the established methods, perineal ultrasound is an easy and cost-effective method of imaging for perianal abscesses and fistulas (**Fig. 24.36**).

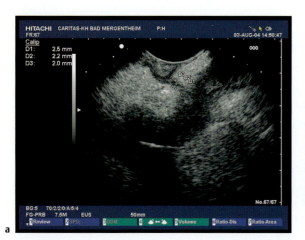 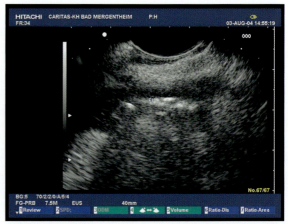

Fig. 24.36a, b Perineal transcutaneous ultrasound is especially effective in demonstrating trans-sphincteral and extrasphincteral locations that are often difficult to demonstrate with endorectal ultrasound. FI, fistula.

References

1. Brugge WR. Endoscopic ultrasonography: the current status. Gastroenterology 1998;115(6):1577–1583.
2. Sailer M, Leppert R, Fuchs KH, Thiede A. Die endorektale Sonographie. Coloproctology 1995;17:149–157.
3. Bhutani MS. Recent developments in the role of endoscopic ultrasonography in diseases of the colon and rectum. Curr Opin Gastroenterol 2007;23(1):67–73.
4. Löhnert M, Dohrmann P, Stoffregen C. Endorektale Sonographie in der Proktologie. In: Braun B, ed. Ultraschalldiagnostik. Lehrbuch und Atlas. Munich: Ecomed; 1990;76–89.
5. Poen AC, Felt-Bersma RJ. Endosonography in benign anorectal disease: an overview. Scand J Gastroenterol Suppl 1999;230:40–48.
6. Hermanek P. Qualitätssicherung in der Onkologie, Diagnose und Therapie maligner Erkrankungen. Kurzgefasste Interdisziplinäre Leitlinie 2000. Munich: Zuckerschwert; 2000.
7. Sailer M, Leppert R, Fuchs KH, Thiede A. Endo-anal sonography in diagnosis of fecal incontinence. [Article in German] Zentralbl Chir 1996;121(8):639–644.
8. Stelzner F. Die anorectalen Fisteln. 3rd ed. Berlin: Springer; 1981.
9. Fritsch H, Brenner E, Lienemann A, Ludwikowski B. Anal sphincter complex: reinterpreted morphology and its clinical relevance. Dis Colon Rectum 2002;45(2):188–194.
10. Sailer M, Bussen D, Fein M, et al. Endoscopic ultrasound-guided transrectal biopsies of pelvic tumors. J Gastrointest Surg 2002;6(3):342–346.
11. Glaser F, Schlag P, Herfarth C. Endorectal ultrasonography for the assessment of invasion of rectal tumours and lymph node involvement. Br J Surg 1990;77(8):883–887.
12. Kuntz C, Glaser F, Buhr HJ, Herfarth C. Endo-anal ultrasound. Indications and results. [Article in German] Chirurg 1994;65(4):352–357.
13. Nielsen MB, Qvitzau S, Pedersen JF, Christiansen J. Endosonography for preoperative staging of rectal tumours. Acta Radiol 1996;37(5):799–803.
14. Akahoshi K, Kondoh A, Nagaie T, et al. Preoperative staging of rectal cancer using a 7.5 MHz front-loading US probe. Gastrointest Endosc 2000;52(4):529–534.
15. Akasu T, Sugihara K, Moriya Y, Fujita S. Limitations and pitfalls of transrectal ultrasonography for staging of rectal cancer. Dis Colon Rectum 1997; 40(10, Suppl):S10–S15.
16. Beynon J, Mortensen NJ, Foy DM, Channer JL, Rigby H, Virjee J. Preoperative assessment of mesorectal lymph node involvement in rectal cancer. Br J Surg 1989;76(3):276–279.
17. Fedyaev EB, Volkova EA, Kuznetsova EE. Transrectal and transvaginal ultrasonography in the preoperative staging of rectal carcinoma. Eur J Radiol 1995;20(1):35–38.
18. Garcia-Aguilar J, Pollack J, Lee SH, et al. Accuracy of endorectal ultrasonography in preoperative staging of rectal tumors. Dis Colon Rectum 2002;45(1):10–15.
19. Herzog U, von Flüe M, Tondelli P, Schuppisser JP. How accurate is endorectal ultrasound in the preoperative staging of rectal cancer? Dis Colon Rectum 1993;36(2):127–134.
20. Katsura Y, Yamada K, Ishizawa T, Yoshinaka H, Shimazu H. Endorectal ultrasonography for the assessment of wall invasion and lymph node metastasis in rectal cancer. Dis Colon Rectum 1992;35(4):362–368.
21. Rafaelsen SR, Kronborg O, Fenger C. Digital rectal examination and transrectal ultrasonography in staging of rectal cancer. A prospective, blind study. Acta Radiol 1994;35(3):300–304.
22. Rifkin MD, Ehrlich SM, Marks G. Staging of rectal carcinoma: prospective comparison of endorectal US and CT. Radiology 1989;170(2):319–322.
23. Sailer M, Leppert R, Bussen D, Fuchs KH, Thiede A. Influence of tumor position on accuracy of endorectal ultrasound staging. Dis Colon Rectum 1997;40(10):1180–1186.
24. Santoro GA, Pastore C, Barban M, DiFalco G. Role of endorectal ultrasound in the management of rectal cancers. Hepato-Gastroenterology 2001;48(SI):CXIX.
25. Yamashita Y, Machi J, Shirouzu K, Morotomi T, Isomoto H, Kakegawa T. Evaluation of endorectal ultrasound for the assessment of wall invasion of rectal cancer. Report of a case. Dis Colon Rectum 1988;31(8):617–623.
26. Frascio F, Giacosa A. Role of endoscopy in staging colorectal cancer. Semin Surg Oncol 2001;20(2):82–85.
27. Hildebrandt U, Klein T, Feifel G, Schwarz HP, Koch B, Schmitt RM. Endosonography of pararectal lymph nodes. In vitro and in vivo evaluation. Dis Colon Rectum 1990;33(10):863–868.
28. Kim HJ, Wong WD. Role of endorectal ultrasound in the conservative management of rectal cancers. Semin Surg Oncol 2000;19(4):358–366.

29. Saitoh N, Okui K, Sarashina H, Suzuki M, Arai T, Nunomura M. Evaluation of echographic diagnosis of rectal cancer using intrarectal ultrasonic examination. Dis Colon Rectum 1986;29(4):234–242.

30. Bipat S, Glas AS, Slors FJM, Zwinderman AH, Bossuyt PMM, Stoker J. Rectal cancer: local staging and assessment of lymph node involvement with endoluminal US, CT, and MR imaging—a meta-analysis. Radiology 2004;232(3): 773–783.

31. Puli SR, Bechtold ML, Reddy JBK, Choudhary A, Antillon MR, Brugge WR. How good is endoscopic ultrasound in differentiating various T stages of rectal cancer? Meta-analysis and systematic review. Ann Surg Oncol 2009;16(2): 254–265.

32. Puli SR, Reddy JBK, Bechtold ML, Choudhary A, Antillon MR, Brugge WR. Accuracy of endoscopic ultrasound to diagnose nodal invasion by rectal cancers: a meta-analysis and systematic review. Ann Surg Oncol 2009;16(5):1255–1265.

33. Giovannoni M, Bernardini D. Biopsie guidée sous echoendoscopie des lésions péri-rectales et peri-coliques. Acta Endosc 1998;28:45–51.

34. Goertz RS, Fein M, Sailer M. Impact of biopsy on the accuracy of endorectal ultrasound staging of rectal tumors. Dis Colon Rectum 2008;51(7):1125–1129.

35. Giovannini M. Endoscopic ultrasonography with a curved array transducer: normal echoanatomy of retroperitoneum. Gastrointest Endosc Clin N Am 1995;5(3):523–528.

36. Sailer M, Leppert R, Kraemer M, Fuchs KH, Thiede A. The value of endorectal ultrasound in the assessment of adenomas, T1- and T2-carcinomas. Int J Colorectal Dis 1997; 12(4):214–219.

37. Doornebosch PG, Bronkhorst PJB, Hop WCJ, Bode WA, Sing AK, de Graaf EJR. The role of endorectal ultrasound in therapeutic decision-making for local vs. transabdominal resection of rectal tumors. Dis Colon Rectum 2008;51(1): 38–42.

38. Zorcolo L, Fantola G, Cabras F, Marongiu L, D'Alia G, Casula G. Preoperative staging of patients with rectal tumors suitable for transanal endoscopic microsurgery (TEM): comparison of endorectal ultrasound and histopathologic findings. Surg Endosc 2009;23(6):1384–1389.

39. Improved survival with preoperative radiotherapy in resectable rectal cancer. Swedish Rectal Cancer Trial. N Engl J Med 1997;336(14):980–987.

40. Kapiteijn E, Marijnen CA, Nagtegaal ID, et al; Dutch Colorectal Cancer Group. Preoperative radiotherapy combined with total mesorectal excision for resectable rectal cancer. N Engl J Med 2001;345(9):638–646.

41. Sauer R, Becker H, Hohenberger W, et al; German Rectal Cancer Study Group. Preoperative versus postoperative chemoradiotherapy for rectal cancer. N Engl J Med 2004; 351(17):1731–1740.

42. Kwok H, Bissett IP, Hill GL. Preoperative staging of rectal cancer. Int J Colorectal Dis 2000;15(1):9–20.

43. Maier A, Fuchsjäger M. Preoperative staging of rectal cancer. Eur J Radiol 2003;47(2):89–97.

44. Giovannini M. What is the role of endo-rectal echography in monitoring of patients operated on for rectal cancer?. [Article in German] Gastroenterol Clin Biol 1998;22(3): 266–268.

45. de Anda EH, Lee SH, Finne CO, Rothenberger DA, Madoff RD, Garcia-Aguilar J. Endorectal ultrasound in the follow-up of rectal cancer patients treated by local excision or radical surgery. Dis Colon Rectum 2004;47(6):818–824.

46. Hünerbein M, Schlag PM. Three-dimensional endosonography for staging of rectal cancer. Ann Surg 1997;225(4): 432–438.

47. Löhnert MS, Doniec JM, Henne-Bruns D. Effectiveness of endoluminal sonography in the identification of occult local rectal cancer recurrences. Dis Colon Rectum 2000;43(4): 483–491.

48. Barnett JL, Hasler WL, Camilleri M; American Gastroenterological Association. American Gastroenterological Association medical position statement on anorectal testing techniques. Gastroenterology 1999;116(3):732–760.

49. Kumar A, Rao SS. Diagnostic testing in fecal incontinence. Curr Gastroenterol Rep 2003;5(5):406–413.

50. Dobben AC, Terra MP, Deutekom M, et al. Anal inspection and digital rectal examination compared to anorectal physiology tests and endoanal ultrasonography in evaluating fecal incontinence. Int J Colorectal Dis 2007;22(7):783–790.

51. Nielsen MB, Hauge C, Pedersen JF, Christiansen J. Endosonographic evaluation of patients with anal incontinence: findings and influence on surgical management. AJR Am J Roentgenol 1993;160(4):771–775.

52. Law PJ, Kamm MA, Bartram CI. Anal endosonography in the investigation of faecal incontinence. Br J Surg 1991;78(3): 312–314.

53. Eckardt VF, Jung B, Fischer B, Lierse W. Anal endosonography in healthy subjects and patients with idiopathic fecal incontinence. Dis Colon Rectum 1994;37(3):235–242.

54. Sultan AH, Kamm MA, Hudson CN, Thomas JM, Bartram CI. Anal-sphincter disruption during vaginal delivery. N Engl J Med 1993;329(26):1905–1911.

55. Oberwalder M, Connor J, Wexner SD. Meta-analysis to determine the incidence of obstetric anal sphincter damage. Br J Surg 2003;90(11):1333–1337.

56. Christiansen J, Roed-Petersen K. Clinical assessment of the anal continence plug. Dis Colon Rectum 1993;36(8): 740–742.

57. Abbasakoor F, Nelson M, Beynon J, Patel B, Carr ND. Anal endosonography in patients with anorectal symptoms after haemorrhoidectomy. Br J Surg 1998;85(11):1522–1524.

58. Marshall M, Halligan S, Fotheringham T, Bartram C, Nicholls RJ. Predictive value of internal anal sphincter thickness for diagnosis of rectal intussusception in patients with solitary rectal ulcer syndrome. Br J Surg 2002;89(10):1281–1285.

59. Kamm MA. Obstetric damage and faecal incontinence. Lancet 1994;344(8924):730–733.

60. Schäfer R, Heyer T, Gantke B, et al. Anal endosonography and manometry: comparison in patients with defecation problems. Dis Colon Rectum 1997;40(3):293–297.

61. Leppert R, Sailer M, Fuchs KH, Thiede A. Endosonography of anal fistulas and abscesses and their relation with the sphincter complex. Coloproctology 1994;16:327–329.

62. Poen AC, Felt-Bersma RJ, Eijsbouts QA, Cuesta MA, Meuwissen SG. Hydrogen peroxide-enhanced transanal ultrasound in the assessment of fistula-in-ano. Dis Colon Rectum 1998; 41(9):1147–1152.

63. Sailer M, Fuchs KH, Kraemer M, Thiede A. Stepwise concept for treatment of complex anal fistulas. [Article in German] Zentralbl Chir 1998;123(7):840–845, discussion 846.

64. Arulampalam TH, Costa DC, Loizidou M, Visvikis D, Ell PJ, Taylor I. Positron emission tomography and colorectal cancer. Br J Surg 2001;88(2):176–189.

65. Sailer M, Leppert R, Fuchs KH, Thiede A. Endorectal ultrasound for evaluating perirectal processes. [Article in German] Chirurg 1995;66(1):34–39, discussion 39.

66. Rodríguez LV, Terris MK. Risks and complications of transrectal ultrasound guided prostate needle biopsy: a prospective study and review of the literature. J Urol 1998;160(6 Pt 1):2115–2120.

67. Sailer M, Bussen D, Fuchs KH, Thiede A. Endoscopic ultrasound-guided transrectal aspiration of pelvic fluid collections. Surg Endosc 2004;18(5):736–740.

68. McGahan JP, Wu C. Sonographically guided transvaginal or transrectal pelvic abscess drainage using the trocar method with a new drainage guide attachment. AJR Am J Roentgenol 2008;191(5):1540–1544.

69. Sailer M, Bussen D, Leppert R, Fuchs KH, Thiede A. Endosonography of anal carcinomas. Coloproctology 1997;19:84–88.

70. Bartram CI, Burnett JD. Atlas of Anal Endosonography. Oxford: Butterworth-Heinemann; 1991.

71. Magdeburg B, Fried M, Meyenberger C. Endoscopic ultrasonography in the diagnosis, staging, and follow-up of anal carcinomas. Endoscopy 1999;31(5):359–364.

72. Christensen AF, Nielsen MB, Engelholm SA, Roed H, Svendsen LB, Christensen H. Three-dimensional anal endosonography may improve staging of anal cancer compared with two-dimensional endosonography. Dis Colon Rectum 2004;47(3):341–345.

73. Löhnert M, Doniec JM, Kovács G, Schröder J, Dohrmann P. New method of radiotherapy for anal cancer with three-dimensional tumor reconstruction based on endoanal ultrasound and ultrasound-guided afterloading therapy. Dis Colon Rectum 1998;41(2):169–176.

74. Christensen AF, Nyhuus B, Nielsen MB. Interobserver and intraobserver variation of two-dimensional and three-dimensional anal endosonography in the evaluation of recurrent anal cancer. Dis Colon Rectum 2009;52(3):484–488.

III Gastrointestinal Tract

25 Three-Dimensional Endorectal Ultrasound and Rectal Cancer

M. Giovannini

Several studies in the field of endoscopic ultrasound (EUS) technology have reported advantages with three-dimensional (3D) EUS.[1–13] However, most 3D EUS studies have been conducted using catheter-type miniature probe systems.[3,6–9] Some studies have previously reported benefits of a prototype 3D EUS system using a linear-array echoendoscope for 3D guidance of interventional procedures, but the scanning method used in this system has limitations and, as the ultrasound probe was not positioned at the tip of the endoscope, it was difficult to obtain clinically adequate images in the stomach without geometrical distortion.[14–16] A recent study attempted to resolve this problem and maximize the performance of 3D EUS using a linear echoendoscope with a miniature electromagnetic position sensor attached to the tip of the scope, which can be used for freehand scanning in any position.[17] However, the problem with this technique is that the electromagnetic sensor increases the size of the probe. This chapter reports on experience with a totally new 3D EUS software program that works without the need for an electromagnetic sensor and can be used even with electronic radial or linear rectal probes.

Basic Principles of Three-Dimensional Ultrasound

Two types of system have been developed, making use of either a series of two-dimensional (2D) images produced by one-dimensional arrays, or using 2D arrays to produce 3D images directly. Two criteria have to be met to avoid inaccuracies: the relative position and angulation of the acquired 2D images need to be known accurately; and the images have to be acquired rapidly and/or gated to avoid artifacts caused by respiratory, cardiac, and involuntary motion.

Tracked free-hand systems. The operator holds an assembly consisting of the transducer and an attachment, and manipulates it over the anatomy. Two-dimensional images are digitized as the transducer is moved, while meeting two criteria: the precise relative angulation and position of the ultrasound transducer have to be known for each digitized image; and the operator has to ensure that no significant gaps are left when scanning the anatomy.

Three-dimensional reconstruction. The 3D reconstruction process involves generating a 3D image from a digitized set of 2D images. The approach used was the voxel-based volume. The 2D images are built into a 3D voxel-based volume (3D grid) by placing each digitized 2D image into its correct location in the volume. The main advantages of this are that no information is lost during the 3D reconstruction and that a variety of rendering techniques are possible; however, large data files are generated.

Visualization of three-dimensional ultrasound images. The ability to visualize information in the 3D image depends critically on the rendering technique. Three basic methods are used:

- *Surface-based viewing technique.* An operator or algorithm identifies the boundaries of structures in order to create a wire-frame representation. These boundaries are shaded and illuminated, so that surfaces, structures, and organs are visualized.
- *Multiplane viewing techniques* (**Fig. 25.1**).
  - Orthogonal views: three perpendicular planes are displayed simultaneously and can be moved or rotated.
  - Polyhedron: the 3D images are presented as a multiple-sided volume (polyhedron). The appropriate ultrasound image is "painted" onto each face of the polyhedron, which can be manipulated.

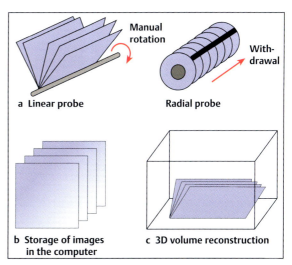

a Linear probe

Radial probe

b Storage of images in the computer

c 3D volume reconstruction

Fig. 25.1a–c The various steps involved in three-dimensional endoscopic ultrasound (3D EUS) scanning using radial or linear echoendoscopes.

- *Volume-based rendering techniques.* The 3D image is projected onto a 2D plane by casting rays through the 3D image. The voxel values intersected by each ray can be multiplied by factors and summed to produce different effects: multiplied by one and then added, to form a radiography-like image; multiplied by factors to produce translucency; or displaying only the voxel with the maximum intensity along each ray.

Results of Three-Dimensional Endorectal Ultrasound in the Literature

Our experience. From May 2003 to March 2004, we conducted 35 3D endorectal ultrasound (ERUS) examinations using this new software program. The indication for EUS was local staging of rectal cancer in all 35 cases. Before 3D ERUS scanning, a standard ERUS examination was performed. Three-dimensional rectal examinations were conducted using a radial electronic rigid probe (Hitachi R 54). The 3D software is included in the new ultrasound scanning machine (Hitachi 6500 or 8000) and allows reconstruction of the 2D EUS pictures in six different scans. The acquisition time is very fast, at around 10–25 seconds. The acquisition time was a function of the number of images recorded.

Thirty-five rectal cancers were assessed using 2D and 3D EUS. All of the tumors were located in the middle and lower part of the rectum, and stenotic tumors were excluded from the study. Three-dimensional EUS was possible in all cases. Two-dimensional EUS data classified the tumor into stages T1N0 (two patients), T2N0 (three patients), T3N0 (15 patients), T3N1 (12 patients) and T4N1 (three patients). Using 2D imaging, it was not possible to establish the degree of involvement of the mesorectum (more or less than 50%) precisely. No differences were found using 3D ERUS for superficial tumors (T1 and T2N0), but in six of the 15 patients staged with T3N0, 3D ERUS identified malignant lymph nodes, which were confirmed surgically in five of the six cases (**Table 25.1**).

By contrast, 3D EUS allowed precise assessment of the extent of infiltration into the mesorectum (**Fig. 25.2**) in all cases and showed quite complete invasion of it in eight cases. These findings were confirmed in all cases by the surgical data. To summarize the findings for rectal cancer: 2D EUS assessed 25 of 35 rectal tumors (71.4%) correctly

with regard to the T and N staging, and 3D EUS increased this result to 31 correct evaluations out of 35 (88.6%).

With regard to the accuracy of 2D and 3D imaging in relation to the T staging (T1–2 versus T3–4), there were no differences (34 of 35 accurate staging findings using both techniques). However, patients staged with 3D imaging as T3N0 developed fewer liver metastases than those classified as T3N0 with 2D imaging (one of nine versus six of 15; 11% versus 40%; $P = 0.002$). This difference was due to the fact that seven of the 15 rectal cancers staged as T3N0 with 2D imaging proved to be pT3N1 in the resected specimens. On the other hand, eight of the 35 patients in whom 3D ERUS showed extensive mesorectal infiltration (more than two-thirds of the thickness of the mesorectum) also developed more metastases (liver or peritoneal carcinomatosis) (four of eight versus seven of 27; 50% versus 26%; $P < 0.001$).

Review of the Literature

Three-dimensional ERUS is a new technique that is still undergoing development. Sumiyama et al.[15,17] recently reported their experience using 3D EUS and an electronic linear probe. They concluded that 3D EUS with a linear-array echoendoscope is accurate and represents a consistent method. They report that 3D EUS facilitates the anatomical interpretation of sonographic images and reduces the procedural difficulty of scanning.

Previous experience with 3D EUS using mechanical miniprobes has been reported for cardiovascular procedures,[18] and using rigid electronic probes for gynecological tumor assessment.[19,20] More recently, results with 3D EUS using mechanical miniprobes have also been published for pancreaticobiliary diseases[3,6,9] and anal diseases.[7]

Our own experience is slightly different, as we are using 3D ERUS with a new software program that allows linear-curved or radial electronic probes to be used, as the software is integrated into the ultrasound system's computer and an external sensor attached to the tip of the EUS scope is not needed. However, the most important question is whether 3D EUS is useful.[21,22]

With regard to the locoregional staging of rectal cancer, several studies have reported interesting results, with better parietal staging,[4,5] accurate staging even in cases of stenotic lesions, and more precise EUS guidance for biopsies.[23] Our own results show that the mesorectal margins are better defined with 3D EUS than with 2D EUS, allowing more accurate parietal staging. This precise definition of mesorectal involvement has a direct impact on therapeutic decision-making, since cancer reaching the margins of the mesorectum is regarded as a T4 lesion, even without the involvement of a pelvic organ.[24] Such lesions have to be treated with preoperative chemoradiotherapy.

More recently, Santoro et al.[25] have evaluated the accuracy of high-resolution 3D endorectal ultrasonography in distinguishing between slight and massive submucosal invasion by early rectal tumors. A total of 142 consecutive patients with clinically possible pT1 rectal cancers underwent 3D endorectal ultrasonography. Slight or massive irregularity of the hyperechoic submucosal layer was considered to characterize uT1 slight or uT1 massive tumors. Treatment was selected on the basis of the ultrasound findings: endoscopic resection or full-thickness transanal local excision was selected for "uT1 slight" lesions, and radical resection was selected for "uT1 massive" tumors. The ultrasound staging was then compared with the histopa-

Table 25.1 Accuracy of three-dimensional endorectal ultrasonography (3D EUS) staging of rectal cancer

	T1/T2N0	T3N0	T3N1	T4N1
2D EUS	5	15	12	3
3D EUS	5	9	18	3
Surgical findings	4	6	22	3

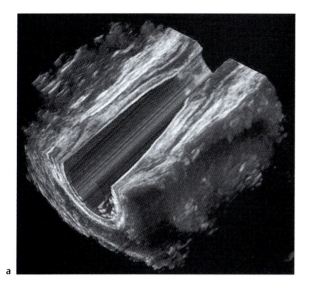

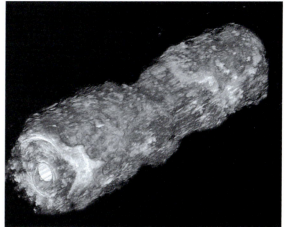

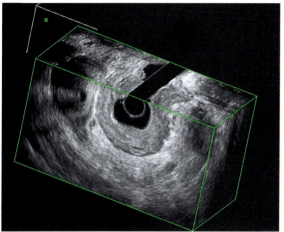

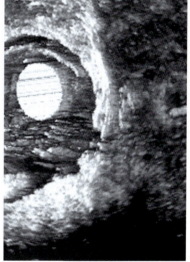

Fig. 25.2a–d a Full 3D reconstruction of the normal rectum and anal canal.
b A 360° 3D image of the normal rectum, with a clear margin of mesorectum.

c A 3D image of T3 rectal cancer, with limited involvement of the mesorectum.
d A 3D image of T4 rectal cancer, with complete involvement of the mesorectum.

thologic staging. A total of 126 patients were included in the final analyses. Three-dimensional endorectal ultrasonography staged 77 lesions as uT0, 25 as uT1 slight, 20 as uT1 massive, and four as uT2. Histologically, adenomas were found in 75 patients and tumor invasion was found in 44 lesions (24 pT1 slight, 16 pT1 massive, four pT2). The overall kappa for the concordance between the ultrasound and histopathologic classifications was 0.81 (95% confidence intervals, 0.72 to 0.89). No invasive carcinomas remained undetected. The depth of invasion was correctly determined in 87.2% of both pT1 slight and pT1 massive lesions. Relative to the full series of 126 patients, the accuracy of this modality for selecting appropriate management was 95.2% (κ 0.84; 95% confidence intervals, 0.71 to 0.96). Adequate surgery was performed in 87.5% of pT1 tumors. Three-dimensional endorectal ultrasonography is useful for assessing the depth of submucosal invasion in early rectal cancer and for selecting therapeutic options.

Conclusions

Three-dimensional ERUS with the new software program described here is currently available and is easy to perform. As there is no need for an external sensor mounted at the tip of the probe, manipulation of the rectal probe is facilitated. Three-dimensional ERUS has a direct therapeutic impact on the pretherapeutic staging of rectal cancer and allows more precise definition of the mesorectal margins, with a direct impact on therapeutic decision-making.

References

1. Kallimanis G, Garra BS, Tio TL, et al. The feasibility of three-dimensional endoscopic ultrasonography: a preliminary report. Gastrointest Endosc 1995;41(3):235–239.
2. Odegaard S, Nesje LB, Molin SO, Gilja OH, Hausken T. Three-dimensional intraluminal sonography in the evaluation of gastrointestinal diseases. Abdom Imaging 1999;24(5):449–451.
3. Kanemaki N, Nakazawa S, Inui K, Yoshino J, Yamao J, Okushima K. Three-dimensional intraductal ultrasonography: preliminary results of a new technique for the diagnosis of diseases of the pancreatobiliary system. Endoscopy 1997; 29(8):726–731.
4. Hünerbein M, Schlag PM. Three-dimensional endosonography for staging of rectal cancer. Ann Surg 1997;225(4):432–438.
5. Ivanov KD, Diavoc CD. Three-dimensional endoluminal ultrasound: new staging technique in patients with rectal cancer. Dis Colon Rectum 1997;40(1):47–50.
6. Tokiyama H, Yanai H, Nakamura H, Takeo Y, Yoshida T, Okita K. Three-dimensional endoscopic ultrasonography of lesions of the upper gastrointestinal tract using a radial-linear switchable thin ultrasound probe. J Gastroenterol Hepatol 1999;14(12):1212–1218.
7. Gold DM, Bartram CI, Halligan S, Humphries KN, Kamm MA, Kmiot WA. Three-dimensional endoanal sonography in assessing anal canal injury. Br J Surg 1999;86(3):365–370.
8. Calleja JL, Albillos A. Three-dimensional endosonography for staging of rectal cancer. Gastrointest Endosc 1998; 47(3):317–318.
9. Marusch F, Koch A, Schmidt U, et al. Routine use of transrectal ultrasound in rectal carcinoma: results of a prospective multicenter study. Endoscopy 2002;34(5):385–390.
10. Liu J, Miller LS, Chung CY, et al. Validation of volume measurements in esophageal pseudotumors using 3D endoluminal ultrasound. Ultrasound Med Biol 2000;26(5):735–741.
11. Chung CY, McCray WH, Dhaliwal S, et al. Three-dimensional esophageal varix model quantification of variceal volume by high-resolution endoluminal US. Gastrointest Endosc 2000;52(1):87–90.
12. Hünerbein M, Ghadimi BM, Gretschel S, Schlag PM. Three-dimensional endoluminal ultrasound: a new method for the evaluation of gastrointestinal tumors. Abdom Imaging 1999;24(5):445–448.
13. Hünerbein M, Gretschel S, Ghadimi BM, Schlag PM. Three-dimensional endoscopic ultrasound of the esophagus. Preliminary experience. Surg Endosc 1997;11(10):991–994.
14. Tamura S, Hirano M, Chen X, et al. Intrabody three-dimensional position sensor for an ultrasound endoscope. IEEE Trans Biomed Eng 2002;49(10):1187–1194.
15. Sumiyama K, Suzuki N, Kakutani H, et al. A novel 3-dimensional EUS technique for real-time visualization of the volume data reconstruction process. Gastrointest Endosc 2002;55(6):723–728.
16. Molin S, Nesje LB, Gilja OH, Hausken T, Martens D, Odegaard S. 3D-endosonography in gastroenterology: methodology and clinical applications. Eur J Ultrasound 1999;10(2-3): 171–177.
17. Sumiyama K, Suzuki N, Tajiri H. A linear-array freehand 3-D endoscopic ultrasound. Ultrasound Med Biol 2003;29(7):1001–1006.
18. Klingensmith JD, Schoenhagen P, Tajaddini A, et al. Automated three-dimensional assessment of coronary artery anatomy with intravascular ultrasound scanning. Am Heart J 2003;145(5):795–805.
19. Ayoubi JM, Fanchin R, Ferretti G, Pons JC, Bricault I. Three-dimensional ultrasonographic reconstruction of the uterine cavity: toward virtual hysteroscopy? Eur Radiol 2002;12(8):2030–2033.
20. Liu JB, Miller LS, Bagley DH, Goldberg BB. Endoluminal sonography of the genitourinary and gastrointestinal tracts. J Ultrasound Med 2002;21(3):323–337.
21. Yoshimoto K. Clinical application of ultrasound 3D imaging system in lesions of the gastrointestinal tract. Endoscopy 1998;30(Suppl 1):A145–A148.
22. Yoshino J, Nakazawa S, Inui K, et al. Surface-rendering imaging of gastrointestinal lesions by three-dimensional endoscopic ultrasonography. Endoscopy 1999;31(7):541–545.
23. Hünerbein M, Dohmoto M, Haensch W, Schlag PM. Evaluation and biopsy of recurrent rectal cancer using three-dimensional endosonography. Dis Colon Rectum 1996; 39(12):1373–1378.
24. Heald RJ, Ryall RD. Recurrence and survival after total mesorectal excision for rectal cancer. Lancet 1986;1(8496):1479–1482.
25. Santoro GA, Gizzi G, Pellegrini L, Battistella G, Di Falco G. The value of high-resolution three-dimensional endorectal ultrasonography in the management of submucosal invasive rectal tumors. Dis Colon Rectum 2009;52(11):1837–1843.

26 Endoscopic Ultrasound of the Colon

C.F. Dietrich, J.C. Mertens

Endoscopic ultrasound (EUS) examination of the colon is possible, particularly using radial scanning techniques with an orthograde endoscopic view. Longitudinal probes in which the endoscopic view is not orthograde are more difficult to use, and this may complicate examinations in certain cases.

Endosonography can be helpful in evaluating submucosal colonic tumors in which the benign or malignant status is unknown. In these cases, the ideal combination of diagnostic methods—such as colonoscopy for precise localization and visualization of the findings and subsequent endosonography (e.g., using instilled water for optimal imaging conditions)—remains a challenge.

Miniprobe technology has proved to be superior to conventional endosonography in the colon (with the exception of the rectum), since tumors or polyps can be visualized, examined, and classified in the same way as in the approach used for esophageal, gastric, and duodenal wall endosonography. Although the place of miniprobe technology has not yet been sufficiently evaluated, it will probably offer a wide range of further indications.

Clinical Relevance

The relevance of flexible endosonography techniques in the lower intestinal tract is a matter of controversy.[1–14] There are as yet no universally accepted indications for endosonography of the colon. In contrast, rectal endosonography using rigid probes is widely used and, in the hands of an experienced examiner, can play an important role in the diagnosis of complicated fistulas and in the staging of rectal carcinomas. In some cases, endosonography may also be helpful for EUS-guided puncture. With further technical improvements and more widespread use of high-frequency miniprobe technology, an extended range of indications for endosonography in the lower gastrointestinal tract can be expected, particularly since lesions can be visualized endoscopically and their intramural and transmural extension can be assessed during the same examination.

The cecal pole and ileocecal valve can be reached with guidance from landmark structures and surrounding organs such as the prostate, seminal vesicle, urinary bladder, psoas muscle, left kidney with hilum, spleen, pancreas, gallbladder, liver, right kidney, and head of the pancreas (**Figs. 26.1, 26.2, 26.3, 26.4, 26.5, 26.6, 26.7, 26.8, 26.9, 26.10, 26.11, 26.12, 26.13, 26.14,** and **26.15**). Fistulas, abscesses, and other pathological transmural findings can be visualized with a high level of sensitivity (**Figs. 26.16** and **26.17**).

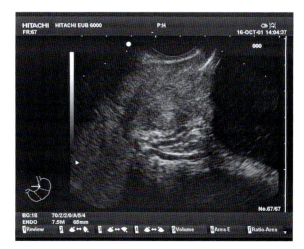

Fig. 26.1 The prostate, with the urethra.

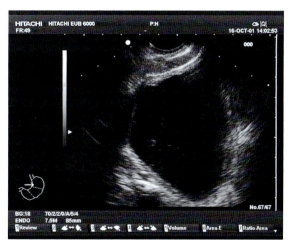

Fig. 26.2 The urinary bladder, with sporadic echoes caused by sediment.

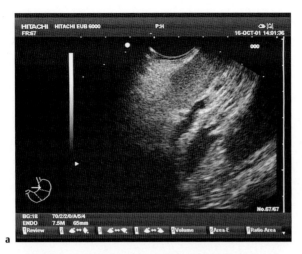
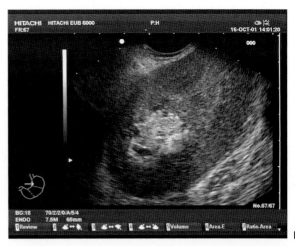

Fig. 26.3a, b a The left kidney, with the vascular hilum.

b The renal parenchyma, as seen from the descending colon.

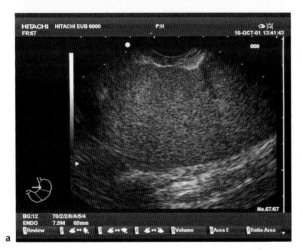
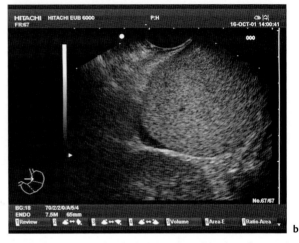

Fig. 26.4a, b The spleen
a With a small amount of physiological perisplenic free fluid toward the kidney.

b With diaphragmatic borders, as seen from the splenic flexure of the colon.

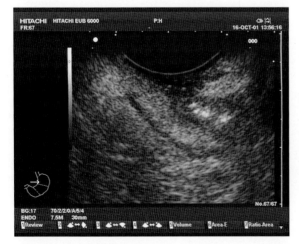
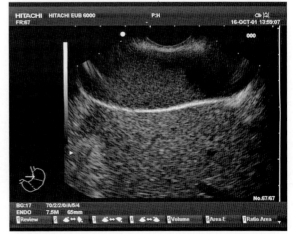

Fig. 26.5 The pancreatic body, with the pancreatic duct, visualized from the transverse colon.

Fig. 26.6 The gallbladder with sludge, visualized from the hepatic (right) flexure of the colon.

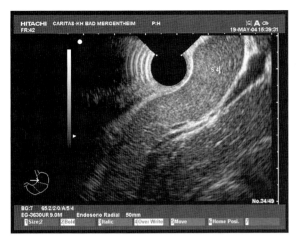

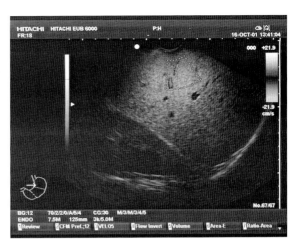

Fig. 26.7 Imaging of the liver from the colon, demonstrating the echogenic borders of the portal vein branches. S4, quadrate lobe.

Fig. 26.8 Imaging of a fatty liver echo texture, including comparison of the parenchymal imaging characteristics of the liver and kidney. It is also possible to assess the vessels using color Doppler imaging.

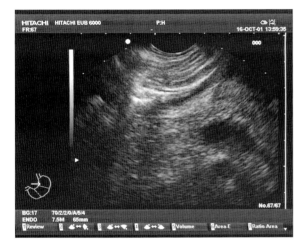

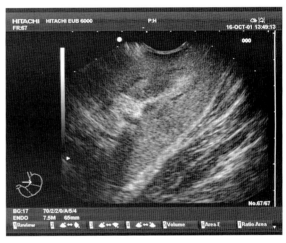

Fig. 26.9 The head of the pancreas, as seen from the ascending colon.

Fig. 26.10 The right kidney, as seen from the ascending colon.

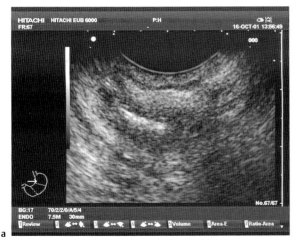

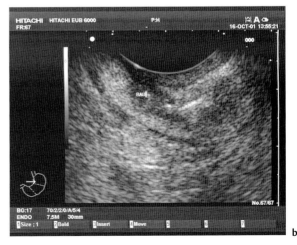

a

b

Fig. 26.11a, b a The ileocecal valve.

b With the orifice of the terminal ileum. BAU, Bauhin valve (ileal papilla).

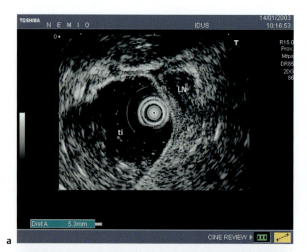

a

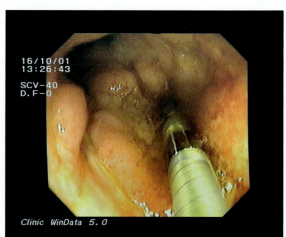

b

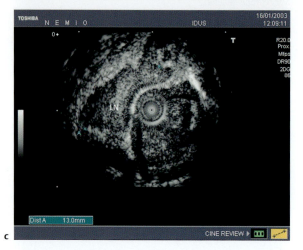

c

Fig. 26.12a–c a The terminal ileum (ti), examined with miniprobe ultrasound, with visualization of small (physiological) lymph nodes (LN) in the immediate vicinity.

b, c Pathological lymph nodes due to Crohn disease (**b**, endoscopic image; **c**, miniprobe image).

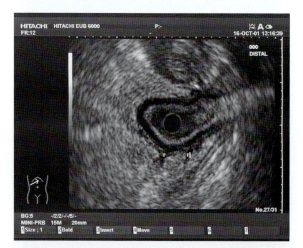

Fig. 26.13 A fistula in a patient with Crohn disease. There is a transmural inflammatory reaction, with a blind-ending fistula (F). Fissural ulcerations corresponding to the endoscopic image were visible, the transmural size of which was only able to be evaluated with miniprobe endosonography.

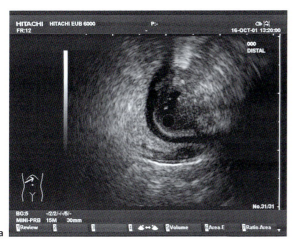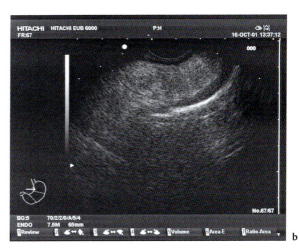

Fig. 26.14a, b Imaging of a fistula with a surrounding transmural inflammatory mesenteric reaction, with echogenic air outside the intestinal wall.

a Miniprobe imaging.
b Conventional endosonography.

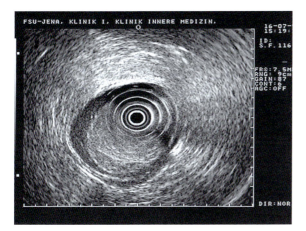

Fig. 26.15 A lipoma in the transverse colon. As in the upper gastro-intestinal tract, submucosal tumors can be assigned to a specific layer of the intestinal wall—for example, the submucosa with lipomas.

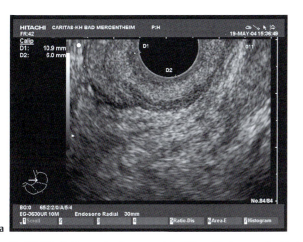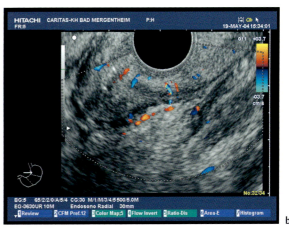

Fig. 26.16a, b Hemorrhagic segmental colitis, with circumscribed ischemic thickening in the right colon.

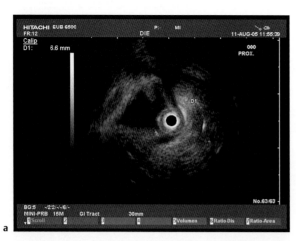
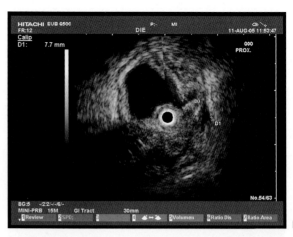

a   b

Fig. 26.17a, b Diverticula (between the markers) visualized using miniprobe endosonography.

References

1. Ahmad NA, Kochman ML, Long WB, Furth EE, Ginsberg GG. Efficacy, safety, and clinical outcomes of endoscopic mucosal resection: a study of 101 cases. Gastrointest Endosc 2002;55(3):390–396.
2. Bhutani MS, Nadella P. Utility of an upper echoendoscope for endoscopic ultrasonography of malignant and benign conditions of the sigmoid/left colon and the rectum. Am J Gastroenterol 2001;96(12):3318–3322.
3. Dietrich CF, Lembcke B, Seifert H, Caspary WF, Wehrmann T. Ultrasound diagnosis of penicillin-induced segmental hemorrhagic colitis [Article in German] Dtsch Med Wochenschr 2000;125:755–760.
4. Giovannini M, Bernardini D, Seitz JF, et al. Value of endoscopic ultrasonography for assessment of patients presenting elevated tumor marker levels after surgery for colorectal cancers. Endoscopy 1998;30(5):469–476.
5. Hirata N, Kawamoto K, Ueyama T, Iwashita I, Masuda K. Endoscopic ultrasonography in the assessment of colonic wall invasion by adjacent diseases. Abdom Imaging 1994;19(1):21–26.
6. Hizawa K, Suekane H, Aoyagi K, Matsumoto T, Nakamura S, Fujishima M. Use of endosonographic evaluation of colorectal tumor depth in determining the appropriateness of endoscopic mucosal resection. Am J Gastroenterol 1996; 91(4):768–771.
7. Hünerbein M, Handke T, Ulmer C, Schlag PM. Impact of miniprobe ultrasonography on planning of minimally invasive surgery for gastric and colonic tumors. Surg Endosc 2004;18(4):601–605.
8. Lew RJ, Ginsberg GG. The role of endoscopic ultrasound in inflammatory bowel disease. Gastrointest Endosc Clin N Am 2002;12(3):561–571.
9. Okada N, Hirooka Y, Itoh A, et al. Cholecystocolonic fistula preoperatively diagnosed by endoscopic ultrasound of the colon. J Gastroenterol Hepatol 2005;20(10):1621–1624.
10. Sasaki Y, Niwa Y, Hirooka Y, et al. The use of endoscopic ultrasound-guided fine-needle aspiration for investigation of submucosal and extrinsic masses of the colon and rectum. Endoscopy 2005;37(2):154–160.
11. Stergiou N, Haji-Kermani N, Schneider C, Menke D, Köckerling F, Wehrmann T. Staging of colonic neoplasms by colonoscopic miniprobe ultrasonography. Int J Colorectal Dis 2003;18(5):445–449.
12. Tsuga K, Haruma K, Fujimura J, et al. Evaluation of the colorectal wall in normal subjects and patients with ulcerative colitis using an ultrasonic catheter probe. Gastrointest Endosc 1998;48(5):477–484.
13. Watanabe F, Honda S, Kubota H, et al. Preoperative diagnosis of ileal lipoma by endoscopic ultrasonography probe. J Clin Gastroenterol 2000;31(3):245–247.
14. Waxman I, Saitoh Y, Raju GS, et al. High-frequency probe EUS-assisted endoscopic mucosal resection: a therapeutic strategy for submucosal tumors of the GI tract. Gastrointest Endosc 2002;55(1):44–49.

IV Lung and Mediastinum

27 Mediastinum from the Esophagus

C.F. Dietrich, M. Hocke, F.J.F. Herth

Endoscopic ultrasound (EUS) diagnostic techniques are extremely valuable in the mediastinum, but this has not yet been fully exploited in everyday clinical practice. It is not possible to evaluate the mediastinum adequately using only one method of examination; instead, a combination of endoscopic methods (e.g., bronchoscopy), radiographic methods (e.g., conventional techniques, computed tomography, magnetic resonance imaging), surgical methods (e.g., mediastinoscopy, thoracoscopy, thoracotomy), and ultrasound methods is necessary.

Conventional radiography is undoubtedly important at the start of diagnostic work-up in the mediastinal region. The upper and anterior mediastinum can be seen adequately with *transthoracic mediastinal ultrasonography,* which is easily performed and also allows targeted aspiration of tumors to obtain histological confirmation of the suspected diagnosis.[1–5] However, examination of the aortic lymph nodes and lymph-node groups in the lower and posterior mediastinum is not adequate with this method. *Computed tomography* (CT) allows the mediastinum to be examined accurately, but aspiration and collection of histological specimens from structures deep in the mediastinum require a separate procedure. *Transesophageal endoscopic ultrasonography* allows examination of the posterior mediastinum, as well as visualization and targeted aspiration of even the smallest structures in this area. On the other hand, the examination of pretracheal and paratracheal structures using endoscopic ultrasonography is not adequate (with the exception of the 2 L and 4 L nodes). *Transbronchial endoscopic ultrasonography* shows signs of being a promising method, but so far has only been used in a few centers and has not yet been fully evaluated.

The diagnostic confirmation of mediastinal tumors and staging of bronchial carcinoma are therefore still dependent on mediastinoscopy, video-assisted thoracoscopy, and thoracotomy and mediastinotomy if necessary. Each of these methods only has a limited range of indications. Coordinating the application of the methods is even more difficult, since ultrasound techniques are not yet fully developed in the field of pneumology. Transesophageal EUS is often carried out by gastroenterologists, and interdisciplinary collaboration may be inadequate. A further disadvantage is that there is a relatively small number of pneumology centers in Europe in comparison with the USA, for example.

Anatomy

The mediastinum is a complex space in which the lymph nodes of the upper mediastinum, the aortic lymph nodes, the lymph nodes of the lower mediastinum, and the pulmonary lymph nodes have to be distinguished. The pulmonary lymph nodes (hilar, interlobar, lobar, segmental, and subsegmental) are known as the N1 lymph nodes; the mediastinal and subcarinal lymph nodes as the N2 lymph nodes; and the supraclavicular and scalene lymph nodes as the N3 lymph nodes. The mediastinal lymph nodes are classified in accordance with the Mountain and Dresler system,[6] which is adapted from an earlier classification by Tsuguo Naruke.

The paratracheal lymph-node groups (level 2 L and 4 L; L = left), the lymph-node groups in the aortopulmonary window (level 5), the subcarinal (level 7), and in particular the paraesophageal lymph nodes (level 8), can be viewed and punctured with real-time visualization. This is also possible in part for the lymph nodes in the region of the inferior pulmonary ligament (level 9). The same is true of metastases in the left adrenal gland, determining the prognosis in up to 5% of cases.[7]

Lymph-node levels 1, 2 R, 3, and 4 R (R = right), as well as 6, are not able to be assessed in most patients with normal-sized lymph nodes, due to interference from the larger airways (**Fig. 27.1**). EUS imaging may be possible in patients with larger lymphomas.

It has been shown that CT, which simply determines the size of mediastinal lymph nodes, is inadequate, with an accuracy level of 50–80%. The longitudinal position of the lymph nodes in the mediastinum is the critical factor, as this means that the lymph nodes can only be imaged from the side or at an angle. This is the reason for the notable inaccuracy of CT for determining the size of the lymph nodes. Endoscopic ultrasonography is able not only to assess the criteria relative to size, but also changes pertaining to the echo pattern, architecture, and localized infiltration.

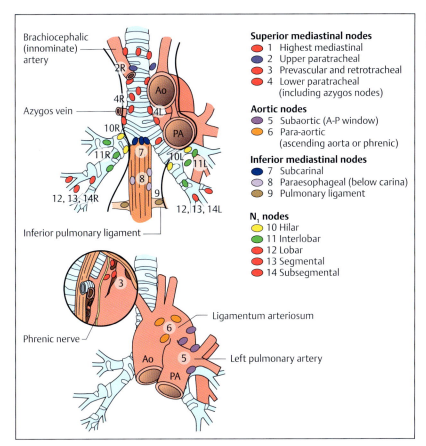

Brachiocephalic (innominate) artery

Azygos vein

Inferior pulmonary ligament

Phrenic nerve

Ligamentum arteriosum

Left pulmonary artery

Superior mediastinal nodes
1 Highest mediastinal
2 Upper paratracheal
3 Prevascular and retrotracheal
4 Lower paratracheal (including azygos nodes)

Aortic nodes
5 Subaortic (A-P window)
6 Para-aortic (ascending aorta or phrenic)

Inferior mediastinal nodes
7 Subcarinal
8 Paraesophageal (below carina)
9 Pulmonary ligament

N_1 nodes
10 Hilar
11 Interlobar
12 Lobar
13 Segmental
14 Subsegmental

Examination Techniques

■ General

Radial and linear instruments are available for transesophageal endoscopic ultrasonography in the mediastinum, but the radial technique does not allow aspiration, and the longitudinal scanner is therefore preferable from the pneumological point of view. Aspiration specimens obtained with EUS can be assessed using either cytology or molecular biology.

When enlarged lymph nodes are present, detection is also easier. When lymph nodes are detected, the lymph node (or an adrenal lesion) that is considered to be the most distant should be biopsied first, to avoid spreading malignant cells from local lymph nodes to more distant ones.

Prerequisites. Esophagogastroduodenoscopy (EGD) should be carried out before EUS in order to exclude stenosis and minimize the risk of perforation by the relatively inflexible EUS instrument. Extra care should be taken in inserting the instrument into the middle esoph-

agus if a traction diverticulum is suspected and during passage through the gastroesophageal junction, where there is an increased risk of perforation due to aggressive forward movement. The explanation of the procedure given to the patient should be the same as for any endoscopic procedure in the upper gastrointestinal tract, with extra emphasis being given to the increased risk of perforation in comparison with conventional EGD. The patient should be informed about the risk of bleeding and infection (including potentially fatal progressive mediastinitis). The risk of bleeding is small when coagulation is adequate (Quick test > 50%, thrombocytes > 50/nL).

Endoscopic ultrasound examination of the mediastinum can be performed as an outpatient procedure. After it has been explained to the patient, the examination requires 5–20 minutes, depending on the practitioner's level of experience. It has proved helpful to work with a cytologist present during the examination, although this topic is a matter of controversy.

Some authors have found that suction during fine-needle aspiration of lymph nodes increases the bloodiness of the specimen and does not necessarily increase the yield. The aspiration procedure is described elsewhere (see Chapter 10).

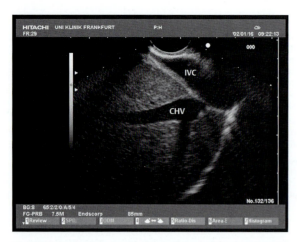

Fig. 27.2 The diaphragm, with the confluence of the hepatic veins (CHV) at the inferior vena cava (IVC).

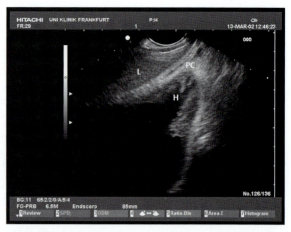

Fig. 27.3 The pericardial cavity (PC) with the left lobe of the liver (L) and tip of the heart (H).

Sedation. Sufficient sedation is extremely important. EUS-guided aspiration should only be carried out with adequate sedation, without cough stimulation or patient movement, as accidental puncture of the heart or large mediastinal vessels has to be avoided. Anesthesia that can be easily controlled is therefore necessary. In our experience, propofol (Diprivan) is more suitable than midazolam for this purpose, but comparative studies on this topic are lacking.

■ Procedure

The instrument is guided into the esophagus with endoscopic visualization. From the upper esophagus (18–20 cm past the incisor line), insertion can continue using either endoscopic or endoscopic ultrasound viewing.

Although orientation may be possible using the surrounding structures while the scope is being inserted, systematic examination starts distally, as control is much better when the scope is withdrawn. When the scope is rotated, the tracheal and bronchial airways ventrally, the echo-free vessels mainly laterally, and the hyperechoic bone structures dorsally can all be used as simple landmarks for orientation.

The systematic examination of the mediastinum starts distally, with the instrument in the cardiac region at the level of the thoracoabdominal junction. In this position, one can identify the liver, hepatic veins, inferior vena cava, heart chambers and heart valves, the left and right ventricular outflow ducts, the ascending aorta, the pulmonary trunk with the pulmonary arteries, and the aortic arch with the aorticopulmonary window. When the endoscope is turned and one orients oneself along the reflexogenic spine, it becomes possible to identify the descending aorta paravertebrally on the left and the azygos vein on the right. Further up, the vessels emerging from the aorta, particu-

larly the cervical vessels (the common carotid artery and jugular vein), the thyroid, and the paratracheal lymphnode groups can be observed from the tracheal bifurcation up to the mouth of the esophagus. The pretracheal lymph nodes are beyond the range of EUS, as they are concealed behind the air-filled trachea. The pneumological examination using EUS is completed by imaging the left adrenal gland and if possible the right adrenal gland (see Chapter 21) and by examining the lymph nodes of the celiac trunk. One can also start assessing the more distally located structures here, with the transduodenal and transgastric part of the examination taking place to begin with. The mediastinal lymph-node groups are examined using the following markers: the echo-free heart chambers and vascular paths; the ventral hyperechoic (air-filled) tracheobronchial system; and the dorsal echogenic bone structures of the spine. Directly next to the esophagus are the periesophageal and paravertebral lymph-node groups. The paracardiac lymph nodes can be found in the immediate neighborhood of the heart. Along the contour of the heart on the upper side of the atrium, the subcarinal lymph nodes can be detected in the tracheobronchial region, and the lymph nodes of the pulmonary ligament are located somewhat further distally.

The course of a typical examination is described in Chapter 2. **Figures 27.2, 27.3, 27.4, 27.5, 27.6, 27.7, 27.8, 27.9, 27.10, 27.11,** and **27.12** focus on the anatomy of the mediastinal vessels using color Doppler imaging and miniprobe ultrasonography of the mediastinum, and showing potential artifacts.

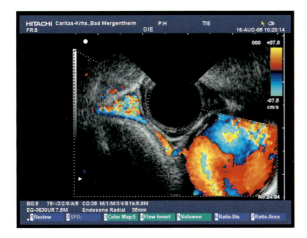

Fig. 27.4 The arterial branches of the aorta can be visualized using color Doppler imaging. The azygos vein can be viewed in its contralateral position on the right in front of the spine. Visualizing the vertebrae (left lower corner of the image) has proved helpful.

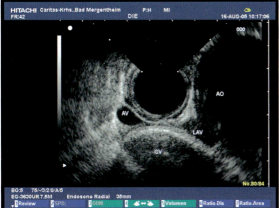

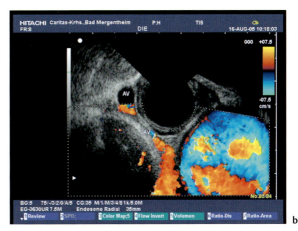

a

b

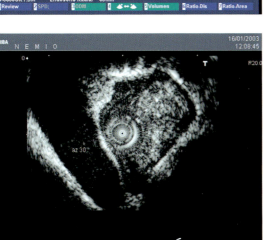

c

Fig. 27.5a–c The azygos vein (AV) can be accurately viewed in its lateral position on the right in front of the spine. Visualizing the aorta (AO) on the left of the cervical vertebrae (CV) has proved helpful.
a The left azygos vein (LAV) is also visible here (B-mode).
b Color Doppler imaging.
c Miniprobe ultrasonography.

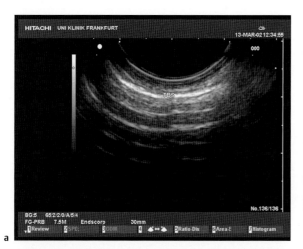
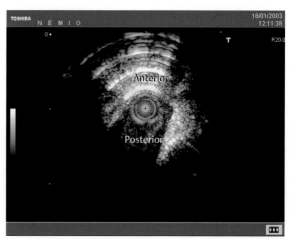

Fig. 27.6a, b The trachea can be imaged with both conventional EUS (**a**) and miniprobe EUS (**b**) by identifying the air echoes ventrally. The lumen is therefore posterior in **b**. TBS, tracheobronchal system.

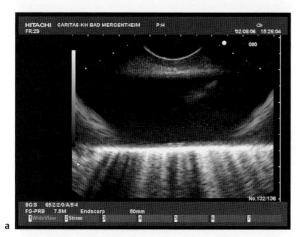
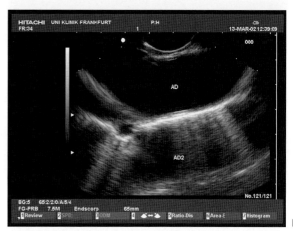

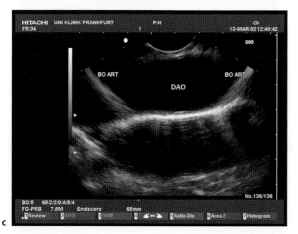

Fig. 27.7a–c The descending aorta (DAO). Due to the extreme differences in acoustic impedance between the blood in the aorta and the surface of the lung, the descending aorta can be imaged in various cross-sections with different artifacts.
a Typical morphology.
b Mirror artifact.
c Arch artifacts (BO ART).

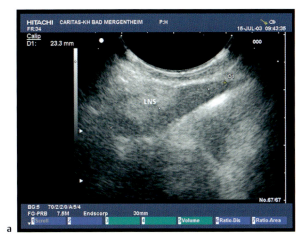

a

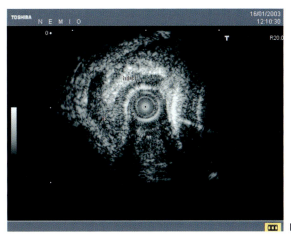

b

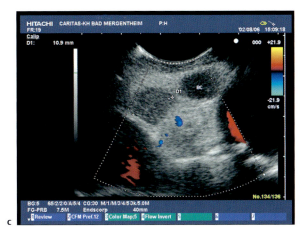

c

Fig. 27.8a–c The subcarinal lymph-node groups on the roof of the left atrium: imaging of the normal lymph-node architecture with a lymph-node sinus (LNS).
a Conventional EUS.
b Miniprobe EUS.
c Pathological lymph nodes often show changes in the architecture, seen here in a patient with bronchial carcinoma (BC).

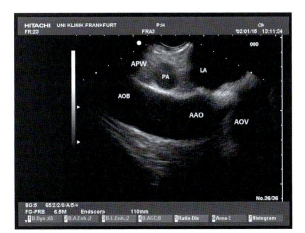

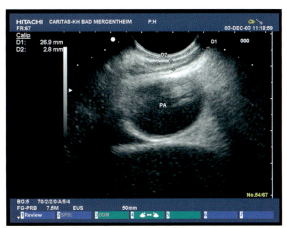

Fig. 27.9 The aortopulmonary window (APW). The left atrium (LA), pulmonary artery (PA), aortic arch (AA), ascending aorta (AAO), and aortic valve (AOV) are also shown. The pulmonary artery separates the aortopulmonary window from the subcarinal lymph-node groups on the roof of the left atrium.

Fig. 27.10 A normal periesophageal lymph node. A very narrow, longitudinally positioned lymph node with normal architecture is shown between the markers. PA, pulmonary artery.

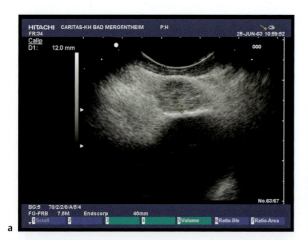

a

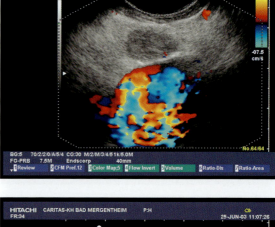

b

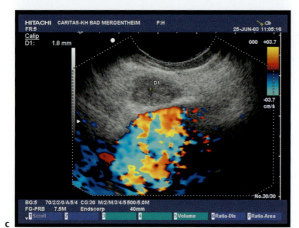

c

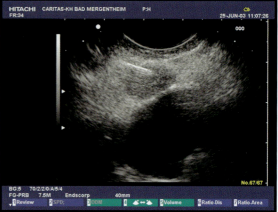

d

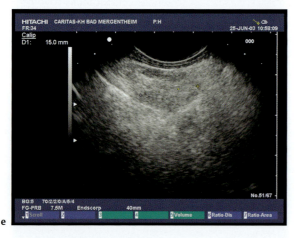

e

Fig. 27.11a–e EUS-guided aspiration. Imaging of a 12-mm lymph node directly adjacent to the aortic arch.
a Conventional EUS.
b Color duplex EUS.
c, d Suspected localized malignant infiltration (**c**), which was aspirated after appropriate sedation (**d**).
e As a result, slight bleeding occurs, producing a change in the echo pattern.

Review of the Literature

Information about the importance of the lymph-node structure in distinguishing between malignant and benign changes in lymph nodes is mainly derived from high-resolution ultrasonography (7.5–12 MHz). Most research has concentrated on the results of cervical lymph-node ultrasonography. Attempts to assess malignancy on the basis of size (malignant > 1 cm), appearance (malignant: round, benign: oval), and internal structure (malignant with no signs of a hilum, benign with identification of a hilum) have shown success rates of 57–94% in various studies.[8–13]

Combining these findings with the use of power Doppler to examine the vascular distribution can improve the accuracy of the diagnosis. In this way, it is possible to observe that benign lymph nodes show hilar vascularization and that malignant lymph nodes usually show vascularization coming from the edge. However, these results, from a study that reported a sensitivity of 92% and a specificity of 100%, need to be tested in further investigations.[14] The criteria may also be easier to image and evaluate with the use of ultrasound contrast enhancement.[15] It would be logical to extend the results to the lymph nodes in the mediastinum and abdominal cavity using high-resolution endoscopic ultrasonography. Initial results from an as yet unpublished study currently being conducted to differentiate between malignant and benign lymph nodes using endoscopic ultrasonography show promising results.

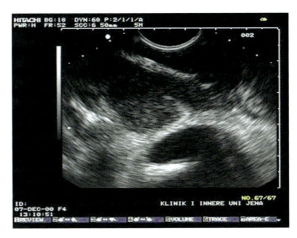

Fig. 27.12 Aspiration of a mediastinal empyema, followed by insertion of a drain via the puncture canal.

■ EUS-Guided Fine-Needle Aspiration in the Mediastinum

Indications and results. The diagnosis and mediastinal staging of lung cancer is by far the most common indication for guided fine-needle aspiration (EUS-FNA) in pulmonary medicine. For mediastinal staging, most studies have been conducted in selected patients with enlarged or positron-emission tomography–positive nodes. The sensitivity (range 72–100%), specificity (range 88–100%), negative predictive value (range 39–100%), and accuracy (77–100%) have been reported (**Table 27.1**). In the three studies performed in patients without enlarged nodes, sensitivities of between 35% and 61% and accuracies of between 76% and 89% have been reported for mediastinal staging.[16–18] The lower accuracy in small nodes may be due to sampling errors, technical difficulty in sampling small nodes, or the fact that nodes with a normal sonographic appearance are simply not biopsied.[19] It has been suggested that EUS-FNA can be used as a re-staging method after induction chemoradiotherapy, and accuracy rates of 83% and 86% have been reported for this.[20,21]

EUS-FNA offers a minimally invasive alternative to surgical staging, as it can prevent 70% of scheduled mediastinoscopies.[22–24] Thanks to its complementary diagnostic reach, the addition of EUS to mediastinoscopy improves staging[25] and therefore reduces the number of futile thoracotomies.[26]

EUS-FNA has a yield of 82%[27–29] in assessing granulomas in patients with suspected sarcoidosis. Patients with sarcoidosis often present with multiple, clustered, well-demarcated nodes,[27] which are frequently well vascularized.[28] EUS-FNA provides an alternative to bronchoscopy and peripheral lung biopsies (which involve a risk of hemoptysis and pneumothorax) and should be performed if available before a mediastinoscopy.

EUS-FNA can also be used for the mediastinal staging for extrathoracic tumors—for example, for suspected mediastinal metastases from breast carcinoma or renal carcinoma.[29]

Bronchogenic and paraesophageal cysts can be visualized well with EUS.[30] EUS-FNA of mediastinal nodes is considered safe, as no serious complications have been reported. However, FNA of cystic mediastinal lesions should be avoided due to the risk of mediastinitis.[30,31]

■ Non-Small Cell Lung Cancer

The problem. In patients with non-small cell lung cancer (NSCLC) who undergo surgery, the procedure may be futile due to advanced mediastinal disease in up to 50% of cases. This is particularly important in up to 25% of patients who are found to have normal-sized lymph nodes (< 1 cm) on chest CT. Up to 15% of operations for NSCLC result in exploratory thoracotomies without tumor resection; in addition, up to 35% of the operations are unsuccessful due to postoperative tumor recurrence.

The treatment of NSCLC is stage-dependent. Surgical resection is considered if no spread outside the lung is found (stages I and II). Induction chemotherapy followed by resection is considered in patients with ipsilateral mediastinal lymph-node disease (stage IIIA). Chemotherapy or chemoradiotherapy are considered if contralateral mediastinal lymphadenopathy or distant metastases are present (stages IIIB and IV).

Table 27.1 Results of real-time transesophageal ultrasound-guided fine-needle aspiration in mediastinal lymph-node staging in patients with (suspected) lung cancer

Author	Patients	Sensitivity	Specificity	PPV	NPV	Accuracy
Silvestri[33]	27	89	100	100	82	93
Gress[34]	24	93	100	100	90	96
Williams[35]	82	87	100	100	73	90
Fritscher-Ravens[36]	153	92	100	100	92	95
Wallace[37]	107	87	100	100	68	90
Wiersema[38]	33	100	88	96	100	97
Larsen[39]	79	92	100	100	89	91
Fritscher-Ravens[40]	33	88	100	100	89	91
Annema[25]	36	93	100	100	80	94
Kramer[30]	81	72	100	100	39	77
Savides[41]	59	96	100	100	97	98
Wallace[a16]	69	61	98	94	79	83
Leblanc[a17]	72	35	100	100	73	76
Annema[23]	100	76	97	92	91	91
Eloubeidi[42]	93	93	100	100	96	97
Annema[25]	215	91	100	100	74	93
Tournoy[24]	67	100	100	100	100	100
Fernandez-Esparrach[a18]	47	50	100	100	88	89

Data are presented as n or %. PPV, positive predictive value; NPV, negative predictive value.
[a] Lymph nodes, short axis, 1 cm.

Lymph-node staging. When a tumor has been histologically confirmed and is thought to be potentially operable, lymph-node staging is required in order to examine the contralateral mediastinal lymph-node groups (the patient is considered to be inoperable if these are positive).

Imaging methods. Chest radiography, thoracic CT, and bronchoscopy are the main imaging methods and are a prerequisite for further investigations (such as EUS, mediastinoscopy, and video-assisted thoracoscopy).

EUS. The advantage of EUS over CT is that it provides an opportunity to assess the fine lymph-node structure through the echo patterns. Localized malignant lymph-node infiltrations can be recognized more easily using EUS, even when CT produces negative results.

EUS-FNA after induction chemotherapy. EUS-FNA appears to be indicated for down-staging evaluation after induction chemotherapy. In one study, 19 consecutive patients with NSCLC and confirmed ipsilateral or subcarinal lymph-node metastases who had been treated with induction chemotherapy underwent mediastinal re-staging using EUS-FNA. Patients were assessed as having either a partial response or stable disease on the basis of sequential CT scans of the thorax. When EUS-FNA re-staged the mediastinum as showing no regional lymph-node metastases (N0), surgical resection of the tumor with lymph-node sampling or dissection was performed. The positive predictive value, negative predictive value, sensitivity, specif-

icity, and accuracy were 100%, 67%, 75%, 100%, and 83%, respectively, showing that EUS-FNA is an accurate method for re-staging of mediastinal lymph nodes after induction chemotherapy in patients with NSCLC. EUS-FNA appears to be able to identify a subgroup of down-staged patients who may benefit from further surgical treatment.

Limitations and prospects. Most of the studies discussed above were retrospective rather than consecutive and included only selected patients. No blinding was used in comparisons between EUS-FNA, mediastinoscopy, and transbronchial aspiration. Most of the published results are from expert centers.

Mediastinoscopy. Mediastinoscopy is regarded as the gold standard for mediastinal staging, and recently published guidelines recommend invasive mediastinoscopy (with a complication rate of 2–3%) before resection with curative intent is carried out. However, mediastinoscopy is limited to the anterior mediastinum (with examination of the pretracheal and paratracheal lymph-node groups) and N2–3 disease is found in up to 15% of patients who undergo thoracotomy after negative mediastinoscopy findings.

Diagnostic Work-Up

• Chest radiography, thoracic CT, and bronchoscopy should be carried out in all patients using the best available equipment.

- EUS of the mediastinum, including potential fine-needle aspiration of lymph nodes, should be used as a secondary diagnostic method if it is not possible to classify peripheral tumors using bronchoscopy (with transbronchial biopsy).
- Mediastinoscopy, covering the anterior mediastinum, and EUS-FNA, covering the posterior mediastinum, have been regarded as complementary. However, there have been no studies actually comparing the two methods with a controlled and blinded design. Mediastinoscopy is indicated for enlarged lymph nodes in groups 2 and 4. The prevascular and retrotracheal lymph-node group 3 and the N1 groups require supplementary examination procedures.
- Transthoracic puncture can be done using CT or transthoracic ultrasonography.
- It has been postulated that transbronchial miniprobe EUS might be helpful for lymph-node staging in patients in whom N1 groups are affected.

Prospects and Limitations

The limitations of EUS examination of the mediastinum and fine-needle aspiration are especially clear in the case of the pretracheal and right-sided paratracheal lymph-node groups (2 R, 4 R), which are often affected, since air in the tracheobronchial tree makes the ultrasound examination impossible. Transesophageal mediastinal EUS and mediastinoscopy are complementary in the area of the pretracheal lymph-node groups, since mediastinoscopy offers in particular a good approach to the pretracheal and paratracheal lymph-node groups, which cannot be assessed adequately with EUS. EUS examination of the mediastinum has advantages for evaluating periesophageal, subcarinal, and aortopulmonary lymph-node groups, in addition to the region around the pulmonary ligament.

Conclusions

Radial and linear instruments are available for transesophageal EUS of the mediastinum, but the radial technique does not allow puncture procedures. Longitudinal scanners are therefore preferable for pneumological purposes. The lymph nodes in the aortopulmonary window, subcarinal nodes, and nodes in the paraesophageal region can be examined with EUS-FNA. This is also possible with some of the lymph nodes in the region of the inferior pulmonary ligament and left paratracheal region. Lymph-node levels 1, 2 R, 3, 4 R, and 6 are not always able to be assessed, due to interference from the larger airways. The left adrenal gland should always be examined as well, as it determines the prognosis in up to 5% of cases.

References

1. Dietrich CF, Braden B, Wagner TOF. Thorax- und Lungensonographie. Dt Aerzteblatt 2000;97:A103–A110.
2. Dietrich CF, Hirche TO, Schreiber D, Wagner TO. Sonographie von pleura und lunge. [Article in German] Ultraschall Med 2003;24(5):303–311.
3. Dietrich CF, Chichakli M, Bargon J, et al. Mediastinal lymph nodes demonstrated by mediastinal sonography: activity marker in patients with cystic fibrosis. J Clin Ultrasound 1999;27(1):9–14.
4. Dietrich CF, Viel K, Braden B, Caspary WF, Zeuzem S. Mediastinal lymphadenopathy: an extrahepatic manifestation of chronic hepatitis C? [Article in German] Z Gastroenterol 2000;38(2):143–152.
5. Dietrich CF, Liesen M, Buhl R, et al. Detection of normal mediastinal lymph nodes by ultrasonography. Acta Radiol 1997;38(6):965–969.
6. Mountain CF, Dresler CM. Regional lymph node classification for lung cancer staging. Chest 1997;111(6):1718–1723.
7. Dietrich CF, Wehrmann T, Hoffmann C, Herrmann G, Caspary WF, Seifert H. Detection of the adrenal glands by endoscopic or transabdominal ultrasound. Endoscopy 1997; 29(9):859–864.
8. Ahuja A, Ying M. An overview of neck node sonography. Invest Radiol 2002;37(6):333–342.
9. Vassallo P, Wernecke K, Roos N, Peters PE. Differentiation of benign from malignant superficial lymphadenopathy: the role of high-resolution US. Radiology 1992;183(1): 215–220.
10. Vassallo P, Edel G, Roos N, Naguib A, Peters PE. In-vitro high-resolution ultrasonography of benign and malignant lymph nodes. A sonographic-pathologic correlation. Invest Radiol 1993;28(8):698–705.
11. Hajek PC, Salomonowitz E, Turk R, Tscholakoff D, Kumpan W , Czembirek H. Lymph nodes of the neck: evaluation with US. Radiology 1986;158(3):739–742.
12. van den Brekel MW, Castelijns JA. Imaging of lymph nodes in the neck. Semin Roentgenol 2000;35(1):42–53.
13. van den Brekel MW, Castelijns JA, Stel HV, Golding RP, Meyer CJ, Snow GB. Modern imaging techniques and ultrasound-guided aspiration cytology for the assessment of neck node metastases: a prospective comparative study. Eur Arch Otorhinolaryngol 1993;250(1):11–17.
14. Ariji Y, Kimura Y, Hayashi N, et al. Power Doppler sonography of cervical lymph nodes in patients with head and neck cancer. AJNR Am J Neuroradiol 1998;19(2):303–307.
15. Schade G. Experiences with using the ultrasound contrast medium Levovist in differentiation of cervical lymphomas with color-coded duplex ultrasound. [Article in German] Laryngorhinootologie 2001;80(4):209–213.
16. Wallace MB, Ravenel J, Block MI, et al. Endoscopic ultrasound in lung cancer patients with a normal mediastinum on computed tomography. Ann Thorac Surg 2004;77(5): 1763–1768.
17. Leblanc JK, Devereaux BM, Imperiale TF, et al. Endoscopic ultrasound in non-small cell lung cancer and negative mediastinum on computed tomography. Am J Respir Crit Care Med 2005;172:400–401.

18. Fernández-Esparrach G, Ginès A, Belda J, et al. Transesophageal ultrasound-guided fine needle aspiration improves mediastinal staging in patients with non-small cell lung cancer and normal mediastinum on computed tomography. Lung Cancer 2006;54(1):35–40.

19. Annema JT, Rabe KF. Lung cancer patients with small nodes on CT—what's the next step? Endoscopy 2006;38(Suppl 1): S77–S80.

20. Annema JT, Veseliç M, Versteegh MI, Willems LN, Rabe KF. Mediastinal restaging: EUS-FNA offers a new perspective. Lung Cancer 2003;42(3):311–318.

21. Varadarajulu S, Eloubeidi M. Can endoscopic ultrasonography-guided fine-needle aspiration predict response to chemoradiation in non-small cell lung cancer? A pilot study. Respiration 2006;73(2):213–220.

22. Larsen SS, Krasnik M, Vilmann P, et al. Endoscopic ultrasound guided biopsy of mediastinal lesions has a major impact on patient management. Thorax 2002;57(2): 98–103.

23. Annema JT, Versteegh MI, Veseliç M, Voigt P, Rabe KF. Endoscopic ultrasound-guided fine-needle aspiration in the diagnosis and staging of lung cancer and its impact on surgical staging. J Clin Oncol 2005;23(33):8357–8361.

24. Tournoy KG, Praet MM, Van Maele G, Van Meerbeeck JP. Esophageal endoscopic ultrasound with fine-needle aspiration with an on-site cytopathologist: high accuracy for the diagnosis of mediastinal lymphadenopathy. Chest 2005;128(4):3004–3009.

25. Annema JT, Versteegh MI, Veseliç M, et al. Endoscopic ultrasound added to mediastinoscopy for preoperative staging of patients with lung cancer. JAMA 2005;294(8):931–936.

26. Larsen SS, Vilmann P, Krasnik M, et al. Endoscopic ultrasound guided biopsy performed routinely in lung cancer staging spares futile thoracotomies: preliminary results from a randomised clinical trial. Lung Cancer 2005;49(3): 377–385.

27. Annema JT, Veseliç M, Rabe KF. Endoscopic ultrasound-guided fine-needle aspiration for the diagnosis of sarcoidosis. Eur Respir J 2005;25(3):405–409.

28. Fritscher-Ravens A, Sriram PV, Topalidis T, et al. Diagnosing sarcoidosis using endosonography-guided fine-needle aspiration. Chest 2000;118(4):928–935.

29. Wildi SM, Judson MA, Fraig M, et al. Is endosonography guided fine needle aspiration (EUS-FNA) for sarcoidosis as good as we think? Thorax 2004;59(9):794–799.

30. Kramer H, Koëter GH, Sleijfer DT, van Putten JW, Groen HJ. Endoscopic ultrasound-guided fine-needle aspiration in patients with mediastinal abnormalities and previous extrathoracic malignancy. Eur J Cancer 2004;40(4):559–562.

31. Wildi SM, Hoda RS, Fickling W, et al. Diagnosis of benign cysts of the mediastinum: the role and risks of EUS and FNA. Gastrointest Endosc 2003;58(3):362–368.

32. Annema JT, Veseliç M, Versteegh MI, Rabe KF. Mediastinitis caused by EUS-FNA of a bronchogenic cyst. Endoscopy 2003;35(9):791–793.

33. Silvestri GA, Hoffman BJ, Bhutani MS, et al. Endoscopic ultrasound with fine-needle aspiration in the diagnosis and staging of lung cancer. Ann Thorac Surg 1996;61(5): 1441–1445, discussion 1445–1446.

34. Gress FG, Savides TJ, Sandler A, et al. Endoscopic ultrasonography, fine-needle aspiration biopsy guided by endoscopic ultrasonography, and computed tomography in the preoperative staging of non-small-cell lung cancer: a comparison study. Ann Intern Med 1997;127(8 Pt 1):604–612.

35. Williams DB, Sahai AV, Aabakken L, et al. Endoscopic ultrasound guided fine needle aspiration biopsy: a large single centre experience. Gut 1999;44(5):720–726.

36. Fritscher-Ravens A, Sriram PV, Bobrowski C, et al. Mediastinal lymphadenopathy in patients with or without previous malignancy: EUS-FNA-based differential cytodiagnosis in 153 patients. Am J Gastroenterol 2000;95(9): 2278–2284.

37. Wallace MB, Silvestri GA, Sahai AV, et al. Endoscopic ultrasound-guided fine needle aspiration for staging patients with carcinoma of the lung. Ann Thorac Surg 2001;72(6): 1861–1867.

38. Wiersema MJ, Vilmann P, Giovannini M, Chang KJ, Wiersema LM. Endosonography-guided fine-needle aspiration biopsy: diagnostic accuracy and complication assessment. Gastroenterology 1997;112(4):1087–1095.

39. Larsen SS, Krasnik M, Vilmann P, et al. Endoscopic ultrasound guided biopsy of mediastinal lesions has a major impact on patient management. Thorax 2002;57(2): 98–103.

40. Fritscher-Ravens A, Davidson BL, Hauber HP, et al. Endoscopic ultrasound, positron emission tomography, and computerized tomography for lung cancer. Am J Respir Crit Care Med 2003;168(11):1293–1297.

41. Savides TJ, Perricone A. Impact of EUS-guided FNA of enlarged mediastinal lymph nodes on subsequent thoracic surgery rates. Gastrointest Endosc 2004;60(3):340–346.

42. Eloubeidi MA, Cerfolio RJ, Chen VK, Desmond R, Syed S, Ojha B. Endoscopic ultrasound-guided fine needle aspiration of mediastinal lymph node in patients with suspected lung cancer after positron emission tomography and computed tomography scans. Ann Thorac Surg 2005;79(1): 263–268.

28 Endobronchial Ultrasound with Miniprobe Radial Scanning

F.J.F. Herth, N. Kahn, R. Eberhardt

In the bronchi, the endoscopist's view is restricted to the lumen and internal surface of the airways. Intramural processes and those adjacent to the airways can only be assessed using indirect signs. The clinical staging of lung cancer corresponds to pTNM in only 60% of cases. For these reasons, there was a need to improve the tools available for endoscopic diagnosis. As external mediastinal ultrasonography and transesophageal endosonography were insufficient for the imaging of mediastinal structures, there was a need for a different solution involving the use of miniaturized probes of the type used for endoscopic ultrasonography (EUS)[1] and cardiovascular endosonography, preliminary experience with which had been reported in endovascular sonography of the pulmonary artery to exclude tumor invasion.[2]

Miniprobes: General Considerations

During the 1990s, miniaturized probes with a frequency of 7.5 MHz began to be used. Probes with 12 and 20 MHz also became available later. The first probes had a diameter of 3 mm, with a mechanical single-element transducer at the tip rotating at ≈ 400 rpm and producing a 360° image perpendicular to the axis. Due to the large diameter of the probe, it was mainly used during rigid bronchoscopy, with a metallic tube serving as a guide. To achieve better contact with the tracheobronchial wall, a latex balloon was attached at the tip of the probe, which was filled with sterile water via a side port. Later, models with a diameter of 2.5 mm became available that were capable of being introduced via biopsy channels at least 2.8 mm in diameter in regular flexible fiberscopes. These have been available commercially since 1999 (Olympus UM-2 R/3 R, with an MH-240 driving unit and EU-M20 and 30 processors). In addition, dedicated balloon catheters are available that can be attached to the probe at the connector for the driving unit (Olympus UM-BS20-26 R) (**Fig. 28.1**).

A special feature is the O-ring at the tip, which fits to a notch at the tip of the probe (Olympus UM-BS20-26 R). When the balloon is overinflated or pressure is exerted due to coughing, the tip slips off the probe, preventing rupture with fragments dislodging into the lung. This comparatively simple device meets three requirements for optimal imaging: firstly, 20-MHz probes, with their high resolution, can be used; secondly, as the water in the balloon in front of the transducer shifts the focus to

the periphery, the depth of penetration is sufficient for imaging the surrounding mediastinal structures; and thirdly, the balloon provides complete circular contact with the airway wall, which is essential for orientation.

Handling of Miniprobes

■ Storage and Preparation

Miniprobes are fragile and have to be handled very delicately. The transducer and connecting driving wire are protected from friction inside the plastic sheath by applying a gel solution. As this is not completely air-sealed, small air bubbles may collect in front of the transducer and interfere with the image. The devices should therefore be stored in a hanging position, with the connector upward and the tip of the probe downward. If a bubble has collected in front of the transducer, the catheter should be held ≈ 40 cm proximal from its tip and the end should be gently rotated like a lasso, so that the centrifugal force drives the gel toward the tip and the bubble travels

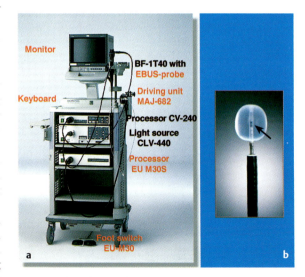

Fig. 28.1a, b a The complete miniprobe system.
b The miniprobe is introduced via the biopsy channel of a video bronchoscope. The probe is armed with a balloon catheter. The grayish mechanical rotating transducer can be seen inside the balloon (arrow).

proximally. After the probe has been inserted into the balloon catheter and fixed at the connector, the balloon catheter should be completely filled with sterile water until drips appear at the distal end. Saline solution should not be used, as the salt may crystallize on the tip of the probe and interfere with the ultrasonic signal. After filling of the catheter, the O-ring of the balloon is slipped onto the groove on the tip of the catheter. This can be achieved with the fingertip or with the help of a dedicated rubber device. Exerting too much force on the tip, which results in bending or even kinking of the tip, should be avoided. The balloon is then refilled. If a few air bubbles are still observed, the balloon is kept with its tip downward, so that the air collects at the end of the catheter. The air is evacuated by suctioning the water from the balloon with the syringe. This should always be held in such a way that the air is above the fluid and is not flushed back into the catheter.

■ Application

The miniprobes should always be used with bronchoscopes that have an appropriate biopsy channel at least 2.8 mm in diameter when applied with the balloon sheath. We prefer to use a little medical silicone on the tip before insertion. During introduction, the assistant should apply suction to completely evacuate the balloon, preventing dislocation from the tip or damage due to friction within the biopsy channel. The probe should never be advanced when the tip of the endoscope is in a sharply bent position. It should also not be activated then, as the transducer may be fixed while the wire is still rotating and could therefore shear off. Force should never be used while advancing the probe, neither when there is resistance against the tip nor by pushing the probe forcefully sideways against the wall. Inside stenoses and in the periphery as well, the probe should never be advanced using force, as the tip easily becomes kinked in this way. The balloon should never be overinflated. Particularly when the probe is being advanced inside narrowing airways or if the patient coughs, the balloon's safety feature will not work with overinflation, as the O-ring is not able to slip off; in this case, the balloon may fracture and latex fragments may be lost inside the lung.

Technique of Endoscopic Bronchial Ultrasonography

The miniprobes are inserted through the biopsy channel of flexible scopes with a diameter of at least 2.8 mm. Precise placement is performed with endoscopic visualization, and once the balloon is in place, it is filled with sterile

water until firm contact with the wall is established. Adequate contact is confirmed by a complete circular image of the bronchial wall and the surrounding structures. The development of the image can be compared to a sunrise, in which all of the structures gradually become visible. With the patient under local anesthesia, complete inflation of the balloon is possible in bilaterally ventilated lungs after sufficient preoxygenation, up to the main bronchi and even the trachea. Complete obstruction of a remaining main bronchus after contralateral resection, or resection of the trachea, can therefore be tolerated for up to 2 minutes with sufficient sedation. If necessary, the bronchoscope can be introduced via a larynx mask. In these cases, general anesthesia may be preferable, as it can provide additional time for imaging of the mediastinal structures. In our view, this procedure is well justified due to the useful additional information that can be obtained. We have never observed barotrauma during complete obstruction, since according to our measurements even with high-frequency jet ventilation, the pressure distal to the balloon during filling rapidly drops to zero after complete inflation. If the patient is not able to tolerate complete obstruction at all, the balloon can be partially filled and applied with semicircular contact.

■ Imaging Artifacts

Motion artifacts with irregular rotation were observed when early probes were used inside calibration phantoms, causing considerable distortion of the circumferential sector images—whereas the radial distances were measured correctly, as reported with other systems. However, the image construction is still slow enough for respiratory motion to create artifacts. As these are not synchronous, they can be readily differentiated from pulsations. Most frequently, a multiple ring reflection is caused by the strong echo of the balloon. As the airways are surrounded by strongly reflecting structures, multiple reflex echoes and mirror and comet artifacts are observed in endoscopic bronchial ultrasonography (EBUS), as in other applications. This applies in particular to the adjacent lung surface, vertebral column, calcified cartilage, and lymph nodes. Triangular distortion of lymph nodes and attenuation of the outer contours in echogenic structures is also very common with 20-MHz probes. Air bubbles in the balloon can cause shadows or image distortions resembling a "rabbit's ear" (**Fig. 28.2**).

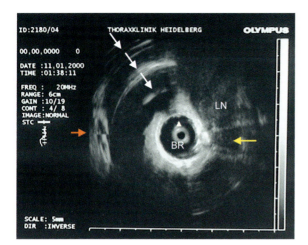

Fig. 28.2 Artifacts in bronchial imaging. *Rotation artifact:* on the left, in the 9-o'clock position, there is an interruption in the contour of the wall and the adjacent pulmonary artery (red arrow). In this position, the image is refreshed after one circulation of the transducer. If the structures have in the meantime been displaced by breathing, pulsation, or movement of the bronchoscope, the interruption can be observed. *Repeat echoes:* in the 11-o'clock position, there is insufficient contact between the balloon and the bronchial wall. The strong echo from the balloon is repeatedly reflected in quarter-circles (three arrows). *Shadows due to air:* also in the 11-o'clock position, small bubbles have collected inside the balloon (arrowhead). These are causing the triangular shadow, in which the structures are lost. However, the strong echoes from the balloon are still visible. Another shadow is seen in the 3-o'clock position (yellow arrow), where a bronchial branch is emerging and the air inside is reflecting the ultrasound and causing the shadow. *Fading:* as the lower energy from the 20 MHz is dissipating inside the tissue by dispersion and absorption, the external boundary of the lymph node (LN) is not visible.

■ Sonographic Anatomy

In animals and in resected human specimens, we have observed a seven-layered structure in the central airways in vitro. This is in contrast to the findings of other groups, who have described three layers, or more recently five,[3,4] in some cases due to the use of probes with a lower resolution. The first (innermost) layer, the mucosa, has a highly echogenic structure that is mostly confluent with the echo of the balloon and only becomes visible with high magnification. The second layer has low echogenicity and represents the submucosa. In normal conditions, it can be easily differentiated from the mucosa and from the third layer, the strongly reflecting internal surface of the cartilage, which we term "endochondrium." The spongiform internal structure of the cartilage, the fourth layer, is hypoechoic again, whereas a fifth hyperechoic layer represents the external surface of the cartilage (perichondrium). It is a little-known fact that the central airways are surrounded by a double layer of loose and dense connective tissue, representing the sixth (hypodense) and seventh (hyperdense) ultrasonic layers (**Fig. 28.3**). This seven-lay-

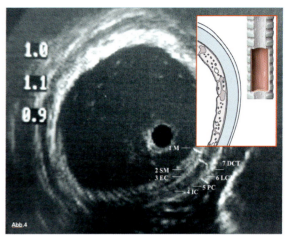

Fig. 28.3 The structure of the wall of the central airways. At high magnification, the seven-layered structure is clearly visible with the 20-MHz probe. The three layers of cartilage, consisting of endochondrium (EC), an internal spongiform structure (IC), and perichondrium (PC), are accompanied by mucosa (M) and submucosa (SM) on the inside and loose connective tissue (LCT) and dense connective tissue (DCT) on the outside. The anatomical illustration shows the high resolution provided by the ultrasound image, at less than 1 mm.

ered structure has been confirmed in another prospective experimental study.[5]

In vivo, the complex structure can be only seen with high magnification, whereas at medium and low-powered magnification, the delicate layers are confluent with the strong echo from the supporting cartilages. At the dorsal membranous wall and in the periphery distal to the lobar bronchi, the structure only consists of three layers. The layered structure is not visible with the 7.5-MHz ultrasound bronchoscope.

Orientation within the mediastinum is difficult. This is mainly due to the complex anatomy, as well as to motion artifacts and pulsation, but it is also due to the very unusual planes that are present. The plane of the circumferential image of the miniprobe is perpendicular to the axis of the probe. While the planes inside the trachea are comparable to those in horizontal computed tomography (CT) images, following the oblique course of the airways, the images tilt more and more as one follows the main bronchi until a coronary plane is reached in the distal left main bronchus, or even an inverse horizontal plane on entering the apical segments of the upper lobes.

For orientation, it is useful to recognize key anatomical structures and their relationship to the airways and to each other, rather than to observe the position of the probe. Familiarity with the anatomy is essential for orientation. The image has to be set accordingly, so that landmark structures that are found only ventral or dorsal to the bronchus, such as the esophagus or pulmonary artery, are in the correct position. It is helpful to place the tip of the bronchoscope close to the balloon, or even better to

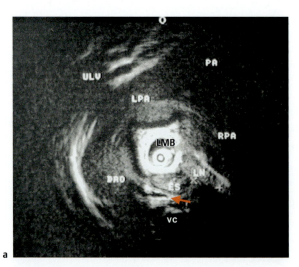

a

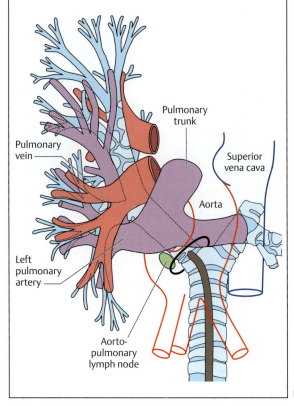

b

Fig. 28.4a, b Mediastinal anatomy

a The typical ultrasound anatomy of the proximal left main bronchus (LMB) and surrounding structures. Dorsally lies the esophagus (ES, above the red arrow); to the right of the esophagus, there is a borderline lymph node (LN); on the left lie the descending aorta (DAO) and the beginning of the aortic arch. Behind the esophagus and in front of the vertebral column (VC), an intercostal artery is crossing to the right (red arrow). Ventrally, the main pulmonary artery (PA) and its left (LPA) and right (RPA) branches are visible. On the left, the pulmonary upper lobe vein (ULV) crosses towards the left atrium. O marks the 12 o'clock position.

b The diagram illustrates the anatomy and the ultrasound plane (reproduced with permission of Wang et al.[6]).

look inside the balloon and follow the motion of the probe on the ultrasound image, while the tip of the bronchoscope is flexed up and down. Once the sagittal orientation is set and the EBUS image is adjusted with the scroll ball on the keyboard, right and left orientation can be set accordingly, with lateral motion being observed on the ultrasound image and the reverse key being used if necessary.

Vessels are easily recognized by their low echogenicity and by pulsations; arteries and veins differ in characteristic ways. However, in the periphery the variations are so complex that this may become impossible. Observation of the pulse oximeter is often helpful. Lymph nodes are easily differentiated by their comparatively higher echogenicity.

As filling of the balloon catheter with water shifts the focus more distally, even with the 20-MHz probes the depth of penetration can be up to 5 cm. Thus, the left atrium and mitral valve can frequently be seen from the left main bronchus. Near the bifurcation, the main pulmonary artery and its branching into the left and right main arteries can be seen ventrally. Dorsally, the descending aorta, the multilayered structure of the esophagus, and the vertebral column are clear landmarks for orientation. The aortopulmonary window can be inspected and approached from the left main bronchus (**Fig. 28.4**).[6]

Ventral to the right main bronchus, the right pulmonary artery is always found, crossed by the azygos vein, which can often be followed as far as its confluence with the vena

cava, which is situated beside the root of the aorta. Slightly more proximally, at the level of the tracheobronchial angle, the esophagus is seen crossing to the left, accompanied by the azygos vein, which crosses forward at the right toward the vena cava. Pathological soft-tissue structures are easily differentiated from these structures. Further distally, in the intermediate bronchus, the pulmonary artery and pulmonary vein are found ventrally. At the level of the middle lobe bronchus, the segmental artery for the apical segment of the lower lobe (S6) can be seen crossing laterally beside the intermediate bronchus, whereas the bright reflection of the adjacent pleura of S6 is a significant dorsal landmark.

In the periphery, conditions are less favorable, as the surrounding air is strongly reflective and thus frequently prevents detailed analysis of the bronchial wall and adjacent vessels. Despite this, some Japanese authors have even succeeded in analyzing the alveolar structures with EBUS.[7] However, solid and cystic structures are clearly demarcated against the hyperechoic lung structure by their lower echogenicity. EBUS is thus useful for guiding biopsy procedures in these lesions.

Clinical Results

In a prospective study including 648 patients, we demonstrated that EBUS has a very low complication rate and only adds an average of 6.3 minutes per bronchoscopy, with 18.9 minutes for the whole procedure.[8] Complications were rare and minor; 5% of the patients required additional oxygen. Transient minor arrhythmias were observed in 18 of 103 patients (17%) who underwent blockage of the left main bronchus by the balloon. Rarely, minor bleeding occurred during placement of the probe inside the periphery of the lung. In addition, the study confirmed the cost-effectiveness of the procedure, with re-sterilization and reuse of the probes being possible as long as they resisted the mechanical stress.[9] EBUS is now reimbursed in the USA. However, the system is also cost-effective in Europe, in view of the more invasive and expensive procedures that the procedure makes it possible to avoid. We have conducted prospective studies to validate EBUS for various indications.[10–13] The results have been confirmed by other authors and demonstrate that EBUS is comparable with other procedures and in many instances even superior.

Staging of Lung Cancer

The purpose of staging is to provide precise classification in accordance with the TNM system as a rational basis for treatment. The bronchoscopic criteria for tumor spread are documented in the recent UICC classification.[14] Small, radiographically invisible tumors have to be located in individuals who are at risk or have positive sputum cytology. The decision on whether to carry out treatment is taken on the basis of tumor spread and the depth of infiltration into the layers of the bronchial wall. The decision also depends on the histological assessment of biopsy specimens. Lymph-node involvement in hilar and mediastinal nodes can be assessed using transbronchial needle aspiration (TBNA). In addition to the size and extent of the lesion, its internal structure and relationship to mediastinal structures are of interest. Metastasis can also involve the parabronchial mediastinal structures, central airways, lung, and pleura. EBUS provides useful information, particularly in regions that are not directly visible through the bronchoscope.

Primary lung cancer: endobronchial extent. *Early cancer* was until recently considered to be radiographically invisible. This has changed since the introduction of endobronchial ultrasonography. It is known from earlier radiographic studies that only 75% of bronchographically visible tumors are radiographically detectable.[15] Radiographically invisible tumors included lesions that had already penetrated into the deeper layers of the wall. In several patients referred to our institution for endobronchial treatment of supposedly early cancer, transmural invasion and even local lymph-node involvement were detected that had escaped all previous diagnostic procedures.

By pathological definition, early cancer is limited to the bronchial wall, whereas in-situ carcinoma does not cross the lamina propria. In all cases of macroscopic alteration of the mucosa, alterations in the texture were identified on endosonography. Depending on the extent of infiltration, the wall is thickened and the architecture is altered. As has been reported for other tumors, hyperechoic structures were found, although hypoechoic structures were more frequent. Extensive submucosal tumor spread and even infiltration beyond the cartilage is sometimes detected with EBUS even in macroscopically intact mucosa. When there are no signs of infiltration of the deeper layers or lymph-node involvement, tumors of this type that are limited to the bronchial wall can be treated with curative intent using endoscopic methods.[16]

With the development of autofluorescence bronchoscopy for detection of tumors that are invisible with white-light bronchoscopy, there has been renewed interest in early detection. Extinction of autofluorescence can be also caused by benign lesions such as inflammation, granuloma, scars, and dysplasia. We have shown that analyzing the structure of the wall with EBUS improves the specificity significantly and can clarify the nature of a lesion with a high degree of reliability.[17] In our experience, correlation with the histology was improved from 58% to 92% (**Fig. 28.5**).

Despite the curative potential of endoscopic treatment modalities using electrocautery or photodynamic therapy (PDT), the relapse rate reported in the literature is as high as 50%.[15,18] This has been attributed to failure of treatment. Since the introduction of EBUS, we have shown that cancers detected using autofluorescence have often penetrated the deeper layers of the wall and are not really early lesions. This has been confirmed by Miyazu et al.,[19] who showed that all tumors that were found to be limited to the internal layers of the bronchial wall using both autofluorescence and EBUS were associated with long-term complete remission after PDT. This proves that EBUS is currently the only reliable method for precise staging of localized early cancer. In the future, therefore, screening using molecular cytodiagnosis in the sputum, blood, or swabs from the buccal mucosa, along with localization using autofluorescence and local staging with EBUS, will be the three pillars of early detection and local minimally invasive treatment for central early lung cancer.[20]

Local T staging of advanced lung cancer. Computed tomography is still the gold standard for the diagnosis of local tumor spread. However, clinical staging is confirmed by surgery in only 60–70% of cases.[21] In locally advanced cancer, EBUS also provides important information to support treatment decisions. In patients with complete

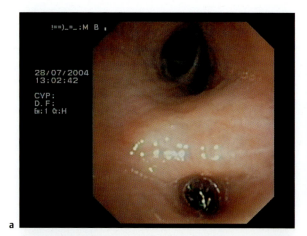

a

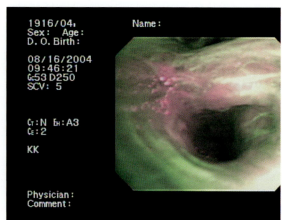

b

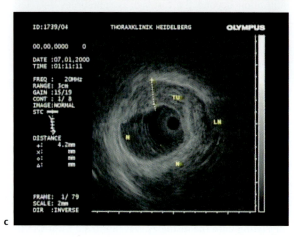

c

Fig. 28.5a–c Early cancer

a The carina of the left apical lower lobe segment is widened in comparison with the distal segments, and the light reflex is irregular (white-light imaging).

b With blue-light autofluorescence (AFI System, Olympus, Tokyo, Japan), the true submucosal extent of the lesion is visible from the magenta discoloration in comparison with the normal greenish color.

c It is only with endobronchial ultrasound that the true intramural extent of the tumor (TU) becomes visible—4.2 mm in comparison with the normal wall (N) of 1.5 mm—as well as a 1-cm lymph node (LN). Histological assessment of a deep biopsy identified a squamous cell cancer that was beginning to penetrate but was still limited to the bronchial wall. In accordance with the ultrasound findings, the tumor was treated with curative intent by bronchoscopic brachytherapy, as the patient was not able to undergo surgery following right-sided pneumonectomy.

obstruction of the airway, we have been able to localize the base and surface of the occluding tumor, diagnose the extent to which the tumor has penetrated into the wall and into the mediastinum, and assess whether the distal airways were patent. Particularly for the surgical strategy, it is essential to know the precise intended resection lines. Involvement of the main bronchi, main carina, or trachea requires more extensive resection and frequently precludes operability. A combination of autofluorescence and EBUS also proved useful here for detecting submucosal tumor spread. In particular, the potential to diagnose involvement of the pulmonary vessels influences decisions regarding intervention.[22] Perfusion of the lung can be shut down by the Euler–Liljestrand reflex even when the pulmonary artery is patent. Usually, one then has to exclude organic obstruction using conventional or CT angiography, as endoscopic obliteration in this case would merely increase dead-space ventilation. Passing through the stenosis with the miniprobe enabled us to diagnose infiltration of the pulmonary artery (**Fig. 28.6**) and also made it possible to see whether the bronchi distal to the stenosis were patent. In some patients, application of the ultrasound bronchoscope can provide additional quantitative information on blood flow, using the Doppler function.

Mediastinal infiltration: trachea, pulmonary artery, esophagus, large vessels. Diagnosis of infiltration of the large mediastinal vessels—the aorta, vena cava, and main pulmonary artery—is crucial and can be difficult using radiographic methods. Tumors located in the trachea, left main bronchus, and left hilum are located in the close vicinity of the esophagus, and we have been able to detect direct infiltration using EBUS in several cases (**Fig. 28.7**).

In addition, tumor invasion of the aortic arch, descending aorta, and main pulmonary artery can be diagnosed from the main bronchi and the trachea. Infiltration of these structures usually precludes surgical procedures. However, if there is a distinct sonographic interface between the tumor and these structures, operability is possible, as has been confirmed in many of our patients. Particularly with miniprobes, infiltration of the external layers of the trachea and main bronchi can be reliably diagnosed and distinguished from impression without infiltration. In a prospective study, CT was only found to have a sensitivity of 25% and a specificity of 80% (accuracy 51%) in comparison with EBUS, which had an accuracy of 94%, a sensitivity of 89%, and a specificity of 100%.[10] The 7.5-MHz resolution provided by the ultrasound bronchoscope is insufficient for this purpose.

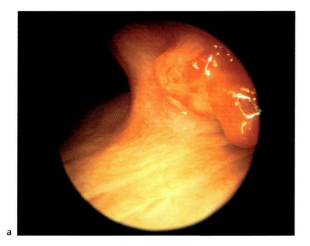

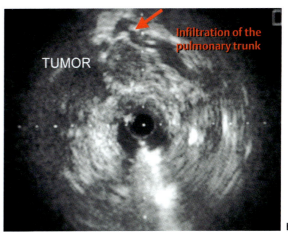

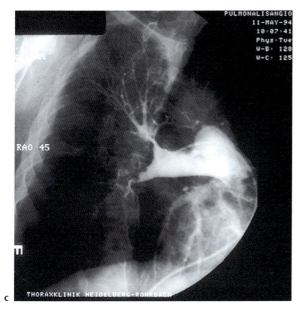

Fig. 28.6a–c Infiltration of the pulmonary artery.
a On bronchoscopy, the left upper lobe bronchus is seen to be obstructed by a tumor.
b On ultrasonography, the upper lobe artery is seen to be invaded by the tumor and almost completely obstructed.
c This finding was confirmed on angiography. We now rely on endobronchial ultrasound and no longer carry out conventional or computed-tomographic angiography for confirmation.

EBUS-guided biopsies of lymph nodes. The relationship between extraluminal lymph nodes and tumors and the airways is easily visualized using EBUS. Once a target lesion has been identified, the probe is removed and TBNA can be performed. Although radial EBUS facilitates guided biopsies, it is limited by the absence of real-time sampling. The reported diagnostic yield with radial EBUS-guided TBNA is 72–86%,[23–26] and this guided procedure has been shown to improve diagnostic rates over "blind" conventional TBNA in mediastinal lymph node stations 2 and 4.

EBUS-guided biopsies of peripheral lung lesions. Radial EBUS can be used to guide biopsies of peripheral lung lesions, and it increases the diagnostic yield of transbronchial lung biopsies of smaller lesions (< 20–30 mm). Diagnostic sensitivities of 61–80%, independent of the size of the lesions, have been reported using peripheral radial EBUS probes.[11,27–34] However, the reported data show wide variability in the level of expertise and experience of the operators participating. It is also not possible to combine data, due to variations in the use of guide sheaths, fluoroscopy, and biopsy methods such as forceps biopsy, brushing, and needle aspiration.

Despite this, EBUS appears to be capable of overcoming variables that affect the diagnostic yield, such as the presence of the CT bronchus sign, underlying disease, and a lobar location.[28] EBUS-guided transbronchial lung biopsy without fluoroscopic guidance has also been shown to be safe and effective.[11,19,30,33,35]

EBUS-guided biopsy of peripheral lung lesions is relatively uncomplicated. The transducer probe is inserted through a guide sheath into the bronchus in which the lesion is suspected on the basis of preprocedural radiological imaging. Normal air-filled alveoli produce a whitish snowstorm image, with "comet-tail" artifacts. Peripheral

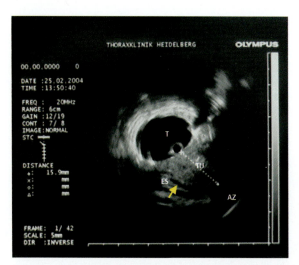

Fig. 28.7 Infiltration of the esophagus. The dorsal wall of the trachea (T) has been infiltrated by an extensive tumor (TU), and the layer structure has been disrupted. The tumor is penetrating the esophagus (ES) and has disrupted its structure as well. Whether or not the azygos vein (AZ) is also involved is not clear from the 20-MHz ultrasound image, as the depth of penetration is not sufficient.

lung lesions are usually hypoechoic. Ultrasound features indicating malignancy are the presence of a continuous margin around the lesion, heterogeneous echogenicity, and an absence of linear air bronchograms.[36] A combination of these features further increases the positive predictive value for malignancy.[37]

When sonographic images of peripheral lesions are seen all around the probe on the screen, the probe can be considered to be situated inside the target. The transducer is then removed, and regular biopsy forceps are used to take biopsies through the guide sheath. Biopsies of lesions in which the probe is positioned inside the lesion have been shown to have higher diagnostic rates than when the probe is adjacent to the lesion, and the optimum number of biopsies is reported to be approximately five specimens.[28] Endobronchial washing and brushing specimens can be obtained in a similar manner.

Needle aspiration in addition to forceps biopsy may increase the diagnostic yield further, particularly if the transducer probe cannot be redirected in such a way that it is located inside rather than adjacent to the peripheral lung lesion. Successful biopsy of small and fluoroscopically invisible nodules is also possible, with diagnostic rates of 70%.[30] It may be more difficult and time-consuming to locate these small peripheral lung lesions, but if they can be found on EBUS, then the diagnostic yield appears to be unaffected by the size of the lesion. Double-hinged curettes and electromagnetic navigation bronchoscopy can be used to navigate the EBUS probes into such peripheral lung lesions, further improving the diagnostic yield.[31,32,35]

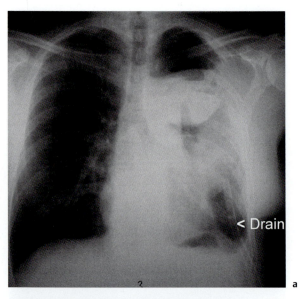

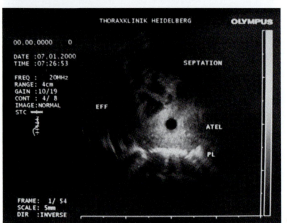

Fig. 28.8a, b A septated pleural effusion after surgery.
a Pulmonary radiograph after resection of the upper lobe due to squamous cell cancer. Despite suction with drainage, the lung is still partially collapsed, and the apical segment of the lower lobe is infiltrated.
b Endobronchial ultrasound shows an extensive septated effusion (EFF), which has not been drained, and the lung is atelectatic (ATEL). The visceral pleura (PL) shows strong echoes. This situation usually has to be treated using video-assisted thoracoscopy.

Pleura and neighboring organs. If there is an acoustic window due to atelectasis, or a fluid collection close to the bronchi, the pleura and neighboring structures—such as solid structures in the visceral, mediastinal, and parietal pleura, or on the pericardium—can be visualized (**Fig. 28.8**).

EBUS is particularly useful for diagnosing infiltration of the esophagus by tumors of the central airways. In these cases, surgery is no longer feasible in most instances, and bronchoscopic interventions also have to be carried out very cautiously, since there is a very high risk of esophagobronchial fistulas after extensive laser resection and additional radiotherapy, for example. In these cases, simultaneous exploration of the esophagus with the miniprobe is very useful.

EBUS in Therapeutic Bronchoscopy

The value of EBUS in decision-making and in guiding treatment applications was mentioned above. In our institution, 20% of all bronchoscopies conducted include therapeutic procedures. In 48% of these interventions, ultrasound provides useful additional information, which has strategic importance for the planning of the procedure in 43% of cases.[13] Exploration of central airway stenoses with EBUS to assess the extent and cause of the lesion and its relation to surrounding structures is helpful in decision-making regarding the appropriate technique—for example, mechanical dilation, laser resection, argon plasma coagulation, or stenting—and for checking the effectiveness of the treatment during the follow-up period. Before the resection of granulomas and scars, precise evaluation of their thickness and vascularization is important in order to avoid perforation or hemorrhage.

Particularly in potentially curative bronchoscopic treatment of localized malignancies using photodynamic therapy or brachytherapy, precise diagnosis of the extension of the lesions into the bronchial wall is essential for success. EBUS is superior to all other imaging modalities in this context for analyzing the delicate layers of the tracheobronchial wall. Complications in the healing of anastomoses after bronchoplastic procedures can be difficult to recognize using bronchoscopy alone, and it can be difficult to differentiate between edema with superficial necrosis of the mucosa and incipient dehiscence. EBUS is useful here for checking the integrity of the bronchial layers and particularly for assessing the adjacent pulmonary artery. Thus, in cases of local abscess formation with peribronchial fluid collections, the decision on whether or not to carry out a surgical intervention can be taken before hemoptysis signals fatal hemorrhage.

EBUS in Pediatric Bronchoscopy

EBUS has also proved to be useful in many instances in pediatric bronchoscopy, as conventional imaging in small patients can be even less reliable due to motion artifacts and restrictions on radiation exposure.[38] In 412 children (3% of all patients), with a median age of 4.2 years, whom we examined between January 1998 and December 2001, EBUS was used in 140 cases (34%)—almost equivalent to the frequency in adults. The indications included analysis of structures in stridor and intermittent dyspnea, which

especially in these patients can be caused by vascular malformations such as pulmonary slings. The authors detected 11 of these, in some cases even after cardiovascular exploration had been negative. Solid lesions, perforating lymph nodes, atelectasis, and pneumonia were among the other indications. Children tolerated EBUS as well as adults did, and the time required for the examination was not longer.

Training and Learning Curve in EBUS

By comparison, EBUS is more difficult to learn and apply than many other bronchoscopic techniques. This is due in the first place to a general lack of training in ultrasound among most bronchoscopists, who have only very recently started to learn the handling of the devices and the interpretation of ultrasound images. Secondly, the application is more demanding, as the airways cannot be occluded for a longer period, and especially in patients receiving local anesthesia, the time available for the examination is short and the procedure has to be repeatedly interrupted. Finally, the anatomy of the airways and mediastinum is very complex, and orientation is difficult. This is the why the use of EBUS is only becoming more widespread very slowly. Training in the theory of the procedure through reading, lectures, digital media, and attendance at a 1-week course in a training center may be useful for obtaining anatomical orientation and taking the initial steps in interpreting the images. Posters illustrating the anatomy and the corresponding ultrasound images, including the location of lymph nodes, are available for this purpose, and digital media (CDs and DVDs) are available for interactive learning. This needs to be intensified through personal practical experience in patients, for which ≈ 50 procedures are necessary. According to Falcone et al.,[39] 20 procedures are necessary for image interpretation, and sufficient expertise was gained after 6–24 months, depending on the frequency of examinations—illustrating the difficulty of this method in comparison with other techniques. The development of interactive virtual training models could be very effective in shortening the learning curve, since at present neither training in phantom models nor in animal models is capable of replacing experience in real patients.

Cost-Effectiveness

As with all new procedures, cost-effectiveness is an important issue in EBUS as well. In the United States, EBUS is reimbursed as a separate procedure. For Europe, we carried out a cost assessment using the example of lymph-node staging. The costs involved in the acquisition and

Table 28.1 Various applications of endobronchial ultrasound probes

	Miniprobe	Puncture scope
Range	+++ (Central/lung)	++ (Central)
Maneuverability	+++	++
Orientation	+++	+
Layers	+++	Negative
Lymph nodes	++ (80–90%)	+++ (95–100%)
Mediastinum	+	+++
Vessels	++ (small)	+++ (Doppler)
Lung	+++ (75%)	Negative
Stenosis	+++	Negative
Intervention	Peripheral navigation	Central control

depreciation of the equipment, costs for the physician and staff, and the costs of the disposable materials amount to approximately € 138 (US$ 187) per procedure (excluding costs for bronchoscopy, which are the same for all calculation models). If 100 patients with enlarged lymph nodes undergo mediastinoscopy for preoperative staging, the total costs amount to € 162 000 (US$ 2 190 000), calculated on the basis of € 1620 (US$ 2190) per procedure. If staging is performed, including conventional CT-guided TBNA, the costs can be calculated as follows: the costs for disposables, needles, staff, and pathologist amount to € 57 (US$ 77). Calculating an accuracy rate of 60% (an optimistic figure), 40 patients will need additional mediastinoscopy. Thus, the total costs will amount to € 70 500 (US$ 95 292) (100 × € 57 for TBNA and 40 × € 1620 for mediastinoscopy). Improving the results of TBNA to 80% using EBUS, 100 × € 57 for TBNA have to be added to 100 × € 138 for EBUS. Since with this strategy only 20 patients would need additional mediastinoscopy (20 × € 1620), the total is € 51 900 (US$ 70 152).[40] This demonstrates that EBUS-guided TBNA is the most cost-effective strategy for lymph-node staging. Since reimbursement in Germany, for example, is currently in accordance with a system aimed at further rationalization of resources, it can be expected that EBUS-guided TBNA will continue to be applied more extensively.

Conclusions and Future Prospects

EBUS with miniprobes is currently being performed in some 100 institutions throughout the world, and the results have been largely consistent. EBUS is beginning to replace other methods for several indications, as it has proved to be superior. These include the staging of early lung cancer and TBNA. Currently, the new ultrasonic endoscope is attracting wide attention, and this will increase the use of EBUS, as the technology is more similar to what

bronchoscopists are used to handling. However, it should be borne in mind that the two methods are complementary rather than competing (**Table 28.1**).

EBUS using the miniprobe is superior for analyzing the delicate structures of the bronchial wall to detect early cancer and invasion by mediastinal lesions. This can make it possible to avoid inappropriate bronchoscopic treatment and futile surgery. Stenoses can be passed to allow precise staging. Peripheral lesions can be located and biopsied to allow histological assessment without the need for fluoroscopy. Unnecessary surgical resections of benign lesions might be avoided in this way in many cases.

Further developments might include higher resolution, with 30-MHz ultrasonography to analyze vascularization (e.g., after bronchoplastic procedures or in patients with inflammation and neoplastic neovascularization). With regard to the use tissue analysis and computerized image analysis, color-coded tissue characterization using algorithms quantified with a learning vector might become useful and could increase the sensitivity and specificity in detecting early central and peripheral cancer and lymph-node metastasis.

It can be expected that increasing numbers of small pulmonary lesions will be detected with CT screening for peripheral lesions. A large number of these will be benign and will not require intervention. In this context, EBUS could play an important role in guiding diagnostic procedures and helping in decision-making through image analysis.

It is also possible that endobronchial ultrasonography could be applied using higher focused energies for thermal ablation and noncontact destruction of lesions. This could include early central lesions, as well as peripheral nodular lesions in the lung. As the EBUS image changes depending on the water content, computerized analysis of impedance changes in EBUS images could then serve to check the effectiveness of treatment.

In conclusion, EBUS has now become potentially just as important as endoscopic ultrasonography in the esophagus, although it is not yet as widely used. Currently, however, it is complementing the existing armamentarium of diagnostic and therapeutic tools in bronchoscopy, and in many respects it is already replacing less effective technologies. Diagnostic and therapeutic decisions can be assisted with EBUS directly during bronchoscopy, without the need for further time-consuming and costly procedures.

References

1. Koga T, Ogata K, Hayashida R, Hattori R. Usefulness of transluminal ultrasonography in the evaluation of bronchial stenosis secondary to tuberculosis. J Jpn Soc Bronch 1994; 16:477–482.
2. Frank N, Holzapfel P, Wenk A. Neue Endoschall Minisonde in der täglichen Praxis. Endosk Heute 1994;3:238–244.

3. Hürter T, Hanrath P. Endobronchial sonography in the diagnosis of pulmonary and mediastinal tumors. [Article in German] Dtsch Med Wochenschr 1990;115(50): 1899–1905.

4. Hürter T, Hanrath P. Endobronchial sonography: feasibility and preliminary results. Thorax 1992;47(7):565–567.

5. Netter FH. Atlas of human anatomy, 2nd ed. Summit, NJ: Novartis Pharmaceuticals; 1998.

6. Wang KP, Mehta AC, Turner JF, eds. Flexible Bronchoscopy. 2nd ed. Malden, MA: Blackwell; 2004.

7. Omori S, Takiguchi Y, Hiroshima K, et al. Peripheral pulmonary diseases: evaluation with endobronchial US initial experience. Radiology 2002;224(2):603–608.

8. Herth F, Becker HD, Manegold C, Drings P. Endobronchial ultrasound (EBUS)—assessment of a new diagnostic tool in bronchoscopy for staging of lung cancer. Onkologie 2001; 24(2):151–154.

9. Becker HD. Options and results in endobronchial treatment of lung cancer. Minim Invasive Ther Allied Technol 1996; 5:165–178.

10. Herth F, Ernst A, Schulz M, Becker H. Endobronchial ultrasound reliably differentiates between airway infiltration and compression by tumor. Chest 2003;123(2):458–462.

11. Herth FJ, Becker HD, Ernst A. Ultrasound-guided transbronchial needle aspiration: an experience in 242 patients. Chest 2003;123(2):604–607.

12. Herth FJ, Ernst A, Becker HD. Endobronchial ultrasound-guided transbronchial lung biopsy in solitary pulmonary nodules and peripheral lesions. Eur Respir J 2002;20(4): 972–974.

13. Herth F, Becker HD, LoCicero J III, Ernst A. Endobronchial ultrasound in therapeutic bronchoscopy. Eur Respir J 2002; 20(1):118–121.

14. Mountain CF. Revisions in the international system for staging lung cancer. Chest 1997;111(6):1710–1717.

15. Naidlich DP. Staging of lung cancer. Controversy: computed tomography versus bronchoscopic needle aspiration: pro computed tomography. J Bronchol 1996;3:73.

16. Becker HD. Endobronchial ultrasound—a new perspective in bronchology. [Article in German] Ultraschall Med 1996;17(3):106–112.

17. Herth F, Becker HD, LoCicero J, Ernst A. Endobronchial ultrasound improves classification of suspicious lesions detected by autofluorescence bronchoscopy. J Bronchol 2003;10:249–252.

18. Ono R, Suemasu K, Matsunaka T. Bronchoscopic ultrasonography in the diagnosis of lung cancer. Jpn J Clin Oncol 1993;23(1):34–40.

19. Miyazu Y, Miyazawa T, Kurimoto N, Iwamoto Y, Kanoh K, Kohno N. Endobronchial ultrasonography in the assessment of centrally located early-stage lung cancer before photodynamic therapy. Am J Respir Crit Care Med 2002; 165(6):832–837.

20. Lam S, Becker HD. Future diagnostic procedures. Chest Surg Clin N Am 1996;6(2):363–380.

21. Basset O, Sun Z, Mestas JL, Gimenez G. Texture analysis of ultrasonic images of the prostate by means of co-occurrence matrices. Ultrason Imaging 1993;15(3):218–237.

22. Herth F, Becker HD. Endobronchial ultrasound of the airways and the mediastinum. Monaldi Arch Chest Dis 2000;55(1):36–44.

23. Shannon JJ, Bude RO, Orens JB, et al. Endobronchial ultrasound-guided needle aspiration of mediastinal adenopathy. Am J Respir Crit Care Med 1996;153(4 Pt 1): 1424–1430.

24. Plat G, Pierard P, Haller A, et al. Endobronchial ultrasound and positron emission tomography positive mediastinal lymph nodes. Eur Respir J 2006;27(2):276–281.

25. Herth F, Becker HD, Ernst A. Conventional vs endobronchial ultrasound-guided transbronchial needle aspiration: a randomized trial. Chest 2004;125(1):322–325.

26. Herth FJ, Becker HD, Ernst A. Ultrasound-guided transbronchial needle aspiration: an experience in 242 patients. Chest 2003;123(2):604–607.

27. Paone G, Nicastri E, Lucantoni G, et al. Endobronchial ultrasound-driven biopsy in the diagnosis of peripheral lung lesions. Chest 2005;128(5):3551–3557.

28. Yamada N, Yamazaki K, Kurimoto N, et al. Factors related to diagnostic yield of transbronchial biopsy using endobronchial ultrasonography with a guide sheath in small peripheral pulmonary lesions. Chest 2007;132(2):603–608.

29. Yoshikawa M, Sukoh N, Yamazaki K, et al. Diagnostic value of endobronchial ultrasonography with a guide sheath for peripheral pulmonary lesions without X-ray fluoroscopy. Chest 2007;131(6):1788–1793.

30. Herth FJ, Eberhardt R, Becker HD, Ernst A. Endobronchial ultrasound-guided transbronchial lung biopsy in fluoroscopically invisible solitary pulmonary nodules: a prospective trial. Chest 2006;129(1):147–150.

31. Kikuchi E, Yamazaki K, Sukoh N, et al. Endobronchial ultrasonography with guide-sheath for peripheral pulmonary lesions. Eur Respir J 2004;24(4):533–537.

32. Asahina H, Yamazaki K, Onodera Y, et al. Transbronchial biopsy using endobronchial ultrasonography with a guide sheath and virtual bronchoscopic navigation. Chest 2005; 128(3):1761–1765.

33. Koh MS, Tee A, Wong P, Antippa P, Irving LB. Advances in lung cancer diagnosis and staging: endobronchial ultrasound. Intern Med J 2008;38(2):85–89.

34. Shirakawa T, Imamura F, Hamamoto J, et al. Usefulness of endobronchial ultrasonography for transbronchial lung biopsies of peripheral lung lesions. Respiration 2004;71(3): 260–268.

35. Eberhardt R, Anantham D, Ernst A, Feller-Kopman D, Herth F. Multimodality bronchoscopic diagnosis of peripheral lung lesions: a randomized controlled trial. Am J Respir Crit Care Med 2007;176(1):36–41.

36. Lie CH, Chao TY, Chung YH, Wang JL, Wang YH, Lin MC. New image characteristics in endobronchial ultrasonography for differentiating peripheral pulmonary lesions. Ultrasound Med Biol; 2009;35(3):376–381.

37. Kuo CH, Lin SM, Chen HC, Chou CL, Yu CT, Kuo HP. Diagnosis of peripheral lung cancer with three echoic features via endobronchial ultrasound. Chest 2007;132(3):922–929.

38. Herth FJ, Eberhardt R. Actual role of endobronchial ultrasound (EBUS). Eur Radiol 2007;17(7):1806–1812.

39. Falcone F, Fois F, Grosso D. Endobronchial ultrasound. Respiration 2003;70(2):179–194.

40. Kunst PWA, Eberhardt R, Herth FJF. Combined EBUS real time TBNA and conventional TBNA are the most cost-effective means of Lymph node staging. J Bronchol 2008;15: 17–20.

29 Endobronchial Ultrasound

F.J.F. Herth, R. Eberhardt

Pathological evaluation of mediastinal lymph nodes in lung cancer is essential for accurate staging and planning of effective treatment.[1] Locoregional spread involves mediastinal lymph-node involvement, and this is a major determinant of surgical resectability. Despite the advances in surgical treatment and multimodality treatment, lung cancer is still the leading cause of death from malignant diseases worldwide. Accurate staging of the disease is important not only in order to determine the prognosis, but also to decide on the most suitable treatment plan for both operable and inoperable patients with non-small cell lung cancer (NSCLC). During the staging process, accurate mediastinal lymph-node staging is one of the important factors that affect the management of patients. Conventional imaging methods available for evaluating the mediastinum, such as computed tomography (CT), are inaccurate in the diagnosis of mediastinal lymph-node metastasis.[2] Positron-emission tomography (PET) has been reported to increase the diagnostic yield.[3]

The increasing use of minimally invasive techniques and day-case procedures has renewed interest in the use of transbronchial needle aspiration (TBNA) for mediastinal lymph-node staging. Conventional TBNA relies on "blind" needle puncture, guided by static CT scans. The technique is highly operator-dependent, and reported sensitivities vary widely, between 15% and 78%.[4] Higher yields are noted from the subcarinal station and when lymphadenopathy is present. However, due to the discouraging results that many operators obtain during their initial experience with the technique, recent surveys have shown that only 25% of pulmonologists use TBNA.[5,6]

Endobronchial ultrasound (EBUS) using a radial probe is an imaging technique capable of detecting even small mediastinal lymph nodes.[7] However, imaging alone is inaccurate. Tissue confirmation of suspected malignant lymphadenopathy is therefore required, especially before surgical resection. Various invasive and noninvasive methods have been used to obtain tissue confirmation. In particular, endoscopic ultrasound–guided fine-needle aspiration (EUS-FNA) is a well-known modality with a high yield for tissue sampling of the mediastinum.

Lymph-Node Staging

In favorable conditions, lymph nodes can be detected with EBUS down to a size of 2–3 mm, and the internal structure (sinuses and folliculi) as well as small lymph vessels can be analyzed. The results of transbronchial needle aspiration (TBNA) can be significantly improved using endosonographic localization of lymph nodes, with a sensitivity of up to 85%.[8] This is especially true for positions in which reliable landmarks on the CT are missing—for example, in high and low paratracheal locations. Herth et al.[9] investigated the results of EBUS-guided TBNA in comparison with conventional TBNA. In this randomized study, the authors confirmed that the yield of EBUS-guided TBNA is higher than that of conventional TBNA (85% versus 66%). In an additional analysis of the lymph-node stations, they showed that particularly in locations that lack endoscopic landmarks (lymph-node stations 2, 3, and 4 in the Mountain and Dresler scheme[10]), the detection technique is helpful for increasing the yield. On the other hand, it was also demonstrated that when there are enlarged subcarinal nodes, conventional TBNA has the same yield as TBNA after EBUS detection.[7]

Since the development of the EBUS-TBNA scope, the use of miniprobes for TBNA guidance has dramatically declined.

Description of the EBUS-TBNA Endoscope and Needle

The flexible ultrasonic bronchoscope (Olympus XBF-UC40P; Olympus, Tokyo, Japan) (**Fig. 29.1**) has an outer diameter of the insertion tube of 6.7 mm, with a working length of 550 mm (total length 870 mm). The instrument has a small, curved linear-array electronic transducer 10 mm long located at the distal end of the endoscope in front of a 30° oblique forward viewing fiberoptic lens (with an angle of view of 80°) (**Fig. 29.2**). The diameter of the distal end of the endoscope with the transducer is 6.9 mm. The angulation range of the distal end of the endoscope is 160° upward and 90° downward. The endoscope has a biopsy channel of 2 mm. The ultrasonic frequency is 7.5 MHz, with a penetration depth of 4–5 cm. The depth of imaging can be adjusted from 2 to 9 cm at 1-cm intervals. The scanning direction is parallel to the longitudinal

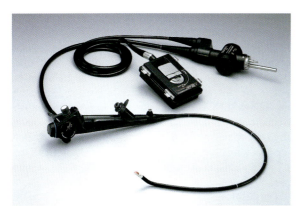

Fig. 29.1 The linear-array ultrasound bronchoscope (Olympus BF-UC40F-OL5; Olympus Ltd., Tokyo, Japan).

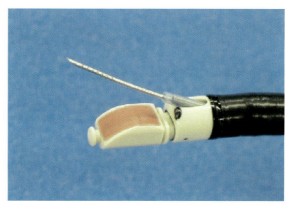

Fig. 29.2 The needle is extended through the working channel and exits obliquely.

axis of the endoscope, with a scanning angle of 50°. This allows full ultrasonic monitoring of a needle when inserted via the biopsy channel during scanning. The endoscope can either be connected to an Olympus ultrasound processor (Olympus EU-121 C2000) or to an Aloka ultrasound scanner. A balloon, which can be filled with water, can be mounted around the transducer for better ultrasonic coupling with the bronchial wall. The ultrasound images can be frozen, and the size of lesions can be measured in two dimensions by placing cursors. The system also has a Doppler mode.

A dedicated 22-gauge needle (Olympus NA-201SX-4022) was developed for carrying out transbronchial aspiration (**Fig. 29.3**). The inner diameter of the needle is nearly equal to that of a conventional 21-gauge needle, which allows sampling of histological cores in some cases. The needle is also equipped with an internal sheath, which is withdrawn after the bronchial wall has been passed, avoiding contamination during EBUS-TBNA. The needle can be visualized through the lenses and on the ultrasound image.

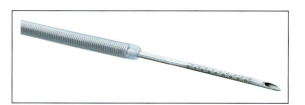

Fig. 29.3 The 22-gauge needle

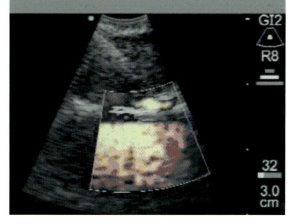

Fig. 29.4 Checking the vessels during a puncture procedure. The needle is visible within the lymph node.

Procedure

The ultrasonic bronchoscope is introduced to the area of interest via an endotracheal tube under visual guidance and with the patient under local anesthesia, usually as an outpatient procedure. The bronchoscope is inserted orally, with additional sedation usually with 2 mg midazolam. Patients have to be monitored for electrocardiography, pulse oximetry, and blood pressure if an anesthesiologist is not present. Images can be obtained by directly contacting the probe or by attaching a balloon to the tip and inflating it with saline. Since the balloon is designed not to overinflate, it will not occlude the central airway. No experiences of technical difficulties using the balloon have been reported.

When a lesion is outlined, the needle is introduced via the endoscope's biopsy channel. Power Doppler imaging is used immediately before the biopsy to avoid unintended puncture of vessels between the wall of the bronchi and the lesion (**Fig. 29.4**). With real-time ultrasonic guidance, the needle is inserted into the lesion. Suction is applied with a syringe, and the needle is moved back and forth inside the lesion, as in the EUS-FNA procedure (**Figs. 29.5** and **29.6**).

Results

Real-time EBUS-TBNA has been shown to have a higher diagnostic yield in mediastinal staging than blind TBNA and may be comparable in sensitivity to cervical mediastinoscopy.[11,12] The pooled diagnostic sensitivity is 90% and the specificity is 100%, but the false-negative rate remains high at ≈ 20%.[13] Combined analysis of the available data is not possible due to differing prevalences of malignancy, variations in the size of the lymph nodes targeted, the use of preprocedural imaging methods such as positron-emission tomography, the number of needle passes used, the varying levels of expertise of the endoscopists participating, and the availability of on-site cytology.

Even without the availability of rapid on-site cytology, diagnostic yields of 88–100% have been reported with real-time EBUS-TBNA.[14–17] Despite the encouraging results of the diagnostic yield, the high false-negative rates make it mandatory for all negative results to be followed up either clinically or with further testing using alternative modalities such as mediastinoscopy, in order to confirm that the results are true negatives. If on-site cytology is used, the majority of true-negative aspirates have moderate to abundant lymphocyte yields, suggesting that lymphocyte numbers are a marker for the adequacy of samples.[18]

The histological staging of a normal mediastinum on the basis of CT scans—for example, when there is lymphadenopathy < 10 mm—is also feasible.[19,20] In addition, the dedicated 22-G EBUS-TBNA needle is capable of taking samples that are sufficient for genetic and molecular analysis (e.g., for epidermal growth factor receptor mutations).[21] Restaging of the mediastinum after neoadjuvant chemotherapy has been less successful, with a reported diagnostic sensitivity of only 76% and a negative predictive value that remains at 20%.[22]

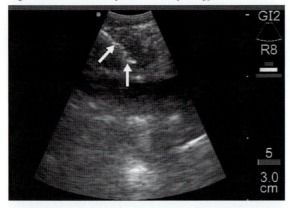

Fig. 29.5 Puncture of an 8-mm lymph node in position 4R. The needle (arrows) is visible within the node.

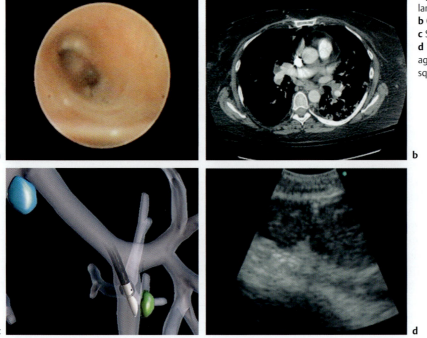

Fig. 29.6a–d a Endoscopic view of enlarged nodes in 11 L.
b Computed tomography.
c Schematic view.
d Endoscopic bronchial ultrasound image. Cytological proof of N3-positive squamous cell cancer was obtained.

EBUS-TBNA in Combination with EUS-FNA

Four papers have been published describing the combined approach. Again, Herth et al.[23] showed that the sensitivity and specificity of the combined techniques led to the same results as a routine mediastinoscopy. A recent study[24] has reported promising results with regard to the combination of EUS-FNA and EBUS-TBNA. EUS-FNA and EBUS-TBNA were compared for lung cancer staging in 33 patients with an established diagnosis of NSCLC (n = 20) or for diagnosis of suspected malignant lesions in the mediastinum in patients with suspected lung cancer (n = 13). The diagnoses were verified in 27 of 31 patients either by thoracotomy (n = 9) or through clinical follow-up (n = 18). A total of 119 lesions were sampled using EUS-FNA (n = 59) and EBUS-TBNA (n = 60). With regard to the results with the combined approach (EUS-FNA + EBUS-TBNA), in 28 of 31 patients in whom a final diagnosis was obtained in relation to the evaluation of cancer involving the mediastinum, 20 patients were found to have mediastinal involvement, whereas no mediastinal metastases were found in eight patients. The accuracy of EUS-FNA and EBUS-TBNA, in combination, for diagnosing mediastinal cancer was 100% (95% CI, 83% to 100%). The authors concluded that EUS-FNA and EBUS-TBNA appear to be complementary methods.

In the most recent trial,[25] Herth et al. examined whether the two procedures can be performed with a single EBUS bronchoscope. A total of 150 consecutive patients with presumptive evidence of NSCLC underwent mediastinal staging with EBUS-TBNA and EUS-FNA through a single linear ultrasound bronchoscope. The sensitivity was 89% for EUS-FNA and 91% for EBUS-TBNA. The combined approach had a sensitivity of 96% and negative predictive value of 95%—values higher than with either approach alone.

Other Applications

EBUS-TBNA has also been shown to be useful in diagnostic areas other than lung cancer. In patients with clinically suspected lymphoma, the reported diagnostic sensitivity is 91%.[26] For demonstrating noncaseating granulomatous inflammation, EBUS-TBNA has a diagnostic yield for sarcoidosis of 85–94%.[27–29] If more tissue specimens are needed for histological analysis, it is even possible to insert a 1.15-mm miniforceps through the EBUS scope and past the airway wall via a needle puncture in order to obtain real-time guided forceps biopsies of mediastinal lymph nodes.[30]

EBUS-TBNA has also been used successfully to obtain biopsy specimens in centrally located paratracheal and peribronchial tumors, with a diagnostic sensitivity of 82–94%.[31,32] In addition, real-time guided EBUS-TBNA has been used therapeutically to drain mediastinal and bronchogenic cysts, relieving central airway obstruction.[33,34]

Conclusion

Endobronchial ultrasonography has been widely available for more than 7 years. A growing body of good-quality research studies support the view that it has a significant role to play in airway assessment and procedural guidance. A further step in technological development has been made with the introduction of the EBUS-TBNA scope.

The results of the trials show that there is a high diagnostic yield for the correct prediction of lymph-node staging in patients with lung cancer in comparison with other modalities. Moreover, EBUS-TBNA avoids many invasive procedures. In addition, there were no complications during any of the procedures. EBUS-TBNA is a minimally invasive procedure with a high diagnostic rate, and many patients can benefit from the procedure. EBUS-TBNA should be considered in the staging of mediastinal lymph nodes as well as in the diagnosis of lung cancer.

The combined approach with EUS-FNA and EBUS-TBNA may be able to replace more invasive methods for evaluating patients with lung cancer in whom there are suspected hilar or mediastinal metastases, as well as for evaluating unknown mediastinal or hilar lesions.

References

1. Spira A, Ettinger DS. Multidisciplinary management of lung cancer. N Engl J Med 2004;350(4):379–392.
2. Sihoe AD, Yim AP. Lung cancer staging. J Surg Res 2004; 117(1):92–106.
3. Toloza EM, Harpole L, Detterbeck F, McCrory DC. Invasive staging of non-small cell lung cancer: a review of the current evidence. Chest 2003; 123(1, Suppl)157S–166S.
4. Mehta AC, Kavuru MS, Meeker DP, Gephardt GN, Nunez C. Transbronchial needle aspiration for histology specimens. Chest 1989;96:1268–1272.
5. Prakash UB, Offord KP, Stubbs SE. Bronchoscopy in North America: the ACCP survey. Chest 1991;100(6):1668–1675.
6. Haponik EF, Shure D. Underutilization of transbronchial needle aspiration: experiences of current pulmonary fellows. Chest 1997;112(1):251–253.
7. Herth F, Becker HD, Ernst A. Conventional vs endobronchial ultrasound-guided transbronchial needle aspiration: a randomized trial. Chest 2004;125(1):322–325.
8. Herth F, Becker HD. Endobronchial ultrasound of the airways and the mediastinum. Monaldi Arch Chest Dis 2000; 55(1):36–44.

9. Herth F, Hecker E, Hoffmann H, Becker HD. Endobronchial ultrasound for local tumour and lymph node staging in patients with centrally growing lung cancer. [Article in German] Ultraschall Med 2002;23(4):251–255.

10. Mountain CF, Dresler CM. Regional lymph node classification for lung cancer staging. Chest 1997;111(6):1718–1723.

11. Wallace MB, Pascual JM, Raimondo M, et al. Minimally invasive endoscopic staging of suspected lung cancer. JAMA 2008;299(5):540–546.

12. Ernst A, Anantham D, Eberhardt R, Krasnik M, Herth FJ. Diagnosis of mediastinal adenopathy-real-time endobronchial ultrasound guided needle aspiration versus mediastinoscopy. J Thorac Oncol 2008;3(6):577–582.

13. Detterbeck FC, Jantz MA, Wallace M, Vansteenkiste J, Silvestri GA; American College of Chest Physicians. Invasive mediastinal staging of lung cancer: ACCP evidence-based clinical practice guidelines (2nd edition). Chest 2007; 132(3, Suppl):202S–220S.

14. Krasnik M, Vilmann P, Larsen SS, Jacobsen GK. Preliminary experience with a new method of endoscopic transbronchial real time ultrasound guided biopsy for diagnosis of mediastinal and hilar lesions. Thorax 2003;58(12):1083–1086.

15. Yasufuku K, Chiyo M, Sekine Y, et al. Real-time endobronchial ultrasound-guided transbronchial needle aspiration of mediastinal and hilar lymph nodes. Chest 2004; 126(1):122–128.

16. Rintoul RC, Skwarski KM, Murchison JT, Wallace WA, Walker WS, Penman ID. Endobronchial and endoscopic ultrasound-guided real-time fine-needle aspiration for mediastinal staging. Eur Respir J 2005;25(3):416–421.

17. Herth FJF, Eberhardt R, Vilmann P, Krasnik M. EBUS-TBNA: a new device for endoscopic transbronchial real time ultrasound guided biopsy for diagnosis and staging of mediastinal lymph nodes. Thorax 2006;61(9):795–8.

18. Alsharif M, Andrade RS, Groth SS, Stelow EB, Pambuccian SE. Endobronchial ultrasound-guided transbronchial fine-needle aspiration: the University of Minnesota experience, with emphasis on usefulness, adequacy assessment, and diagnostic difficulties. Am J Clin Pathol 2008;130(3):434–443.

19. Herth FJ, Ernst A, Eberhardt R, Vilmann P, Dienemann H, Krasnik M. Endobronchial ultrasound-guided transbronchial needle aspiration of lymph nodes in the radiologically normal mediastinum. Eur Respir J 2006;28(5):910–914.

20. Herth FJ, Eberhardt R, Krasnik M, Ernst A. Endobronchial ultrasound-guided transbronchial needle aspiration of lymph nodes in the radiologically and positron emission tomography-normal mediastinum in patients with lung cancer. Chest 2008;133(4):887–891.

21. Nakajima T, Yasufuku K, Suzuki M, et al. Assessment of epidermal growth factor receptor mutation by endobronchial ultrasound-guided transbronchial needle aspiration. Chest 2007;132(2):597–602.

22. Herth FJ, Annema JT, Eberhardt R, et al. Endobronchial ultrasound with transbronchial needle aspiration for restaging the mediastinum in lung cancer. J Clin Oncol 2008;26(20):3346–3350.

23. Herth FJ, Lunn W, Eberhardt R, Becker HD, Ernst A. Transbronchial versus transesophageal ultrasound-guided aspiration of enlarged mediastinal lymph nodes. Am J Respir Crit Care Med 2005;171(10):1164–1167.

24. Vilmann P, Krasnik M, Larsen SS, Jacobsen GK, Clementsen P. Transesophageal endoscopic ultrasound-guided fine-needle aspiration (EUS-FNA) and endobronchial ultrasound-guided transbronchial needle aspiration (EBUS-TBNA) biopsy: a combined approach in the evaluation of mediastinal lesions. Endoscopy 2005;37(9):833–839.

25. Herth FJF, Ernst A, Krasnik M, Kahn N, Eberhardt R. Combined Endoesophageal-Endobronchial Ultrasound-Guided, Fine-Needle Aspiration of Mediastinal Lymph Nodes through a Single Bronchoscope in 150 Patients with Suspected Lung Cancer. Chest 2010;138(4):790–794.

26. Kennedy MP, Jimenez CA, Bruzzi JF, et al. Endobronchial ultrasound-guided transbronchial needle aspiration in the diagnosis of lymphoma. Thorax 2008;63(4):360–365.

27. Oki M, Saka H, Kitagawa C, et al. Real-time endobronchial ultrasound-guided transbronchial needle aspiration is useful for diagnosing sarcoidosis. Respirology 2007;12(6):863–868.

28. Wong M, Yasufuku K, Nakajima T, et al. Endobronchial ultrasound: new insight for the diagnosis of sarcoidosis. Eur Respir J 2007;29(6):1182–1186.

29. Garwood S, Judson MA, Silvestri G, Hoda R, Fraig M, Doelken P. Endobronchial ultrasound for the diagnosis of pulmonary sarcoidosis. Chest 2007;132(4):1298–1304.

30. Herth FJ, Morgan RK, Eberhardt R, Ernst A. Endobronchial ultrasound-guided miniforceps biopsy in the biopsy of subcarinal masses in patients with low likelihood of non-small cell lung cancer. Ann Thorac Surg 2008;85(6):1874–1878.

31. Tournoy KG, Rintoul RC, van Meerbeeck JP, et al. EBUS-TBNA for the diagnosis of central parenchymal lung lesions not visible at routine bronchoscopy. Lung Cancer 2009; 63(1):45–49.

32. Nakajima T, Yasufuku K, Fujiwara T, et al. Endobronchial ultrasound-guided transbronchial needle aspiration for the diagnosis of intrapulmonary lesions. J Thorac Oncol 2008; 3(9):985–988.

33. Nakajima T, Yasufuku K, Shibuya K, Fujisawa T. Endobronchial ultrasound-guided transbronchial needle aspiration for the treatment of central airway stenosis caused by a mediastinal cyst. Eur J Cardiothorac Surg 2007;32(3):538–540.

34. Dhand S, Krimsky W. Bronchogenic cyst treated by endobronchial ultrasound drainage. Thorax 2008;63(4):386.

V Additional Applications

30   EUS-Guided Neurolysis of the Celiac Plexus

S. Hollerbach

Celiac plexus neurolysis has been used since 1950 to treat severe visceral pain syndromes. In the initial clinical studies, dorsal and paraspinal routes or transabdominal techniques with fluoroscopic guidance were used to access the region of the celiac trunk. These techniques were mainly used in large treatment centers to treat intractable pain caused by pancreatic carcinoma, and sometimes in chronic pancreatitis. However, because of the high level of expertise and specialization required to carry out such invasive procedures safely in patients, the techniques did not come into widespread use outside a few tertiary care centers. Alternative surgical methods also never became treatment options, as they were even more invasive and were not an attractive option for use in terminally ill groups of patients. With the advent of various highly effective and potent analgesic drugs and anesthetics, interest in developing additional invasive methods of treating cancer pain declined even further. However, when computed tomography (CT) techniques were further refined during the 1980s, interest among clinicians gradually returned to the issue of celiac plexus neurolysis (**Fig. 30.1a**).

Since then, a few specialized pain centers have reported clinical "success rates" in the range of 60–85 % with CT-guided interventions in uncontrolled open studies, although evidence from controlled studies is still lacking. A significant risk of a few but serious side effects and complications associated with percutaneous plexus block interventions, including paraplegia and pneumothorax, was encountered with CT-guided techniques, which is one of the major reasons for continuing efforts since the mid-1990s to develop novel techniques such as endoscopic ultrasound (EUS)-guided plexus neurolysis (EUS-CPN). This approach always appeared attractive, as it has the advantages that it is carried out with the patient in intravenous sedation and is considerably less invasive, since very fine needles are used (22–25 G) with direct ultrasound visualization, very close to the anatomical structures that indicate the location of the celiac plexus—the neural ganglionic structures of which are not visible themselves with any imaging methods (**Fig. 30.1b**).

However, the clinical effectiveness of this novel interventional EUS technique has still not yet been confirmed in randomized and controlled clinical studies. The initial studies and uncontrolled clinical studies currently in progress[1–4] have provided encouraging results with regard to the feasibility and safety of EUS-CPN in this setting. Technical success was reported in 50–90 % of cases, with reduced analgesic requirements and stabilization of the pain. The clinical effectiveness may be greater when alcohol is injected bilaterally than when injected centrally, relative to the supposed position of the celiac plexus under EUS vision.[4] Relevant side effects of EUS-CPN include transient diarrhea, hypotension, and rare cases of infection and bleeding. No randomized controlled clinical studies have

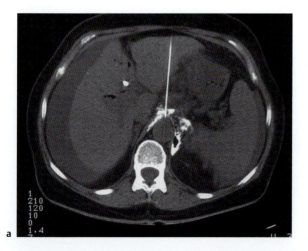

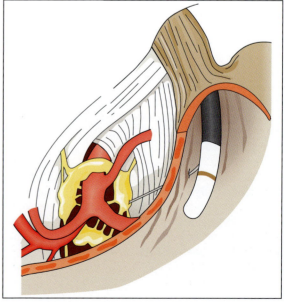

Fig. 30.1a, b a Computed tomography-guided celiac plexus neurolysis.
b Endoscopic ultrasound-guided celiac plexus blockade, showing some of the anatomical landmarks.

Table 30.1 Indications for diagnostic and therapeutic endoscopic ultrasound-guided fine-needle aspiration (EUS-FNA)

Diagnosis and/or local staging
Mediastinal lymphomas (bronchial carcinoma, Hodgkin lymphoma, non-Hodgkin lymphoma, tuberculosis, sarcoidosis)
Mediastinal tumors (bronchial carcinoma, germ cell tumor, thymoma, metastases, inflammatory pseudotumors, etc.)
Mediastinal abscess (perforating abscess, tuberculosis), fluid collections in the posterior mediastinum
Pathological lesions in the thyroid and parathyroid[a]
N/M1A staging of esophageal carcinoma
Intramural esophageal tumors
Submucosal tumors in the esophagus, stomach, and duodenum
Diagnosis of the type and N/M staging of tumors, metastases, lymph nodes, abscesses, and fluid collections in the peritoneum and retroperitoneum
Diagnosis of periampullary tumors and malignant pancreatic tumors (including N and local M staging)
Diagnosis of pathological lesions in the left lobe of the liver and central segments of the liver and hilar region (metastases, hepatocellular carcinoma, cholangiocarcinoma, adenoma, hilar lymph nodes, abscesses)
Diagnosis of lesions in the left adrenal gland (metastases, adenomas, multiple endocrine neoplasia, tuberculosis)
Circumscribed lesions of the spleen (non-Hodgkin lymphoma, Hodgkin disease, metastases)
Therapy
Celiac plexus block (neurolysis) for pain treatment in pancreatic and papillary carcinoma, as well as chronic pancreatitis
EUS-targeted drainage treatment for pancreatic pseudocysts (with stent placement)
EUS-targeted drainage treatment in cholestasis[a] and accessible dilated bile ducts (with stent placement)
EUS-guided endoscopic mucosal resection
EUS-guided intratumoral fine-needle injection therapy

[a] If these procedures are not easier with EUS-FNA, percutaneous access is also possible.

been published on the topic to date; an attempt was made in German centers, but failed to obtain ethics approval. Consequently, no sham-controlled, randomized studies are currently available that support a major role for this attractive technique as a standard procedure of care in clinical oncology. However, a recent "meta-analysis"[5] of eight uncontrolled studies concluded that EUS-guided CPN is safe and offers additional benefit for pain relief in some patients with cancer, although its use in chronic pancreatitis cannot be generally recommended as yet.

Minimally invasive interventional therapeutic endosonography has in the meantime emerged as an established technique. With the advent of improved endoscopic technology and the development of longitudinal scanners, it became possible some 20 years ago to combine ultrasonography and endoscopy in such a way that ultrasound-guided transmural needle interventions (biopsies) became possible during the same endoscopy session. This method has the unique advantage that even small and previously inaccessible pathological lesions (≤5 mm) can be reached with EUS guidance even if they are located in the posterior mediastinum, around the cardia, the cranial retroperitoneum, the adrenal glands, the hilum of the liver, the pancreatic region, and the rectum.[6–10] These techniques were initially used only to obtain EUS-guided fine-needle aspiration (FNA) biopsies for diagnostic purposes, but today they are increasingly being used for transvisceral therapeutic procedures.[1,2,5,11,12] The variety of options available and the fact that the complication rate is relatively low

makes EUS-guided interventions particularly attractive. However, EUS-guided interventions are technically highly demanding, and considerable endoscopic and ultrasound training is needed to carry out procedures of this type safely. Skill and expertise in EUS-guided interventions are necessary before these rather delicate methods can be safely conducted in patients. **Table 30.1** provides an overview of the current routine and experimental indications for diagnostic and therapeutic uses of EUS-FNA.

This chapter provides an overview of one of the earliest interventional applications of EUS-guided therapy: celiac plexus neurolysis (EUS-CPN) for the treatment of severe visceral pain in malignant disease, using injection therapy. It should be borne in mind that this form of treatment is largely supportive, although it can make a significant contribution to a comprehensive and interdisciplinary approach to pain management in malignant disease. It helps the clinician control pain in patients with end-stage disease and adds valuable nonpharmacological options. As mentioned, however, there is still a lack of prospective and controlled clinical studies.

Prerequisites for EUS-Guided Celiac Plexus Neurolysis and Other Treatments

The effectiveness of therapeutic EUS depends on a variety of different factors:

- *General experience and skill.* One of the most important prerequisites for carrying out EUS-guided treatments successfully is excellent endoscopic skills, with full mastery of all of the conventional endoscopic techniques using straight-viewing and side-viewing endoscopes, including esophagogastroduodenoscopy and endoscopic retrograde cholangiopancreatography. In addition, comprehensive training in interventional transcutaneous sonography, including fine-needle puncture and drainage techniques, is needed in order to meet the high requirements for interventional therapeutic EUS.
- *Specialized endosonography skills.* Endoscopic ultrasonography with fine-needle aspiration (EUS-FNA) is probably one of the most technically demanding and training-intensive endoscopic examination procedures. Experience with at least 250–300 previous endosonographic examinations, including fine-needle biopsies, is needed to ensure that treatments in this field are administered safely and successfully in routine clinical conditions in patients.
- *Cost-effectiveness.* Interventional EUS for routine use in an endoscopy department generally involves substantial costs, including the high initial investment and installation costs and expenses for repair procedures, as well as additional costs for accessory materials such as puncture needles and other appliances. These additional materials are usually much more expensive than any of the catheters and needles used for percutaneous procedures. Depending on the type of needle used and local price negotiations, the cost of a biopsy or injection needle as a single-use device can amount to € 150–300 (US$ 203–405). On top of this, costs for sedatives and anesthetics, cytology and/or histology, and microbiology have to be taken into account, representing an additional € 50–150 (US$ 68–203), depending on the severity and type of disease and procedure. With therapeutic interventions, even higher total costs have to be calculated (between approximately € 850 (US$ 1149) and € 1500 (US$ 2027) per drainage procedure) if metal stents are not inserted; metal stents can increase the cost up to a total of € 1500–2500 (US$ 2027–3379). Finally, the amount of time and the numbers of staff needed for demanding procedures such as these mean that the use of the techniques outside specialized care centers, with reasonable numbers of patients with special needs, is questionable and unattractive. In general, only specialized clinical care centers dealing with a significant number of complex gastroenterology and oncology cases, which also offer a wide range of minimally

invasive visceral surgical procedures per year, should consider installing therapeutic EUS facilities in order to qualify as centers of expertise. Any other institutions would need to weigh up the benefits of such niche techniques carefully against the medical and financial risks, since basic endosonographic problems can be reasonably assessed with radial-scanning echoendoscopes, allowing appropriate selection of patients with special medical needs who can still be referred to secondary or tertiary care centers for therapeutic EUS.

Indications for Therapeutic EUS

Several new applications for interventional EUS techniques are in principle feasible and are currently being investigated. Only a few therapeutic EUS techniques have yet made their way into prospective clinical studies that allow preliminary evidence-based conclusions to be drawn (**Table 30.1**). Clinically approved therapeutic EUS techniques currently include:

- EUS-CPN to achieve better control of chronic visceral pain in patients with pancreatic and periampullary carcinoma and other types of retroperitoneal tumor (clinical efficacy ≈ 50–80 %, depending on the definition of the outcome; however, further research is still required).
- EUS-guided drainage of pancreatic pseudocysts and necroses, including one-step placement of stents and drainage catheters
- EUS-guided drainage of obstructed bile ducts in the left liver lobe or from the duodenal bulb, as an alternative to percutaneous transhepatic cholangiographic drainage (PTCD)
- EUS-guided drainage of obstructed pancreatic ducts and placement of transpapillary pancreatic guide wires (experimental)

Other experimental therapeutic EUS options and techniques include:

- EUS-guided intratumoral injection therapy with cytotoxic agents (local chemotherapy), immunomodulators (e.g., mixed allogenic lymphocyte populations or lectins, TNF-erade), and other agents
- EUS-guided radiofrequency ablation of tumors (pancreas, liver metastasis, retroperitoneal tumors)
- EUS-guided local laser ablation therapy or photodynamic therapy

Contraindications to Therapeutic EUS

In general, EUS-FNA applications are considered to be safe. Most of the contraindications are therefore only relative, but the benefits need to be carefully weighed up against the potential risks in each individual patient affected by the relative contraindications. The most frequent complications are listed in **Table 30.2**. Diagnostic puncture biopsies with fine needles (19–25 G) are generally safe, while therapeutic procedures involve a small but considerable risk of side effects, particularly in severely ill patients with multiple risk factors such as severe coagulopathy. The contraindications to diagnostic fine-needle injection (FNI) therapy (e.g., for celiac plexus neurolysis and other therapeutic procedures) are:

- Lack of informed consent from the patient
- Poor clinical status of the patient (Karnofsky index < 70%)
- Large vessels blocking the needle path
- Lack of visualization of the needle tip
- Severe coagulopathy (Quick test < 30%, thrombocyte count < 40 000)

Table 30.2 General complications of endoscopic ultrasound-guided fine-needle aspiration (EUS-FNA)

Complications	Frequency (approx.)
Cervical perforation	0.03%
Other types of perforation	Only in high-grade stenosis (caution required)
Significant bacteremia (solid processes)	< 0.05%
Infections (cystic processes)	Up to 10% (antibiotic prophylaxis required)
Significant extraluminal hemorrhage[a]	1.3%
Mild transient pancreatitis (only in pancreatic fine-needle aspiration)	0.5%
Aspiration	0.2%

[a] Literature reports all describe bleeding as resolving spontaneously, without the need for therapeutic interventions.

Materials

■ Echoendoscopes

There are at present different manufacturers producing echoendoscopes that allow diagnostic and therapeutic EUS procedures. These consist exclusively of longitudinal-scanning endoscopes with a biopsy channel (longitudinal convex-array scanners).

Pentax-Hitachi (Hitachi Medical Corporation Tokyo, Japan; Pentax Europe Ltd., Hamburg, Germany) has the longest record with longitudinal EUS and produces several ranges of digital video echoendoscopes for diagnostic and therapeutic interventions. These dedicated endoscopes have an oblique-viewing 60° lens with a longitudinal echo transducer at the tip of the scope. The working channels for biopsies have different sizes (2.0 or 3.2 mm). The electronic curved-array transducer produces a sectorlike 120° image along the longitudinal scope axis that allows fully EUS-guided interventional maneuvers under full vision. The transducer frequency can be switched between 5 and 10 MHz. A water-filled balloon around the tip of the instrument enhances contact between the ultrasound beam and the mucosal surfaces and minimizes disturbing air reflexes within the gastrointestinal tract. All of the endoscopes are equipped with a color Doppler device and continuous-wave Doppler to facilitate the analysis of vascular structures.

Fujinon. Another manufacturer of longitudinal echoendoscopes with working channels for biopsies is Fujinon, which produces a dedicated combined echoendoscope and integrated digital ultrasound unit (Fujinon Europe Ltd., Willich, Germany). The flexibility and local resolution provided by this device is very good, including the biopsy channel, which features an elevator. The current clinical performance of this novel device is good to excellent and there is hope that further enhancements will become available in the near future.

Olympus (Olympus Europe Ltd., Hamburg, Germany) has long experience in the field and has developed a wide range of different radial and longitudinal echoendoscopes, including digital radial scanners and longitudinal scopes that contain large working channels for therapeutic maneuvers. These endoscopes maintain the same high solid-state standards as those of the conventional endoscopes the company produces. The digital video scopes will soon be part of the company's successful high-resolution 180 video series and have working channels ranging from 2.8 to 3.8 mm for therapeutic applications. They all incorporate color Doppler units. The longitudinal puncture endoscopes manufactured by Olympus are all equipped with an elevator that facilitates introduction of the biopsy needle under ultrasound guidance, within certain limits.

The specific choice of interventional EUS equipment to be used certainly depends on many different factors, including individual preferences, previous experience, the local ultrasound and endoscope equipment available, and the financial options at one's disposal. For instance, there are differences between the manufacturers' products with regard to ultrasound resolution, flexibility, and appliances, but also in terms of mechanical properties and electronic endoscope quality. These factors need to be individually weighed up against each other to reach a final decision relative to the available budget. Successful EUS procedures are certainly also highly dependent on the operator's skills

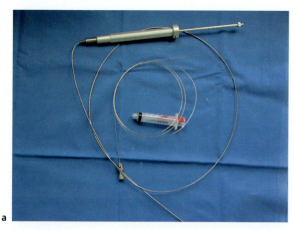

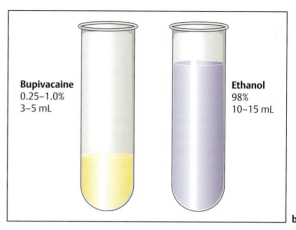

Fig. 30.2a, b Materials required for EUS-guided celiac plexus neurolysis (EUS-CPN).

a Standard Hancke–Vilmann biopsy needle, including the piston, protective sheath, stylet and needle, and Luer aspiration syringe. **b** Injection solutions.

and experience, while the endoscope facilities and ultrasound applications are clearly of secondary importance.

■ Materials for Therapeutic EUS Procedures

Various commercially available needle systems can be used to carry out EUS-guided fine-needle injections for celiac plexus neurolysis. At present, a wide range of different needle systems is available on the medical product market. The main players in this field are the companies GIP/Medi-Globe Ltd. (Achenmühle, Germany), Cook (Cook Endoscopy, Winston-Salem, North Carolina, USA), and Olympus. However, successful treatment is possible with almost any of the products available, and in many cases it is the price of the needle that determines preferences in an individual EUS department. The least expensive needle currently available is the Hancke–Vilmann metal needle (Medi-Globe), which consists of a metal needle made of stainless steel (170 cm/0.8 mm, 22 gauge). It has a metal stylet, a reusable metal spiral sheath, and a grip with a piston (**Fig. 30.2**) to guide the needle tip properly. Numerous pioneering clinical studies have been conducted using this needle, which has been the standard in EUS-FNA for many years now. For therapeutic applications, however, a similar 19-G needle is available, for example, for pancreatic pseudocyst drainage procedures. This needle has a larger lumen and is also practical for injection therapy, while the price is still the lowest on the market due to the reusable outer parts. However, there are problems in that the visibility of these needles is in some cases very limited, while the outer sheath is rather rigid.

Other diagnostic and therapeutic needle systems at higher prices are available in different sizes and styles (19–25 G) from GIP, Cook, and Olympus. The Olympus needles are solid-state metal ones (22 G) that can be

used for diagnostic EUS-FNA and injection treatments such as plexus neurolysis. They have fair-to-good visibility in tissue and are rather flexible, while the price is considerable. Cook supplies a wide range of specialized and dedicated diagnostic and therapeutic needles (e.g., the 22-G EchoTip EUS needles, the 19-G EchoTip needle, and the 25-G EchoTip needle), and has also developed a novel dedicated cutting needle for histological purposes (the 19-G Quick-Core EUSN-19-QC). The company has also developed the only specially designed spray needle for celiac plexus neurolysis, with multiple side holes and a diameter of 20 G (EchoTip EUSN-20-CPN). The GIP needles (Sonotip II) are very similar to the Cook needles. However, good though these needles may be, there is no scientific evidence as yet that the high cost of these appliances is justified by their individual performance status, which remains to be demonstrated in ongoing clinical studies in several EUS centers around the world. In addition, it has not been shown that the spray needle fares better than conventional injection needles for EUS-CPN.

Injectant solutions are required for celiac plexus neurolysis. These consist of a local anesthetic and absolute alcohol solution for final and permanent neurolysis, with an amount of 5–15 mL of a commercially available local anesthetic—procaine benzylpenicillin (novocaine), lidocaine, or mepivacaine and lauromacrogol 400 (Scandicain)—which is followed by 20–30 mL of absolute alcohol (98 % ethanol). **Figure 30.2** shows the equipment and solutions required for EUS-guided celiac plexus neurolysis (CPN).

Celiac Plexus Neurolysis

■ Preparation for the Procedure

The patient should be placed in the left lateral decubitus position, as recommended for conventional esophagogastroduodenoscopy (EGD) procedures. However, in some cases it can be helpful to rotate the patient's body toward the abdomen during the EUS intervention, to provide a better overview of the celiac plexus region. Topical anesthetic sprays are strongly recommended (e.g., with lignocaine/Xylocaine) to ensure event-free endoscope insertion. Intervenous sedative medication should always be administered to facilitate the EUS procedure. The recommended agents are the same as those used for standard EGD and colonoscopy procedures, including midazolam (Dormicum, 5–10 mg), propofol (Diprivan, 50–200 mg), and/or pethidine (Dolantin, 25–75 mg). Additional use of hyoscine butylbromide (Buscopan) or atropine can only be recommended in exceptional cases—for instance, when the duodenal bulb cannot be reached easily or if cramps and spasms inhibit the insertion of the scope into the second part of the duodenum. Monitoring devices for continuous measurement of blood pressure and pulse oximetry are mandatory to ensure safe surveillance of vital signs during echoendoscopy in all cases. If high-risk patients are being examined (e.g., patients with concomitant severe respiratory and cardiovascular problems) portable or stationary electrocardiography (ECG) monitors should be used as well. Facilities for continuous oxygen administration via nasal or oral probes or masks during endoscopic procedures are essential, and oxygen should be administered even during episodes of slight hypoxemia.

The side-viewing echoendoscope is then introduced under proper sedation, with minimal pressure during pharyngeal and laryngeal passage into the esophagus. In routine conditions, 2.5–5.0 mg midazolam is recommended, and this should be combined with bolus administration of propofol in boluses of 30–50 mg with continuous monitoring of oxygenation and blood pressure. Alternatively, 25–50 mg pethidine can be used, particularly in countries that do not permit the use of propofol for this indication. Several countries restrict the use of propofol to endoscopy units with physicians present who have formal training in intensive-care treatment, since the agent is an intravenous anesthetic that can potentially cause severe respiratory depression and hypoventilation, including life-threatening hypoxia, if not administered correctly. However, with the necessary experience, careful bolus administration, and continuous patient monitoring, we have found that propofol is very helpful and safe in our experience. We therefore strongly recommend the combination of low-dose midazolam and propofol as the sedation method of choice in most cases, particularly if EUS-guided therapy is planned or scheduled.

Antibiotic prophylaxis. In accordance with standard endocarditis prevention guidelines, prophylactic antibiotics should be administered before the EUS intervention in all patients who have an increased risk of endocarditis or other systemic infections (artificial valve, valvular stenoses or insufficiencies, shunts). In addition, if cystic lesions are being punctured during EUS-FNA or EUS-FNI, antibiotic prophylaxis should also be administered intravenously. Recommended single antibiotic substances include amoxicillin, ampicillin, piperacillin, ceftriaxone, and cefuroxime. Before administration, however, the individual risk situation should be assessed and the choice of antibiotics should be tailored to the specific situation, as recommended in the current endocarditis prevention guidelines.

Prophylaxis in EUS-FNI. Intravenous antibiotics should be administered prophylactically before EUS-FNI if there is an increased risk of endocarditis and/or if spontaneous bacterial peritonitis has to be avoided. Suitable antibiotics include ampicillin, amoxicillin, or ceftriaxone. It is not known whether administration of proton-pump inhibitors (PPIs) is helpful in preventing ulcer complications after therapeutic EUS procedures. However, in the absence of solid data, we would currently recommend avoiding PPI administration in severely ill patients, if clinically feasible, as the agents could theoretically increase bacterial overgrowth.

■ Procedure

Using an echoendoscope with a linear transducer, the region at the root of the celiac ganglion, arising just cephalad and anterior to the celiac artery, can be reached in most patients (**Fig. 30.3**). The echoendoscope is pulled back just below the cardia, ≈ 40–45 cm from the incisors, and placed a few centimeters below the phrenic hiatus, with the transducer curved posteriorly against the stomach wall. After this position has been achieved, either a 22-G diagnostic FNA needle (or a specially designed 20-G spray needle with side holes) is introduced through the endoscope's working channel and carefully inserted through the stomach wall. With close observation of the tip of the needle, the operator advances the needle under direct vision until the wall of the common celiac trunk is just touched, and the scope is then withdrawn 3–5 mm on reaching the arterial wall. In cases of doubt or uncertainty, the needle position can also be visualized by injecting contrast agents for fluoroscopy (**Fig. 30.4**). Before anything is injected, aspiration should be applied to exclude intravascular positioning of the needle tip, for example, in the celiac artery. The best results are achieved when the injection starts ≈ 2 mm cephalad to the celiac trunk, to spread the injection agent widely in the soft tissue surrounding the retroperitoneal region. This procedure requires considerable skill and should only be performed

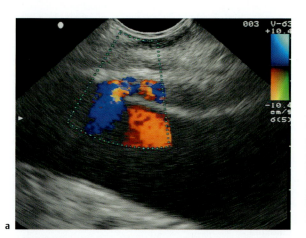

a

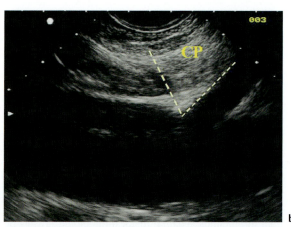

b

Fig. 30.3a, b Endosonographic appearance of the target region for EUS-guided celiac plexus neurolysis (EUS-CPN).
a Identification of the celiac trunk with color duplex ultrasound scanning, and positioning of the longitudinal transducer above the abdominal aorta.

b The presumed anatomical position of the major celiac plexus (CP) ganglion network, indicated by the triangular line. The tip of the injection needle is also visible.

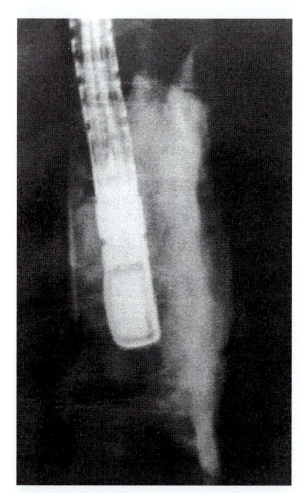

Fig. 30.4 Fluoroscopic image of the celiac trunk and its surroundings after EUS-guided fine-needle injection of contrast material before celiac plexus neurolysis. The wide distribution of the injection fluid is well demonstrated.

by experienced EUS interventionists. Subsequently, 10–15 mL bupivacaine (0.25%) is instilled for local anesthesia on both sides of the celiac axis, whenever anatomically possible, by repositioning the endoscope and needle. This injection is extremely important in order to avoid severe local pain after administration of the neurolytic agent (absolute alcohol).

The utmost care should be taken to keep the tip of the needle away from the arterial wall, to prevent significant complications such as arterial bleeding and embolization during the injection. Subsequently, 10–15 mL 98% ethanol (absolute alcohol) is injected first and the injection is then repeated after repositioning of the EUS instrument by angling the tip by ≈ 90°. When the alcohol is injected under ultrasound vision, the image of the needle becomes increasingly blurred, as the injectant solution produces highly echogenic cloudlike ultrasound artifacts (**Fig. 30.5**). The treatment should therefore be administered rapidly as a bolus injection to both application sides of the celiac trunk, and the procedure should be terminated immediately after the end of the injection. There have been some uncontrolled reports suggesting that bilateral injection is more effective than central injection, but this conclusion still awaits confirmation in randomized trials.

The EUS-CPN procedure can be carried out on an outpatient basis, as it rarely causes any lasting side effects. Celiac plexus neurolysis can also be undertaken at the end of a diagnostic tumor-staging procedure for pancreatic carcinomas. In this case, the procedure is preceded by morphological EUS staging of the tumor and locoregional lymph-node staging, in combination with diagnostic EUS-FNA, to allow histological assessment of the tumor, followed by the EUS-CPN procedure as described above.

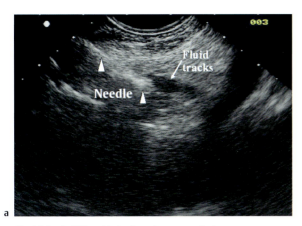
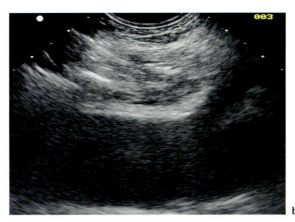

Fig. 30.5a, b EUS-guided celiac plexus neurolysis.
a The celiac plexus is located directly cephalad and anterior to the celiac trunk arteries as they emerge from the aorta. The EUS-guided fine needle is carefully introduced and advanced close to the wall of the celiac trunk.

b The local anesthetic agent is then sprayed or injected, followed by injection of the absolute alcohol, which is sprayed or injected in equal aliquots on both sides of the celiac trunk.

■ Problems and Complications

Most EUS-guided therapeutic interventions are still regarded as experimental. In addition to the general risks and side effects of standard endoscopy, therefore, the specific procedure-related risks associated with EUS-guided treatments have to be assessed before the treatment. If it is performed correctly, EUS-guided celiac plexus neurolysis usually only causes mild complications such as transient diarrhea or mild local tenderness. However, a few individual cases of major complications have been reported, including pancreatic abscess, arteriovenous malformations, and bleeding, which suggests that careful clinical observation is absolutely mandatory after all interventional measures. EUS-guided treatments are extremely safe when administered by experienced interventional endoscopists, with careful technique and the use of safe injection materials, although there are as yet only limited data for safety assessments. Our experience in more than 50 patients treated with EUS-FNI is positive; only three of the patients (1.5%) developed mild, transient, and self-limiting complications, and no severe complications requiring interventional treatment developed. **Table 30.2** lists the published types and frequency of potential complications related to EUS-FNI.

■ Postinterventional Measures

In principle, all EUS-guided interventions can take place in an outpatient setting. However, postinterventional in-hospital surveillance should be considered in patients with a high risk of complications, for example, patients with coagulation disorders or severe respiratory and cardiac problems. In view of the favorable safety profile of EUS-guided interventions such as EUS-FNA and EUS-FNI, severe complications occur extraordinarily rarely if the techniques are applied correctly. In all routine cases of EUS-FNI, surveillance after the intervention follows the general principles for diagnostic and therapeutic outpatient endoscopy with the use of sedatives and anesthetics. The patients should fast for at least 1 hour after the intervention due to the use of local anesthetics and potential nausea or vomiting. Depending on the duration, dosage, and depth of the sedation used, adequate clinical monitoring of patients after endoscopic interventions must include careful clinical monitoring (observation, repeated measurements of blood pressure and pulse rate, oximetry). When sedatives or anesthetics are administered, the patient must be instructed not to drive a vehicle for 24 hours. In addition, the patient must be absent from work and should have no responsibility for major business activities on the day of the operation, and prior consent should be obtained to ensure this. High-risk patients and those in whom difficult EUS-guided interventions are planned should be offered an in-hospital procedure with overnight observation.

References

1. Wiersema MJ, Wiersema L. Endosonography-guided celiac plexus neurolysis (EUS-CPN). Gastrointest Endosc 1996;44: 656–662.
2. Will U, Burmester E, Erk J. Normal anatomy and landmarks. In: Rösch T, Will U, Chang KJ, eds. Longitudinal endosonography: atlas and manual for use in the upper gastrointestinal tract. Berlin: Springer; 2001:2:22–55.
3. Levy MJ, Topazian MD, Wiersema MJ, et al. Initial evaluation of the efficacy and safety of endoscopic ultrasound-guided direct Ganglia neurolysis and block. Am J Gastroenterol 2008;103(1):98–103.
4. Sahai AV, Lemelin V, Lam E, Paquin SC. Central vs. bilateral endoscopic ultrasound-guided celiac plexus block or neurolysis: a comparative study of short-term effectiveness. Am J Gastroenterol 2009;104(2):326–329.
5. Puli SR, Reddy JB, Bechtold ML, Antillon MR, Brugge WR. EUS-guided celiac plexus neurolysis for pain due to chronic pancreatitis or pancreatic cancer pain: a meta-analysis and systematic review. Dig Dis Sci 2009;54(11):2330–2337 Epub ahead of print.
6. Vilmann P, Hancke S, Henriksen FW, Jacobsen GK. Endoscopic ultrasonography-guided fine-needle aspiration biopsy of lesions in the upper gastrointestinal tract. Gastrointest Endosc 1995;41(3):230–235.
7. Caletti G, Fusaroli P, Bocus P. Endoscopic ultrasonography. Digestion 1998;59(5):509–529.
8. Wiersema MJ, Vilmann P, Giovannini M, Chang KJ, Wiersema LM. Endosonography-guided fine-needle aspiration biopsy: diagnostic accuracy and complication assessment. Gastroenterology 1997;112(4):1087–1095.
9. Giovannini M, Seitz JF, Monges G, Perrier H, Rabbia I. Fine-needle aspiration cytology guided by endoscopic ultrasonography: results in 141 patients. Endoscopy 1995;27(2): 171–177.
10. Hollerbach S, Klamann A, Topalidis T, Schmiegel W. Endoscopic ultrasonography–guided biopsy (EUS-FNA) aids in the diagnosis of chronic pancreatitis. Endoscopy 2001; 33:824–831.
11. Chang KJ, Nguyen PT, Thompson JA, et al. Phase I clinical trial of allogeneic mixed lymphocyte culture (cytoimplant) delivered by endoscopic ultrasound-guided fine-needle injection in patients with advanced pancreatic carcinoma. Cancer 2000;88(6):1325–1335.
12. Pfau PR, Chak A. Endoscopic ultrasonography. Endoscopy 2002;34(1):21–28.

31   EUS-Guided Biliary Drainage

E. Burmester, J. Niehaus

Endoscopic retrograde cholangiography (ERCP) with stenting of the bile duct is a well-established procedure for palliative treatment of malignant pancreaticobiliary strictures.[1,2] In 5–10 % of cases, it is not possible to obtain access to the bile duct and place a stent, due to previous surgical procedures such as gastrectomy with Roux-en-Y anastomosis, Billroth II surgery, or Whipple resection. Other reasons may include failed bile duct cannulation, infiltrations of the papilla of Vater, complete stenosis of the common bile duct, obstruction of the pylorus or duodenum in tumor infiltration, and anatomic variations such as upside-down stomach. When ERCP fails, percutaneous transhepatic biliary drainage (PTBD) has so far been the alternative method and is successful in 90 % of the patients.[3–6] However, PTBD can be associated with complications such as bleeding, peritonitis, cholangitis, infections, hemobilia, and injuries to the adjacent lung and pleura. If subsequent internal drainage fails, it leads to a significant impairment of quality of life, and the patient has to accept long-term external biliary drainage. Endoscopic ultrasound (EUS)-guided internal biliary drainage is a potential alternative in these cases.

Technique

As in other EUS-guided interventions, use of a therapeutic linear echoendoscope with a working channel of 3.7–3.8 mm and an Albarrán is strongly recommended in EUS-guided biliary drainage (e.g., Hitachi EG-3870-UTK, EG3830-UT, Olympus GF-UCT140-AL5, Fujinon EG-530UT). The procedure is carried out under endosonographic and fluoroscopic control. Administering prophylactic antibiotics reduces the risk of cholangitis, especially if the procedure fails.

The access route to the bile duct system depends on the anatomy:

- Normal anatomy *or* Billroth I resection: common bile duct *or* left hepatic duct (**Fig. 31.1**)
- Billroth II resection or gastrectomy: left hepatic duct (**Fig. 31.2**)

The technical success of the procedure is greater if the shortest route to the dilated duct is chosen; the water-filled balloon on the transducer can sometimes be used to stabilize the position of the device after needle puncture.

In normal anatomy or after Billroth I resections, the transducer can be placed either at the level of the cardia for the left hepatic duct or in the duodenum for the common bile duct, depending on the site of infiltration. In Billroth II anatomy, transgastric EUS, or in cases of gastrectomy transjejunal EUS, provides excellent imaging of the dilated intrahepatic ducts in the left liver lobe in patients

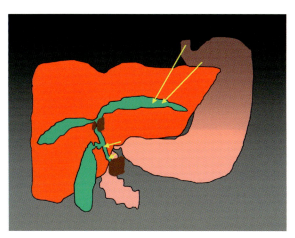

Fig. 31.1 Normal anatomy, showing possible access routes for EUS-guided biliary drainage (arrows).

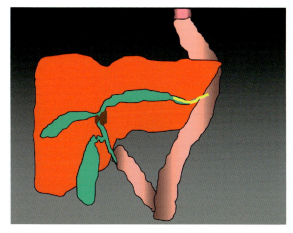

Fig. 31.2 A possible access route for EUS-guided biliary drainage following gastrectomy.

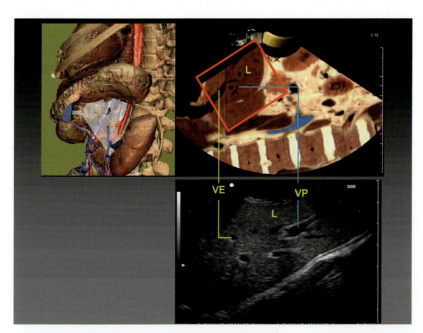

Fig. 31.3 EUS meets Voxel-MAN. The transducer is directed toward the left liver lobe (L), with visualization of the portal vein (VP) and hepatic veins (VE).

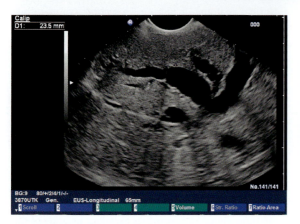

Fig. 31.4 EUS, showing dilation of the left intrahepatic bile duct.

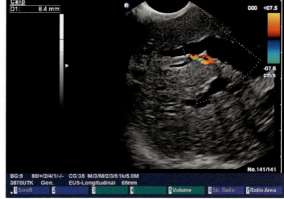

Fig. 31.5 Color Doppler, showing a dilated left intrahepatic duct and the portal vein.

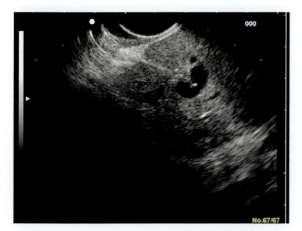

Fig. 31.6 EUS: puncture of the bile duct with a 19-gauge needle.

with biliary obstruction (**Figs. 31.3** and **31.4**). The EUS transducer has to be placed at the level of the cardia.

To reduce the risk of bleeding, puncture should be carried out with color Doppler ultrasound imaging in order to avoid interposed vessels (**Fig. 31.5**). A 19-gauge aspiration needle (EchoTip Ultra Echo-19, Wilson-Cook; EZ Shot 19 G, Olympus Medical) is inserted into the dilated bile duct through the gastric or intestinal wall (**Fig. 31.6**). After removal of the stylet and bile aspiration, contrast medium is injected to obtain a cholangiogram (**Fig. 31.7**). Particularly in patients with Klatskin tumors, complete imaging of the intrahepatic ducts is necessary in order to obtain information about the location of the stenosis or occlusion, the length of the stenosis, the involvement of both ducts, or whether it is possible to reach the duodenum via a guide wire.

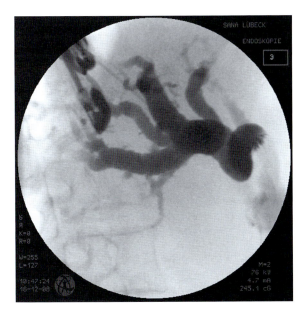

Fig. 31.7 Fluoroscopy: puncture of the left hepatic duct.

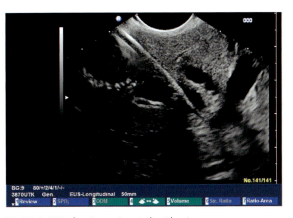

Fig. 31.8 EUS, showing an inserted guide wire.

A 0.035-inch guide wire is inserted into the bile duct via the needle (Hydra Jagwire 0.035, Boston Scientific; Tracer Metro Guide 0.035 inch, Cook-Medical; Nitinol 0.035, MTW). To reduce the risk of wire dislocation, it is recommended to insert as much as possible of the wire into the duct (**Figs. 31.8** and **31.9**). In patients with normal anatomy or Billroth I resection, an attempt should always be made to pass the guide wire into the duodenum across the biliary stricture, with subsequent rendezvous ERCP drainage. In all other cases, the wire is placed at the level of the bile duct bifurcation.

After placement of the guide wire under fluoroscopy, it is often difficult to pass the gastrointestinal wall without dilation of the transmural tract. The tract should therefore be opened with an ERCP cannula or with a needle-knife, cystotome (6 Fr or 8 Fr), bile duct bougie (6 Fr), or a dilating balloon (4–6 mm). If a needle-knife or cystotome is used, electrocoagulation should be strongly limited to the gastrointestinal wall in order to avoid any ultrasound artifacts in the liver parenchyma, which can significantly reduce the ultrasound image quality and may ultimately lead to failure.

A 5–7-cm long, 8.5-Fr or 10-Fr biliary standard plastic stent (**Figs. 31.10** and **31.11**) or a self-expanding covered metal stent (**Figs. 31.12, 31.13,** and **31.14**) (e.g., Wallstent RX biliary endoprosthesis, Boston Scientific; 9 Fr biliary stent, Leufen) is inserted through the gastrointestinal tract into the bile duct. To avoid biliary peritonitis, uncovered metal stents are not recommended.

In principle, two main methods of drainage can be considered:

• Stenting of the stenosis without a fistula between the bile duct and the stomach or intestine. This is preferable

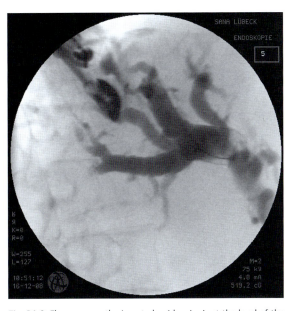

Fig. 31.9 Fluoroscopy: the inserted guide wire is at the level of the bile duct bifurcation.

in patients with normal anatomy and Billroth I resection if the rendezvous maneuver fails.
• Stenting of the fistula between the bile duct and the stomach or intestine without passage of the tumor stenosis. This is preferable in all patients with complete obstruction of the bile duct or after Billroth II resection or gastrectomy.

The final result after stenting should be checked with abdominal ultrasound (**Figs. 31.15** and **31.16**) and laboratory blood tests.

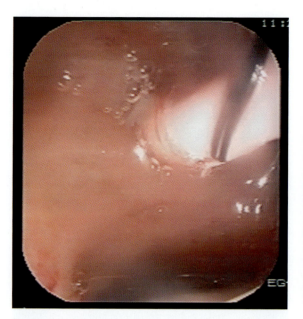

Fig. 31.10 Endoscopic view of the correct positioning of the stent just before the fistulotome is retrieved.

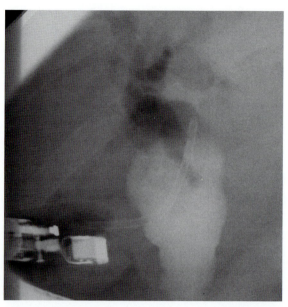

Fig. 31.11 Radiograph showing aerobilia and correct positioning of the stent.

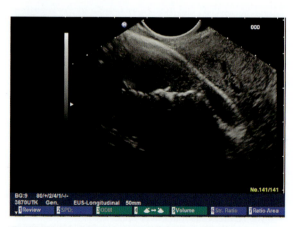

Fig. 31.12 EUS, showing an inserted self-expanding stent.

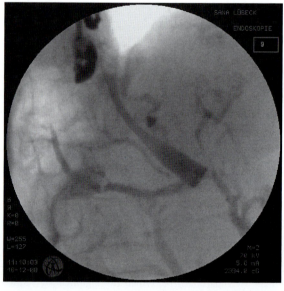

Fig. 31.13 Fluoroscopic image of the inserted metal stent.

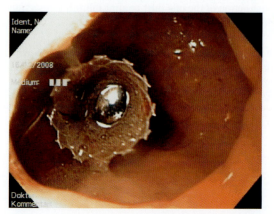

Fig. 31.14 Endoscopy: the distal part of the self-expanding metal biliary stent, at the level of the cardia.

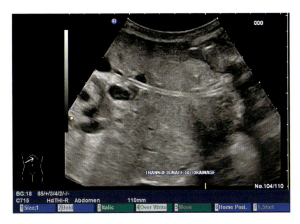

Fig. 31.15 Abdominal ultrasound: a plastic stent has been inserted into the left liver lobe.

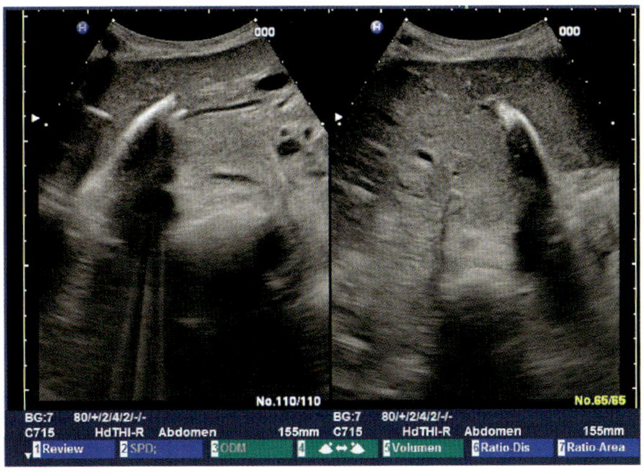

Fig. 31.16 Abdominal ultrasound: a self-expanding metal stent has been inserted into the left liver lobe.

Discussion

EUS is a well-established diagnostic tool in the diagnosis of gastrointestinal wall diseases and in diseases of organs adjacent to the alimentary tract. Linear endoscopic ultrasound has developed from use in interventional diagnostic indications such as EUS-guided fine-needle aspiration (EUS-FNA) to therapeutic interventional EUS-guided indications such as drainage of pancreatic pseudocysts, celiac plexus neurolysis, injections of antitumor agents, and treatment for pancreatic cystic lesions.

In 1996, Wiersema et al.[7] reported the first case of EUS-guided cholangiography. In 2001, Giovannini et al.[8] described the first EUS-guided drainage procedure using a two-step technique in the bile duct in a patient with pancreatic cancer and failed cannulation of the bile duct with ERCP. In 2003, Burmester et al.[9] published four cases of successful EUS-guided cholangiodrainage using a one-step technique, in a modification of the one-step technique described by Seifert et al.[10] for the drainage of pancreatic pseudocysts. In 2004, Mallery et al.[11] reported an EUS-guided rendezvous procedure in three of six patients for biliary and pancreatic stenting. There have been similar reports on successful EUS-guided biliary drainage in malignant diseases, with technical success rates ranging from 90% to 100%, clinical success rates of 75–100%, and a low complication rate (0–18%) in ≈ 100 patients.[12–24,29] The complications observed include pain, bleeding, cholangitis, cholecystitis, bile leakage, biloma, hemobilia, and pneumoperitoneum. Kahaleh et al.[25] in 2006 and Tarantino et al.[26] in 2008 also included benign conditions in which ERCP had failed in their series.

There have as yet been no controlled randomized studies comparing PTBD with EUS-guided biliary drainage. The technique has certain limitations, which need to be noted and discussed. In patients with Billroth II resection and gastrectomy, the procedure can only be used if the left hepatic duct is dilated; patients with isolated obstruction of the right hepatic duct are still candidates for PTBD. Interposed ascites may increase the risk for biliary peritonitis. The procedure is not indicated in patients with coagulopathy, as passage into the liver and dilation of the gastrointestinal tract increases the rate of bleeding. Stent migration is a potentially severe complication, especially if the stent migrates out of the gastrointestinal wall; this is less likely in patients who have undergone surgical resection.

The technical accessories currently available for these interventions need to be improved in order to avoid failures due to insufficient stiffness of the needles when there is a long distance between the wall and the duct, and to reduce the risk of shearing off the covering of the guide wire at the tip of the needle during guide-wire manipulation. Several issues still have to be clarified regarding the best access route, the best methods of dilation, the optimal stent design (plastic or self-expanding metal stents) and replacement procedures. Only a few authors have described repeat interventions, although all reported a high rate of technical success.[17,24,26,29,30]

The published data therefore suggest that the procedure should be restricted to patients with inoperable malignant diseases in whom ERCP has failed, and to centers with a high level of experience in interventional ERCP and EUS.[21,27,28]

Conclusions

Endoscopic ultrasound-guided biliary drainage appears to be a good alternative to PTBD when ERCP has failed in the palliative treatment of patients with malignant biliary obstruction, particularly those who have undergone gastrectomy or Billroth II resection. The main advantage of the technique is the proximity of the transducer to the dilated extrahepatic or intrahepatic duct, which allows direct EUS-guided puncture under color Doppler control and primary internal drainage. One-step EUS-guided drainage with therapeutic linear echoendoscopes is technically feasible and low-risk. As the numbers of patients requiring the treatment can be expected to be low, the procedure should be restricted to centers with a high level of experience in interventional ERCP and EUS.

References

1. Schöfl R. Diagnostic endoscopic retrograde cholangiopancreatography. (review) Endoscopy 2001;33(2):147–157.
2. Fogel EL, Sherman S, Devereaux BM, Lehman GA. Therapeutic biliary endoscopy. (review) Endoscopy 2001; 33(1):31–38.
3. McPherson SJ, Gibson RN, Collier NA, Speer TG, Sherson ND. Percutaneous transjejunal biliary intervention: 10-year experience with access via Roux-en-Y loops. Radiology 1998; 206:665–672.
4. Perry LJ, Stokes KR, Lewis WD, Jenkins RL, Clouse ME. Biliary intervention by means of percutaneous puncture of the antecolic jejunal loop. Radiology 1995;195(1):163–167.
5. Beissert M, Wittenberg G, Sandstede J, et al. Metallic stents and plastic endoprostheses in percutaneous treatment of biliary obstruction. Z Gastroenterol 2002;40(7):503–510.
6. Born P, Rösch T, Sandschin W, Weiss W. Arterial bleeding as an unusual late complication of percutaneous transhepatic biliary drainage. Endoscopy 2003;35(11):978–979.
7. Wiersema MJ, Sandusky D, Carr R, Wiersema LM, Erdel WC, Frederick PK. Endosonography-guided cholangiopancreatography. Gastrointest Endosc 1996;43(2 Pt 1):102–106.
8. Giovannini M, Moutardier V, Pesenti C, Bories E, Lelong B, Delpero JR. Endoscopic ultrasound-guided bilioduodenal anastomosis: a new technique for biliary drainage. Endoscopy 2001;33(10):898–900.
9. Burmester E, Niehaus J, Leineweber T, Huetteroth T. EUS-cholangio-drainage of the bile duct: report of 4 cases. Gastrointest Endosc 2003;57(2):246–251.
10. Seifert H. Interventional therapeutic endosonography: current status. In: Rösch T, Will U, Chang KJ, eds. Longitudinal endosonography. 1st ed. Heidelberg: Springer; 2001: 157–163.
11. Mallery S, Matlock J, Freeman ML. EUS-guided rendezvous drainage of obstructed biliary and pancreatic ducts: Report of 6 cases. Gastrointest Endosc 2004;59(1):100–107.
12. Giovannini M, Dotti M, Bories E, et al. Hepaticogastrostomy by echo-endoscopy as a palliative treatment in a patient with metastatic biliary obstruction. Endoscopy 2003; 35(12):1076–1078.
13. Kahaleh M, Yoshida C, Kane L, Yeaton P. Interventional EUS cholangiography: A report of five cases. Gastrointest Endosc 2004;60(1):138–142.
14. Püspök A, Lomoschitz F, Dejaco C, Hejna M, Sautner T, Gangl A. Endoscopic ultrasound guided therapy of benign and malignant biliary obstruction: a case series. Am J Gastroenterol 2005;100(8):1743–1747.
15. Yamao K, Sawaki A, Takahashi K, Imaoka H, Ashida R, Mizuno N. EUS-guided choledochoduodenostomy for palliative biliary drainage in case of papillary obstruction: report of 2 cases. Gastrointest Endosc 2006;64(4):663–667.
16. Will U, Meyer F, Schmitt W, Dollhopf M. Endoscopic ultrasound-guided transesophageal cholangiodrainage and consecutive endoscopic transhepatic Wallstent insertion into a jejunal stenosis. Scand J Gastroenterol 2007; 42(3): 412–415.
17. Bories E, Pesenti C, Caillol F, Lopes C, Giovannini M. Transgastric endoscopic ultrasonography-guided biliary drainage: results of a pilot study. Endoscopy 2007;39(4): 287–291.
18. Ang TL, Teo EK, Fock KM. EUS-guided transduodenal biliary drainage in unresectable pancreatic cancer with obstructive jaundice. JOP 2007;8(4):438–443.
19. Shami VM, Kahaleh M. Endoscopic ultrasonography (EUS)-guided access and therapy of pancreatico-biliary disorders: EUS-guided cholangio and pancreatic drainage. Gastrointest Endosc Clin N Am 2007;17(3):581–593, vii–viii.
20. Fujita N, Noda Y, Kobayashi G, et al. Histological changes at an endosonography-guided biliary drainage site: a case report. World J Gastroenterol 2007;13(41):5512–5515.
21. Püspök A. Biliary therapy: are we ready for EUS-guidance? Minerva Med 2007;98(4):379–384.
22. Fujita N, Noda Y, Kobayashi G, et al. Temporary endosonography-guided biliary drainage for transgastrointestinal deployment of a self-expandable metallic stent. J Gastroenterol 2008;43(8):637–640.
23. Itoi T, Itokawa F, Sofuni A, et al. Endoscopic ultrasound-guided choledochoduodenostomy in patients with failed endoscopic retrograde cholangiopancreatography. World J Gastroenterol 2008;14(39):6078–6082.
24. Will U. Therapeutic endosonography. [Article in German] Z Gastroenterol 2008;46(6):555–563.
25. Kahaleh M, Hernandez AJ, Tokar J, Adams RB, Shami VM, Yeaton P. Interventional EUS-guided cholangiography: evaluation of a technique in evolution. Gastrointest Endosc 2006;64(1):52–59.
26. Tarantino I, Barresi L, Repici A, Traina M. EUS-guided biliary drainage: a case series. Endoscopy 2008;40(4):336–339.
27. Itoi T, Yamao K; EUS 2008 Working Group. EUS 2008 Working Group document: evaluation of EUS-guided choledochoduodenostomy (with video). Gastrointest Endosc 2009; 69(2, Suppl):S8–S12.
28. Savides T, Varadarajulu S, Palazzo L. EUS 2008 Working Group document: evaluation of EUS-guided hepaticogastrostomy. Gastrointest Endosc 2009;69(2):S8–S12.
29. Yamao K, Bhatia V, Mizuno N, et al. EUS-guided choledochoduodenostomy for palliative biliary drainage in patients with malignant biliary obstruction: results of long-term follow-up. Endoscopy 2008;40(4):340–342.
30. Niehaus J, Burmester E, Leineweber T, Huetteroth T. EUS-cholangio-drainage of the bile duct: report of 4 cases. Gastrointest Endosc 2003;57(2):246–251 .

32 Laparoscopic Ultrasound Scanning

P. Vilmann, C. Ortiz-Moyano

Intraoperative ultrasound scanning has been in use for more than 40 years, and its value for detecting lesions in the pancreas, liver, and retroperitoneum is well documented. During the past 10–15 years, diagnostic laparoscopy and laparoscopic surgery have replaced many of the open procedures. This has led to an increasing need to find a substitute for the tactile feedback that manual palpation provides during open surgery. Recent technology has provided specially designed ultrasound probes that can pass through standard laparoscopic trocars in order to perform intra-abdominal as well as intrathoracic examinations and ultrasound-guided interventions (**Table 32.1**). Laparoscopic ultrasound scanning (LUS) represents a significant technical improvement in diagnostic laparoscopy and therapeutic laparoscopic interventions. This chapter provides a description of the procedure and the instruments used for LUS, with special focus on a new-generation LUS probe designed for LUS-guided interventions, as well as a review of the literature.

Equipment

The dedicated LUS probes currently available use electronic transducers with a linear or convex array mounted on a rigid or a flexible tip on the instrument. Movement of the flexible tip is controlled by a steering wheel located on the instrument's shaft. Depending on the manufacturer, the tip can be moved in either two or four directions (**Table** **32.1**). The frequency is either fixed at 5.0–7.5 MHz or variable, ranging from 4 or 5 MHz to 10 MHz. The new laparoscopic probes have additional features such as power Doppler and color Doppler. This is especially valuable for differentiating between vascular structures and tubular structures in which there is no flow, such as the common bile duct.

Only one manufacturer (B-K Medical, Herlev, Denmark) offers an ultrasound unit that can be fully integrated into the laparoscopic rack. A remote control that operates the different ultrasonic functions is also available from the company. It is of course important for the operator to be able to control the ultrasound features personally instead of having a second person manipulating the ultrasound console. The laparoscopic image and the ultrasound image should preferably be superimposed (picture-in-picture). This option is important, because the movement of the transducer has to be coordinated with the real-time ultrasound image.

Adequate sterilization has been one of the limitations of laparoscopic LUS. The transducers do not tolerate heating to more than 50–55 °C. Until recently, cleaning has therefore either been carried out using disinfection with glutaraldehyde or similar detergents, or alternatively, gas sterilization. Others have used sterile plastic coverings. However, none of these methods has been perfect. Recently, materials have been developed for the probes that allow Sterrad or Sterris sterilization (Advanced Sterilization Products, Irvine, California, USA) without damaging the transducers.

Table 32.1 Laparoscopic ultrasound probes

Manufacturer	Frequency range (MHz)	Shaft diameter (mm)	Color Doppler	Flexible tip	Biopsy facility
ATL	5.0–9.0		Yes	Yes (4-way)	No
Aloka (SSD 1700)	4.0–10.0		Yes	Yes (2-way)	No
Aloka (UST 5222 L-7.5)	7.5	10	No	No	No
B-K Medical (8666)	5.0–10	Fits into a 12-mm port	Yes	Yes (4-way)	Yes
Esaote Biomedica (LP13, AU4)	7.5–10.0	Fits into a 10-mm port	Yes	Yes (4-way)	No
Hitachi	5.0–7.5		Yes	Yes (4-way)	No
Hitachi (EUP-OL531)	5.0–10.0	11.8	Yes	Yes (4-way)	Yes
Siemens (LAP8–4)	4.0–8.0	10	Yes	Yes (4-way)	No
Toshiba	7.0		Yes	Yes (4-way)	No
Toshiba (PVM-787LA)	5.0–9.0	14.8	Yes	No	Yes
Olympus (MH-300)	7.5	?	?	Yes	No

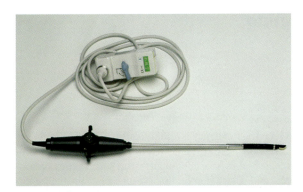

Fig. 32.1 The laparoscopic ultrasound probe without its biopsy covering (Hitachi OL-531).

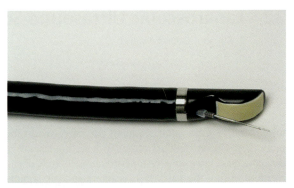

Fig. 32.2 The transducer is electronic, with a scanning angle of 60° and a lateral and slightly oblique forward view.

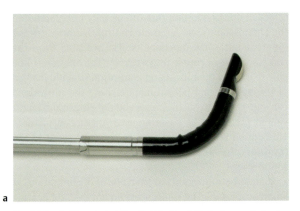

a

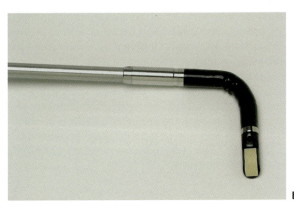

b

Fig. 32.3a, b Mounted at the flexible tip of the instrument, the transducer can be moved 90° up or down and left or right.

The diameter of the probes is up to 1 cm, so that they can be introduced into the abdominal cavity through a standard trocar with a diameter of either 10 mm or 12 mm. There are at present only three manufacturers that provide biopsy facilities with the laparoscopic probe. The B-K probe was the first on the market. The biopsy channel is not fully integrated into the shaft of the probe. A flexible channel passes outside parallel to the probe, ending in a hole near the transducer.[1,2] This means that a needle has to pass a flexible sheath that is not supported by the probe and that the tip of the needle has to be directed into an inlet near the transducer when a biopsy is needed. This maneuver is somewhat cumbersome, and this may be the reason why this procedure has not come into widespread use. The second company offering biopsy facilities with their probe is Toshiba (PVM-787LA). However, this probe is stiff, with a forward-viewing transducer and a diameter of 24 mm.[3] The probe is primarily produced for radiofrequency ablation (RF) of liver lesions. Only one company has the biopsy channel fully integrated into a probe (Hitachi OL-531), with the probe being introduced via a standard trocar (**Fig. 32.1**).

This probe was recently developed by the present author (P.V.) and the Hitachi company in collaboration. It has a diameter of 11.8 mm and fits into a 12-mm port. The total length of the instrument is 67 cm and the length of the insertion tube is 42 cm. The transducer is electronic, with a scanning angle of 60° and a lateral and slightly oblique forward view (**Fig. 32.2**).

The curve radius is 10 mm. The central frequency is 7.5 MHz, with a bandwidth of 5–10 MHz. The transducer mounted at the flexible tip of the instrument can be moved 90° up or down and left or right (**Fig. 32.3**). A removable metal needle cover case around the body of the probe shaft forms a biopsy channel with a diameter of 3.2 mm (**Figs. 32.4** and **32.5**). The biopsy channel can be reduced to 2.4 mm with a mountable inner plastic tube (**Figs. 32.6** and **32.7**), allowing use of a modified 22-gauge or 19-gauge aspiration biopsy needle (SonoTip II, Medi-Globe Ltd., Achenmühle, Germany) (**Fig. 32.8**). When it is not reduced, the biopsy channel allows the introduction of a standard-sized radiofrequency needle. The probe can be connected to a Hitachi ultrasound scanner (EUB-6500 or EUB-8500) with power and color Doppler facilities. The probe can be fully sterilized with Sterrad (H_2O_2 plasma) and ethylene oxide (ETO) gas sterilization.

Laparoscopic ultrasound-guided biopsy has hitherto been a difficult and cumbersome procedure using the

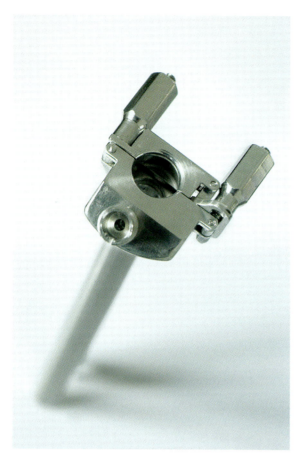

Fig. 32.4 A removable metal needle cover case around the body of the probe shaft forms a biopsy channel with a diameter of 3.2 mm. The image shows a proximal and oblique image of the metal cover, with a view into the biopsy channel inlet.

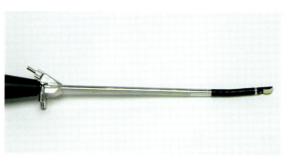

Fig. 32.5 The metal cover is locked onto the probe shaft, and the transducer is ready for a laparoscopic ultrasonic examination with biopsy of a lesion.

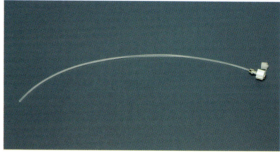

Fig. 32.6 The biopsy channel can be reduced to 2.4 mm with an inner plastic tube.

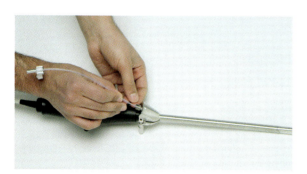

Fig. 32.7 The inner plastic tube being introduced via the inlet on the metal cover.

probes available on the market. The biopsy procedure with the new probe can be performed without difficulty during routine laparoscopic scanning. The probe also allows radiofrequency ablation of hepatic lesions during laparoscopic ultrasound scanning. A needle is at present under construction (the HiTT-Flex monopolar radiofrequency needle, compatible with the Elektrotom HiTT 106 ablation system; Berchtold Ltd., Tuttlingen, Germany) (**Fig. 32.9**). The construction of the new laparoscopic probe for guided interventions is a fresh advance toward minimally invasive procedures for primary diagnosis, staging, and treatment guided by laparoscopic ultrasound scanning.

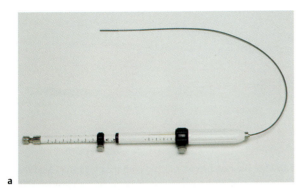

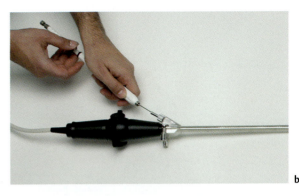

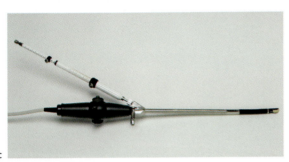

Fig. 32.8a–c a A prototype modified 22-gauge aspiration biopsy needle (SonoTip II, Medi-Globe Ltd., Achenmühle, Germany).
b The needle is introduced via the biopsy inlet of the laparoscopic probe.
c The needle is now mounted on the laparoscopic probe, ready for a biopsy to be taken.

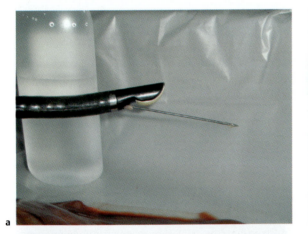

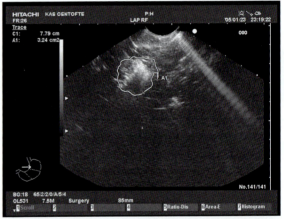

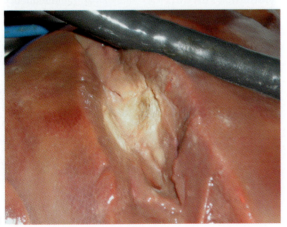

Fig. 32.9a–c The probe also allows radiofrequency ablation of hepatic lesions during laparoscopic ultrasound scanning.
a The radiofrequency needle (HiTT-Flex) has been introduced.
b The image shows the burning effect visible during radiofrequency ablation of the liver in a swine model.
c The necrosis seen after laparoscopic ultrasound-guided radiofrequency ablation in the liver.

Examination Procedure

The procedure is carried out with the patient under general anesthesia. Several examination procedures have been described. The presetting of the image direction is, as usual, with distal to the right and proximal to the left in the ultrasound image. This provides images very similar to the endoscopic ultrasound (EUS) images obtained with linear transducers. The access site for the laparoscope and probe is selected depending on the indications for the examination. Most frequently, a supraumbilical or infraumbilical access site is chosen for the laparoscope itself. Some authors favor access via the right upper abdominal quadrant for the second port when the liver and hepatobiliary region have to be examined. Others use a port in the left upper quadrant. The aim is to obtain good access and to examine the region or organ in question in two directions. This can be accomplished by switching ports between the laparoscope and the probe. For the staging of upper gastrointestinal cancer, the present authors prefer the left upper quadrant and the supraumbilical port (**Fig. 32.10**).

This provides good access to the left liver lobe, the region of the cardia, the hepatoduodenal ligament in a longitudinal scanning direction, and the pancreas in horizontal section. The aorta and the celiac vessels can be seen from the umbilical port, and the right liver lobe can be examined as well. LUS has to be conducted in a systematic way, including all segments of the liver, the hepatoduodenal ligament, and the celiac trunk and superior mesenteric artery. The intra-abdominal examination follows the same principles as transcutaneous ultrasonography.

The images obtained during LUS are frequently excellent, with optimum scanning conditions, due to the close proximity to the intra-abdominal organs (**Fig. 32.11**).

Generally, the contact technique is used to scan solid organs such as the liver. In the upper abdomen, the liver is usually also used as an acoustic window for more deeply located structures. Better image quality is sometimes obtained with indirect scanning through a saline solution. This method improves discrimination of individual wall layers and offers higher resolution in the transducer's focal zone. When the liver is scanned, the transducer is placed directly on the left or right liver lobe. The liver is scanned systematically by moving the probe over all segments while simultaneously following it optically with the laparoscope, manipulated by an assistant (**Fig. 32.12**).

The caudal parts of the liver should be examined from both the anterior and posterior surface. This is important, as small lesions just under the liver capsule can easily be missed due to their close proximity to the transducer. The location, number, and size of hepatic lesions must be

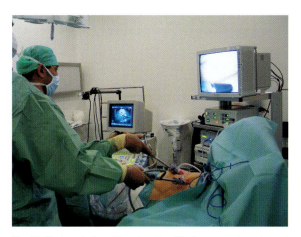

Fig. 32.10 A typical working situation. The laparoscopic probe and the laparoscope have been introduced via two ports. The ultrasound scanner and the laparoscopic rack are seen, and the images are visible simultaneously.

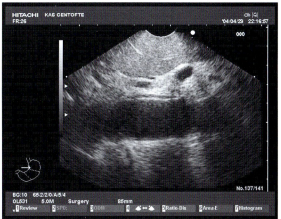

a

b

Fig. 32.11a, b The images obtained during laparoscopic ultrasonography are frequently excellent, with optimum scanning conditions due to close proximity to the intra-abdominal organs.

a A laparoscopic ultrasound image of the aorta with the celiac trunk, seen with color Doppler.
b A view of the aorta with the celiac trunk and the left gastric artery just below part of the left liver lobe.

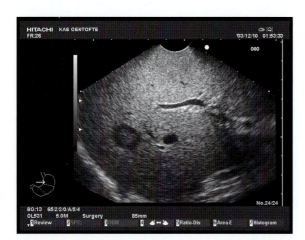

Fig. 32.12 A hepatic metastasis ≈ 10 mm in size in the right liver lobe.

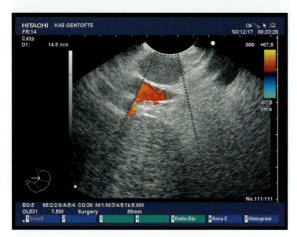

Fig. 32.13 A 14.5-mm hypoechoic lymph node in the retroperitoneum in a patient with gastric cancer.

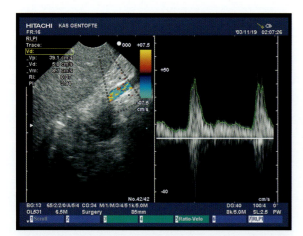

Fig. 32.14 Color Doppler examination is extremely valuable. The image shows a duplex scan of an abdominal vessel with color Doppler, pulsed Doppler, and B-mode scanning.

documented. Relevant anatomic structures such as the portal and hepatic veins and bile ducts can be visualized. The segmental anatomy of the liver can be delineated and the relation of the tumor to these structures allows assessment of the extent of resection and the amount and function of the remaining liver tissue. The structures of the porta hepatis can be best assessed (in longitudinal section) when the probe is introduced through the left subcostal trocar and placed on segment IV of the liver. The distal part of the common bile duct is identified by positioning the transducer directly on the hepatoduodenal ligament. The stomach can be visualized by direct-contact scanning, or using the liver as an acoustic window. Acoustic shadowing of the posterior wall of the stomach and the pancreas can be avoided by aspiration of air and if necessary instillation of 300–500 mL saline solution through a nasogastric tube into the stomach. The branches of the celiac axis, portal vein, superior mesenteric artery, and aorta are displayed in transverse sections from the left subcostal trocar. Lymph nodes along these vessels are classified in accordance with the TNM classification (**Fig. 32.13**).

Metastatic lymph-node involvement is characterized by a hypoechoic pattern, round shape, and well-delineated boundaries. Color Doppler examinations can be helpful in delineating the vascular anatomy and distinguishing vessels from lymph nodes (**Fig. 32.14**).

Biopsy of lymph nodes is always relevant if a biopsy confirming malignancy will alter the management of the patient.

Biopsy Procedure

Until recently, LUS-guided biopsy was if not impossible, then at least cumbersome. The needle had to be introduced through the anterior abdominal wall, and freehand guidance of the transducer had to be used.[4–6] Alternatively, as with the B-K probe, the needle has to pass through an exterior floppy biopsy sheath before the biopsy maneuver is started.[2,7] With the new LUS probe from Hitachi, the procedure has become simple and easy. After a lesion is outlined, the needle is simply introduced via the biopsy inlet of the probe and firmly connected to the Luer-lock biopsy inlet (see **Fig. 32.8b**, **c**). The stylet is withdrawn a few millimeters. The needle can then be advanced under ultrasound guidance directly into the lesion (**Fig. 32.15a**). The stylet is removed completely, and a vacuum is applied to the needle. To-and-fro movements are made, still with ultrasound guidance (**Fig. 32.15b–e**).

The entire biopsy instrument is then removed, and the material is expelled onto glass slides and smeared for cytological evaluation. At present, only needles for fine-needle biopsy have been developed for this probe, but a Tru-Cut histological needle is commercially available for the B-K probe. It is only a matter of time before a histo-

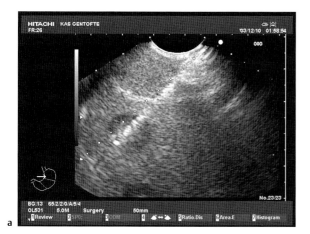

a

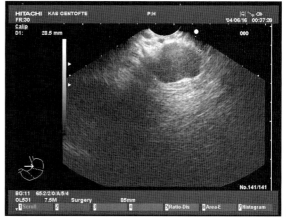

b

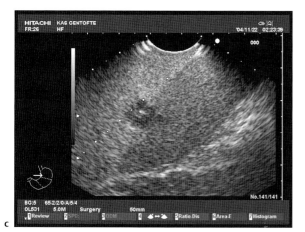

c

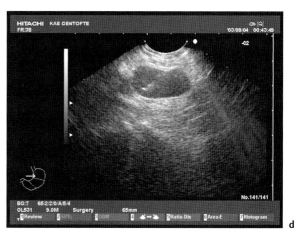

d

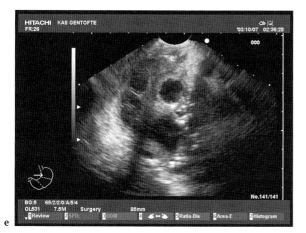

e

Fig. 32.15a–e The biopsy needle is introduced and a guided biopsy of a hepatic metastasis is taken.

a Note the deflections from the needle just below the needle guide line.

b A suspicious hypoechoic lesion in the left adrenal gland in a patient with gastric cancer. The laparoscopic ultrasound (LUS)-guided biopsy revealed malignant cells, and the patient was ultimately staged as having incurable disease (M1).

c LUS-guided biopsy of a hypoechoic hepatic metastasis 7 mm in size.

d LUS-guided biopsy of an enlarged suspicious lymph node in the retroperitoneum in a patient with cancer of the gastric cardia.

e A cystic neoplasm in the tail of the pancreas. The biopsy confirmed malignancy. The multiple cysts inside the solid tumor are notable.

logical needle becomes available for the Hitachi probe as well. In a single case in which fine-needle biopsy was not sufficient, the authors used the Tru-Cut needle designed for the B-K probe together with the OL-531 probe (**Fig. 32.16**). However, it should be emphasized that for safety reasons this is not at present recommended before a dedicated histological needle has been manufactured (the main risk being transducer damage).

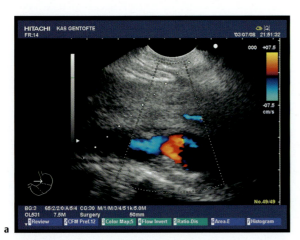
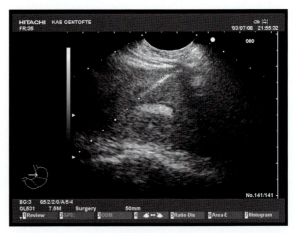

Fig. 32.16a, b A laparoscopic ultrasound (LUS) image in a patient with retroperitoneal fibrosis.
a There is a hypoechoic, thickened rim of fibrosis compressing the aorta, seen in color Doppler mode.

b An LUS-guided histological needle biopsy was taken, demonstrating fibrosis.

Review of the Literature

■ Staging of Gastrointestinal Cancers

Patients with upper gastrointestinal cancer frequently present at an advanced stage of the disease in which curative treatment is not possible. The prognosis in gastrointestinal cancer is poor, but it is closely related to the TNM stage of the tumor. It is therefore mandatory to evaluate the preoperative stage carefully to avoid unnecessary and futile surgery in patients with disseminated disease, and to select patients with locally advanced disease who may benefit from neoadjuvant chemoradiotherapy before surgical resection.

Endoscopic ultrasound scanning has proved to be significantly more accurate for assessing the TN staging preoperatively in comparison with transabdominal ultrasonography, computed tomography (CT), and magnetic resonance imaging (MRI). However, the method has some limitations. EUS is not capable of detecting metastases in the right liver lobe, superficial liver metastases, or peritoneal carcinosis. In addition, if impassable stenotic tumors are present in the esophagus or stomach, the staging evaluation is insufficient.

Laparoscopy in combination with LUS has been shown to allow excellent staging and resectability evaluation of gastrointestinal cancers in comparison with other imaging modalities such as CT, transabdominal ultrasound, and MRI. This superiority has been thoroughly documented, and if LUS is combined with EUS, the rate of futile operations such as unnecessary exploratory laparotomy can be reduced from 30–40% down to less than 5%.[8–11]

There appears to be some variance in the clinical impact of LUS staging depending on the cancer evaluated.[12] According to van Dijkum et al.,[12] in a study including more than 400 patients, laparoscopic staging avoided laparotomy in 20% of the patients: 5% of those with an esophageal tumor, 20% of those with a gastroesophageal junction tumor, 15% of those with a periampullary tumor, 40% of those with a proximal bile duct tumor, 35% of those with a liver tumor, and 40% of those with a pancreatic body or tail tumor.

■ LUS in Esophagogastric Cancer

The presence of liver metastases, malignant ascites, or peritoneal carcinosis and specific cases of invasion of adjacent organs (stage T4) in patients with esophageal and gastric cancer are in most centers regarded as a contraindication for major surgical resections. Laparoscopy with laparoscopic ultrasound scanning has been shown to add significant staging information to the preoperative evaluation of patients with cancer of the stomach and gastric cardia, whereas the added value in patients with cancer of the middle and upper esophagus is more limited.[13–16] The reported accuracy of LUS in the evaluation of resectability is in the range of 50–100%.[9–11] The impact on therapy is such that laparotomies can be avoided in 25–63% of patients examined with LUS.[9,12–17] In many of the publications, LUS-guided biopsy was not possible.[15] Our own results with the new LUS probe show that LUS-guided biopsy adds significant staging information.[69] Of a total of 175 patients with esophagogastric cancer undergoing LUS, 19 (11%) underwent LUS-guided FNA after a significant lesion was found. The LUS-guided FNA confirmed distant metastasis in 14 of the 19 patients, resulting in a change of the clinical management for these 14 patients (8%). There were no adverse effects due to LUS or LUS-guided FNA.

Table 32.2 Laparoscopy and laparoscopic ultrasonography in the staging of regional and distant metastases in esophageal, gastric, and cardia carcinoma

First author (ref.)	Lesion	Location	Patients (n)	Sensitivity (%)	Specificity (%)	Accuracy (%)
Stein 1997[13]	Esophagus and cardia	Celiac axis	127	67	92	
Romijn 1998[15]	Esophagus and cardia	Distant metastases	60	81	100	
Hulscher 2000[14]	Gastric cardia	Distant metastases	48	79		
Lavonius 2002[18]	Gastric tumors	Distant metastases	37	63	100	83

Table 32.3 Studies combining laparoscopy and laparoscopic ultrasonography to assess unresectability in pancreatic and ampullary tumors

First author (ref.)	Patients (n)	Sensitivity (%)	Specificity (%)	PPV (%)	NPV (%)	Accuracy (%)
Durup Scheel-Hincke 1999[9]	35	86	100	100	80	
Minnard 1998[25]	90	98	100	100	98	
Merchant and Conlon 1998[29]	90	91		100	98	
Catheline 1999[24]	26	94				80.7
Pietrabissa 1999[27a]	50	94	80			87
Jimenez 2000[30]	125	97				
Schachter 2000[20]	67	100	88	89	100	
Menack 2001[22]	27	77	100	100	90	
Taylor 2001[26]	51	67	100	100	91	92

[a] Vascular invasion. NPV, negative predictive value; PPV, positive predictive value.

In a large study by Stein et al.,[13] laparoscopy and LUS yielded a 24% rate of relevant new findings not seen with standard preoperative staging modalities in patients with cancer of the esophagus or cardia. Laparoscopy including LUS is at present considered mandatory in the preoperative staging evaluation of patients with locally advanced carcinoma of the distal esophagus or gastroesophageal junction who are being considered for neoadjuvant therapy or primary resection (**Table 32.2**).[13–15,18]

■ LUS in Pancreatic Cancer

Carcinoma of the pancreas is associated with a dismal prognosis, with an overall 5-year survival rate of ≈ 5%. At the time of diagnosis, pancreatic cancer is a disseminated disease in the majority of cases. Pancreatic cancer either spreads by invading adjacent structures and organs, or sends metastases to the lymph nodes, peritoneum, liver, or lungs. The only chance of cure is surgery. Exact staging prior to treatment decisions is therefore paramount in order to avoid futile laparotomies in incurable patients. A variety of image modalities are at present available in the evaluation of pancreatic cancer. However, none of these is sufficiently accurate as single methods. To date, dynamic contrast-enhanced CT has been the preoperative imaging modality of choice. However, when CT is used in the evaluation of resectability, about half of the patients undergo exploratory surgery because disseminated disease is detected, preventing radical resection. The sensitivity and positive predictive value of CT in defining resectability are only 75% and 38%, respectively.[19] Improvements in assessing resectability are seen when laparoscopy is used, and 24–40% of patients deemed to have resectable disease at CT have been demonstrated to have incurable disease at laparoscopy. Endoscopic ultrasound scanning appears to be comparable to multiple-slice CT in the evaluation of vascular infiltration, but may be preferable due to the biopsy facilities available if disseminated disease is outlined, either in the form of suspicious lymph nodes or small liver metastases. LUS has been shown to improve pancreatic carcinoma staging over laparoscopy alone, providing additional surgical information in 14–25% of cases.[20–28] In a study by Taylor et al.[26] including 51 patients, LUS prevented unnecessary extensive surgery in 53% of patients deemed resectable by CT. Another study in 214 patients[12] showed that LUS resulted in a change in the decision regarding surgical intervention in 40% of the patients.

LUS has also been shown to be valuable for the detection of insulinomas, with subsequent laparoscopic resection or enucleation.[28]

There is no doubt that LUS represents an advance in the evaluation of pancreatic lesions (**Table 32.3**).[9,20,22,24–30]

Table 32.4 Diagnostic values for laparoscopic ultrasonography for detecting bile duct calculi during laparoscopic cholecystectomy

First author (ref.)	Patients (n)	Sensitivity (%)	Specificity (%)	PPV (%)	NPV (%)
Birth 1998[35]	518	83.3	100	100	99.2
Thompson 1998[36]	360	90	100	100	98.4
Machi 1999[37]	100	88.9	100	100	98.9
Kimura 1999[38]	184	82.4	100		
Siperstein 1999[39]	300	96.2	100	100	99.6
Tranter 2001[40]	367	92	100	100	98
Tranter 2003[41]	135	96	100	100	98
Catheline 2002[42]	900	80	99	89	99

NPV, negative predictive value; PPV, positive predictive value.

LUS in Colonic Cancer

Laparoscopic colectomy has developed rapidly as a minimally invasive method in colonic surgery, reducing the stress response usually seen after an open surgical procedure. However, one of the limitations of laparoscopy is the inability to palpate organs and tissue with this modality. LUS has been described as the only real alternative to manual exploration.[31–34] Despite full preoperative staging with transabdominal ultrasound and CT, intraoperative ultrasonography has been shown to find additional liver metastases in 10–30% of patients with cancer of the colon. Theoretically, LUS should therefore be able to add valuable staging information in patients scheduled for laparoscopic colonic resection. Several studies have focused on LUS in the detection of liver metastases in patients with colonic cancer, but only one study has evaluated the role of LUS in the complete TNM staging of colorectal cancer.[31] In the study by Goletti et al.,[31] the therapeutic program was changed thanks to laparoscopy and LUS in 33% of cases. The added value of LUS was 12%. The accuracy of T staging was 97%. LUS had a sensitivity in the detection of hepatic metastases of 100%, compared with 63% and 75% with preoperative radiographic methods and laparoscopy, respectively. Nodal metastases were diagnosed with a sensitivity of 94%, compared with 18% in preoperative staging and 6% with laparoscopy, but the method had a low specificity of 53% and an overall accuracy of 72%—comparable with the evaluation of lymph-node metastases with EUS imaging in most other gastrointestinal cancers. However, no LUS-guided biopsies were taken, and this might potentially change the low specificity obtained with imaging alone, as when EUS-guided fine-needle aspiration is used in upper gastrointestinal cancers.

LUS in Gallstone Disease

Intraoperative cholangiography (IOC) has traditionally been used to detect choledocholithiasis during open and laparoscopic cholecystectomy. An additional benefit of IOC is the definition of the biliary anatomy it provides, which makes it possible to detect anomalies and potentially avoid bile duct injury during surgery. However, there are some limitations with the method, and IOC is not possible in several situations, either due to contraindications (e.g., pregnancy) or difficult cannulations.[24] Several studies have been published describing the value of LUS in the detection of stones in the common bile duct (**Table 32.4**).[35–45] The sensitivity of the method for detecting common bile duct (CBD) stones lies in the range of 80–96% (**Table 32.4**). According to the studies, LUS is comparable with IOC and as such may replace or at least be able to serve as an adjunct to IOC in the evaluation of the biliary tree during laparoscopic cholecystectomy.

In a large prospective study including 900 patients,[42] the combination of IOC and LUS was found to have a sensitivity of 95% and a specificity of 98%. In another prospective, single-blinded study[41] including 135 patients, the bile ducts were satisfactorily identified using LUS and IOC in 131 and 121 cases, respectively. The sensitivity of LUS for detecting CBD stones was 96%, in comparison with 86% with IOC, while the specificity values were 100% and 99%, respectively. In a randomized comparative study in 518 patients, the overall accuracy of LUS for identifying unsuspected CBD stones was 99.2%, in comparison with 98.9% with IOC.[35] The conclusion of these studies is that LUS is equal to or superior to IOC for detecting CBD stones during laparoscopic cholecystectomy. An additional benefit of LUS is that the time required for the procedure is approximately half of that needed for IOC.[35,37]

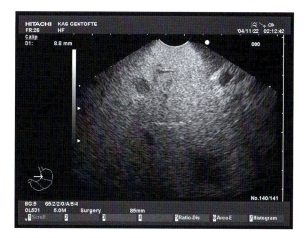

Fig. 32.17 A small hepatic metastasis detected during a staging procedure. The lesion had not been seen with conventional image modalities before the LUS examination. The LUS-guided biopsy revealed malignant cells.

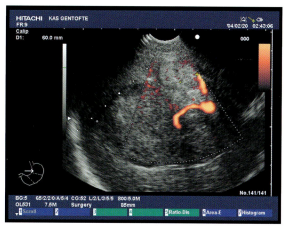

Fig. 32.18 Color Doppler examination of a 6-cm malignant tumor in the right lobe of the liver.

Table 32.5 Diagnostic values for laparoscopic ultrasonography in assessing the resectability of primary liver tumors and metastases

First author (ref.)	Lesions	Patients (n)	Sensitivity (%)	Specificity (%)	Accuracy (%)
Callery 1997[46]	HBP malignancies	50	96	92	
Barbot 1997[47]	Liver tumors	23	100	40	
Rahusen 1999[33]	Colorectal cancer and lesions in the liver	50	89		
Jarnagin 2001[48]	HBP malignancies	186	97		
Lo 2000[49]	HCC	184	59.6	100	89.4
Milsom 2000[32]	Colorectal cancer and lesions in the liver	77	95		

HBP, hepatobiliary and pancreatic; HCC, hepatocellular carcinoma.

■ LUS in Liver Disease

The use of LUS to examine the liver has become an important part of surgical oncology, especially for the screening of metastatic lesions (**Fig. 32.17**). In patients in whom there is already a known liver malignancy, whether primary or metastatic, however, LUS has also been effective in detecting previously unrecognized additional malignant foci within the hepatic parenchyma (**Fig. 32.18**). In patients scheduled for liver resection, LUS can detect possible unresectability or incurability and thereby avoid futile laparotomies (**Table 32.5**).[32,33,46–57] In addition to this, LUS is used to guide the surgical procedure. Limited hepatic resections are possible laparoscopically, and LUS can be helpful in locating the lesion and confirming resectability, as well as during the resection. In recent years, the indications for the resection of hepatic metastases have changed toward a more aggressive approach, with local or segmental resection for multiple lesions even in patients with bilobar disease. A better understanding of liver anatomy and familiarity with intraoperative ultrasonography has led to a practical, segment-oriented approach to hepatic resections.[52] The use of local ablation techniques such

as radiofrequency ablation and microwave ablation may further extend the options for curative surgical treatment.

In a study by de Castro et al.[52] including 84 patients with 33 primary liver tumors and 51 secondary liver tumors, resectability was correctly predicted with LUS in 72 % of the patients. LUS found additional lesions not seen on preoperative CT in 36 % of the patients with primary liver malignancies. Additional lesions were found with LUS in 25 % of patients with secondary liver malignancies.

In a study by Montorsi et al.[58] including 68 patients with primary liver cancer, additional information was found in 57 %, including new hepatocellular cancer nodules in different hepatic segments and an adrenal metastasis in 22 % of the cases. In another study by Foroutani et al.,[51] LUS detected all 201 tumors seen on preoperative CT and detected 21 additional lesions in 11 patients. It appears from this study that small lesions in particular are liable to be overlooked with CT. In a study by Lo et al.,[49] the addition of LUS avoided exploratory laparotomies in 31 of 52 patients (60 %) with unresectable disease that had not been detected in preoperative studies.

LUS has also been reported to be helpful in the detection and subsequent management of hepatic cysts with laparoscopic deroofing.[57]

◼ Miscellaneous Applications of LUS

LUS has also been used in gynecological, urological, laparoscopic, and thoracoscopic procedures.[59–61] Laparoscopic surgery is increasingly being used in the management of patients with gynecologic malignancies.[59,60] LUS can be used either to detect ovarian tumors during laparoscopy, to assist with the surgical resection, or to localize pelvic and para-aortic lymph nodes in patients with cervical carcinomas. In a study by Cheung et al.,[60] the sensitivity and specificity of LUS in detecting pelvic lymph-node metastases were 91% and 100%, respectively. The authors concluded that the LUS procedure was simple, easy to learn, and highly sensitive.

In urology, LUS appears to be a promising adjunct to four current procedures: difficult pelvic lymphocele marsupialization, renal cyst decortications, nephrolithotomy and other forms of renal stone surgery, and cryotherapy or radiofrequency therapy of renal masses.[61]

The role of ultrasound scanning during video-assisted thoracic surgery has been evaluated in a study by Piolanti et al.[62] Thoracoscopic ultrasonography was performed with an LUS probe in 35 patients in order to localize pulmonary nodules suspected of malignancy. In 37 of 40 lesions (sensitivity 93%), ultrasonography was able to locate lesions preoperatively detected by CT. In addition, ultrasonography also located two nodules not visualized with helical CT. Eighteen nodules were not visible or palpable at the thoracoscopic examination and were only identified with thoracoscopic ultrasonography. Further studies are needed before final conclusions can be drawn.

◼ LUS-Guided Therapy

LUS-guided therapy has been primarily reported in the treatment of hepatic lesions such as primary hepatocellular carcinomas (HCC) and hepatic metastases. The treatment options have been either ethanol injection, microwave coagulation, cryoablation, or radiofrequency ablation.[63–68] Most authors prefer radiofrequency ablation, due to the potentially larger coagulation size. Patients treated with radiofrequency ablation have long-term survival rates that are comparable to those in patients treated with hepatectomy. Although most of the patients can be treated percutaneously, there are some cases in which percutaneous ultrasound guidance is not appropriate. Laparoscopic access allows easier detection and more accurate targeting of the tumor in comparison with percutaneous access and can minimize complications. It is therefore an attractive treatment modality for localized hepatocellular carcinoma and hepatic metastases. In addition, the method is favorable in terms of the length of hospital stay and with regard to cost-effectiveness, as it is completed in a single session.[65] Lesions located in the sub-

phrenic area of hepatic segment VIII (right posterior medial segment) or segment III (left anterior lateral segment) may often be difficult to demonstrate using percutaneous ultrasonography. Tumors located adjacent to the gallbladder may cause serious complications when treated percutaneously. Caution may be required with other tumors located on the surface of the liver or protruding from the liver surface in order to avoid injuring the peritoneum or adjacent organs. Although a laparoscopic approach for local ablation plays an important role in treating hepatic lesions near the liver surface, precise targeting of ablation has been difficult using conventional linear ultrasound probes. One problem has been the lack of LUS probes with proper needle-guiding facilities. Most studies of LUS-guided radiofrequency ablation have therefore used an indirect method of guidance, with needle insertion via a route different from that of the LUS probe.

In a study by Noguchi et al.[67] including 51 patients with HCC, the survival after treatment with laparoscopic ablation was 95.2% after 1 year and 82.4% after 3 years. The tumor stage was a significant prognostic factor ($P < 0.0001$). There were no local recurrences within 6 months of the treatment in the successfully treated patients.

In another study by Machi et al.[66] including 46 patients, both hepatic metastases and HCCs were treated using percutaneous (81 lesions), laparoscopic (14 lesions), and open surgical approaches (109 lesions). Local tumor recurrence at the radiofrequency ablation site was diagnosed in 18 of 204 tumors (8.8%) during a mean follow-up period of 20.5 months. The risk factors for local recurrence included large tumor size and major vessel invasion. The recurrence rates for tumors less than 4 cm, 4–10 cm, and over 10 cm, and for those with vascular invasion, were 3.3%, 14.7%, 50%, and 47.8%, respectively. Ten of 18 tumors recurring locally were re-treated with radiofrequency ablation, and eight of them showed no further recurrence. The authors concluded that ultrasound-guided radiofrequency ablation is a relatively safe, well-tolerated, and versatile treatment option that offers excellent local control of primary and metastatic liver tumors. The appropriate use of percutaneous, laparoscopic, and open surgical radiofrequency ablation is beneficial in the management of patients with liver tumors in a variety of situations.

There appears to be a clear need for safe and accurate needle guidance during LUS in patients with liver lesions. We have tested the Hitachi LUS probe (OL-531) with a semiflexible radiofrequency needle in a porcine model and were able to insert the needle via the channel without any problems and to create a coagulation necrosis (see **Fig. 32.9**). Other needle systems are currently being developed, and it is expected that LUS-guided radiofrequency ablation of liver lesions will become a standard option as a minimally invasive approach in a selected group of patients with malignant liver lesions in the near future.

References

1. Mortensen MB, Durup J, Pless T, et al. Initial experience with new dedicated needles for laparoscopic ultrasound-guided fine-needle aspiration and histological biopsies. Endoscopy 2001;33(7):585–589.

2. Durup Scheel-Hincke J, Mortensen MB, Pless T, Hovendal CP. Laparoscopic four-way ultrasound probe with histologic biopsy facility using a flexible tru-cut needle. Surg Endosc 2000;14(9):867–869.

3. Hozumi M, Ido K, Hiki S, et al. Easy and accurate targeting of deep-seated hepatic tumors under laparoscopy with a forward-viewing convex-array transducer. Surg Endosc 2003; 17(8):1256–1260.

4. Santambrogio R, Podda M, Zuin M, et al. Safety and efficacy of laparoscopic radiofrequency ablation of hepatocellular carcinoma in patients with liver cirrhosis. Surg Endosc 2003;17(11):1826–1832.

5. Berber E, Garland AM, Engle KL, Rogers SJ, Siperstein AE. Laparoscopic ultrasonography and biopsy of hepatic tumors in 310 patients. Am J Surg 2004;187(2):213–218.

6. Ido K, Nakazawa Y, Isoda N, et al. The role of laparoscopic US and laparoscopic US-guided aspiration biopsy in the diagnosis of multicentric hepatocellular carcinoma. Gastrointest Endosc 1999;50(4):523–526.

7. Mortensen MB, Durup J, Pless T, et al. Initial experience with new dedicated needles for laparoscopic ultrasound-guided fine-needle aspiration and histological biopsies. Endoscopy 2001;33(7):585–589.

8. Rau B, Hünerbein M, Schlag PM. Is there additional information from laparoscopic ultrasound in tumor staging? Dig Surg 2002;19(6):479–483.

9. Durup Scheel-Hincke J, Mortensen MB, Pless T, Hovendal CP. Laparoscopic ultrasonography—a method for staging of upper gastrointestinal cancer. Eur J Ultrasound 1999; 9(2): 177–184.

10. Olsen AK, Bjerkeset OA. Laparoscopic ultrasound (LUS) in gastrointestinal surgery. Eur J Ultrasound 1999;10(2-3):159–170.

11. Tang CN, Siu WT, Ka-Wah-Li M. Use of diagnostic laparoscopy and laparoscopic ultrasound in the management of upper gastrointestinal malignancy. Ann Coll Surg HK 2001;5:19–24.

12. Nieveen van Dijkum EJ, de Wit LT, van Delden OM, et al. Staging laparoscopy and laparoscopic ultrasonography in more than 400 patients with upper gastrointestinal carcinoma. J Am Coll Surg 1999;189(5):459–465.

13. Stein HJ, Kraemer SJ, Feussner H, Fink U, Siewert JR. Clinical value of diagnostic laparoscopy with laparoscopic ultrasound in patients with cancer of the esophagus or cardia. J Gastrointest Surg 1997;1(2):167–172, discussion 72–73.

14. Hulscher JB, Nieveen van Dijkum EJ, de Wit LT, et al. Laparoscopy and laparoscopic ultrasonography in staging carcinoma of the gastric cardia. Eur J Surg 2000;166(11):862–865.

15. Romijn MG, van Overhagen H, Spillenaar Bilgen EJ, Ijzermans JN, Tilanus HW, Laméris JS. Laparoscopy and laparoscopic ultrasonography in staging of oesophageal and cardial carcinoma. Br J Surg 1998;85(7):1010–1012.

16. Flett ME, Lim MN, Bruce D, Campbell SH, Park KG. Prognostic value of laparoscopic ultrasound in patients with gastroesophageal cancer. Dis Esophagus 2001;14(3-4):223–226.

17. Tsioulias GJ, Wood TF, Chung MH, Morton DL, Bilchik A. Diagnostic laparoscopy and laparoscopic ultrasonography optimize the staging and resectability of intraabdominal neoplasms. Surg Endosc 2001;15(9):1016–1019.

18. Lavonius MI, Gullichsen R, Salo S, Sonninen P, Ovaska J. Staging of gastric cancer: a study with spiral computed tomography, ultrasonography, laparoscopy, and laparoscopic ultrasonography. Surg Laparosc Endosc Percutan Tech 2002;12(2):77–81.

19. Giger U, Schäfer M, Krähenbühl L. Technique and value of staging laparoscopy. Dig Surg 2002;19(6):473–478.

20. Schachter PP, Avni Y, Shimonov M, Gvirtz G, Rosen A, Czerniak A. The impact of laparoscopy and laparoscopic ultrasonography on the management of pancreatic cancer. Arch Surg 2000;135(11):1303–1307.

21. Kwon AH, Inui H, Kamiyama Y. Preoperative laparoscopic examination using surgical manipulation and ultrasonography for pancreatic lesions. Endoscopy 2002;34(6): 464–468.

22. Menack MJ, Spitz JD, Arregui ME. Staging of pancreatic and ampullary cancers for resectability using laparoscopy with laparoscopic ultrasound. Surg Endosc 2001;15(10): 1129–1134.

23. Koler AJ, Lilly MC, Arregui ME. Suprapancreatic and periportal lymph nodes are normally larger than 1 cm by laparoscopic ultrasound evaluation. Surg Endosc 2004;18(4): 646–649.

24. Catheline JM, Turner R, Rizk N, Barrat C, Champault G. The use of diagnostic laparoscopy supported by laparoscopic ultrasonography in the assessment of pancreatic cancer. Surg Endosc 1999;13(3):239–245.

25. Minnard EA, Conlon KC, Hoos A, Dougherty EC, Hann LE, Brennan MF. Laparoscopic ultrasound enhances standard laparoscopy in the staging of pancreatic cancer. Ann Surg 1998;228(2):182–187.

26. Taylor AM, Roberts SA, Manson JM. Experience with laparoscopic ultrasonography for defining tumour resectability in carcinoma of the pancreatic head and periampullary region. Br J Surg 2001;88(8):1077–1083.

27. Pietrabissa A, Caramella D, Di Candio G, et al. Laparoscopy and laparoscopic ultrasonography for staging pancreatic cancer: critical appraisal. World J Surg 1999;23(10): 998–1002, discussion 1003.

28. Jaroszewski DE, Schlinkert RT, Thompson GB, Schlinkert DK. Laparoscopic localization and resection of insulinomas. Arch Surg 2004;139(3):270–274.

29. Merchant NB, Conlon KC. Laparoscopic evaluation in pancreatic cancer. Semin Surg Oncol 1998;15(3):155–165.

30. Jimenez RE, Warshaw AL, Fernandez-Del Castillo C. Laparoscopy and peritoneal cytology in the staging of pancreatic cancer. J Hepatobiliary Pancreat Surg 2000;7(1):15–20.

31. Goletti O, Celona G, Galatioto C, et al. Is laparoscopic sonography a reliable and sensitive procedure for staging colorectal cancer? A comparative study. Surg Endosc 1998; 12(10):1236–1241.

32. Milsom JW, Jerby BL, Kessler H, Hale JC, Herts BR, O'Malley CM. Prospective, blinded comparison of laparoscopic ultrasonography vs. contrast-enhanced computerized tomography for liver assessment in patients undergoing colorectal carcinoma surgery. Dis Colon Rectum 2000;43(1):44–49.

33. Rahusen FD, Cuesta MA, Borgstein PJ, et al. Selection of patients for resection of colorectal metastases to the liver using diagnostic laparoscopy and laparoscopic ultrasonography. Ann Surg 1999;230(1):31–37.

34. Hartley JE, Kumar H, Drew PJ, et al. Laparoscopic ultrasound for the detection of hepatic metastases during laparoscopic colorectal cancer surgery. Dis Colon Rectum 2000; 43(3): 320–324, discussion 324–325.

35. Birth M, Ehlers KU, Delinikolas K, Weiser HF. Prospective randomized comparison of laparoscopic ultrasonography

using a flexible-tip ultrasound probe and intraoperative dynamic cholangiography during laparoscopic cholecystectomy. Surg Endosc 1998;12(1):30–36.

36. Thompson DM, Arregui ME, Tetik C, Madden MT, Wegener M. A comparison of laparoscopic ultrasound with digital fluorocholangiography for detecting choledocholithiasis during laparoscopic cholecystectomy. Surg Endosc 1998; 12(7):929–932.

37. Machi J, Tateishi T, Oishi AJ, et al. Laparoscopic ultrasonography versus operative cholangiography during laparoscopic cholecystectomy: review of the literature and a comparison with open intraoperative ultrasonography. J Am Coll Surg 1999;188(4):360–367.

38. Kimura T, Umehara Y, Yoshida M, Sakuramachi S, Kawabe A, Suzuki K. Laparoscopic ultrasonography and operative cholangiography prevent residual common bile duct stones in laparoscopic cholecystectomy. Surg Laparosc Endosc Percutan Tech 1999;9(2):124–128.

39. Siperstein A, Pearl J, Macho J, Hansen P, Gitomirsky A, Rogers S. Comparison of laparoscopic ultrasonography and fluorocholangiography in 300 patients undergoing laparoscopic cholecystectomy. Surg Endosc 1999;13(2): 113–117.

40. Tranter SE, Thompson MH. Potential of laparoscopic ultrasonography as an alternative to operative cholangiography in the detection of bile duct stones. Br J Surg 2001; 88(1): 65–69.

41. Tranter SE, Thompson MH. A prospective single-blinded controlled study comparing laparoscopic ultrasound of the common bile duct with operative cholangiography. Surg Endosc 2003;17(2):216–219.

42. Catheline JM, Turner R, Paries J. Laparoscopic ultrasonography is a complement to cholangiography for the detection of choledocholithiasis at laparoscopic cholecystectomy. Br J Surg 2002;89(10):1235–1239.

43. Kelly SB, Remedios D, Lau WY, Li AK. Laparoscopic ultrasonography during laparoscopic cholecystectomy. Surg Endosc 1997;11(1):67–70.

44. Santambrogio R, Bianchi P, Opocher E, Verga M, Montorsi M. Prevalence and laparoscopic ultrasound patterns of choledocholithiasis and biliary sludge during cholecystectomy. Surg Laparosc Endosc Percutan Tech 1999;9(2): 129–134.

45. Catheline JM, Turner R, Rizk N, Barrat C, Buenos P, Champault G. Evaluation of the biliary tree during laparoscopic cholecystectomy: laparoscopic ultrasound versus intraoperative cholangiography: a prospective study of 150 cases. Surg Laparosc Endosc 1998;8(2):85–91.

46. Callery MP, Strasberg SM, Doherty GM, Soper NJ, Norton JA. Staging laparoscopy with laparoscopic ultrasonography: optimizing resectability in hepatobiliary and pancreatic malignancy. J Am Coll Surg 1997;185(1):33–39.

47. Barbot DJ, Marks JH, Feld RI, Liu JB, Rosato FE. Improved staging of liver tumors using laparoscopic intraoperative ultrasound. J Surg Oncol 1997;64(1):63–67.

48. Jarnagin WR, Bach AM, Winston CB, et al. What is the yield of intraoperative ultrasonography during partial hepatectomy for malignant disease? J Am Coll Surg 2001;192(5): 577–583.

49. Lo CM, Fan ST, Liu CL, et al. Determining resectability for hepatocellular carcinoma: the role of laparoscopy and laparoscopic ultrasonography. J Hepatobiliary Pancreat Surg 2000;7(3):260–264.

50. Potter MW, Shah SA, McEnaney P, Chari RS, Callery MP. A critical appraisal of laparoscopic staging in hepatobiliary and pancreatic malignancy. Surg Oncol 2000;9(3):103–110.

51. Foroutani A, Garland AM, Berber E, et al. Laparoscopic ultrasound vs triphasic computed tomography for detecting liver tumors. Arch Surg 2000;135(8):933–938.

52. de Castro SM, Tilleman EH, Busch OR, et al. Diagnostic laparoscopy for primary and secondary liver malignancies: impact of improved imaging and changed criteria for resection. Ann Surg Oncol 2004;11(5):522–529.

53. Grobmyer SR, Fong Y, D'Angelica M, Dematteo RP, Blumgart LH, Jarnagin WR. Diagnostic laparoscopy prior to planned hepatic resection for colorectal metastases. Arch Surg 2004;139(12):1326–1330.

54. D'Angelica M, Fong Y, Weber S, et al. The role of staging laparoscopy in hepatobiliary malignancy: prospective analysis of 401 cases. Ann Surg Oncol 2003;10(2):183–189.

55. Lo CM, Lai EC, Liu CL, Fan ST, Wong J. Laparoscopy and laparoscopic ultrasonography avoid exploratory laparotomy in patients with hepatocellular carcinoma. Ann Surg 1998;227(4):527–532.

56. Catheline JM, Champault G. Ultrasonographic laparoscopy of the liver. [Article in German] Chirurgie 1999;124(5): 568–576.

57. Schachter P, Sorin V, Avni Y, et al. The role of laparoscopic ultrasound in the minimally invasive management of symptomatic hepatic cysts. Surg Endosc 2001;15(4): 364–367.

58. Montorsi M, Santambrogio R, Bianchi P, et al. Laparoscopy with laparoscopic ultrasound for pretreatment staging of hepatocellular carcinoma: a prospective study. J Gastrointest Surg 2001;5(3):312–315.

59. Helin HL, Kirkinen P. Laparoscopic ultrasonography during conservative ovarian surgery. Surg Endosc 2000;14(2): 161–163.

60. Cheung TH, Yang WT, Yu MY, Lo WK, Ho S. New development of laparoscopic ultrasound and laparoscopic pelvic lymphadenectomy in the management of patients with cervical carcinoma. Gynecol Oncol 1998;71(1):87–93.

61. Matin SF, Gill IS. Laparoscopic ultrasonography. J Endourol 2001;15(1):87–92.

62. Piolanti M, Coppola F, Papa S, Pilotti V, Mattioli S, Gavelli G. Ultrasonographic localization of occult pulmonary nodules during video-assisted thoracic surgery. Eur Radiol 2003; 13(10):2358–2364.

63. Santambrogio R, Podda M, Zuin M, et al. Safety and efficacy of laparoscopic radiofrequency ablation of hepatocellular carcinoma in patients with liver cirrhosis. Surg Endosc 2003;17(11):1826–1832.

64. Kim RD, Nazarey P, Katz E, Chari RS. Laparoscopic staging and tumor ablation for hepatocellular carcinoma in Child C cirrhotics evaluated for orthotopic liver transplantation. Surg Endosc 2004;18(1):39–44.

65. Nagae G, Ido K, Isoda N, Sato S, Kita H, Sugano K. Laparoscopic ablation therapy for hepatocellular carcinoma. Dig Endosc 2005;17:1–8.

66. Machi J, Uchida S, Sumida K, et al. Ultrasound-guided radiofrequency thermal ablation of liver tumors: percutaneous, laparoscopic, and open surgical approaches. J Gastrointest Surg 2001;5(5):477–489.

67. Noguchi O, Izumi N, Nishimura Y, et al. Laparoscopic ablation therapy for hepatocellular carcinoma: clinical significance of a newly developed laparoscopic sector ultrasonic probe. Dig Endosc 2003;15:179–184.

68. Ido K, Isoda N, Sugano K. Microwave coagulation therapy for liver cancer: laparoscopic microwave coagulation. J Gastroenterol 2001;36(3):145–152.

69. Hassan H, Vilmann P, Sharma V, Holm J. Initial experience with a new laparoscopic ultrasound probe for guided biopsy in staging of upper gastrointestinal cancer. J. Surg Endosc 2009;23:1552–1558.

33 Hot Topics in Interventional EUS

U. Will, F. Meyer

The range of interventional endoscopic ultrasound (EUS) techniques has expanded enormously during the last 10 years, and there has been growing interest throughout the world in novel interventional approaches using EUS. The combination of endoscopy with the tissue differentiation facilities possible with ultrasound, along with interventional options, means that various surgical procedures can be avoided and that potentially dangerous interventions can be carried out with greater safety.[1] In addition to outlining EUS-guided treatment for pancreatic pseudocysts, abscesses and necroses, the aims in this overview of the topic are:

- To describe novel techniques for EUS-guided internal drainage of the biliary and pancreatic ducts
- To emphasize and critically discuss the relevance of these techniques in everyday clinical practice, with a review of recent literature references

EUS-Guided Drainage of Pancreatic Pseudocysts, Abscesses, and Necroses

Pseudocysts are frequent complications in patients with acute or chronic pancreatitis. Before every endoscopic intervention, these locular fluid collections with a capsule-like margin surrounding them and with no epithelial layer need to be distinguished from neoplastic, cystic pancreatic lesions. This can be achieved by correlating the clinical symptomatology, EUS morphology, and laboratory and cytological analysis of the cyst fluid. With its outstanding capacity for tissue differentiation in local imaging in comparison with other imaging procedures, along with integrated color-coded Doppler ultrasonography and the option for targeted fine-needle aspiration, EUS has the advantage that it allows precise classification of the various types of pancreatic cysts and lesions.[2–5] Cystic neoplasms have a different sonomorphology in comparison with pancreatic pseudocysts. In addition to solid polycyclic tumors growing on the intraluminal side and indicated by wall thickening, enlarged intracystic septa can be detected, and atypical vascular patterns can also be displayed using color-coded Doppler ultrasound. Uncomplicated pseudocysts are commonly characterized by a flat wall with no fluid signals and an echo-free or slightly echogenic and homogeneous fluid. Sequestra and necroses in complicated pseudocysts mostly consist of sediment, and no vessels can be detected with color-coded ultrasound. In

these cases, the cystic fluid often has a mixed echogenic and inhomogeneous appearance. If there is any doubt about the specific entity present on the basis of the EUS morphology, primary EUS-guided internal drainage should be avoided and the cystic fluid should be sampled using EUS-guided fine-needle aspiration (EUS-FNA) for cytologic examination, laboratory analysis (for carcinoembryonic antigen, CA19-9, and lipase), and microbiological analysis.[2,6–13] A detection rate in the range of 75–95% for cystic neoplasia has been reported with EUS-FNA and cystic fluid analysis.

With regard to treatment for pseudocysts, endoscopic internal drainage should only be carried out with symptomatic cysts.[5,14–16,60] If a transpapillary drain cannot be placed and if the classic bulging sign is absent, conventional endoscopic drainage is not possible.[15] EUS can precisely depict the local relationship between pseudocysts and the gastric or duodenal wall. Intramural or periluminal vessels that may bleed during interventions can be detected and avoided when a drain is being placed. EUS-guided drainage is not appropriate for impressions on the wall of the stomach or small intestine. Numerous EUS-based techniques for internal drainage of cysts and abscesses have been reported in the literature and cannot be discussed here in detail.[1,5,15–19] In recent years, a simple and reproducible technique with a low complication rate has been established, which is preferred by the majority of endoscopic ultrasonographers and is described below.

Puncture is carried out after EUS examination at a site in which needle penetration will not affect high-risk anatomic structures—for example, when there are no vessels along the puncture track and when the transluminal distance to the cyst is very short. Intervention with fluoroscopic guidance is recommended, firstly to allow the position of the endoscope to be identified before puncture and secondly to allow a guide wire to be introduced after puncture with a 19-G needle. Knowing the endoscope's position is important to allow the endoscopist to carry out subsequent interventions easily, such as transgastric endoscopic debridement in infected necroses. A heavily angled EUS instrument can make subsequent transgastric repeat interventions considerably more difficult. Following EUS-guided puncture of the cyst, the further approach has to be decided in accordance with the clinical symptoms, EUS morphology, and the consistency of the cystic fluid. If there is a noninfectious cyst with clear cystic fluid and an echo-free pattern, an 8.5-Fr or 10-Fr prosthesis can be placed after a wire-guided cystostomy using a diathermy knife. If possible, pigtail prostheses should be

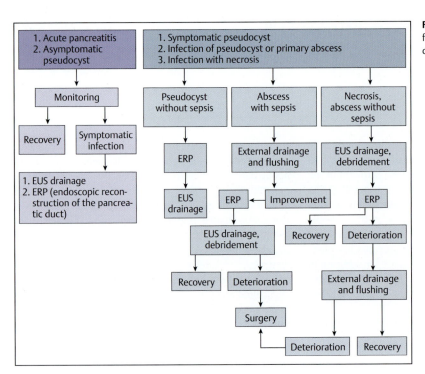

Fig. 33.1 A logical treatment algorithm for patients with pancreatic pseudocysts, abscesses, and necroses.

used in order to avoid dislocation of the prosthesis. If there is any evidence of an infectious cyst or even an abscess, the ostium of the cystogastroenterostomy can be dilated atraumatically up to a diameter of 10–20 mm with a dilation balloon via the guide wire, which is still in place. To keep the cystoenterostomy open and maintain access to the abscess or necrotic cavity, placement of two or three (8.5–10-Fr) pigtail drains is recommended. Introducing a nasogastric rinsing tube along with percutaneous external rinsing drainage, which is comfortable for the patient, can accelerate the removal of adherent necrotic sequestra in case of infected necroses, minimizing the number of endoscopic interventions needed.

There have as yet been no controlled studies on the results with this type of combined approach. A survey of members of the American Society of Gastrointestinal Endoscopy (ASGE) on the value and importance of EUS in the treatment of pseudocysts showed that only 70% of American endoscopists and 59% of non-American endoscopists use EUS with diagnostic intent before endoscopic drainage of pseudocysts or cysts.[20] This was a surprising finding, as it has been shown in numerous studies that conventional endoscopic drainage of a pseudocyst is only successful in 40–57% of cases (or even zero, for cysts in the pancreatic tail), while drainage is successfully achieved in 75–97% of cases, independent of the cyst site, when EUS is used.[1,2,17–19,21–33] In a comparative study by Varadarajulu et al.,[17] a primary endoscopic attempt to place a drain failed in 23 of 53 patients. Subsequent EUS-guided drainage was successful in all of the patients.

With improved training for gastroenterologists in the field of interventional EUS, along with the convincing success rates achieved and reported at the major EUS centers, EUS-guided drainage of cysts, abscesses, and encapsulated necroses has become the preferred method of treatment. In addition to providing better differentiation between pseudocysts and cystic neoplasia with color-coded Doppler ultrasound and FNA, EUS makes it possible to treat peripancreatic fluid collections with a low complication rate and expands the endoscopic treatment options available for patients with abscesses or necroses. **Table 33.1** lists the results of large case series on EUS-guided drainage of pseudocysts, abscesses, and encapsulated necroses.

The complication rates are low (0–21%). In addition to hemorrhage and cystic infections (3–15%), perforations have been reported after balloon dilation or endoscopic debridement.[1,14,16,25] The long-term clinical success rate of 90% reported in recent studies shows that EUS-guided management is a reasonable approach in the treatment of peripancreatic fluid collections.

The central role that EUS plays in the treatment of pseudocysts, abscesses, and necroses is indicated in **Fig. 33.1**. The recognized treatment methods depend on the specific diseases and clinical symptoms, leading to a treatment algorithm that can be varied in accordance with the clinical course.

Table 33.1 Results of EUS-guided drainage of pseudocysts, abscesses, and pancreatic necroses (in chronological order)

First author, ref.	Patients (n)	Technique	Drainage of:	Success rate	Complications	Clinical long-term success
Pfaffenbach[21] (1998)	11	EUS-guided	Pancreatic cyst	91%	0%	80%
Giovannini[18] (2001)	35	EUS-guided	Pancreatic cyst, Abscess	Pancreatic cyst 100%, Abscess 80%	3%	93%, 89%
Vosoghi[22] (2002)	14	EUS	Pancreatic cyst	93%	7%	93%
Dohmoto[23] (2003)	47	Transpapillary EUS (n = 5) and conventional	Pancreatic cyst	89%	2%	86%
Seewald[24] (2005)	13	EUS-guided	Abscess, Necrosis	76.9%	30.8%	84.6%
Kahaleh[25] (2006)	99	EUS-guided (n = 46), Conventional (n = 53)	Pancreatic cyst	84%, 91%	19%, 18%	N.d.
Hookey[26] (2006)	116	Transpapillary (n = 15), Conventional (n = 60), Combined (n = 41) (EUS-guided 44%)	Pancreatic cyst, Abscess, Necrosis	93.6%, 88.9%, 25%, Total 87.9%	11%	84.5%
Krüger[27] (2006)	35	EUS-guided	Pancreatic cyst, Necrosis	88%	0%	88%
Seewald[24] (2005)	8	EUS-guided	Pancreatic cyst, Abscess	100%	0%	0%
Ahlawat[28] (2006)	11	EUS-guided	Pancreatic cyst	82%	0%	22%
Charnley[29] (2006)	13	EUS-guided	Necrosis	92% (69% patients with percutaneous or surgical drainage were included)	0%	N.d.
Will[19] (2006)	27	EUS-guided, Ultrasound	Pancreatic cyst, Abscess, Necrosis	94%	11%	92%
Antillon[30] (2006)	33	EUS-guided	Pancreatic cyst, Abscess	94%	15%	97%
Lopes[31] (2007)	51	EUS-guided	Pancreatic cyst, Abscess	94%	3%	82%
Papachristou[32] (2007)	53	Conventional EUS-guided (n = 8)	Necrosis	81%	21%	
Varadarajulu[17] (2007)	53	Conventional (n = 30), EUS (n = 21)	Pancreatic cyst, Abscess	Conventional 53%, EUS 100%	4%	N.d.
Voermans[1] (2007)	25	EUS	Necrosis	100%	7%	93%
Barthet[33] (2008)	50	EUS (n = 28), Conventional (n = 13), Transpapillary (n = 8)	Pancreatic cyst	98%	18% (mortality 0.5%)	96%
Will[59] (2011)	147	EUS, Ultrasound, ERP	Pancreatic cyst, Necrosis, Abscess	97%	9.6% (mortality 0.7%)	96.2%

EUS, endoscopic ultrasound; N.d., no data.

Table 33.2 Results of transintestinal EUS-guided cholangiodrainage (EUCD)

First author, ref.	Patients (n)	Stent type	Drainage success rate	Complications	Clinical long-term success
Burmester[39] (2003)	4	Plastic stent	75%	0%	N.d.
Bories[37] (2007)	11	7 plastic stents 3 SEMS	90%	18% (biloma, n = 1; cholangitis, n = 1)	90% (repeat interventions, n = 2)
Püspök[40] (2005)	6	5 plastic stents 1 SEMS	100%	16% (cholecystitis, n = 1)	N.d.
Will[56] (2007)	10	4 plastic stents 5 SEMS	90%	12.5% (bleeding, n = 1; cholangitis, n = 1)	80%
Kahaleh[42] (2006)	23	11 plastic stents 10 SEMS	91%	17% (bleeding, n = 1; pneumoperitoneum, n = 2; biliary leakage, n = 1)	78%
Tarantino[41] (2008)	9	7 plastic stents 1 metal stent	100%	0%	100% (repeat intervention, n = 1)
Will[58] (2009)	24	5 plastic stents 14 metal stents	75% (18 of 24 patients)	17% (mortality 4%; cholecystitis, n = 3; hemobilia, n = 1)	94% (repeat intervention, n = 1; change of metal/ plastic stent)

N.d., no data; SEMS, self-expanding metallic stent.

EUS-Guided Biliary Drainage

Percutaneous cholangiographic drainage (PTCD) is used in most gastroenterological centers as an alternative in patients in whom endoscopic retrograde cholangiography (ERC) has failed due to malignant obstructive diseases. In addition to having a higher complication rate in comparison with endoscopic retrograde cholangiopancreatography (ERCP), PTCD is unable to achieve external or internal drainage in all cases.[34–36] Solely external drainage disturbs the patient's physical integrity, which can become a substantial psychological problem in those with advanced or metastatic malignant disease and limited life expectancy, in addition to the disadvantage of a permanent loss of bile. The basic aim is to achieve adequate, permanent, and if possible internal drainage of the biliary tree as part of a palliative therapeutic approach in patients with malignant, incurable disease and obstructive, tumor-induced jaundice. The treatment should be associated with a low complication rate and should not require any further repeat interventions during the patient's life. The results of large case series have shown that EUS-guided cholangiodrainage (EUCD) is a treatment method that is capable of achieving these aims.[19,25,37,61] The first EUS-guided cholangiography procedure was reported by Wiersema et al. in 1996,[38] and the first larger case series on EUS-guided cholangiodrainage was published by Burmester et al. in 2003.[39] Larger case series in recent years have shown that a technical success rate with EUCD in the range of 75–100%, along with low complication rates (0–18%), can be achieved[19,25,37,39–43] (**Table 33.2**). However, there is still a lack of controlled and randomized studies compar-

ing EUCD with PTCD and ERCP. The groups of patients treated in the case series are very heterogeneous. While Bories et al.[37] and Will et al.[43] only treated patients with advanced malignant disease, Kahaleh et al.[42] and Tarantino et al.[41] also included patients with benign diseases. This makes meaningful comparison of the long-term results difficult.

The studies show that EUCD is indicated in patients with obstructive cholestatic disease in whom ERCP and internal drainage cannot be achieved for anatomic reasons or due to progressive tumor growth (following a previous gastrectomy, Whipple procedure, tumor-induced gastric outlet syndrome, previous hepaticojejunostomy, or inability to introduce the catheter into the papilla). Two EUS-guided approaches are in principle possible:

- If the papilla can be reached with the duodenoscope, but the bile duct cannot be catheterized, a rendezvous procedure with ERC is preferable.
- If the papilla cannot be reached, primary transintestinal EUCD can be used.

With the rendezvous technique, the dilated bile duct is punctured with a 19-G needle toward the papilla; subsequently, a 0.035-inch guide wire is advanced through the papilla into the duodenal lumen. After a change to a duodenoscope has been made, further interventions are then carried out over the guide wire.

Direct EUCD can be achieved via two routes:

- Extrahepatic transintestinal puncture and drainage of the bile duct (**Fig. 33.2a, b**)
- Transintestinal transhepatic puncture and drainage of a peripheral segment of the bile duct in the left hepatic lobe (**Fig. 33.3a, b**)

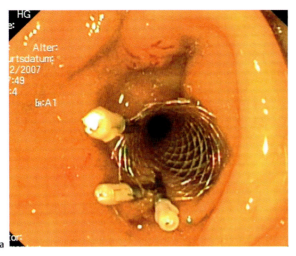
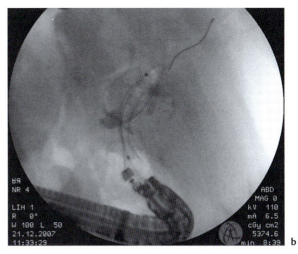

Fig. 33.2a, b In a patient with unresectable pancreatic carcinoma and jaundice, with a distal occlusion, transgastric extrahepatic drainage of the bile duct was carried out. The prosthesis was fixed with metal clips to prevent stent migration.

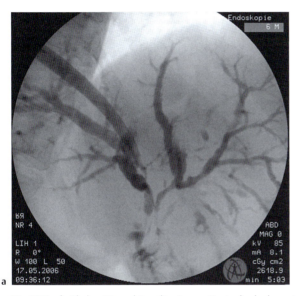
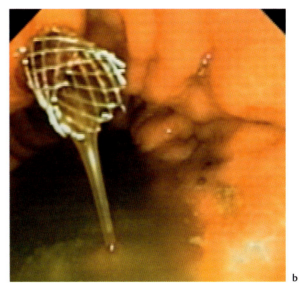

Fig. 33.3a, b Cholangitis and jaundice in a patient who had previously undergone hepaticojejunostomy due to a Klatskin tumor, with recurrent tumor growth at the anastomosis. Transgastric transhepatic drainage was carried out, and a covered Wallstent was placed.

After puncture and cholangiography, the access site is dilated using bougies or balloons for the bile duct, and plastic prostheses or covered metal stents are subsequently placed. The decision in favor of a specific approach and drainage procedure is taken in accordance with the anatomic situation, the accessible bile duct on longitudinal EUS, and the patient's underlying disease.

Personal experience and the literature data currently available suggest that EUCD can be regarded as an elegant approach with a low complication rate that provides a technical and clinical success rate (indicated by adequate internal drainage of bile) of more than 80%. The range of complications includes cholangitis, stent migration, and biliary leakage, reported with a frequency of 15–17%. At present, EUCD must still be regarded as an experimental procedure that should only be carried out by highly experienced interventional EUS examiners in large gastroenterology centers.[44,45]

However, there are still several open questions and aspects that are currently unclear:

1. Should EUCD performed only in patients with obstructive jaundice due to malignant tumor growth, or also in patients with benign conditions?
2. At which point is EUCD reasonable in the treatment algorithm—primarily after unsuccessful ERC, or after PTCD, or even before PTCD in each case?

3. Which access route is safest—transhepatic, with drainage of the intrahepatic segments of the bile duct, or drainage of the extrahepatic part of the bile duct via an extrahepatic access site?
4. Which is the best access method and which is feasible—atraumatic, using bougies and balloon dilation, or traumatic, with high-frequency diathermy?
5. Which type of stent is preferable—covered metal or plastic?
6. Should stents be changed periodically, and if yes, what are the most appropriate time intervals?

The advantages of EUCD that are emerging in current case series, in terms of patient comfort and morbidity rates in comparison with PTCD, have yet to be confirmed in randomized studies, and it is not at present possible to give a general recommendation in favor of EUCD when ERC has failed.

EUS-Guided Drainage of the Pancreatic Duct (EUPD)

The main cause of pain in patients in whom a dilated pancreatic duct is found and a malignant tumor has also been definitively excluded is intraductal hypertension due to stenotic segments or total or subtotal obstruction of the duct.[46] Pathogenetically, the underlying diseases include chronic pancreatitis with ductal stenoses, obstruction by calcifications and pancreaticolithiasis, and ductal ruptures. In addition, an inflammatory stenosis of the papilla, anatomic variations (pancreas divisum) and stenosis following previous surgical interventions may also be responsible for the retention of pancreatic juice in the duct.[47] The aim of pain management for these patients is to achieve endoscopic or surgical drainage of the pancreatic duct. Success rates of 70–90% have been reported in endoscopic and surgical studies.[48–54] The chances of achieving successful endoscopic transpapillary drainage of the pancreatic duct are limited when there are anatomic variants (such as pancreas divisum) or after Billroth II procedures and gastrointestinal reconstruction using a Roux-en-Y jejunal loop. Treatment of obstructive pancreatitis in the residual pancreatic tissue after a previous resection of the pancreatic head can also be difficult when there is a stenotic anastomosis or a chronic pancreaticocutaneous fistula. Repeated surgical interventions are often the last option to improve the situation for the patient.

According to the initial results from large case series, EUS-guided pancreatography with extended EUPD can be regarded as an appropriate option for achieving drainage of the dilated pancreatic duct system in patients with obstructions of the pancreatic duct and unsuccessful transpapillary drainage.[47,55–57] Before EUPD, adequate diagnostic measures should be carried out to definitively

exclude malignant tumor lesions. If there is any doubt, exploratory laparotomy is indicated in order to clarify the histologic diagnosis, to allow consideration of pylorus-preserving cephalic pancreaticoduodenectomy in case of malignant tumor growth if required, or alternatively to allow a duodenum-preserving cephalic pancreatic resection if possible as the treatment of choice in patients with symptomatic chronic pancreatitis and a residual pancreatic duct.[50] In the largest series reporting transintestinal EUS-guided drainage of the pancreatic duct, five of 36 patients were diagnosed as having malignant lesions during the follow-up period.[47] This underlines the need to ensure that EUPD is correctly indicated.

There are two basic options when carrying out EUPD:
- If the papilla of Vater can be reached with the endoscope, but the pancreatic duct cannot be catheterized and/or the stenosis cannot be passed, a rendezvous procedure is initially preferable.
- If the papilla cannot be reached, primary transintestinal EUS-guided drainage is chosen.

The pancreatic duct is usually punctured using a rendezvous technique from the antrum or duodenal bulb. After puncture with a 19-G needle, a 0.035-inch guide wire is introduced and pulled out of the minor or major papilla (**Fig. 33.4a–c**). After the endoscopic instrument has been exchanged for a therapeutic duodenoscope and the wire protruding from the orifice of the papilla has been caught, endoscopic retrograde pancreatography (ERP) is performed in the usual way. If the papilla cannot be reached or if the guide wire cannot be pulled out of the papilla, transduodenal or transgastric drainage of the pancreatic duct is carried out (**Fig. 33.5a–c**). While puncture of the pancreatic duct and subsequent pancreatography are successful in nearly 100% of cases, placement of a drain is not always possible. A technical success rate in the range of 25–91% has been reported in four case series. The reported techniques used to create a pancreaticointestinostomy before placement of the drain have included use of a diathermy knife, various bougies and balloons, and a stent retriever. The groups of patients studied have also varied widely, so that direct comparison of the results in reports with small case numbers is not possible. The reported complication rates have been in the range of 14–25%. In addition to hemorrhage, pseudocysts, perforations, and pancreatitis have been described. There have been no cases of intervention-associated mortality in any of the series (**Table 33.3**). Long-term clinical success rates of 69–80% have been reported, which are comparable with rates achieved after transpapillary and surgical drainage.[50,53,54] Stent migration and stent occlusion have been reported as potential problems during the long-term course in up to 55% of cases, requiring repeat interventions.[47]

Personal experience and the literature data currently available suggest that EUPD can be regarded as an alternative approach for achieving drainage of a dilated

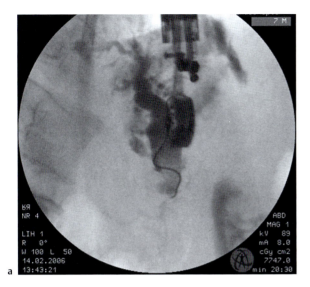
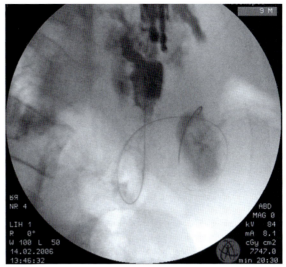

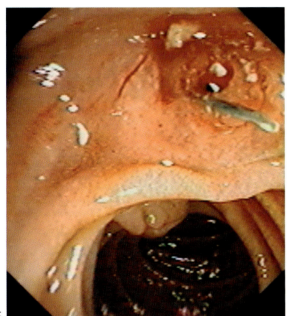

Fig. 33.4a–c EUS-guided drainage of the pancreatic duct using the rendezvous technique in a patient with pancreas divisum. Transgastric puncture was carried out with a 19-G needle, and a guide wire was introduced and pulled out of the minor papilla.

Table 33.3 Results of transintestinal EUS-guided drainage of the pancreatic duct (EUPD)

First author (ref.)	Patients (n)	Technical success of drainage	Complications	Clinical long-term success
Will[43] (2007)	14	69%	15%	78%
Mallery[55] (2004)	4	25%	25%	N.d.
Kahaleh[42] (2006)	13	76%	15%	69%
Tessier[47] (2007)	36	91.6%	14%	69%
Will[58] (2009)	27	70.8%	25%	75%

N.d., no data.

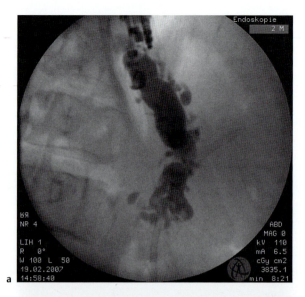

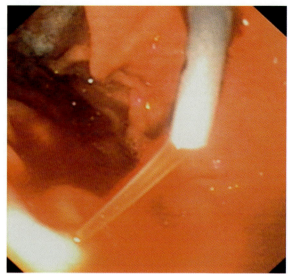

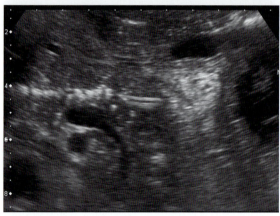

Fig. 33.5a–c Transgastric EUS-guided drainage of the pancreatic duct in a patient with chronic pancreatitis.
a Transgastric pancreatography.
b Stenting.
c Ultrasound control.

pancreatic duct system that is not accessible via the conventional endoscopic route. In particular, high-risk patients (with liver cirrhosis or portal hypertension), patients with previous surgical procedures, and those with persistent pancreaticocutaneous fistulas or stenoses at the anastomotic site with a residual pancreatic duct are suitable candidates for this specific approach. Like EUCD, EUPD must still be regarded as an experimental procedure that should only be carried out by experienced and well-trained interventional endoscopic ultrasonographers in large gastroenterology and endoscopy centers.

There are still several open questions with EUPD:

1. What is the appropriate timing for EUPD: before or only after surgical intervention for chronic pancreatitis?
2. Can EUPD with the rendezvous technique always be recommended if feasible, or is initial use of the transintestinal route also acceptable?
3. Which is the best technique in the transintestinal approach to the pancreatic duct—atraumatic, using bougies and balloon dilation, or traumatic, with high-frequency diathermy and a retriever?
4. Which type or design of stent is preferable—a covered metal stent or a plastic stent?
5. When should stents be exchanged, and what are the most appropriate time intervals?
6. When do functional pancreaticointestinal fistulas develop, or does this happen at all?

EUPD can be regarded as a potentially successful and complementary procedure in comparison with ERP in a selected group of patients in order to achieve endoscopic drainage of the pancreatic duct in cases of obstruction. It will probably not be possible to carry out randomized studies on a similar basis to those comparing ERP with surgical intervention in patients with chronic pancreatitis. Further results from prospective studies will therefore have to be awaited before conclusive assessments of the indications, technical and clinical success rates, complication rates, and outcome can be made and recommendations on the appropriate use of EUPD can be provided.

References

1. Voermans RP, Veldkamp MC, Rauws EA, Bruno MJ, Fockens P. Endoscopic transmural debridement of symptomatic organized pancreatic necrosis (with videos). Gastrointest Endosc 2007;66(5):909–916.
2. Scheiman JM. Management of cystic lesions of the pancreas. J Gastrointest Surg 2008;12(3):405–407.
3. Lee CJ, Scheiman J, Anderson MA, et al. Risk of malignancy in resected cystic tumors of the pancreas < or = 3 cm in size: is it safe to observe asymptomatic patients? A multi-institutional report. J Gastrointest Surg 2008;12(2):234–242.
4. Khalid A, Brugge W. ACG practice guidelines for the diagnosis and management of neoplastic pancreatic cysts. Am J Gastroenterol 2007;102(10):2339–2349.
5. Fockens P. EUS in drainage of pancreatic pseudocysts. Gastrointest Endosc 2002; 56(4, Suppl):S93–S97.
6. Wu H, Yan LN, Cheng NS, Zhang YG, Ker CG. Role of cystic fluid in diagnosis of the pancreatic cystadenoma and cystadenocarcinoma. Hepatogastroenterology 2007;54(79):1915–1918.
7. Wang Y, Gao J, Li Z, Jin Z, Gong Y, Man X. Diagnostic value of mucins (MUC1, MUC2 and MUC5AC) expression profile in endoscopic ultrasound-guided fine-needle aspiration specimens of the pancreas. Int J Cancer 2007;121(12):2716–2722.
8. Attasaranya S, Pais S, LeBlanc J, McHenry L, Sherman S, DeWitt JM. Endoscopic ultrasound-guided fine needle aspiration and cyst fluid analysis for pancreatic cysts. JOP 2007;8(5):553–563.
9. Aljebreen AM, Romagnuolo J, Perini R, Sutherland F. Utility of endoscopic ultrasound, cytology and fluid carcinoembryonic antigen and CA 19-9 levels in pancreatic cystic lesions. World J Gastroenterol 2007;13(29):3962–3966.
10. Shami VM, Sundaram V, Stelow EB, et al. The level of carcinoembryonic antigen and the presence of mucin as predictors of cystic pancreatic mucinous neoplasia. Pancreas 2007;34(4):466–469.
11. Linder JD, Geenen JE, Catalano MF. Cyst fluid analysis obtained by EUS-guided FNA in the evaluation of discrete cystic neoplasms of the pancreas: a prospective single-center experience. Gastrointest Endosc 2006;64(5):697–702.
12. van der Waaij LA, van Dullemen HM, Porte RJ. Cyst fluid analysis in the differential diagnosis of pancreatic cystic lesions: a pooled analysis. Gastrointest Endosc 2005;62(3):383–389.
13. Ryu JK, Woo SM, Hwang JH, et al. Cyst fluid analysis for the differential diagnosis of pancreatic cysts. Diagn Cytopathol 2004;31(2):100–105.
14. Jacobson BC, Baron TH, Adler DG, et al; American Society for Gastrointestinal Endoscopy. ASGE guideline: The role of endoscopy in the diagnosis and the management of cystic lesions and inflammatory fluid collections of the pancreas. Gastrointest Endosc 2005;61(3):363–370.
15. Baillie J. Pancreatic pseudocysts (Part I). Gastrointest Endosc 2004;59(7):873–879.
16. Baillie J. Pancreatic pseudocysts (Part II). Gastrointest Endosc 2004;60(1):105–113.
17. Varadarajulu S, Wilcox CM, Tamhane A, Eloubeidi MA, Blakely J, Canon CL. Role of EUS in drainage of peripancreatic fluid collections not amenable for endoscopic transmural drainage. Gastrointest Endosc 2007;66(6):1107–1119.
18. Giovannini M, Pesenti C, Rolland AL, Moutardier V, Delpero JR. Endoscopic ultrasound-guided drainage of pancreatic pseudocysts or pancreatic abscesses using a therapeutic echo endoscope. Endoscopy 2001;33(6):473–477.
19. Will U, Wegener C, Graf KI, Wanzar I, Manger T, Meyer F. Differential treatment and early outcome in the interventional endoscopic management of pancreatic pseudocysts in 27 patients. World J Gastroenterol 2006;12(26):4175–4178.
20. Yusuf TE, Baron TH. Endoscopic transmural drainage of pancreatic pseudocysts: results of a national and an international survey of ASGE members. Gastrointest Endosc 2006;63(2):223–227.
21. Pfaffenbach B, Langer M, Stabenow-Lohbauer U, Lux G. Endosonography controlled transgastric drainage of pancreatic pseudocysts. [Article in German] Dtsch Med Wochenschr 1998;123(48):1439–1442.
22. Vosoghi M, Sial S, Garrett B, et al. EUS-guided pancreatic pseudocyst drainage: review and experience at Harbor-UCLA Medical Center. MedGenMed 2002;4(3):2.
23. Dohmoto M, Akiyama K, Lioka Y. Endoscopic and endosonographic management of pancreatic pseudocyst: a long-term follow-up. Rev Gastroenterol Peru 2003;23(4):269–275.
24. Seewald S, Groth S, Omar S, et al. Aggressive endoscopic therapy for pancreatic necrosis and pancreatic abscess: a new safe and effective treatment algorithm (videos). Gastrointest Endosc 2005;62(1):92–100.
25. Kahaleh M, Shami VM, Conaway MR, et al. Endoscopic ultrasound drainage of pancreatic pseudocyst: a prospective comparison with conventional endoscopic drainage. Endoscopy 2006;38(4):355–359.
26. Hookey LC, Debroux S, Delhaye M, Arvanitakis M, Le Moine O, Devière J. Endoscopic drainage of pancreatic-fluid collections in 116 patients: a comparison of etiologies, drainage techniques, and outcomes. Gastrointest Endosc 2006;63(4):635–643.
27. Krüger M, Schneider AS, Manns MP, Meier PN. Endoscopic management of pancreatic pseudocysts or abscesses after an EUS-guided 1-step procedure for initial access. Gastrointest Endosc 2006;63(3):409–416.
28. Ahlawat SK, Charabaty-Pishvaian A, Jackson PG, Haddad NG. Single-step EUS-guided pancreatic pseudocyst drainage using a large channel linear array echoendoscope and cystotome: results in 11 patients. JOP 2006;7(6):616–624.
29. Charnley RM, Lochan R, Gray H, O'Sullivan CB, Scott J, Oppong KE. Endoscopic necrosectomy as primary therapy in the management of infected pancreatic necrosis. Endoscopy 2006;38(9):925–928.
30. Antillon MR, Shah RJ, Stiegmann G, Chen YK. Single-step EUS-guided transmural drainage of simple and complicated pancreatic pseudocysts. Gastrointest Endosc 2006;63(6):797–803.
31. Lopes CV, Pesenti C, Bories E, Caillol F, Giovannini M. Endoscopic-ultrasound-guided endoscopic transmural drainage of pancreatic pseudocysts and abscesses. Scand J Gastroenterol 2007;42(4):524–529.
32. Papachristou GI, Takahashi N, Chahal P, Sarr MG, Baron TH. Peroral endoscopic drainage/debridement of walled-off pancreatic necrosis. Ann Surg 2007;245(6):943–951.
33. Barthet M, Lamblin G, Gasmi M, Vitton V, Desjeux A, Grimaud JC. Clinical usefulness of a treatment algorithm for pancreatic pseudocysts. Gastrointest Endosc 2008;67(2):245–252.

34. Ferrucci JT Jr, Mueller PR, Harbin WP. Percutaneous trans-hepatic biliary drainage: technique, results, and applications. Radiology 1980;135(1):1–13.

35. Harbin WP, Mueller PR, Ferrucci JT Jr. Transhepatic cholangiography: complications and use patterns of the fine-needle technique: a multi-institutional survey. Radiology 1980;135(1):15–22.

36. Winick AB, Waybill PN, Venbrux AC. Complications of percutaneous transhepatic biliary interventions. Tech Vasc Interv Radiol 2001;4(3):200–206.

37. Bories E, Pesenti C, Caillol F, Lopes C, Giovannini M. Transgastric endoscopic ultrasonography-guided biliary drainage: results of a pilot study. Endoscopy 2007;39(4):287–291.

38. Wiersema MJ, Sandusky D, Carr R, Wiersema LM, Erdel WC, Frederick PK. Endosonography-guided cholangiopancreatography. Gastrointest Endosc 1996;43(2 Pt 1):102–106.

39. Burmester E, Niehaus J, Leineweber T, Huetteroth T. EUS-cholangio-drainage of the bile duct: report of 4 cases. Gastrointest Endosc 2003;57(2):246–251.

40. Püspök A, Lomoschitz F, Dejaco C, Hejna M, Sautner T, Gangl A. Endoscopic ultrasound guided therapy of benign and malignant biliary obstruction: a case series. Am J Gastroenterol 2005;100(8):1743–1747.

41. Tarantino I, Barresi L, Repici A, Traina M. EUS-guided biliary drainage: a case series. Endoscopy 2008;40(4):336–339 Epub ahead of print.

42. Kahaleh M, Hernandez AJ, Tokar J, Adams RB, Shami VM, Yeaton P. Interventional EUS-guided cholangiography: evaluation of a technique in evolution. Gastrointest Endosc 2006;64(1):52–59.

43. Will U, Thieme A, Fueldner F, Gerlach R, Wanzar I, Meyer F. Treatment of biliary obstruction in selected patients by endoscopic ultrasonography (EUS)-guided transluminal biliary drainage. Endoscopy 2007;39(4):292–295.

44. Sherman S. Biliary drainage with endoscopic ultrasound guidance JournalWatch June 22, 2007 [available at: http://www.jwatch.org/].

45. Püspök A. Biliary therapy: are we ready for EUS-guidance? Minerva Med 2007;98(4):379–384.

46. Ebbehøj N, Borly L, Bülow J, et al. Pancreatic tissue fluid pressure in chronic pancreatitis. Relation to pain, morphology, and function. Scand J Gastroenterol 1990;25(10):1046–1051.

47. Tessier G, Bories E, Arvanitakis M, et al. EUS-guided pancreatogastrostomy and pancreatobulbostomy for the treatment of pain in patients with pancreatic ductal dilatation inaccessible for transpapillary endoscopic therapy. Gastrointest Endosc 2007;65(2):233–241.

48. Jimenez RE, Fernandez-Del Castillo C, Rattner DW, Warshaw AL. Pylorus-preserving pancreaticoduodenectomy in the treatment of chronic pancreatitis. World J Surg 2003;27(11):1211–1216.

49. Beger HG, Schlosser W, Friess HM, Büchler MW. Duodenum-preserving head resection in chronic pancreatitis changes the natural course of the disease: a single-center 26-year experience. Ann Surg 1999;230(4):512–519, discussion 519–523.

50. Cahen DL, Gouma DJ, Nio Y, et al. Endoscopic versus surgical drainage of the pancreatic duct in chronic pancreatitis. N Engl J Med 2007;356(7):676–684.

51. Cremer M, Devière J, Delhaye M, Baize M, Vandermeeren A. Stenting in severe chronic pancreatitis: results of medium-term follow-up in seventy-six patients. Endoscopy 1991;23(3):171–176.

52. Gabbrielli A, Pandolfi M, Mutignani M, et al. Efficacy of main pancreatic-duct endoscopic drainage in patients with chronic pancreatitis, continuous pain, and dilated duct. Gastrointest Endosc 2005;61(4):576–581.

53. Rösch T, Daniel S, Scholz M, et al; European Society of Gastrointestinal Endoscopy Research Group. Endoscopic treatment of chronic pancreatitis: a multicenter study of 1000 patients with long-term follow-up. Endoscopy 2002;34(10):765–771.

54. Delhaye M, Arvanitakis M, Verset G, Cremer M, Devière J. Long-term clinical outcome after endoscopic pancreatic ductal drainage for patients with painful chronic pancreatitis. Clin Gastroenterol Hepatol 2004;2(12):1096–1106.

55. Mallery S, Matlock J, Freeman ML. EUS-guided rendezvous drainage of obstructed biliary and pancreatic ducts: Report of 6 cases. Gastrointest Endosc 2004;59(1):100–107.

56. Will U, Fueldner F, Thieme AK, et al. Transgastric pancreatography and EUS-guided drainage of the pancreatic duct. J Hepatobiliary Pancreat Surg 2007;14(4):377–382.

57. Kahaleh M, Hernandez AJ, Tokar J, Adams RB, Shami VM, Yeaton P. EUS-guided pancreaticogastrostomy: analysis of its efficacy to drain inaccessible pancreatic ducts. Gastrointest Endosc 2007;65(2):224–230.

58. Will U, Wanzar C, Gerlach R, Meyer F. Interventional ultrasound-guided procedures in pancreatic pseudocysts, abscesses and infected necroses—Treatment algorithm in a large single-center study. Published online 2011 Ultraschall in Med http://dx.doi.org/10.1055/S-0029-1245949.

59. Will U, Wanzar C, Gerlach R, Meyer F. Ultraschall Med. 2011 Jan 21. [Epub ahead of print] Interventional Ultrasound-Guided Procedures in Pancreatic Pseudocysts, Abscesses and Infected Necroses - Treatment Algorithm in a Large Single-Center Study.

60. Cremer M, Deviere J. Endoscopic management of pancreatic cysts and pseudocysts. [letter] Gastrointest Endosc 1986;32(5):367–368.

61. Yamao K, Bhatia V, Mizuno N, et al. EUS-guided choledochoduodenostomy for palliative biliary drainage in patients with malignant biliary obstruction: results of long-term follow-up. Endoscopy 2008;40(4):340–342.

34 Portal Hypertension and Endoscopic Ultrasound

J.M. Wyse, A.V. Sahai

Anatomical Considerations

Portal hypertension is a pathologic increase in portal venous pressure. It results in a clinical syndrome that may include the development of varices, ascites, and encephalopathy. Although intrinsic liver disease manifesting as cirrhosis is the most common cause in Western countries, presinusoidal portal hypertension due to schistosomiasis is the predominant cause worldwide.[1]

■ Gastroesophageal Varices and Related Vasculature

Gastroesophageal varices have two main inflow tracts, the first being the left gastric or coronary vein, which decompress the portal vein directly (when flow is hepatofugal). The other major route is via the short gastric veins, which decompress the splenic vein at the splenic hilum and are often clinically relevant when splenic vein thrombosis results in isolated fundic varices in the stomach.

One of the most detailed examinations of the venous anatomy of the lower esophagus and upper stomach was reported by Hashizume et al. in 14 cadaver specimens (with portal hypertension in nine cases).[2] The authors demonstrated that, superficially, there are intraepithelial channels that collect and join to form a venous plexus just below the epithelium. The superficial venous plexus and adjacent deep submucosal veins are contiguous from the lower esophagus to the upper stomach and combine to form the endoscopically visible submucosal varices above and below the esophagogastric junction. Finally, adventitial para-esophageal collateral veins connect to the submucosal veins via perforating veins that penetrate through the muscularis propria. These para-esophageal collateral veins have since been classified, using a 20-MHz ultrasound probe, as peri-esophageal collateral veins (peri-ECVs) if they are directly in contact with the muscularis propria, and as para-esophageal collateral veins (para-ECVs) if they are not.[3] An analogous classification for gastric collateral veins (GCVs) into peri-GCVs and para-GCVs has been suggested.

In addition, the study by Hashizume et al. showed that the anterior branch of the left gastric vein forms gastroesophageal varices by directly communicating with submucosal veins (the anterior branch), while the posterior branch of the left gastric vein extends along the outside layer of the esophageal wall across the esophagogastric junction to the aforementioned para-esophageal veins.[2]

In summary, gastroesophageal varices form as a result of a complex but well-described venous circulation.

Diagnosis of Varices

■ Visualization of Esophageal Varices and Gastric Varices

In early studies, endoscopic ultrasonography (EUS) was found to be inferior to upper esophagogastroduodenoscopy (EGD) for detecting esophageal varices.[4–6] This was thought to be due to mechanical compression of esophageal varices by the endoscope and the EUS balloon, as well as the fact that the echoendoscope had a focal length outside the range of the varices.[7] Initially, the maximum reported sensitivity of EUS for esophageal varices was less than 60% relative to EGD. It must be borne in mind that endoscopic grading of varices has been shown to be subject to marked interobserver variability, including variability regarding the presence or absence of red signs.[8] However, when a 20-MHz miniprobe was used, the results were better. Using miniprobes, Miller et al. demonstrated that the mean variceal circumference increased with increasing endoscopic variceal grade, although overall correlation was poor.[8] In contrast, Faigel et al. found that, in comparison with EGD, EUS was similar for detecting esophageal varices (72% versus 74%, respectively).[9] In 2002, Lee et al. compared cirrhotic and dyspeptic (control) individuals.[10] There was good agreement between using EUS and EGD for the endoscopic (luminal) diagnosis of esophageal varices. Using EGD as the gold standard, the sensitivity, specificity, positive predictive value (PPV), and negative predictive value (NPV) of EUS for esophageal varices were each 96%.

EUS appears to be clearly superior to endoscopy for detecting gastric varices.[4–6,9] Using EUS as the gold standard, the sensitivity, specificity, PPV, and NPV of esophagogastroduodenoscopy for gastric varices were 44%, 94%, 78%, and 79%, respectively.[10] Another study reported a sensitivity of 70% with EGD, but the group of patients included had larger varices overall.[11]

In summary, EUS appears to provide similar results to EGD for detecting esophageal varices and is superior to

EGD for detecting gastric varices. The use of higher-frequency miniprobes may improve the performance of EUS with regard to esophageal varices.

Perforating and Collateral Veins

Before the advent of EUS, imaging of the collateral venous system required venography, which is invasive, and/or computed tomography (CT), which has inadequate sensitivity.[10] Although one study demonstrated that multidetector-row CT angiography and EUS were equivalent for fundic gastric collateral varices,[12] CT is still inferior for examining wall thickness and blood flow velocity.[13]

With regard to the esophageal vasculature, Lee et al. detected both peri-ECVs and para-ECVs in two-thirds of cirrhotic patients.[10] The size of the varices correlated positively with the Child–Pugh score and esophageal varix size.[9,10] In addition, 93 % of patients with varices had perforating veins connecting to ECVs, and the remaining two patients had esophageal varices connected to GCVs. All perforators were found within 5 cm above the gastroesophageal junction. However, the sensitivity for perforating veins ranges from 15–100 % in the literature, depending on the technique used and the size of varices.[10,14–16]

With regard to gastric collaterals, Lee et al.[10] found para-GCVs in 81 % of cirrhotic patients and peri-GCVs in 65 %. The number of perforating veins correlated positively with the Child–Pugh score and the sizes of both esophageal varices and gastric varices. Faigel et al. showed that large para-GCVs (> 5 mm) correlated with large para-ECVs (> 5 mm).[9]

Using EUS alone in cirrhotic patients, a diagnosis of portal hypertension could be made on the basis of venous abnormalities with a sensitivity, specificity, PPV, and NPV of 92 %, 95 %, 84 %, and 98 %, respectively.[10] By contrast, diagnosis of portal hypertension with EGD in cirrhotic patients had a sensitivity, specificity, PPV, and NPV of 58 %, 100 %, 100 %, and 89 %, respectively. Another study similarly found that EUS detection of ECVs was 97 % sensitive and 97 % specific for the presence of cirrhosis,[9] while the EGD diagnosis of esophageal varices only had a sensitivity of 74 % for cirrhosis.

In patients without portal hypertension, venous abnormalities were only detectable in 5 % of cases in one study,[10] but 22 % were found to have perigastric collaterals in another.[9] The latter authors argued that small gastric collateral varices may be a normal finding at EUS, but that ECVs signify portal hypertension.

Kakutani et al. identified gastrorenal shunts in patients with gastric varices and reported a 95 % rate of agreement (κ = 0.9) between contrast-enhanced CT and EUS.[17] Two additional shunts found only on EUS were < 5 mm in size. The presence of these shunts may allow balloon-occluded retrograde transvenous obliteration. Bastid et al. subsequently commented that transabdominal Doppler ultrasound should continue to be the first-line examination in assessing these patients.[18]

In summary, EUS can easily visualize ECVs, GCVs, and often perforating veins. The size of the collaterals and the number of perforating veins is associated with the size of the gastroesophageal varices. EUS visualization of varices and/or collateral circulation correlates well with the presence of portal hypertension.

Ectopic Varices

EUS has made it possible to visualize ectopic varices in a variety of locations. Yeh et al. published a case report on duodenal varices.[19] Palazzo et al. reviewed cases of extrahepatic biliary obstruction resulting from biliary varices.[20] Except for a patient who underwent portal venography, each patient had undergone transabdominal ultrasonography and abdominal CT that did not detect the varices. All patients had portal vein thrombosis, which was seen as a solid, echogenic thrombus on EUS. Biliary varices were found both in and around the wall of the common bile duct, as well as in the gallbladder wall. Another case of portal vein thrombosis with choledocholithiasis was reported with biliary varices.[21] Rai et al. suggested that intraductal ultrasound may better visualize biliary varices causing obstructive jaundice.[22] EUS also diagnosed choledochojejunal anastomotic varices following total pancreatectomy.[23]

EUS detection of varices in the lower gastrointestinal tract includes pancolonic varices in a patient with idiopathic portal hypertension,[24] but most commonly involves rectal varices. Dhiman et al. demonstrated submucosal rectal varices that were not visible on endoscopy.[25] More severe rectal varices occurred in patients with large esophageal varices and a history of injection sclerotherapy. There was no correlation between the severity of hemorrhoids and portal hypertension. In another study using endoscopic color Doppler ultrasound (see next section), color flow imaging identified the varices and their afferent vessels in 12 patients with rectal varices.[26] All had a continuous flow wave, except one with a pulsatile component.

In summary, EUS can help identify ectopic varices if the site is endoscopically accessible.

Hemodynamics using Endoscopic Color Doppler Ultrasound (ECDUS)

ECDUS allows hemodynamic examination of blood vessels and displays the direction of flow. It has been shown to enhance EUS imaging of gastroesophageal varices. Sato et al. have published extensively on the use of ECDUS and gastroesophageal varix detection. Color flow images of esophageal varices and esophageal collateral veins, as well as of gastric varices and gastric collateral varices, were obtained in all patients with gastroesophageal varices.[13,27] The wall thickness of gastric varices with red color signs, erosions, or associated bleeding was significantly less than with other gastric varices. The mean flow velocity in gastric varices was also significantly higher in larger varices and in cases with associated bleeding. The authors therefore suggested that flow velocity and wall thickness measurement may be useful for predicting bleeding in patients with gastric varices.[13] However, this has not been confirmed in prospective studies.

As stated, the detection rate for perforating veins in the literature has varied widely, from 15 % to 100 %.[10,14–16] Perforating veins have mostly afferent flow (i. e., toward the submucosal varix), as shown by ECDUS,[3,15,28] and are associated with larger varices.[14,28] Using the galactose-based Doppler-enhancing contrast agent Levovist (Schering, Berlin, Germany), the yield for diagnosing perforating veins improved from 77 % to 97 % and the direction of flow was subjectively assessed more easily.[16] The same group used Levovist to detect recurrent varices, and the sensitivity of ECDUS detection of perforating veins rose from 31 % to 76 %.[15] Levovist also helped improve ECDUS detection of arterial blood flow in esophageal varices.[29] The authors suggest that only afferent perforators (type I) should be targeted with sclerotherapy, and they recommend avoiding efferent (type II) and mixed (type III) perforating veins, which may be serving to partially decompress the gastroesophageal varix.

Wong et al. demonstrated a reproducible continuous venous hum in five patients with gastric varices and in one with pulsatile flow, allowing differentiation from nonvariceal submucosal masses.[30] Gastric varices due to splenic vein thrombosis were described using ECDUS color flow as having "round cardiac and fundal regions at the center," with variceal extension to the greater curvature of the gastric body.[31]

Hino et al. used ECDUS to investigate the left gastric vein and its relation to the formation of gastroesophageal varices.[28] Increased left gastric vein trunk diameter only showed a trend toward association with larger varices, but hepatofugal left gastric vein flow velocity did statistically increase with increasing variceal size. Transabdominal ultrasound has previously shown that flow velocity in the left gastric vein is associated with variceal bleeding.[32] The dominance pattern of the left gastric vein was classified according to the relative sizes of its anterior and posterior branches into an "AD type" for anterior-branch dominance, a "PD type" for posterior branch dominance, and an "ND type" for nondominance (equal branch diameters). The AD type was associated significantly more often with larger variceal size. This was not surprising, as the anterior branch traveled to the esophagogastric junction and ultimately entered varices, whereas the posterior branch traveled via para-ECVs to enter the azygos system, and/or formed a renal shunt. However, the posterior branch may still affect variceal size and bleeding to some

extent via perforating veins originating from the para-ECVs.

Finally, Pontes et al. used an ECDUS balloon to carry out manometry of esophageal varices.[33] The pressure when the Doppler signal disappeared was recorded. Good pressure correlation was observed in an in vitro model. It was possible to measure the esophageal varix pressure in 93 % of cases. This pressure and the portal pressure (estimated using the hepatic vein pressure gradient) correlated significantly ($r = 0.64$).

In summary, hemodynamic assessment with ECDUS has improved our understanding of the pathophysiology of gastroesophageal varices. It appears that the left gastric vein has the greatest impact on variceal formation—mainly through its anterior branch flowing into the area of the esophagogastric junction, but perhaps also via its posterior branch, forming collateral vessels that communicate with gastroesophageal varices, often via afferent-flowing perforating veins.

Nonvariceal Markers of Portal Hypertension and Chronic Liver Disease

It is well known that patients with cirrhosis may have ultrasonographic parenchymal abnormalities such as inhomogeneity, lobularity, irregularity of the liver surface, and prominence of the caudate lobe. Patients with active chronic hepatitis also often have large, benign-appearing perihepatic lymph nodes.

Other indirect signs of portal hypertension include nonvariceal vascular abnormalities and ascites. Although this subject has not been studied specifically in portal hypertension, EUS is likely able to detect very small pockets of ascites and early evidence of variceal congestion that cannot be detected with CT or transcutaneous ultrasound. Small-volume ascites detection has been shown to be feasible in the context of esophageal and gastric cancer.[34,35] These results should apply to ascites in cirrhotic patients as well.

Anecdotally, in patients with proven cirrhosis, the portal vein and splenic vein have been found to be large and tortuous, and there is a noticeable increase in the number of veins around the stomach and especially in the region of the splenic hilum. The true longitudinal dimensions of the spleen may be somewhat difficult to assess with EUS, but obvious splenomegaly is another indirect sign of portal hypertension. In three patients, EUS has also been shown to be able to detect gastric antral vascular ectasia.[36]

As the azygos vein is a key outflow tract for portosystemic shunting, returning blood from gastroesophageal varices to the superior vena cava, the vein's characteristics (size and flow) have been studied as potential indicators of portal hypertension. Azygos blood flow velocity has been validated against a more invasive thermodilution technique.[37,38] In comparison with noncirrhotic individuals, cirrhotic patients have been shown to have increased azygos blood flow velocity[39,40] and an increased vein diameter.[6,9,40] It should be noted that numerous other causes of azygos vein dilation have also been found.[41] Azygos diameter correlated with a deteriorating Child–Pugh score in one study,[9] but not in another.[42] Azygos blood flow has also been shown to increase with declining Child–Pugh grades[42] and with larger gastroesophageal varices.[6] However, changes in azygos blood flow following endoscopic therapy have been less clear. A decrease in azygos blood flow after endoscopic variceal band ligation was demonstrated using magnetic resonance imaging[43] and transesophageal echocardiography.[44] One study using EUS after esophageal variceal injection sclerotherapy reported a decrease in azygos blood flow, but two studies observed no differences.[40]

Nishida et al. used ECDUS to assess the hemodynamic effect of somatostatin and octreotide on azygos blood flow.[38] They showed that the decrease in azygos blood flow induced by both drugs was immediate and transient, with a rebound increase in azygos blood flow seen at 60 minutes after the injection in the somatostatin group. Lee et al. monitored azygos blood flow following pharmacologic intervention with boluses of somatostatin and terlipressin over a 10-minute period.[42] Both drugs caused a reduction in azygos blood flow, but neither reached statistical significance beyond 1 minute.

The thoracic duct diameter has also been examined and was found to be nearly doubled in diameter in cirrhotic individuals in comparison with controls in one study,[9] whereas in another study the duct diameter was increased only in those with ascites and esophageal varices.[45]

In summary, numerous indirect signs of portal hypertension can be detected with EUS, the best studied of which are size and blood flow in the azygos vein. These are likely to remain auxiliary methods of detecting and assessing portal hypertension.

EUS and Variceal Bleeding

■ Predicting the Bleeding Risk

In terms of predicting variceal bleeding, Miller et al. used a 20-MHz probe to examine the total cross-sectional area of esophageal varices.[46] The mean sum of the cross-sectional area differed significantly between those who bled and those who did not. For each increasing square centimeter, the odds ratio for bleeding per month was 6.3. A cut-off value of 0.45 cm^2 provided a sensitivity and specificity for future bleeding of 83% and 75%, respectively. However, the variceal grade did not predict bleeding in this study.

Faigel et al. found that cirrhotic patients with prior gastroesophageal variceal hemorrhage were more likely to have gastric varices, large esophageal collateral varices (> 5 mm), and large gastric collateral varices (> 5 mm) than those without previous bleeding.[9]

Variceal wall tension was examined by Schiano et al., who measured the radius of esophageal varices and the wall thickness successfully, although no correlation between the two was found and the wall tension could therefore not be calculated.[47] Wall tension in esophageal varices has been measured using EUS-guided direct variceal puncture.[48] The 20-MHz miniprobe has also been used to visualize hematocystic spots as "varices on varices."[49] The impact of these techniques on the ability to predict bleeding is still unclear.

In summary, a higher total cross-sectional area in varices, as well as large ECVs and GCVs, appear to portend a higher risk of variceal bleeding.

■ Assessing the Response to Endoscopic Therapy and EUS-Guided Endoscopic Therapy

Much of the literature on EUS-guided endoscopic variceal therapy is concerned with injection sclerotherapy, rather than esophageal variceal band ligation (EVBL). Although injection sclerotherapy is still often used in some countries, a recent American Association for the Study of Liver Diseases/American College of Gastroenterology practice guideline[50] supports the use of either EVBL or injection sclerotherapy *only* in the context of acute variceal bleeding. However, it recommends against the use of injection sclerotherapy for either primary or secondary prophylaxis against esophageal varices and favors EVBL as the endoscopic modality in these cases. The practice guidelines recommend tissue adhesives such as cyanoacrylate in patients with bleeding gastric varices, but list EVBL as an option.

EUS has long been known to be capable of assessing gastroesophageal varices after endoscopic therapy for evidence of complete or partial variceal obliteration.[51] In one study of 35 patients treated with either injection sclerotherapy or EVBL, 17% of those in whom EGD had suggested complete variceal eradication were found to have persistent varices on EUS.[52] Nagamine et al. used a miniprobe to perform "intensive" EVBL in which varices and perforating veins were targeted.[53] Dhiman et al. showed that successful endoscopic variceal obliteration with injection sclerotherapy reduces the number and size of ECVs and the number of GCVs and obliterates perforating veins, in comparison with unsuccessful obliteration.[54] Suzuki et al. carried out EUS after EVBL alone (or with injection sclerotherapy if EVBL failed). Following apparent endoscopic obliteration, 61% of the patients were found to have evidence of persistent esophageal submucosal vessels on EUS, and submucosal cardia varices were identified in all of them. The size of these cardia vessels was predictive of recurrences at a 2-year follow-up examination.[55] Konishi et al. predicted esophageal varix recurrence following EVBL by examining the gastric cardia for varices using EUS. Prior to EVBL, all patients were found to have cardia varices. Following EVBL, the patients with recurrent esophageal varices were more likely to have had more severe perforating veins in the gastric cardia.[11] Leung et al. also studied EUS following EVBL and demonstrated that patients with persistent, large esophageal collateral veins (≥ 5 mm) were more likely to have recurrent esophageal varices and bleeding.[56] Lo et al. showed that ECVs persist significantly more often after EVBL than after injection sclerotherapy, and that they are associated with a greater incidence of esophageal varix recurrence. In both treatment groups, more collaterals were associated with more recurrences, but there was no difference in the bleeding rates.[57]

Irisawa et al. followed up patients treated with endoscopic injection sclerotherapy.[58] In patients with variceal recurrences, perforating veins were both more frequent and larger, and the patients also had more severe *peri*-ECVs. Mild peri-ECVs were seen more often in the group without recurrences. This finding was subsequently confirmed again by the same group.[59] However, no significant differences were observed for *para*-ECVs. The EUS findings 8 months after injection sclerotherapy were shown to be useful for predicting recurrences. The importance of esophageal venous collaterals after injection sclerotherapy in relation to variceal recurrences has also been demonstrated using CT.[60] As stated earlier, blood flow in perforating veins is generally toward the submucosal varix,[3,15] and perforating veins are associated with larger varices.[14] As most perforating veins were found to be joined to peri-ECVs rather than to para-ECVs, it seems plausible that these represent afferent vessels themselves. The authors suggest that para-ECVs may be predominantly efferent.

A recent randomized and controlled trial by de Paulo et al. compared EUS-guided sclerotherapy in esophageal collateral vessels with conventional sclerotherapy.[61] A study by Lahoti et al. differed[62] in that the sclerosant was injected directly into perforating vessels and peri-ECVs and was aimed toward the perforators. Collateral esophageal vessels persisted in one-third of the patients after standard therapy, in comparison with none in the EUS-guided sclerotherapy group. Four of 24 patients who received standard care had recurrences (before 1 year in three cases), while two of 24 patients who underwent EUS-guided sclerotherapy had recurrences after 1 year. However, there were no statistical differences with regard to the recurrence-free survival.

Returning to the left gastric vein, this time in the context of endoscopic therapy, Hino et al.[63] found that left gastric vein flow was significantly lower and that the branching pattern was posterior-dominant or nondominant in patients with fewer esophageal varix recurrences. Kura-

mochi et al. showed that left gastric vein flow velocity ≥ 12 cm/s with the anterior-dominant branching type[64] leads to significantly faster recurrence of esophageal varices.

Similar research has been carried out in patients undergoing gastroesophageal variceal eradication therapy with cyanoacrylate. Iwase et al. demonstrated that cyanoacrylate-treated gastric varices could be followed up using EUS to detect residual flow that was not identifiable endoscopically, and that patients with persistent flow were more likely to bleed.[65] Lee et al. confirmed the usefulness of EUS-guided cyanoacrylate injection for gastric varices that bled by comparing an "on-demand" group with a "repeated injection until obliteration" group.[66] The repeated-injection group had significantly less recurrent bleeding, with a trend toward improved survival. Romero-Castro et al. injected a cyanoacrylate mixture at the level of the perforating veins of gastric varices until obliteration.[67] Neither bleeding nor complications occurred during a mean follow-up period of 10 months. Liao et al. also used EUS to help completely obliterate a partially occluded gastric varix that had become infected.[68]

In summary, endosonographic predictive factors for gastroesophageal varix recurrence following endoscopic therapy are: 1, the presence or recurrence of collateral veins (severe peri-ECVs may play a particularly important role); 2, endoscopically nonvisible submucosal varices (perhaps particularly in the cardia); 3, larger-diameter and more numerous perforating veins (perhaps specifically those showing afferent flow on ECDUS); and 4, an "anterior-dominant" left gastric vein branching pattern with a high flow velocity in the vein.

Future Applications

■ Direct EUS-Guided Portal Pressure Measurement and Venography

Portal hypertension is usually defined indirectly on the basis of an increased hepatic vein pressure gradient (HVPG) above 5–10 mmHg.[69,70] This represents the difference in pressure between the portal vein (estimated using wedged hepatic venous pressure) and the intra-abdominal inferior vena cava (estimated using the free hepatic vein pressure) and requires an invasive radiographic procedure. Varices form when the HVPG exceeds 10 mmHg,[71] and they bleed at > 12 mmHg.[72] A recent study showed that 30 % of pressure tracings from experienced centers were not interpretable.[73] However, when the correct technique is used, there is little variability in HVPG findings, except at lower values.[74] Overall, it is still a safe and accurate technique.[73] In addition, no other less invasive methods of accurately estimating portal hypertension are available,[75] and experts have suggested that less invasive tests may be useful.[76]

During the last 5 years, considerable advances have been made in the technique of EUS-guided portal vein catheterization. The main potential advantages over the above method of measuring HGPV angiographically are: 1, direct measurement of portal vein pressures; 2, diagnosing presinusoidal portal hypertension;[77] 3, simultaneous assessment for gastroesophageal varices both endoscopically and endosonographically during the procedure; and 4, portal venography to assess for thrombosis of the portal venous system.

An initial feasibility study in a swine model compared the transhepatic to the EUS-guided duodenal approach using 22-gauge needles.[78] Transhepatic measurements were achieved in 64% of cases (nine of 14), in comparison with success in 100% of cases (21 of 21) with EUS. High-quality pressure tracings were not achieved in the first three attempts at EUS, but this improved with experience. The mean portal vein pressures, including animals in which portal hypertension had been induced, correlated closely ($r = 0.91$). The transhepatic approach was complicated by severe bleeding, resulting in death in one pig. At autopsy, small subserosal hematomas were found at the EUS puncture site in all of the animals. Among the seven pigs that received anticoagulation and only underwent EUS catheterization, one had a small collection of blood between the portal vein and the duodenum.

Another study in a similar animal model showed that injection of CO_2 provided excellent opacification of all the intrahepatic portal vein branches, the main portal vein, and the splenic vein. No complications, hemodynamic shifts, or hematomas were identified. The authors suggested CO_2 may also reduce contrast-induced nephrologic complications.[79]

The same authors then extended the technique by placing a 5.5-Fr ERCP catheter in the portal vein after a 19-gauge puncture and guide-wire exchange.[80] Portal venography was carried out using either iodinated contrast or CO_2. Continuous portal pressure measurements were obtained. The results were consistent within each animal, although one had elevated pressures, with normal autopsy findings. There were no complications.

EUS may also be able to play a role in the injection of therapeutic agents directly into the portal vein, either to dissolve thrombi or to induce localized atrophy.[77,81] EUS has been shown to allow diagnosis of portal vein thrombosis without venography fairly accurately (sensitivity 81%, specificity 93%, and overall accuracy 89% in comparison with CT-based and surgery-based diagnoses).[82]

In summary, although EUS-guided portal vein catheterization, pressure measurement, and venography appear to be feasible and safe, further research and safety evaluations are needed before they are used in humans, especially in the context of portal hypertension and coagulopathy.

Summary and Conclusions

EUS is an excellent method of detecting the occurrence and recurrence of varices and can simultaneously provide detailed information about the surrounding venous circulation. With further research, EUS may be able to play an important role in predicting variceal bleeding both before and after obliterative endoscopic therapy. The method may also be able to contribute to less invasive direct measurement of portal vein pressure and venography.

References

1. Feldman M, Friedman LS, Brandt LJ, eds. Sleisenger & Fordtran's Gastrointestinal and Liver Disease: Pathophysiology, Diagnosis, Management. 8th ed. Philadelphia: Saunders; 2006.
2. Hashizume M, Kitano S, Sugimachi K, Sueishi K. Three-dimensional view of the vascular structure of the lower esophagus in clinical portal hypertension. Hepatology 1988;8(6):1482–1487.
3. Irisawa A, Obara K, Sato Y, et al. EUS analysis of collateral veins inside and outside the esophageal wall in portal hypertension. Gastrointest Endosc 1999;50(3):374–380.
4. Burtin P, Calès P, Oberti F, et al. Endoscopic ultrasonographic signs of portal hypertension in cirrhosis. Gastrointest Endosc 1996;44(3):257–261.
5. Boustière C, Dumas O, Jouffre C, et al. Endoscopic ultrasonography classification of gastric varices in patients with cirrhosis. Comparison with endoscopic findings. J Hepatol 1993;19(2):268–272.
6. Caletti G, Brocchi E, Baraldini M, Ferrari A, Gibilaro M, Barbara L. Assessment of portal hypertension by endoscopic ultrasonography. Gastrointest Endosc 1990; 36(2,Suppl):S21–S27.
7. Miller L, Abdalla A. The role of endoscopy in the treatment of esophageal varices, 2002-2003. Curr Opin Gastroenterol 2003;19(5):483–486.
8. Miller LS, Schiano TD, Adrain A, et al. Comparison of high-resolution endoluminal sonography to video endoscopy in the detection and evaluation of esophageal varices. Hepatology 1996;24(3):552–555.
9. Faigel DO, Rosen HR, Sasaki A, Flora K, Benner K. EUS in cirrhotic patients with and without prior variceal hemorrhage in comparison with noncirrhotic control subjects. Gastrointest Endosc 2000;52(4):455–462.
10. Lee YT, Chan FK, Ching JY, et al. Diagnosis of gastroesophageal varices and portal collateral venous abnormalities by endosonography in cirrhotic patients. Endoscopy 2002; 34(5):391–398.
11. Konishi Y, Nakamura T, Kida H, Seno H, Okazaki K, Chiba T. Catheter US probe EUS evaluation of gastric cardia and perigastric vascular structures to predict esophageal variceal recurrence. Gastrointest Endosc 2002;55(2):197–203.
12. Willmann JK, Weishaupt D, Böhm T, et al. Detection of submucosal gastric fundal varices with multi-detector row CT angiography. Gut 2003;52(6):886–892.
13. Sato T, Yamazaki K, Toyota J, Karino Y, Ohmura T, Akaike J. Observation of gastric variceal flow characteristics by endo-

scopic ultrasonography using color Doppler. Am J Gastroenterol 2008;103(3):575–580.

14. Choudhuri G, Dhiman RK, Agarwal DK. Endosonographic evaluation of the venous anatomy around the gastroesophageal junction in patients with portal hypertension. Hepatogastroenterology 1996;43(11):1250–1255.

15. Sato T, Yamazaki K, Toyota J, et al. Perforating veins in recurrent esophageal varices evaluated by endoscopic color Doppler ultrasonography with a galactose-based contrast agent. J Gastroenterol 2004;39(5):422–428.

16. Sato T, Yamazaki K, Toyota J, Karino Y, Ohmura T, Suga T. Evaluation of hemodynamics in esophageal varices. Value of endoscopic color Doppler ultrasonography with a galactose-based contrast agent. Hepatol Res 2003;25(1):55–61.

17. Kakutani H, Hino S, Ikeda K, et al. Use of the curved linear-array echo endoscope to identify gastrorenal shunts in patients with gastric fundal varices. Endoscopy 2004; 36(8):710–714.

18. Bastid C, Sahel J. Use of the curved linear-array echo endoscope to identify gastrorenal shunts in patients with gastric fundal varices. Endoscopy 2005;37(4):398, author reply 399.

19. Yeh YY, Hou MC, Lin HC, Chang FY, Lee SD. Case report: successful obliteration of a bleeding duodenal varix using endoscopic ligation. J Gastroenterol Hepatol 1998; 13(6): 591–593.

20. Palazzo L, Hochain P, Helmer C, et al. Biliary varices on endoscopic ultrasonography: clinical presentation and outcome. Endoscopy 2000;32(7):520–524.

21. Umphress JL, Pecha RE, Urayama S. Biliary stricture caused by portal biliopathy: diagnosis by EUS with Doppler US. Gastrointest Endosc 2004;60(6):1021–1024.

22. Rai T, Irisawa A, Takagi T, et al. Intraductal sonography of biliary varices associated with extrahepatic portal vein obstruction. J Clin Ultrasound 2007;35(9):527–530.

23. Levy MJ, Wong Kee Song LM, Kendrick ML, Misra S, Gostout CJ. EUS-guided coil embolization for refractory ectopic variceal bleeding (with videos). Gastrointest Endosc 2008; 67(3):572–574.

24. Francois F, Tadros C, Diehl D. Pan-colonic varices and idiopathic portal hypertension. J Gastrointestin Liver Dis 2007;16(3):325–328.

25. Dhiman RK, Saraswat VA, Choudhuri G, Sharma BC, Pandey R, Naik SR. Endosonographic, endoscopic, and histologic evaluation of alterations in the rectal venous system in patients with portal hypertension. Gastrointest Endosc 1999;49(2):218–227.

26. Sato T, Yamazaki K, Akaike J. Evaluation of the hemodynamics of rectal varices by endoscopic ultrasonography. J Gastroenterol 2006;41(6):588–592.

27. Sato T, Yamazaki K, Toyota J, et al. Usefulness of electronic radial endoscopic color Doppler ultrasonography in esophageal varices: comparison with convex type. J Gastroenterol 2006;41(1):28–33.

28. Hino S, Kakutani H, Ikeda K, et al. Hemodynamic assessment of the left gastric vein in patients with esophageal varices with color Doppler EUS: factors affecting development of esophageal varices. Gastrointest Endosc 2002; 55(4):512–517.

29. Sato T, Yamazaki K, Toyota J, et al. Evaluation of arterial blood flow in esophageal varices via endoscopic color Doppler ultrasonography with a galactose-based contrast agent. J Gastroenterol 2005;40(1):64–69.

30. Wong RC, Farooq FT, Chak A. Endoscopic Doppler US probe for the diagnosis of gastric varices (with videos). Gastrointest Endosc 2007;65(3):491–496.

31. Sato T, Yamazaki K, Akaike J, Toyota J, Karino Y, Ohmura T. Clinical and endoscopic features of gastric varices secondary to splenic vein occlusion. Hepatol Res 2008;38(11): 1076–1082.

32. Matsutani S, Furuse J, Ishii H, Mizumoto H, Kimura K, Ohto M. Hemodynamics of the left gastric vein in portal hypertension. Gastroenterology 1993;105(2):513–518.

33. Pontes JM, Leitão MC, Portela F, Nunes A, Freitas D. Endosonographic Doppler-guided manometry of esophageal varices: experimental validation and clinical feasibility. Endoscopy 2002;34(12):966–972.

34. Lee YT, Ng EK, Hung LC, et al. Accuracy of endoscopic ultrasonography in diagnosing ascites and predicting peritoneal metastases in gastric cancer patients. Gut 2005;54(11): 1541–1545.

35. Sultan J, Robinson S, Hayes N, Griffin SM, Richardson DL, Preston SR. Endoscopic ultrasonography-detected low-volume ascites as a predictor of inoperability for oesophagogastric cancer. Br J Surg 2008;95(9):1127–1130.

36. Avunduk C, Hampf F. Endoscopic ultrasound in the diagnosis of watermelon stomach. J Clin Gastroenterol 1996; 22(2):104–106.

37. Hansen EF, Bendtsen F, Brinch K, Møller S, Henriksen JH, Becker U. Endoscopic Doppler ultrasound for measurement of azygos blood flow. Validation against thermodilution and assessment of pharmacological effects of terlipressin in portal hypertension. Scand J Gastroenterol 2001;36(3): 318–325.

38. Nishida H, Giostra E, Spahr L, Mentha G, Mitamura K, Hadengue A. Validation of color Doppler EUS for azygos blood flow measurement in patients with cirrhosis: application to the acute hemodynamic effects of somatostatin, octreotide, or placebo. Gastrointest Endosc 2001;54(1):24–30.

39. Sukigara M, Matsumoto T, Takeuchi M, et al. Doppler echography for hemodynamic studies of the azygos vein. Surg Endosc 1989;3(1):21–28.

40. Kassem AM, Salama ZA, Rösch T. Endoscopic ultrasonography in portal hypertension. Endoscopy 1997;29(5): 399–406.

41. Shin MS, Ho KJ. Clinical significance of azygos vein enlargement: radiographic recognition and etiologic analysis. Clin Imaging 1999;23(4):236–240.

42. Lee YT, Sung JJ, Yung MY, Yu AL, Chung SC. Use of color Doppler EUS in assessing azygos blood flow for patients with portal hypertension. Gastrointest Endosc 1999;50(1): 47–52.

43. Sugano S, Yamamoto K, Takamura N, Momiyama K, Watanabe M, Ishii K. Azygos venous blood flow while fasting, postprandially, and after endoscopic variceal ligation, measured by magnetic resonance imaging. J Gastroenterol 1999;34(3):310–314.

44. Yokoyama M, Shijo H, Ota K, et al. Effects of endoscopic variceal sclerotherapy on azygos vein blood flow and systemic haemodynamics. J Gastroenterol Hepatol 1996;11(8): 780–785.

45. Parasher VK, Meroni E, Malesci A, et al. Observation of thoracic duct morphology in portal hypertension by endoscopic ultrasound. Gastrointest Endosc 1998;48(6): 588–592.

46. Miller L, Banson FL, Bazir K, et al. Risk of esophageal variceal bleeding based on endoscopic ultrasound evaluation of the

sum of esophageal variceal cross-sectional surface area. Am J Gastroenterol 2003;98(2):454–459.

47. Schiano TD, Adrain AL, Cassidy MJ, et al. Use of high-resolution endoluminal sonography to measure the radius and wall thickness of esophageal varices. Gastrointest Endosc 1996;44(4):425–428.

48. Jackson FW, Adrain AL, Black M, Miller LS. Calculation of esophageal variceal wall tension by direct sonographic and manometric measurements. Gastrointest Endosc 1999;50(2):247–251.

49. Schiano TD, Adrain AL, Vega KJ, Liu JB, Black M, Miller LS. High-resolution endoluminal sonography assessment of the hematocystic spots of esophageal varices. Gastrointest Endosc 1999;49(4 Pt 1):424–427.

50. Garcia-Tsao G, Sanyal AJ, Grace ND, Carey W; Practice Guidelines Committee of the American Association for the Study of Liver Diseases; Practice Parameters Committee of the American College of Gastroenterology. Prevention and management of gastroesophageal varices and variceal hemorrhage in cirrhosis. Hepatology 2007;46(3):922–938.

51. Ziegler K, Gregor M, Zeitz M, Zimmer T, Habermann F, Riecken EO. Evaluation of endosonography in sclerotherapy of esophageal varices. Endoscopy 1991;23(5):247–250.

52. Pontes JM, Leitão MC, Portela FA, Rosa AM, Ministro P, Freitas DS. Endoscopic ultrasonography in the treatment of oesophageal varices by endoscopic sclerotherapy and band ligation: do we need it? Eur J Gastroenterol Hepatol 1995;7(1):41–46.

53. Nagamine N, Ueno N, Tomiyama T, et al. A pilot study on modified endoscopic variceal ligation using endoscopic ultrasonography with color Doppler function. Am J Gastroenterol 1998;93(2):150–155.

54. Dhiman RK, Choudhuri G, Saraswat VA, Agarwal DK, Naik SR. Role of paraoesophageal collaterals and perforating veins on outcome of endoscopic sclerotherapy for oesophageal varices: an endosonographic study. Gut 1996;38(5):759–764.

55. Suzuki T, Matsutani S, Umebara K, et al. EUS changes predictive for recurrence of esophageal varices in patients treated by combined endoscopic ligation and sclerotherapy. Gastrointest Endosc 2000;52(5):611–617.

56. Leung VK, Sung JJ, Ahuja AT, et al. Large paraesophageal varices on endosonography predict recurrence of esophageal varices and rebleeding. Gastroenterology 1997;112(6):1811–1816.

57. Lo GH, Lai KH, Cheng JS, Huang RL, Wang SJ, Chiang HT. Prevalence of paraesophageal varices and gastric varices in patients achieving variceal obliteration by banding ligation and by injection sclerotherapy. Gastrointest Endosc 1999;49(4 Pt 1):428–436.

58. Irisawa A, Saito A, Obara K, et al. Endoscopic recurrence of esophageal varices is associated with the specific EUS abnormalities: severe periesophageal collateral veins and large perforating veins. Gastrointest Endosc 2001; 53(1):77–84.

59. Irisawa A, Obara K, Bhutani MS, et al. Role of para-esophageal collateral veins in patients with portal hypertension based on the results of endoscopic ultrasonography and liver scintigraphy analysis. J Gastroenterol Hepatol 2003;18(3):309–314.

60. Lin CY, Lin PW, Tsai HM, Lin XZ, Chang TT, Shin JS. Influence of paraesophageal venous collaterals on efficacy of endoscopic sclerotherapy for esophageal varices. Hepatology 1994;19(3):602–608.

61. de Paulo GA, Ardengh JC, Nakao FS, Ferrari AP. Treatment of esophageal varices: a randomized controlled trial comparing endoscopic sclerotherapy and EUS-guided sclerotherapy of esophageal collateral veins. Gastrointest Endosc 2006;63(3):396–402, quiz 463.

62. Lahoti S, Catalano MF, Alcocer E, Hogan WJ, Geenen JE. Obliteration of esophageal varices using EUS-guided sclerotherapy with color Doppler. Gastrointest Endosc 2000; 51(3):331–333.

63. Hino S, Kakutani H, Ikeda K, et al. Hemodynamic analysis of esophageal varices using color Doppler endoscopic ultrasonography to predict recurrence after endoscopic treatment. Endoscopy 2001;33(10):869–872.

64. Kuramochi A, Imazu H, Kakutani H, Uchiyama Y, Hino S, Urashima M. Color Doppler endoscopic ultrasonography in identifying groups at a high-risk of recurrence of esophageal varices after endoscopic treatment. J Gastroenterol 2007;42(3):219–224.

65. Iwase H, Suga S, Morise K, Kuroiwa A, Yamaguchi T, Horiuchi Y. Color Doppler endoscopic ultrasonography for the evaluation of gastric varices and endoscopic obliteration with cyanoacrylate glue. Gastrointest Endosc 1995;41(2):150–154.

66. Lee YT, Chan FK, Ng EK, et al. EUS-guided injection of cyanoacrylate for bleeding gastric varices. Gastrointest Endosc 2000;52(2):168–174.

67. Romero-Castro R, Pellicer-Bautista FJ, Jimenez-Saenz M, et al. EUS-guided injection of cyanoacrylate in perforating feeding veins in gastric varices: results in 5 cases. Gastrointest Endosc 2007;66(2):402–407.

68. Liao SC, Ko CW, Yeh HZ, Chang CS, Yang SS, Chen GH. Successful treatment of persistent bacteremia after endoscopic injection of N-butyl-2-cyanoacrylate for gastric varices bleeding. Endoscopy 2007;39(Suppl 1):E176–E177.

69. de Franchis R. Updating consensus in portal hypertension: report of the Baveno III Consensus Workshop on definitions, methodology and therapeutic strategies in portal hypertension. J Hepatol 2000;33(5):846–852.

70. Sanyal AJ, Bosch J, Blei A, Arroyo V. Portal hypertension and its complications. Gastroenterology 2008;134(6):1715–1728.

71. Garcia-Tsao G, Groszmann RJ, Fisher RL, Conn HO, Atterbury CE, Glickman M. Portal pressure, presence of gastroesophageal varices and variceal bleeding. Hepatology 1985;5(3):419–424.

72. Groszmann RJ, Garcia-Tsao G, Bosch J, et al; Portal Hypertension Collaborative Group. Beta-blockers to prevent gastroesophageal varices in patients with cirrhosis. N Engl J Med 2005;353(21):2254–2261.

73. Groszmann RJ, Wongcharatrawee S. The hepatic venous pressure gradient: anything worth doing should be done right. Hepatology 2004;39(2):280–282.

74. Thalheimer U, Mela M, Patch D, Burroughs AK. Targeting portal pressure measurements: a critical reappraisal. Hepatology 2004;39(2):286–290.

75. Huet PM, Pomier-Layrargues G. The hepatic venous pressure gradient: "remixed and revisited". Hepatology 2004; 39(2):295–298.

76. de Franchis R. Evolving consensus in portal hypertension. Report of the Baveno IV consensus workshop on methodology of diagnosis and therapy in portal hypertension. J Hepatol 2005;43(1):167–176.

77. Brugge WR. EUS is an important new tool for accessing the portal vein. Gastrointest Endosc 2008;67(2):343–344.

78. Lai L, Poneros J, Santilli J, Brugge W. EUS-guided portal vein catheterization and pressure measurement in an animal model: a pilot study of feasibility. Gastrointest Endosc 2004;59(2):280–283.

79. Giday SA, Ko CW, Clarke JO, et al. EUS-guided portal vein carbon dioxide angiography: a pilot study in a porcine model. Gastrointest Endosc 2007;66(4):814–819.

80. Giday SA, Clarke JO, Buscaglia JM, et al. EUS-guided portal vein catheterization: a promising novel approach for portal angiography and portal vein pressure measurements. Gastrointest Endosc 2008;67(2):338–342.

81. Matthes K, Sahani D, Holalkere NS, Mino-Kenudson M, Brugge WR. Feasibility of endoscopic ultrasound-guided portal vein embolization with Enteryx. Acta Gastroenterol Belg 2005;68(4):412–415.

82. Lai L, Brugge WR. Endoscopic ultrasound is a sensitive and specific test to diagnose portal venous system thrombosis (PVST). Am J Gastroenterol 2004;99(1):40–44.

Index

Page numbers in *italics* refer to illustrations or tables

DVD Contents

The video topics are numbered to correspond to the chapters in which they appear.

DVD Contents

The video topics are numbered to correspond to the chapters in which they appear.